Repetitive Motion Disorders of the Upper Extremity

American Academy of Orthopaedic Surgeons

Supported by the
National Institute of Arthritis and Musculoskeletal and Skin Diseases

and the
National Institute for Occupational Safety and Health

and the
National Center for Medical Rehabilitation Research, National Institute of Child Health and Human Development

and the
Orthopaedic Research and Education Foundation

and the
Center for VDT & Health Research

and the
Public Health Services Advisory Committee on Employment of Persons With Disabilities

Repetitive Motion Disorders of the Upper Extremity

Edited by
Stephen L. Gordon, PhD
Chief, Musculoskeletal Diseases Branch
National Institute of Arthritis and Musculoskeletal and Skin Diseases
National Institutes of Health
Bethesda, Maryland

Sidney J. Blair, MD, FACS
Professor Emeritus
Department of Orthopedic Surgery
Loyola University Medical Center
Maywood, Illinois

Lawrence J. Fine, MD, Dr PH
Director, Division of Surveillance, Hazard Evaluations and Field Studies
National Institute for Occupational Safety and Health
Cincinnati, Ohio

Workshop Discussion Leaders and Section Editors
Kai-Nan An, PhD
Richard L. Lieber, PhD
Mary Ann Ruda, PhD
Barbara Silverstein, PhD
Robert M. Szabo, MD
Kathryn G. Vogel, PhD

With 157 illustrations

Workshop
Bethesda, Maryland
June 1994

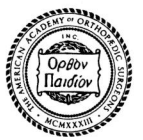

American Academy of Orthopaedic Surgeons
6300 North River Road
Rosemont, IL 60018

Repetitive Motion Disorders of the Upper Extremity
American Academy of Orthopaedic Surgeons

The material presented in *Repetitive Motion Disorders of the Upper Extremity* has been made available by the American Academy of Orthopaedic Surgeons for educational purposes only. This material is not intended to present the only, or necessarily best, methods or procedures for the medical situations discussed, but rather is intended to represent an approach, view, statement, or opinion of the author(s) or producer(s), which may be helpful to others who face similar situations.

Some drugs and medical devices demonstrated in Academy courses or described in Academy print or electronic publications have FDA clearance for use for specific purposes or for use only in restricted settings. The FDA has stated that it is the responsibility of the physician to determine the FDA status of each drug or device he or she wishes to use in clinical practice, and to use the products with appropriate patient consent and in compliance with applicable law.

Furthermore, any statements about commercial products are solely the opinion(s) of the author(s) and do not represent an Academy endorsement or evaluation of these products. These statements may not be used in advertising or for any commercial purpose.

The material contained in this volume was submitted as previously unpublished material, except in the instances in which credit has been given to the source from which some of the illustrative material was derived.

Materials appearing in this book prepared by individuals as part of their official duties as U.S. Government employees are not covered by copyright.

All rights reserved. No part of this publication may be reproduced, stored in a retrieval system, or transmitted, in any form, or by any means, electronic, mechanical, photocopying, recording, or otherwise, without prior written permission from the publisher.

First Edition
Copyright © 1995 by the American Academy of Orthopaedic Surgeons

ISBN 0-89203-143-3

Library of Congress Cataloging-in-Publication Data:

Repetitive motion disorders of the upper extremity / edited by Stephen
  L. Gordon, Sidney J. Blair, Lawrence J. Fine; supported by the
  National Institute of Arthritis and Musculoskeletal and Skin
  Diseases . . . [et al.]. — 1st ed.
     p.   cm.
  Includes bibliographical references and index.
  ISBN 0-89203-143-3
    1. Overuse injuries—Congresses. 2. Arm—Wounds and injuries—
Congresses.   I. Gordon, Stephen L.   II. Blair, Sidney J.
III. Fine, Lawrence J. IV. National Institute of Arthritis and
Musculoskeletal and Skin Diseases (U.S.)
    [DNLM: 1. Arm Injuries—physiopathology—congresses. 2. Arm
Injuries—therapy—congresses. 3. Repetition Strain Injury—
physiopathology—congresses. 4. Repetition Strain Injury—
etiology—congresses. 5. Repetition Strain Injury—therapy—
congresses. 6. Biomechanics—congresses. WE 805 R425 1995]
RD97.6.R47   1995
617.5'7044—dc20
DNLM/DLC   95-9424
for Library of Congress   CIP

American Academy of Orthopaedic Surgeons

Board of Directors, 1995
James W. Strickland, MD, *President*
S. Terry Canale, MD
Charles R. Clark, MD
Paul C. Collins, MD
William C. Collins, MD
Robert D. D'Ambrosia, MD
Kenneth E. DeHaven, MD
Robert N. Hensinger, MD
James H. Herndon, MD
Douglas W. Jackson, MD
Richard F. Kyle, MD
George L. Lucas, MD
David R. Mauerhan, MD
Bernard F. Morrey, MD
Bernard A. Rineberg, MD
D. Eugene Thompson, MD
William W. Tipton, Jr., MD *(ex officio)*

Staff
William W. Tipton, Jr., MD, *Executive Vice-President*
Mark W. Wieting, *Director, Division of Education*
Marilyn L. Fox, PhD, *Director, Department of Publication*
Bruce Davis, *Senior Editor*
Joan Abern, *Associate Senior Editor*
Jane Baque, *Associate Senior Editor*
Lisa Claxton Moore, *Associate Senior Editor*
Loraine Edwalds, *Production Manager*
Kathy Brouillette, *Assistant Production Manager*
Sharon Duffy, *Editorial Assistant*
Sophie Tosta, *Editorial Assistant*
Geraldine Dubberke, *Publications Secretary*
Em Lee Lambos, *Publications Secretary*

Contributors and Participants

Jacqueline Agnew, MPH, PhD*
  Associate Professor
  Johns Hopkins School of Hygiene
    and Public Health
  Baltimore, Maryland

Louis C. Almekinders, MD*†
  Division of Orthopaedic Surgery
  University of North Carolina
  Chapel Hill, North Carolina

Peter C. Amadio, MD*†
  Professor, Orthopaedics
  Consultant, Hand Surgery and
    Orthopaedic Surgery
  Mayo Clinic
  Rochester, Minnesota

David Amiel, PhD*†
  Professor of Orthopaedics
  University of California, San
    Diego
  Department of Orthopaedics
  La Jolla, California

Kai-Nan An, PhD*†
  Director, Biomechanics
    Laboratory
  Department of Orthopedics
  Mayo Clinic and Mayo
    Foundation
  Rochester, Minnesota

Gunnar B. J. Andersson, MD, PhD*†
  Professor and Acting Chairman
  Department of Orthopaedic
    Surgery
  Rush-Presbyterian-St. Luke's
    Medical Center
  Chicago, Illinois

Robert B. Armstrong, PhD*†
  Muscle Biology Laboratory
  Department of Health and
    Kinesiology
  Texas A & M University
  College Station, Texas

Thomas J. Armstrong, PhD*†
  Professor, Department of
    Environmental and Industrial
    Health
  University of Michigan
  Ann Arbor, Michigan

Albert J. Banes, PhD*†
  Professor of Surgery
  Division of Plastic Surgery
  Department of Surgery
  University of North Carolina
  Chapel Hill, North Carolina

Michael Benjamin, PhD*†
  Senior Lecturer, School of
    Molecular and Medical
    Biosciences
  University of Wales
  College of Cardiff
  Cardiff, United Kingdom

Laurence N. Benz, MPT, ECS, OCS*
President
Elizabethtown Physical Therapy, PSC
Elizabethtown, Kentucky

Louis U. Bigliani, MD*
Chief, Shoulder Service
Columbia Presbyterian Medical Center
Associate Professor of Orthopaedic Surgery
College of Physicians and Surgeons
Columbia University
New York, New York

Sidney J. Blair, MD, FACS*†
Professor Emeritus
Department of Orthopedic Surgery
Loyola University Medical Center
Maywood, Illinois

William F. Blair, MD*†
Division of Hand and Microsurgery
Department of Orthopaedic Surgery
University of Iowa Hospitals and Clinics
Iowa City, Iowa

Margit L. Bleecker, MD, PhD*
Director
Center for Occupational and Environmental Neurology
Children's Hospital
Baltimore, Maryland

Scott Boitano, PhD*
Assistant Professor
Department of Anatomy and Cell Biology
University of California, Los Angeles
School of Medicine
Los Angeles, California

Robert C. Bray, MD†
Associate Professor
Department of Surgery
Faculty of Medicine
University of Calgary
Calgary, Alberta, Canada

Brian Brigman, MD†
Department of Surgery
University of North Carolina
Chapel Hill, North Carolina

Thomas D. Brown, PhD†
Director, Biomechanics Laboratory
Orthopedics
University of Iowa
Iowa City, Iowa

Bruce M. Carlson, MD, PhD*†
Chairman, Department of Anatomy and Cell Biology
University of Michigan
Ann Arbor, Michigan

Constance R. Chu, MD†
Orthopaedic Resident
University of California, San Diego
Department of Orthopaedics
La Jolla, California

William P. Cooney III, MD*†
Professor and Consultant
Chair, Division of Hand Surgery
Department of Orthopedics
Mayo Clinic and Mayo Foundation
Rochester, Minnesota

Lars B. Dahlin, MD, PhD†
Associate Professor
Department of Hand Surgery
General Hospital
Lund University
Malmö, Sweden

Bradley Evanoff, MD, MPH*
  Assistant Professor, Department of
    Internal Medicine
  Head, Section of Occupational
    and Environmental Medicine
  Washington University School of
    Medicine
  St. Louis, Missouri

Roger A. Fielding, PhD*†
  Clinical Assistant Professor
  Department of Health Sciences
  Boston University
  Sargent College of Allied Health
    Professions
  Boston, Massachusetts

Lawrence J. Fine, MD, Dr PH*
  Director, Division of Surveillance,
    Hazard Evaluations and Field
    Studies
  National Institute for
    Occupational Safety and Health
  Cincinnati, Ohio

Tom Fischer, PhD†
  Assistant Professor of Medicine
  University of North Carolina
  Chapel Hill, North Carolina

Evan L. Flatow, MD†
  Herbert Irving Associate Professor
    of Orthopaedic Surgery
  Associate Chief, The Shoulder
    Service
  Columbia-Presbyterian Medical
    Center
  New York, New York

Cyril B. Frank, MD†
  Professor
  Department of Surgery
  Faculty of Medicine
  University of Calgary
  Calgary, Alberta, Canada

Jan Fridén, MD, PhD*†
  Associate Professor
  Department of Orthopaedics
  Division of Hand Surgery
  University of Gothenburg
  Gothenburg, Sweden

Robert J. Gatchel, PhD*
  Professor of Psychiatry
  University of Texas Southwestern
    Medical Center at Dallas
  Dallas, Texas

Richard H. Gelberman, MD*
  Massachusetts General Hospital
  Harvard University Medical
    School
  Boston, Massachusetts

Terrence P. Glennon, MD*†
  Assistant Professor
  Baylor College of Medicine
  Department of Physical Medicine
    and Rehabilitation
  Houston, Texas

Barry Goldstein, MD, PhD†
  Assistant Professor
  University of Washington
  Seattle, Washington

Stephen L. Gordon, PhD*
  Chief, Musculoskeletal Diseases
    Branch
  National Institute of Arthritis and
    Musculoskeletal and Skin
    Diseases
  National Institutes of Health
  Bethesda, Maryland

Katharyn A. Grant, PhD†
  Industrial Engineer
  Division of Biomechanical and
    Behavioral Sciences
  National Institute for
    Occupational Safety and Health
  Cincinnati, Ohio

Jung Soo Han, PhD*
Assistant Professor and Director,
   Orthopaedic Research
   Laboratory
Department of Orthopaedics
West Virginia University
Morgantown, West Virginia

David A. Hart, PhD*†
Professor
Departments of Microbiology and
   Infectious Diseases/Medicine
Faculty of Medicine
University of Calgary
Calgary, Alberta, Canada

Robin Herbert, MD*
Assistant Professor
Department of Community
   Medicine
Medical Co-Director, Mount
   Sinai-I.J. Selikoff Occupational
   Health Clinical Center
Mount Sinai Medical School
New York, New York

Stephen P. Heyse, MD, MPH*
Director, Office of Prevention,
   Epidemiology, and Clinical
   Applications
National Institute of Arthritis and
   Musculoskeletal and Skin
   Diseases
National Institutes of Health
Bethesda, Maryland

Benjamin M. Hillberry, PhD*†
Professor of Mechanical
   Engineering
Purdue University
West Lafayette, Indiana

Jay Himmelstein, MD, MPH†
Director, Occupational Health
   Program
UMMC
Worcester, Massachusetts

Peiqi Hu, MD†
Research Fellow, Dermatology
University of North Carolina
Chapel Hill, North Carolina

Joseph P. Iannotti, MD, PhD*†
Associate Professor
Chief, Shoulder Service
University of Pennsylvania
Philadelphia, Pennsylvania

Peter J. Keir, Bsc†
PhD Candidate
Department of Kinesiology
University of Waterloo
Waterloo, Ontario, Canada

Rajeev Kelkar, MS†
Graduate Research Assistant
Orthopaedic Research Laboratory
Columbia University
New York, New York

Wendi A. Latko, ME†
Graduate Research Assistant
University of Michigan
Center for Ergonomics
Ann Arbor, Michigan

W. Thomas Lawrence, MD†
Division Chief, Plastic
   Surgery
Department of Surgery
University of North Carolina
Chapel Hill, North Carolina

Wayne B. Leadbetter, MD*
Clinical Assistant Professor,
   Orthopaedic Surgery
Georgetown University
Washington, District of Columbia

Kwan Hee Lee, MD, PhD*
Research Fellow, Orthopaedic
   Research Laboratory
Health Science Center
South West Virginia University
Morgantown, West Virginia

Joe Lee, MD†
  Orthopaedic Research Resident
  University of California, San Diego
  Department of Orthopaedics
  La Jolla, California

Craig L. Levitz, MD†
  Resident in Orthopaedic Surgery
  Department of Orthopaedics
  Hospital of the University of
    Pennsylvania
  Philadelphia, Pennsylvania

Richard L. Lieber, PhD*†
  Professor of Orthopaedics and
    Bioengineering
  University of California
  VA Medical Centers
  San Diego, California

Dawn A. Lowe, PhD†
  Post-Doctoral Fellow
  Texas A & M University
  College Station, Texas

Göran Lundborg, MD, PhD†
  Professor, Department of Hand
    Surgery
  General Hospital
  Lund University
  Malmö, Sweden

Susan E. Mackinnon*
  Professor of Surgery and
    Occupational Therapy
  Washington University
  School of Medicine
  St. Louis, Missouri

Michael Madison, PhD†
  University of California
  Davis Medical Center
  Department of Orthopaedic
    Surgery
  Sacramento, California

Anne E. Moore, MSc, PEng†
  Centre for Occupational Health
    and Safety
  University of Waterloo
  Waterloo, Ontario, Canada

Bernard F. Morrey, MD†
  Professor and Chairman
  Department of Orthopedics
  Mayo Clinic and Mayo
    Foundation
  Rochester, Minnesota

Van C. Mow, PhD*†
  Professor of Mechanical
    Engineering and Orthopaedic
    Bioengineering
  Director, Orthopaedic Research
    Laboratory
  Columbia University
  New York, New York

Robert P. Nirschl, MD, MS*†
  Orthopedic Director
  Virginia Sports Medicine
    Institute
  Attending Orthopaedic Surgeon
  Arlington Hospital
  Assistant Professor (Clinical)
  Georgetown University
  Arlington, Virginia

Katsuo Nishiyama, PhD, MPH*
  Associate Professor, Department
    of Preventive Medicine
  Shiga University of Medical
    Science
  Otsu, Japan

Ernst M. Noah, MD†
  Microsurgical Research and
    Clinical Fellow
  Eastern Virginia Medical School
  Microsurgical Research Center
  Norfolk, Virginia

Emil Pascarelli, MD*
  Professor of Clinical Medicine
  Columbia University College of
    Physicians and Surgeons
  Connective Tissue Section
  New York, New York

George Piligian, MD*
  Clinical Instructor
  Department of Occupational and
    Environmental Medicine
  Mount Sinai Medical Center
  New York, New York

Roger G. Pollock, MD*†
  Assistant Professor of
    Orthopaedic Surgery
  Columbia-Presbyterian Medical
    Center
  New York, New York

Glenn Pransky, MD, MOccH*†
  Associate Professor
  Department of Family and
    Community Medicine and
    Medicine
  University of Massachusetts
    Medical Center
  Worcester, Massachusetts

Joel M. Press, MD*†
  Medical Director
  Center for Spine, Sports, and
    Occupational Rehabilitation
  Rehabilitation Institute of
    Chicago
  Assistant Professor of Clinical
    Physical Medicine and
    Rehabilitation
  Northwestern University Medical
    School
  Chicago, Illinois

Laura Punnett, ScD†
  Associate Professor
  University of Massachusetts-Lowell
  Department of Work Environment
  Lowell, Massachusetts

Vern Putz-Anderson, PhD*†
  Chief, Psychophysiology and
    Biomechanics Section
  U. S. Department of Health and
    Human Services
  National Institute for
    Occupational Safety and Health
  Cincinnati, Ohio

James R. Ralphs, PhD†
  School of Molecular and Medical
    Biosciences
  University of Wales College of
    Cardiff
  Cardiff, United Kingdom

David Rempel, MD*†
  Assistant Professor of Medicine
  Division of Occupational Medicine
  University of California, San
    Francisco
  San Francisco, California

Leo M. Rozmayn, MD*
  Attending Orthopaedic Hand
    Surgeon
  Shady Grove Adventist Hospital
  Rockville, Maryland

Mary Ann Ruda, PhD*†
  Chief, Cellular and Molecular
    Mechanisms Section
  Neurobiology and Anesthesiology
    Branch
  National Institute of Dental
    Research
  National Institutes of Health
  Bethesda, Maryland

Michael J. Sanderson, PhD†
  Professor
  University of Massachusetts
  Wooster, Massachusetts

Steven L. Sauter, PhD*†
  Chief, Applied Psychology and
    Ergonomics Branch
  Division of Biomedical and
    Behavioral Science
  National Institute for
    Occupational Safety and Health
  Cincinnati, Ohio

H. Ralph Schumacher, Jr, MD*†
  Professor of Medicine
  University of Pennsylvania
  School of Medicine
  Veterans Administration Medical
    Center
  Philadelphia, Pennsylvania

Donald A. Simone, PhD*†
  Assistant Professor, Department of Psychiatry
  Division of Neuroscience Research
  University of Minnesota
  Minneapolis, Minnesota

Steven A. Stiens, MD*†
  Assistant Professor of Rehabilitation
  University of Washington
  Veterans Affairs Medical Center
  Seattle, Washington

Naomi G. Swanson, PhD†
  Chief, Motivation and Stress Research Section
  National Institute for Occupational Safety and Health
  Cincinnati, Ohio

Robert M. Szabo, MD*†
  Professor of Orthopaedic Surgery
  Chief, Hand and Upper Extremity Service
  University of California, Davis
  Davis Medical Center
  Sacramento, California

Julia K. Terzis, MD, PhD, FRCS(C)*†
  Professor, Department of Plastic and Reconstructive Surgery
  Microsurgery Program Director
  Eastern Virginia Medical School
  Microsurgical Research Center
  Norfolk, Virginia

Mari Tsuzaki, DDS, PhD†
  Research Fellow
  Department of Surgery
  University of North Carolina
  Chapel Hill, North Carolina

Eira Viikari-Juntura, MD, DMedSc*†
  Chief Medical Officer
  Finnish Institute of Occupational Health
  Department of Physiology
  Prevention Program on Work-Related Musculoskeletal Disorders
  Helsinki, Finland

Kathryn G. Vogel, PhD*†
  Professor, Department of Biology
  University of New Mexico
  Albuquerque, New Mexico

Gordon L. Warren III, PhD†
  Associate Research Scientist
  Texas A & M University
  College Station, Texas

Richard Wells, MEng, PhD*†
  Associate Professor
  Department of Kinesiology
  Faculty of Applied Health Sciences
  University of Waterloo
  Waterloo, Ontario, Canada

Carol Wilkinson, MD, MSPH*
  Program Director, Corporate Health
  IBM
  Armonk, New York

Savio L-Y Woo, PhD*†
  A.B. Ferguson Professor of Orthopaedics and Vice Chairman for Research
  Professor of Mechanical Engineering
  Musculoskeletal Research Center
  Department of Orthopaedic Surgery
  University of Pittsburgh
  Pittsburgh, Pennsylvania

Michael J. Woods, DO*
  Resident
  National Rehabilitation Hospital
  Washington, District of Columbia

Judith S. Wortman, RN, MA*
Technical Information Specialist
National Institute of Arthritis and Musculoskeletal and Skin Diseases
National Institutes of Health
Bethesda, Maryland

John W. Xerogeanes, MD†
Orthopaedic Resident
University of Pittsburgh
Department of Orthopaedic Surgery
Pittsburgh, Pennsylvania

Hong Xiao, MD†
Research Fellow
Department of Surgery
University of North Carolina
Chapel Hill, North Carolina

Jeffrey L. Young, MD†
Assistant Professor
Department of Physical Medicine and Rehabilitation
Northwestern University Medical School
Chicago, Illinois

* Workshop Participants
† Contributor to Volume

Table of Contents

Section 1 Epidemiologic and Psychologic Laboratory Studies
Section Editor: Barbara Silverstein, PhD

	Overview	3
1	The Role of Physical Stressors in the Development of Hand/Wrist and Elbow Disorders *Eira Viikari-Juntura, MD, DMedSc*	7
2	Epidemiology of Occupational Neck and Shoulder Disorders *Gunnar B. J. Andersson, MD, PhD*	31
3	Work-Related Musculoskeletal Disorders in Computer Keyboard Operation *Laura Punnett, ScD*	43
4	Perceived Exertion as a Function of Physical Effort *Vern Putz-Anderson, PhD* *Katharyn A. Grant, PhD*	49
5	The Relationship Between Workplace Psychosocial Factors and Musculoskeletal Disorders in Office Work: Suggested Mechanisms and Evidence *Steven L. Sauter, PhD* *Naomi G. Swanson, PhD*	65
	Directions for Future Research	77

Section 2 Pathophysiology: Biomechanical Loads
Section Editor: Kai-Nan An, PhD

	Overview	83
6	Physical Stressors: Their Characterization, Assessment, and Relationship With Physical Work Requirements *Thomas J. Armstrong, PhD* *Wendi A. Latko, ME*	87
7	Dynamic Effects of Work on Musculoskeletal Loading *Benjamin M. Hillberry, PhD*	99

8	Applications of Biomechanical Hand and Wrist Models to Work-Related Musculoskeletal Disorders of the Upper Extremity *Richard P. Wells, MEng, PhD* *Peter J. Keir, BSc* *Anne E. Moore, MSc, PEng*	111
9	Musculoskeletal Loading and Carpal Tunnel Pressure *David Rempel, MD*	123
10	The Relationship Between Upper Limb Load Posture and Tissue Loads at the Elbow *Kai-Nan An, PhD* *William P. Cooney III, MD* *Bernard F. Morrey, MD*	133
11	Shoulder Biomechanics and Repetitive Motion *Roger G. Pollock, MD* *Evan L. Flatow, MD* *Louis U. Bigliani, MD* *Rajeev Kelkar, MS* *Van C. Mow, PhD*	145
12	The Biomechanics of Soft Tissue: Normal, Injured, and Healed States *Savio L-Y Woo, PhD* *John W. Xerogeanes, MD*	161
	Directions for Future Research	173

Section 3 Pathophysiology: Connective Tissue
Section Editor: Kathryn G. Vogel, PhD

	Overview	181
13	Functional and Developmental Anatomy of Tendons and Ligaments *Michael Benjamin, PhD* *James R. Ralphs, PhD*	185
14	Fibrocartilage in Tendon: A Response to Compressive Load *Kathryn G. Vogel, PhD*	205
15	Effect of Loading on Metabolism and Repair of Tendons and Ligaments *David Amiel, PhD* *Constance R. Chu, MD* *Joe Lee, MD*	217

16	Tendon Cells of the Epitenon and Internal Tendon Compartment Communicate Mechanical Signals Through Gap Junctions and Respond Differentially to Mechanical Load and Growth Factors *Albert J. Banes, PhD* *Peiqi Hu, MD* *Hong Xiao, MD* *Michael J. Sanderson, PhD* *Scott Boitano, PhD* *Brian Brigman, MD* *Tom Fischer, PhD* *Mari Tsuzaki, DDS, PhD* *Thomas D. Brown, PhD* *Louis C. Almekinders, MD* *W. Thomas Lawrence, MD*	231
17	Inflammatory Processes in Repetitive Motion and Overuse Syndromes: Potential Role of Neurogenic Mechanisms in Tendons and Ligaments *David A. Hart, PhD* *Cyril B. Frank, MD* *Robert C. Bray, MD*	247
18	Morphology and Physiology of Normal Synovium and the Effects of Mechanical Stimulation *H. Ralph Schumacher, Jr, MD*	263
	Directions for Future Research	277

Section 4 Pathophysiology: Muscle
Section Editor: Richard L. Lieber, PhD

	Overview	285
19	Skeletal Muscle Metabolism, Fatigue, and Injury *Richard L. Lieber, PhD* *Jan Fridén, MD, PhD*	287
20	Biomechanical Injury to Skeletal Muscle From Repetitive Loading: Eccentric Contractions and Vibrations *Jan Fridén, MD, PhD* *Richard L. Lieber, PhD*	301
21	The Satellite Cell and Skeletal Muscle Regeneration: The Degeneration and Regeneration Cycle *Bruce M. Carlson, MD, PhD*	313
22	The Role of Inflammatory Processes in Exercise-Induced Muscle Injury: Implications for Changes in Skeletal Muscle Protein Turnover *Roger A. Fielding, PhD*	323

23	Mechanisms in the Initiation of Contraction-Induced Skeletal Muscle Injury *Robert B. Armstrong, PhD* *Gordon L. Warren III, PhD* *Dawn A. Lowe, PhD*	339
	Directions for Future Research	351

Section 5 Pathophysiology: Nerve
Section Editor: Mary Ann Ruda, PhD

	Overview	357
24	Anatomy and Morphology of Upper Extremity Nerves and Frequent Sites of Compression *Julia K. Terzis, MD, PhD, FRCS(C)* *Ernst M. Noah, MD*	359
25	Pathophysiology of Nerve Compression *Göran Lundborg, MD, PhD* *Lars B. Dahlin, MD, PhD*	381
26	Gene Regulation in the Dorsal Root Ganglion in Normal and Pathologic Situations *Mary Ann Ruda, PhD*	399
27	Peripheral Neural Mechanisms of Muscle Pain Resulting From Repetitive Motion and Inflammation *Donald A. Simone, PhD*	407
	Directions for Future Research	415

Section 6 Clinical Issues
Section Editor: Robert M. Szabo, MD

	Overview	419
28	Carpal Tunnel Syndrome as a Work-Related Disorder *Robert M. Szabo, MD* *Michael Madison, PhD*	421
29	De Quervain's Disease and Tenosynovitis *Peter C. Amadio, MD*	435
30	Rehabilitation of Repetitive Motion Disorders of the Wrist *Terrence P. Glennon, MD*	449
31	Cubital Tunnel Syndrome in the Work Environment *William F. Blair, MD*	455
32	Tennis Elbow Tendinosis: Pathoanatomy, Nonsurgical and Surgical Management *Robert P. Nirschl, MD, MS*	467
33	Rehabilitation of Repetitive Trauma at the Elbow *Joel M. Press, MD* *Jeffrey L. Young, MD*	479

34	Overuse Injuries of the Shoulder *Craig L. Levitz, MD* *Joseph P. Iannotti, MD, PhD*	493
35	Cervicobrachial Disorders *Sidney J. Blair, MD, FACS*	507
36	Rehabilitation of the Shoulder After Repetitive Motion Injury *Steven A. Stiens, MD* *Barry Goldstein, MD, PhD*	517
37	Overview of Complete Patient Management in Upper Extremity Repetitive Motion Disorders *Glenn Pransky, MD, MOccH* *Jay Himmelstein, MD, MPH*	539
	Directions for Future Research	551
	Clinical Questions	555
	Index	559

Preface

On June 20-22, 1994, a Workshop on Repetitive Motion Disorders of the Upper Extremity was held in Bethesda, Maryland. It was organized by the National Institute of Arthritis and Musculoskeletal and Skin Disease (NIAMS), National Institutes of Health. Co-sponsors included the National Institute for Occupational Safety and Health (NIOSH), Centers for Disease Control and Prevention; the Orthopaedic Research and Education Foundation; the National Center for Medical Rehabilitation Research, National Institute of Child Health and Human Development, National Institutes of Health; Center for VDT and Health Research; and Public Health Services Advisory Committee on Employment of Persons With Disabilities. This book is based on manuscripts prepared for this workshop and discussions held during the workshop.

The initial impetus to undertake this project began with informal discussion between Sidney J. Blair, MD, FACS, of Loyola University, and myself. We soon added the counsel of Lawrence J. Fine, MD, Dr PH, of NIOSH. Along the way, the three leading organizers and editors had significant help and advice from the section leaders, participants in the workshop, and other members of the scientific and medical community. We greatly appreciate the efforts of all contributors to the workshop and this book.

I would like to thank Marilyn Fox, PhD, Director of the Department of Publications; Lisa Moore and Jane Baque, associate senior editors who were responsible for organizing and managing this project; Bruce Davis, senior editor, who assisted in editing the manuscripts; Loraine Edwalds, production manager, and Kathy Brouillette, assistant production manager, who oversaw the smooth flow of manuscripts through the production process. I would also like to acknowledge the efforts of Sophie Tosta and Sharon Duffy, editorial assistants, and Geraldine Dubberke and Em Lee Lambos, publications secretaries.

The specific phrase "repetitive motion disorders" may be a potential source of concern to some readers of this text. Other descriptors such as "cumulative trauma disorders," "repetitive strain injury," or "overuse injury" are widely found in the scientific literature. Because there are advantages and disadvantages to each of these terms, I have selected, somewhat arbitrarily, "repetitive motion disorders" as the primary term for this text.

The original concept was to have a focus for this project that was different from most of the preceding efforts to gather experts or prepare a text in the field of repetitive motion disorders. Most of these efforts have been directed toward epidemiologic and work environment issues related to identifying and reducing some of the risk factors. Our goal was to review these topics briefly and to emphasize

(1) the pathophysiologic causes of tissue damage and resulting pain and dysfunction and (2) the current clinical approaches to diagnosing and treating these injuries. It is clear throughout this book that recreational and sports activities may act independently or in combination with job activities to produce repetitive motion disorders.

There is overwhelming evidence that the number of reported cases of repetitive motion disorders is rapidly growing. These disorders have become an extremely costly public health issue. Although some individuals believe that the underlying issue may be improper reporting or false claims of a medical problem, the organizers and most of the participants believe that for the vast majority of cases, there is an underlying physiologic insult to one or more of the various tissues involved. Therefore, this book addresses the critical need to understand the pathophysiology of repetitive motion disorders and treat patients effectively.

The scientific expertise of the contributors to this book is very broad. It was the intention of the organizers to cover the assigned topics with a wide spectrum of perspectives from leading basic and clinical scientists. In many cases, more is unknown than known about an issue. Future Research Directions identify many research opportunities in this field. I hope that this book becomes a unique and valuable resource for scientists and practitioners in this field.

STEPHEN L. GORDON, PHD

Section 1

Epidemiologic and Psychologic Laboratory Studies

Section Editor:
Barbara Silverstein, PhD

*Gunnar B. J. Andersson,
   MD, PhD
Katharyn A. Grant, PhD
Laura Punnett, ScD
Vern Putz-Anderson, PhD*

*Steven L. Sauter, PhD
Naomi G. Swanson, PhD
Eira Viikari-Juntura,
   MD, DMedSc*

Overview

Among scientists and in the lay community there has been an increased interest in musculoskeletal disorders of the upper limb associated with repetitive motion and other occupational factors. These disorders primarily affect the soft tissues, including the nerves (eg, carpal tunnel syndrome), tendons (eg, tenosynovitis, peritendinitis, tendinitis, epicondylitis), and muscles (eg, tension neck syndrome).

The term "repetitive motion disorder" may be misleading because, in some instances, it is the absence of motion (eg, static contractions) that appears to be more indicative of the disorders, for example, prolonged static loading of muscles in the neck and shoulder area that stabilize the arm so that precise repetitive motions can be performed (as in data entry tasks).

These repetitive motion disorders represent a continuum from carpal tunnel syndrome, which has both relatively clear diagnostic criteria and pathophysiology, to tension neck syndrome, which is defined primarily by the specific location of pain and has a pathophysiology that is less clearly defined. From a clinical and epidemiologic perspective, some of these upper limb disorders present challenges similar to those of low back pain. In addition, these upper limb disorders are multifactorial with work activities often contributing significantly, but not solely, to their development or exacerbation. Individual, social, and cultural factors sometimes play similarly important roles in their development and whether the affected individual, their employer, and society recognizes or accepts the medical disorder. For example, the workers' compensation system in some states considers carpal tunnel syndrome as a potentially work-related condition, whereas in other states it does not. Health belief models may contribute to when, where, and how these disorders materialize. Different countries have different health care systems and avenues for recognizing these disorders, making international comparisons difficult. Repetitive activities from nonoccupational pursuits, such as racquetball, may also contribute or aggravate these conditions. There has been considerable controversy recently in the scientific literature and in society at large about the relative importance of repetitive motion and other occupational factors in the etiology of these conditions.[1,2]

The national surveillance data from the United States Department of Labor Bureau of Labor Statistics (BLS) showed that more than 60% of new occupational illnesses in 1992 were associated with repetitive motion.[3] In both the BLS and in workers' compensation state systems, the number of occupational injuries far exceeds the number of occupational diseases. In these surveillance data sources, however, the last several years have shown a sharp increase in the incidence of repetitive-related disorders, such as carpal tunnel syndrome. In the BLS system, the overall national rate increased from 5 cases per 10,000 workers in 1982 to 44 per 10,000 workers in 1992. In BLS and workers' compensation systems, the highest rates generally occur in the industries with a substantial amount of repetitive work. In 1992, the BLS reported that meatpacking plants had the highest incidence (1,395 cases per 10,000 workers), followed by automobile manufacturing (860 cases per 10,000 workers). More recently, there has been an increased incidence in "safe industries" in which data entry jobs predominate; for example, 5% of the cases of repetitive motion disorders reported to BLS were in key entry jobs. This movement may be related to the rapid computerization of the American work force. Less than 25% of workers used computers on their jobs in 1984, but by 1994, more than 47% of workers used computers.

Although there have been clinical reports of musculoskeletal disorders related to repetitive motion from as early as Ramazzini (1713), epidemiologic studies of associations between primarily work factors and these disorders of the upper limb have been relatively recent; that is, in the past 20 years. Although these musculoskeletal disorders have been reported in athletes and hobbyists, the epidemiologic studies have involved primarily the work environment (eg, manufacturing, office environment, construction, agriculture).

This section of the book is primarily focused on a review of epidemiologic studies that have contributed to our current understanding of the role of occupational factors in these disorders. Most epidemiologic studies of these disorders have considered almost exclusively the physical attributes of work, such as the number of wrist movements per hour; however, psychosocial factors are increasingly recognized as important factors to be investigated as well. As a result, a review of psychosocial factors has been included. The epidemiologic perspective of this section is enhanced by a summary of laboratory and field studies of workers' perceptions of what are "acceptable" working exposures because these psychophysical studies contribute to the understanding of these disorders.

Several common limitations of these epidemiologic studies are apparent. Because most epidemiologic studies involve a large number of subjects who are actively employed and because most of these disorders cannot be diagnosed with laboratory methods, epidemiologic case definitions based on questionnaires such as the Nordic Questionnaire have been utilized.[4] Detailed exposure assessment of all aspects of the physical work environment using accurate quantitative methods are not common in these studies. Some studies have attempted to address these common limitations by using electrodiagnostic techniques to measure median and ulnar nerves, and electromyographic techniques to define disease endpoints and better characterize exposure. Few studies devoted equal resources to measure the psychosocial and physical factors of work.

Eira Viikari-Juntura, MD, DMedSc, reviews the epidemiology of neck and shoulder disorders and their association with work-related activities. In some countries and industries, shoulder disorders have been reported to be second only to back injuries in terms of seeking medical care and workers' compensation. The importance of static as well as repetitive loading of tissues is addressed. Gunnar B. J. Andersson, MD, PhD, addresses the physical risk factors of work associated with neck and shoulder disorders. Laura Punnett, ScD, focuses on the emerging problem of upper limb disorders among video display unit (VDU) operators, including, but not limited to, duration and speed of keying activities. Steven L. Sauter, PhD, and Naomi G. Swanson, PhD, address one of the critical issues for epidemiologists regarding exposure assessment methods: are there surrogates for direct measurement of exposure that can be used to predict "safe" levels of exposure? Vern Putz-Anderson, PhD, and Katharyn A. Grant, PhD review the evidence for psychosocial causal mechanisms for upper limb disorders, focusing on the office work environment.

Although there are many areas for further research, associations between different work activities and upper limb musculoskeletal disorders are reasonably strong and consistent. From a public health perspective of prevention, there is enough information to begin to reduce these risk factors with engineering and administrative controls while the research continues.

References

1. Silverstein BA, Fine LJ: Cumulative trauma disorders of the upper extremity: A preventive strategy is needed. *J Occup Med* 1991;33:642–644.
2. Hadler NM: Cumulative trauma disorders: An iatrogenic concept. *J Occup Med* 1990;32:38–41.
3. *Occupational Injuries and Illnesses in the United States, 1992.* Washington, DC, U.S. Department of Labor, Bureau of Labor Statistics, 1994, gov doc no L2.2:OC1/153.
4. Kuorinka I, Jonsson B, Kilbom A, et al: Standardised Nordic questionnaires for the analysis of musculoskeletal symptoms. *Appl Ergonomics* 1987;18:233–237.

Chapter 1

The Role of Physical Stressors in the Development of Hand/Wrist and Elbow Disorders

Eira Viikari-Juntura, MD, DMedSc

Introduction

The earliest epidemiologic studies on work-related upper limb disorders date back to the 1950s.[1] Before that time, most articles described cases or case series of different disorders.[2,3] In the 1970s, various research groups started to develop methods to assess local physical work load[4] and assess diagnostic criteria of different disorders.[5] The validity of these assessment methods became a focus as late as in the 1980s.[6–10] This means that the validity aspects of assessment methods have been considered only in relatively recent epidemiologic studies.

Workers with upper limb problems show a variety of conditions, from clearly diagnosable peritendinitis or carpal tunnel syndrome (CTS) to ill-defined regional or generalized pain. Most epidemiologic studies have been conducted on specific tendon or nerve disorders. This may be considered an advantage because the results can then be discussed in relation to the pathomechanisms, which are fairly well known for these disorders. On the other hand, focusing research on the epidemiology and pathomechanisms of previously less known conditions may help to clarify the problems of the workers with these disorders and guide in their prevention.

In this article, I will review epidemiologic studies addressing the role of physical factors in the causality of work-related upper limb disorders. The internal validity of the studies will be assessed, including possible bias in the selection of the study populations and the validity of the assessment of the outcome and exposure. The following factors are considered in discussing causality: temporal relationship, strength of association, exposure-effect relationship, consistency of results, and biologic plausibility. Conditions that have been extensively studied will be emphasized, such as carpal tunnel syndrome (CTS), tenosynovitis and peritendinitis, epicondylitis, but other potentially work-related conditions will be discussed as well. Hand-arm vibration syndrome will not be included in this review.

Carpal Tunnel Syndrome, Other Nerve Entrapments, and Compression Neuropathies

Carpal Tunnel Syndrome

CTS is the most commonly studied work-related upper limb disorder. In their recent review on CTS studies with clinically defined outcome, Hagberg and associates[11] discuss 15 cross-sectional and six case-referent studies. Some cross-sectional studies with a reference group have been listed in Table 1 and some case-referent studies are listed in Table 2. Both cross-sectional and case-referent studies have assessed the prevalence of CTS among working populations, mostly with several years of seniority in the job. The workers in manually strenuous jobs therefore represent survivor populations, which tends to dilute the associations observed.

Of the six cross-sectional studies listed in Table 1, three based the diagnosis of CTS on electrodiagnostic examination, and the other three based diagnosis on symptoms and clinical tests. Case definition based on clinical tests is subject to considerable misclassification, because no clinical test has proved valid, if electrodiagnosis is considered the gold standard.[10] Only two studies[13,15] mention blinding those who assessed the subjects. Misclassification may be considerable also when electrodiagnostic tests are used, if age, finger temperature, and anthropometry are not considered.[22] All of these misclassifications are most likely nondifferential and tend to dilute the observed associations between the disease and physical work load.

With the exception of a small subgroup from the normal population in the study of deKrom and associates,[21] the cases in the case referent studies were seeking medical care for CTS and, in two studies, the cases had undergone CTS surgery (Table 2). Such catchment of cases may cause a referral bias in the estimation of the etiologic role of work load.[23] deKrom and associates[21] attempted to determine whether the odds ratios might have been biased using the case population of primarily hospital patients. They also performed the analysis on the small subgroup of the cases detected in a cross-sectional study among a normal population sample. The odds ratios for the physical work load factors seemed to be of similar direction and magnitude for this subgroup, suggesting no referral bias in their study.

Most cross-sectional and case-referent studies have considered current physical work load, and many of them have also considered length of employment in the current job. One case-referent study also considered also the subjective estimation of cumulative exposure for some risk factors,[20] and another study attempted to estimate the average duration of exposure per week during 5 years preceding the interview.[21] When based on subjective assessment, the perception of symptoms and disability may affect the assessment, resulting in differential misclassification.

In the cross-sectional studies, current exposure was assessed differently in different studies: by job title,[12] by job type assessed by an expert,[14,15] by generic risk factors assessed by the researchers,[16] by job title and job checklists,[17] and by video and electromyographic recordings of some workers per job and extrapolating the results to all subjects in the job.[13] The magnitude of the associations between CTS and physical load factors seems to be greatest for the studies with the most accurate method of assessment of work load.

As both cross-sectional and case-referent studies have assessed the prevalence of CTS, the temporal relationships between the physical work load factors and the onset of the disease are not known. An effort to include only diseases that had an onset since the worker first started the job under study was used in two of the studies,[13,16] but recall bias may invalidate this method. No prospective longitudinal studies on the role of physical factors in the etiology of CTS have been reported.

High risk of developing CTS was observed for grinders as an occupational group and for work tasks that demanded high force and repetition. In the case-referent studies, cumulative exposure to vibration from tools,[20] and to work with flexed and extended wrist[21] showed an exposure-effect relationship. The results of most of the studies are consistent, especially with regard to the effects of generic risk factors, such as forcefulness,[13,16] repetitiveness,[13,15,16] and vibration.[13,20] Activities in nonneutral wrist postures were associated with CTS in studies by deKrom and associates[21] and Barnhart and associates[15] but not in the study by Silverstein and associates.[13] Likewise, Armstrong and Chaffin[18] associated pinch force with CTS, but deKrom and associates[21] and Silverstein and associates[13] did not. In studies contrasting occupations or occupational groups, low odds ratios may be due to weak contrasts between occupations with regard to physical work load[12] or misclassification of exposure.[14]

The median nerve is compressed in the carpal canal when the canal is narrow either congenitally or as a result of a narrowing process later in life; eg, new bone formation on a fractured carpal bone or growth of carpal ganglion. Thickening of the contents of the carpal canal (as in flexor tenosynovitis) and accumulation of fluid in the tissues (as during pregnancy) may increase the carpal canal pressure and cause median nerve compression. Armstrong and associates[24] demonstrated in cadavers that the histologic changes in the flexor tendons and the median nerve (synovial membrane hyperplasia, median nerve epineural density and arteriole muscular wall hypertrophy) are at their maximum at the carpal canal, suggesting that flexor tendons have a possible role in the genesis of CTS. Median nerve dysfunction may result directly, after compression of the nerve, or indirectly, through ischemia. Carpal canal pressure is increased by loading of the flexor profundus tendons, especially of the second and third fingers; the increase is potentiated when the wrist is flexed.[25] It is biologically plausible, therefore, that non-neutral wrist postures and forceful gripping and pinching may cause CTS. Gripping on a vibrating tool increases the grip force,[26] which is likely to be the mechanism through which low-frequency vibration may cause CTS.[27]

Given the abundance of papers on CTS in the literature, the number of qualified epidemiologic studies considering physical factors is small. The evidence on the role of some physical factors (eg, forcefulness of grip and repetitive motions of the hand) is fairly consistent. It is also evident from Tables 1 and 2 that there are no published studies among heavily exposed populations showing negative results.

A more detailed description of the patterns of force levels and their distribution over the work day has not been used in any epidemiologic study. Opinions differ whether such detailed information is possible to collect and utilize.[28,29] However, it would be feasible to study the induction times for various types of work sufficient to cause the disease and the latency in the manifestation of the disease.[23,30] Because no prospective follow-up studies have been conducted on CTS that consider occupational status and level of physical work load, the natural course of the disorder is not well known. For example, it is not known whether people can adapt to certain levels of physical stress after an initial disease episode, nor is it known whether a chronic underlying condition (eg, thickening of the flexor tendons) continues to produce and exacerbate symptoms at relatively low stress levels.

A considerable proportion of CTS sufferers are treated surgically. In most cases, the immediate and long-term results have been reported to be good.[31] Yet, a study among workers in a meat packing plant reported results that were not as good with 52% returning to work after 1 year.[32] Likewise, in the study by Adams and associates,[31] workers in high-risk occupations were less likely to return to their previous jobs than were workers in medium-to low-risk oc-

Table 1 Cross-sectional studies on carpal tunnel syndrome

Study Population	Outcome	Exposure
162 female garment workers, 73 hospital workers	Nocturnal pain, numbness or tingling in the median nerve innervated area of the hand; 2 of the following 3 additional criteria had to be met: weakness in gripping or pinching, alleviation by absence from work, aggravation by household work or other nonoccupational tasks; positive Tinel's or Phalen's test	Garment work (stitching, finishing, underpressing), floor work, shipping, others (operation of fusing machine, etc), hospital work (nurses, physical therapists, technicians, administrative employees)
652 industrial workers, 358 men and 294 women	Pain, numbness, or tingling in the median nerve distribution of the hand with nocturnal exacerbation more than 20 times or lasting more than 1 week in the previous year; onset of symptoms since on current job; positive Tinel's sign or Phalen's test; cervical root, thoracic outlet, pronator teres syndrome, rheumatoid arthritis and traumatic onset excluded	39 jobs allocated to 4 exposure categories based on video and EMG recordings of 3 workers/job: low force-low repetitive (LOF-LOR), low force-high repetitive (LOF-HIR), high force-low repetitive (HIF-LOR), high force-high repetitive (HIF-HIR)
471 industrial employees, gender not reported	Maximum latency difference of 0.4 ms or greater for 8 sensory latencies assessed in consecutive 1-cm segments of the median nerve	Occupations classified into 5 categories according to estimated amount of resistance and rate of repetition: administrative/clerical (I), keyboard operator (II), assembly (III), general plant (IV), grinder (V)
173 ski manufacturing workers: 48 men and 58 women in repetitive jobs, 43 men and 24 women in nonrepetitive jobs	Prevalence of CTS using the following 3 case definitions: 1) median-ulnar sensory latency difference > 0.5 ms 2) as above plus positive Phalen's test or Tinel's sign 3) median-ulnar sensory latency difference > 0.5 ms plus positive Phalen's test or Tinel's sign, or history of CTS symptoms	Jobs classified into repetitive and nonrepetitive. Repetitive jobs involved repeated or sustained flexion, extension, or ulnar deviation of the wrist by 45°; radial deviation by 30°; or use of pinch grip
207 frozen food factory workers, 67 men and 140 women	Numbness, pain, or tingling in the fingers innervated by the median nerve and positive Tinel's sign or Phalen's test. Onset of symptoms since in current job, systemic disease and traumatic onset ruled out	Classification of workers into 3 groups according to the ergonomic risks of the shoulders and upper limbs: low repetition and low force (group I), high repetition or high force (group II), high repetition and high force (group III); video recordings performed on 1 worker per group
240 industrial workers: 103 with median nerve symptoms in the hand ("symptomatic hand" group), 137 with no symptoms in the hand ("asymptomatic hand" group); 105 control subjects in administrative and professional positions	Median sensory and motor amplitudes and distal latencies, median-ulnar sensory latency difference	Industrial and nonindustrial (control) job; industrial jobs further classified based on checklists according to repetitiveness, forcefulness, mechanical stress, pinch grip, and wrist deviation

* EMG, electromyography
† RR, rate ratio; OR, odds ratio

Adjustment	Exposed Prevalence		Referents' Prevalence		Risk (RR)	95% CI	Reference
None	6.8		5.5		1.2	0.4-3.8	Punnett et al 1985[12]
Age, gender, plant, years on job	HIF-LOR	1.9	LOF-LOR	0.6	unadj. RR:[+] 1.6	0.2-17.2	Silverstein et al 1987[13]
	LOF-HIR	2.1	LOF-LOR	0.6	3.3	0.4-27.5	
	HIF-HIR	5.6	LOF-LOR	0.6	8.0	1.4-44.9	
	HIF-LOR	1.9	LOF-LOR	0.6	adj. OR:[+] 1.8	0.2-20.6	
	LOF-HIR	2.1	LOF-LOR	0.6	2.7	0.3-28.4	
	HIF-HIR	5.6	LOF-LOR	0.6	15.5	1.7-141.5	
Age	Group II	27	Group I	28	1.0	0.5-2.0	Nathan et al 1988[14]
	Group III	47	Group I	28	1.7	1.3-2.3	
	Group IV	38	Group I	28	1.4	1.0-1.9	
	Group V	61	Group I	28	2.2	1.3-3.6	
Age, gender	Case definition 1	34		19	1.9	1.0-3.6	Barnhart et al 1991[15]
	Case definition 2	15		3	4.0	1.0-15.8	
	Case definition 3	33		18	1.6	0.8-3.2	
None	HIF or HIR, men	6.9	LOF and LOR, men	3.1	2.2	0.2-22.0	Chiang et al 1993[16]
	HIF or HIR, women	18.0	LOF and LOR, women	13.8	1.3	0.5-3.5	
	HIF and HIR, men	0.0	LOF and LOR, men	3.1	2.6	1.0-7.3	
	HIF and HIR, women	36.4	LOF and LOR, women	13.8			
Age, height, skin temperature, and dominant index finger circumference	No classification of nerve conduction values. All median sensory amplitudes were smaller and distal latencies longer among the "asymptomatic hand" group than among the control group. Within the industrial population, median sensory amplitudes smaller, and distal latencies longer among the "symptomatic hand" group than among the "asymptomatic hand" group. A similar difference according to forcefulness of job.						Stetson et al 1993[17]

Table 2 Case-referent studies on carpal tunnel syndrome

Case Definition	Referents	Exposure	Adjustment	Risk (OR)	95% CI	Reference
18 female sewing machine workers with a history of CTS (history of numbness or pain in the area of the hand innervated by the median nerve, or CTS surgery, or positive Phalen's test, or thenar atrophy)	18 women in the same jobs as the cases with no history, symptoms or signs of CTS	Hand and wrist postures by cinematography, estimation of forearm flexor force in various wrist and hand postures by EMG	None	The cases tended to use pinch grip more often and to exert more force in pinch grip than the controls. The cases also tended to use nonneutral wrist postures more frequently and to exert more force in these postures than the controls		Armstrong and Chaffin 1979[18]
16 workers in an aircraft company receiving compensation benefits for the treatment of CTS (plant medical diagnosis) plus 14 cases with CTS who had not received workers' compensation benefits, for a total of 27 women and 3 men	3 referents per case matched for gender selected randomly from the same company	Use of low-frequency vibrating tools and repetitive motion tasks of the wrists determined by job title, years on the job	Years on the job, use of low-frequency vibrating tools, repetitive motion tasks of the wrist, history of gynecologic surgery	Years on the job 0.9 Use of vibr. tools 7.0 Rep. motion tasks 2.1	0.8-1.0 3.0-17 0.9-5.3	Cannon et al 1981[19]
34 hospital patients (all men) for whom CTS surgery had been performed (clinical diagnosis and electrodiagnostic verification)	2 referents matched for gender, age and operation year from other surgical patients from the same hospital (1 surgery for bladder disease, 1 surgery for varicose veins); 2 additional referents matched for age and gender from the general population of the hospital's catchment area	Years worked with hand-held vibrating tools, years worked with repetitive movements of the wrist, years with tasks causing great loads on the wrist, assessed by telephone interview	None (matched for gender and age)	1-20 years vibrating tools 2.7 > 20 years vibrating tools 4.8 1-20 years rep. movements 1.5 > 20 years rep. movements 4.6 1-20 years heavy loads 1.7 > 20 years heavy loads 2.1	1.1-6.7 1.5-15.6 0.5-4.4 1.8-11.9 0.7-3.9 0.8-5.5	Wieslander et al 1989[20]
28 CTS cases from a population survey plus 128 consecutive CTS patients from a hospital (altogether 25 men and 131 women). CTS diagnostic criteria: tingling, pain and/or numbness in the median nerve innervated fingers at least twice a week, usually waking up at night plus abnormal median nerve conduction at the wrist (distal motor latency > 4.5 msec, median ulnar nerve distal sensory latency difference > 0.4 msec)	Random population sample of 164 men and 483 women.	Activities with flexed wrist, extended wrist, extended and flexed wrist in combination, and pinch grasp 0-5 years ago (hours per week based on interview). Similar recording of typing hours.	Gender, age	1-7 hours flexed wrist 1.5 8-19 hours flexed wrist 3.0 20-40 hours flexed wrist 8.7 1-7 hours extended wrist 1.4 8-19 hours extended wrist 2.3 20-40 hours extended wrist 5.4 Activities with extended and flexed wrist in combination, pinch grasp, and typing hours not associated with CTS	1.3-1.9 1.8-4.9 3.1-24.1 1.0-1.9 1.0-5.2 1.1-27.4	deKrom et al 1990[21]

cupations (61% versus 75%). These results suggest that workers in hand-intensive tasks may have difficulty coping with their tasks after CTS surgery.

One reason for this may be the alterations in the biomechanical conditions in the wrist during gripping as a consequence of the incision of the volar ligament. The results of a small study of patients treated surgically for CTS suggest that the transverse carpal arch is widened due to surgery and that the extent of widening is associated with the loss of grip strength.[33] This means that a patient who has been treated surgically for CTS has to use a higher proportion of his or her maximal voluntary contraction during gripping in a given task than he or she did before surgery. Assuming that the patient returns to his or her previous work tasks, the relative force requirements will be increased. Carefully conducted studies considering the functional status of the hand before and after surgery and the demands of the work on the hand are needed to give more information about the effects CTS surgery has on the performance of the hand.

Other Nerve Entrapments

The median nerve may be trapped in the forearm, causing the anterior interosseous syndrome, and in several locations at the elbow, causing the pronator syndrome. The ulnar nerve may be trapped in the cubital tunnel in the elbow and in Guyon's canal in the proximal palm. The radial nerve may be trapped at the lateral aspect of the proximal forearm, causing the radial tunnel syndrome or the posterior interosseous nerve syndrome.[34]

Specific movements have been associated with the occurrence of certain entrapment neuropathies, such as forceful pronations with the pronator syndrome,[35] elbow flexions and extensions with the cubital tunnel syndrome,[34] and repetitive movements of the wrist and forearm with the radial tunnel syndrome[34] and the posterior interosseous nerve entrapment.[36] The vast majority of such information has been based on observations of cases or case series and no properly designed epidemiologic study attempting to evaluate the relative role of occupational and individual factors has been reported. In the study by Stetson and associates,[17] ulnar sensory amplitudes (wrist-digit IV, wrist-digit V, wrist-midpalm) were smaller and distal latencies longer in the asymptomatic industrial population than in the control population, suggesting that manually strenuous tasks had an effect on distal ulnar nerve function. Different kinds of tumors, ganglions, tight fibrotic bands of muscles, aberrant courses of nerves, and trauma have often been mentioned as the primary causes for these entrapments.[34]

Compression Neuropathies

In addition to entrapment neuropathies, compression neuropathies are fairly common in the ulnar nerve at Guyon's canal. Ulnar nerve compression symptoms have been associated with compression from the knife in deboning work of meat packers.[37] The median nerve may be compressed in the wrist by poorly fitting gloves and in the palm by tools or levers.[38]

Tendon Disorders

Case series of tenosynovitis and peritendinitis in the wrist and forearm region have been described in the literature since the beginning of this century.[2,3,39,40] Although these disorders have been the focus of interest for such a long time, it is noteworthy that so few studies have been undertaken using modern epidemiologic principles and validated exposure and outcome measures (Table 3).

The assessment of the outcome presents a major problem in epidemiologic studies on tenosynovitis and peritendinitis. There is no feasible way of objectively measuring the existence or the severity of the disease. A clinical diagnosis of tenosynovitis or peritendinitis is probably valid at an acute stage of the disease when clearly distinguishable swelling may be observed or crepitation is present. Such a condition is not very common among working populations.[6] Therefore, some investigators have used softer criteria in order to find a sufficient number of subjects with a diagnosable disorder in a cohort study.[41,42] The validity of such diagnoses is largely unknown. No case-referent studies have been reported on tendon disorders.

The wide range in the prevalence rates of tenosynovitis or peritendinitis in the studies listed in Table 3 may be explained by differences in study population characteristics and occupational exposure or by the differences in the diagnostic criteria used and the poor interexaminer consistency between most items in the physical examination.[45,46] With strict diagnostic criteria, the prevalence of these diseases may be fairly low, even in highly exposed subjects.[6,7] Although two of the studies[7,42] used detailed information on physical exposure, this information was extrapolated based on the evaluation of only some of the workers on each job, and therefore individual differences in working techniques were not considered.

Most studies listed in Table 3 show strong associations between manually strenuous tasks and tenosynovitis or peritendinitis. In the cross-sectional studies, high repetitiveness of work movements and the use of high forces appeared as risk factors. The exception was the study by Kuorinka and Koskinen,[42] in which cycle time was not a risk factor, and only the total work load tended to be associated with muscle tendon syndrome. The authors suggested that one reason for this may have been that the cycle time did not always seem to be associated with the speed of work movements. Use of a more accurate measure of repetitiveness, fundamental cycles in the analysis might have revealed stronger associations. Furthermore, job rotation may have caused error in individual exposure assessments. Finally, differences in the tasks between the workers may not have been large enough to cause differences in the prevalence of the outcome. Kurppa and associates[44] based their case definition on a diagnosis made during the worker's visit to a doctor's office. A difference in illness behavior, that is, a greater proneness of the afflicted workers with strenuous tasks than those with less strenuous tasks to seek medical advice most likely contributed to the high incidence rate ratios.[47]

The absence of evidence for an association between nonneutral wrist postures and tendon disorders is noteworthy in the only study in which this was specifically assessed. In the study by Kurppa and associates,[44] the packers worked in a cold environment, which may partially explain the extra risk of packers when compared with sausage makers.

None of the studies listed in Table 3 addressed the temporal relationships between the exposure and the disease. According to the analyses of clinical case series of tenosynovitis and peritendinitis[3,48] and the cases of peritendinitis in one epidemiologic study,[6] most of the afflictions are preceded by a change in work exposure (resumption of activities after a leave or a change in the quantity or quality of work) or trauma. An induction period of some days to some weeks from the onset of the exposure to the manifestation of the disease has been reported.[3,6] The prognosis of acute tenosynovitis and peritendinitis is usually favorable, and the symptoms resolve in most cases in from 1 to 2 weeks.[44]

Occupational health physicians do see workers with chronic tendon problems, but the nature and course of such problems has been poorly described in the literature.

Under working conditions the tendons are exposed to tensile loads and compressive loads either extrinsically or intrinsically. Intrinsic compressive forces arise when loaded tendons pass around deviated joints. The tendons respond to tensile loads by elongation, which is reversible within certain load-rest levels. Beyond these limits, one may observe "accumulated" creep,[49] the significance of which regarding the pathogenesis of tendon-related disorders is not known.[50] Moore[50] suggests that under physiologic conditions, tendon fibril disruption is more likely caused by compressive loads than by tensile loads. The existing knowledge on the responses by the tissues to mechanical loads suggests that it is biologically plausible that repetitive tendon loading together with nonneutral wrist and finger postures are important risk factors of tendon disorders. Peritendinitis is believed to occur when fatigue of the muscle or direct trauma cause circulatory disturbances and edema in the muscle and paratenon.[50]

The maximal voluntary contraction of the muscles is reduced in a cold environment.[51] The muscles must use a higher proportion of their maximal voluntary contraction for a given task in a cold environment than would be needed for the same task in a warm environment; ie, the relative force demands are increased. Tenosynovitis has also been reported to occur by a cold injury mechanism after sudden exposure to temperatures clearly below 0° C.[52]

Although there seems to be little controversy in the literature that strenuous manual tasks may be causal factors in the development of tenosynovitis and peritendinitis of the wrist and forearm region, knowledge about the role of physical factors is almost entirely on a qualitative level. Knowledge on exposure-effect relationships is urgently needed. The contribution of wrist and hand postures and cold environment needs further exploration. Valid objective methods for case definition would be of great value for epidemiologists.

Epicondylitis

The six studies on epicondylitis listed in Table 4 have used fairly consistent criteria to define the disease. Most of the studies[41,43,44,54] have assessed exposure according to occupational title and no study assessed generic risk factors by validated methods. The results of these studies are conflicting, however. Some of the cross-sectional studies suggest an association between strenuous manual tasks and epicondylitis,[16,41,43] and others do not.[53,54] Four studies had low statistical power.[16,41,43,54] Some studies clearly dealt with survivor populations.[43,54]

An interesting result was observed in the study of Chiang and associates.[16] The prevalence of epicondylitis associated with increasing repetitiveness and forcefulness of work was statistically significant when only those who had been in their current job less than 12 months were considered. A similar trend was observed among those who had been in their job for 12 to 60 months, but a reverse trend was observed among those employed for more than 60 months. One explanation for this could be that in this study population, workers with epicondylitis had left the job. Accordingly, a prospective study among a cohort of new workers in hand-intensive tasks might provide interesting information on the association between physical stressors and epicondylitis. The incidence rate ratios of epicondylitis between workers in strenuous and nonstrenuous jobs were higher in the study of Kurppa and associates[44] than in any rate ratios

Table 3 Epidemiologic studies on tenosynovitis or peritendinitis of the wrist-forearm region

Study Population	Outcome	Exposure	Adjustment
152 female assembly-line packers, 133 female shop assistants	Prevalence of muscle-tendon syndrome (tenosynovitis or peritendinitis of the wrist-forearm): local ache, pain during movement, tenderness, weakness in gripping	Operating hard bread sawing and packing machines, finishing of packages, some job rotation (assembly line packers) (video recordings showed repetitive motions of the hands and fingers up to 25,000 cycles per day, static muscle work of forearm muscles, extreme postures of the fingers and deviations of the wrist, lifting); physically light work performed when standing (shop assistants, cashiers excluded)	None
90 female and 3 male scissor makers	Prevalence of muscle-tendon syndrome (tenosynovitis or peritendinitis of the wrist-forearm)	8 tasks classified according to dominating characteristic (inspection or manipulation), cycle time, and wrist deviation index, based on observations and video recordings of 1 to 10 workers per task; total work load during the investigation year recorded individually as pieces handled	None
90 meatcutters, 72 construction foremen	Prevalence of tenosynovitis (local pain during movement, swelling, weakness in finger movements)	Meatcutter's work in slaughterhouses or food processing industry	None
574 industrial workers, 287 men and 287 women	Prevalence of cumulative trauma disorders, consisting primarily of tendon related disorders and CTS, fulfilling the following criteria: pain numbness or tingling lasting > 1 week or occurring > 20 times in the previous year, no traumatic onset, no related systemic disease, onset since in current job, characteristic signs of muscle, tendon, or peripheral nerve lesions, differential diagnostics considered	39 jobs allocated to 4 exposure categories based on video and EMG recordings of at least 3 workers/job: low force-low repetitive (LOF-LOR), low force-high repetitive (LOF-HIR), high force-low repetitive (HIF-LOR), high force-high repetitive (HIF-HIR)	Age, gender, plant, years on job
102 male meatcutters (248 person years [py]), 107 female sausage makers (220 py), 118 female packers (253 py), and 141 men (334 py) and 197 women (456 py) in nonstrenuous tasks	Incidence (rate per 100 py) of tenosynovitis or peritendinitis in the wrist or forearm based on visits to doctor during a follow-up of 31 months	Cutting of veal (appr. 1,200 kg per day) or pork (appr. 3,000 kg per day) (meatcutters); spraying the sausages and hanging them on bars (sausage makers); peeling sausages, inserting them into slicing machine, setting the slices into packages, setting packages on a conveyer belt, collecting finished packages into bags; room temperature 8° to 10° C (packers); nonstrenuous tasks included primarily office work	None, same gender and similar age structure between groups compared

Exposed Prevalence or Incidence (%)	Referents' Prevalence or Incidence (%)	Risk (RR)	95% CI	Reference

Muscle-tendon syndrome 56
Tenosynovitis
  Extensors 44
  Flexors 18
Peritendinitis
  Extensors 26
  Flexors 17
Right hand more often than left affected, bilateral involvement in 31% of cases. Both extensor and flexor sides affected in 19% of cases
	Muscle-tendon syndrome 14
	Tenosynovitis
	  Extensors 6
	  Flexors 8
	Peritendinitis
	  Extensors 4
	  Flexors 3
	Left hand more often than right affected, bilateral involvement in 6% of cases, Both extensor and flexor sides affected in 0% of cases
		4.1
		
		7.3
		2.5
		
		6.8
		5.7
			2.8-6.0
			
			4.3-12.5
			1.3-4.7
			
			3.3-14.3
			2.4-13.7
				Luopajärvi et al 1979[41]

Prevalence of muscle tendon syndrome 18%. No statistically significant differences in prevalence according to dominating job characteristic, cycle time or wrist deviation index. Tendency of workers with muscle-tendon syndrome to have a higher total work load than those without				Kuorinka and Koskinen 1979[42]
4.5	0.0			Roto and Kivi 1984[43]

Men
  HIF-LOR 1
  LOF-HIR 2
  HIF-HIR 15
Women
  HIF-LOR 17
  LOF-HIR 8
  HIF-HIR 25
Men and women
  HIF-LOR 7
  LOF-HIR 7
  HIF-HIR 20
	Men
	  LOF-LOR 0
	  LOF-LOR 0
	  LOF-LOR 0
	Women
	  LOF-LOR 3
	  LOF-LOR 3
	  LOF-LOR 3
	Men and women
	  LOF-LOR 2
	  LOF-LOR 2
	  LOF-LOR 2
		(unadj. RR:)
		5.3
		2.7
		7.8
		(adj OR:)
		5.2
		3.3
		29.1
			
			1.4-19.5
			0.7-11.4
			2.5-24.3
			
			1.1-25.0
			0.7-15.9
			5.9-142.7
				Silverstein et al 1986[7]

Meatcutters 13 Sausage makers 17 Packers 25	Nonstrenuous jobs, men 1 Nonstrenuous jobs, women 1 Nonstrenuous jobs, women 1	14.0 25.6 38.5	5.7-34.4 11.7-56.1 19.2-77.5	Kurppa et al 1991[44]

Table 4 Epidemiologic studies on humeral epicondylitis

Study Population	Outcome	Exposure
152 female assembly line packers, 133 female shop assistants	Prevalence of lateral and medial epicondylitis (local pain during rest or active movements, tenderness at the lateral/medial epicondyle on palpation, pain during resisted extension/flexion of the wrist and fingers with the elbow extended)	See Table 3
90 meatcutters, 72 construction foremen	Prevalence of lateral or medial epicondylitis (local tenderness, pain during resisted extension/flexion of the wrist and fingers, decreased hand grip power)	Meatcutter's work in slaughterhouses or food processing industry
540 workers in an engineering industry (494 men and 52 women, 340 blue-collar workers and 200 white-collar workers)	Prevalence of lateral epicondylitis (lateral elbow pain, pain on palpation at the lateral epicondyle, pain increase on wrist extension against resistance)	Estimated elbow stress according to job title
102 male meatcutters, 107 female sausage makers, 118 female packers, and 141 men and 197 women in nonstrenuous tasks	Prevalence of lateral and medial epicondylitis in three clinical cross-sectional studies (tenderness to palpation at the lateral/medial epicondyle and pain at the same epicondyle in resisted extension/flexion of the wrist and fingers with the elbow extended)	Cutting of veal (approx. 1200 kg/day) or pork (approx. 3000 kg/day) (meatcutters); spraying the sausages and hanging them on bars (sausage makers); peeling sausages, inserting them into slicing machine, setting the slices into packages, setting packages on a conveyer belt, collecting finished packages into bags; room temperature 8° to 10° C (packers); nonstrenuous tasks included primarily office work
102 male meatcutters (248 person years [py]), 107 female sausage makers (220 py), 118 female packers (253 py) and 141 men (334 py) and 197 women (456 py) in nonstrenuous tasks	Incidence of lateral or medial epicondylitis based on visits to doctor during a follow-up of 31 months (case definition as above)	Same as in the study of Viikari-Juntura et al[54]
207 workers in 8 fish processing plants, 67 men and 140 women	Prevalence of lateral or medial epicondylitis (local tenderness, pain in resisted extension or flexion of the wrist and fingers, decreased hand grip strength)	Groups I-III are defined as in Table 1

Adjustment	Exposed Prevalence or Incidence (%)	Referents' Prevalence or Incidence (%)	Risk (RR)	95% CI	Reference
None	Epicondylitis 5.3 Lateral 2.6 Medial 3.3	Epicondylitis 2.3 Lateral 2.3 Medial 0.0	2.6 1.2	0.8-9.0 0.3-5.1	Luopajärvi et al 1979[41]
None	8.9	1.4	6.4	1.0-40.9	Roto and Kivi 1984[43]
None	Blue-collar wkrs 5 Elbow stress not associated with occurrence of epicondylitis	White-collar workers 11	0.5	0.3-0.9	Dimberg 1987[53]
None (same gender and similar age structure between groups compared)	Epicondylitis 0.8 Lateral 0.6 Medial 0.2 (meatcutters, sausage makers, packers)	Epicondylitis 0.8 Lateral 0.5 Medial 0.3 (workers in nonstrenuous tasks)			Viikari-Juntura et al 1991[54]
None (same gender and similar age structure between groups compared)	Meatcutters 6 Sausage makers 11 Packers 7	Nonstrenuous jobs, men 1 Nonstrenuous jobs, women 1 Nonstrenuous jobs, women 1	7.1 10.3 6.4	2.5-20.5 4.7-22.3 2.7-15.1	Kurppa et al 1991[44]
None	Group II 15 Men 10 Women 17 Group III 21 Men 33 Women 18	Group I 10 Men 6 Women 14 Group I 10 Men 6 Women 14	 1.7 1.2 5.3 1.3	 0.3-9.2 0.4-3.4 1.0-28.5 0.4-4.7	Chiang et al 1993[16]

from other studies. In this study, case definition was based on visits to a doctor. It is plausible that forceful and repetitive exertions of the forearm muscles can cause epicondylitis, however, the epidemiologic evidence, is limited.

Bone and Joint Pathology

In their extensive review on radiologically assessed bone and joint pathology in the hands and arms of workers using vibrating tools, Gemne and Saraste[27] mention four types of pathology: exostosis at the sites of tendon insertion, osteoarthrosis, special types of pathology (eg, Kienböck's disease [lunate malacia] and pseudarthrosis of the scaphoid), and cysts and vacuoles.

Based on epidemiologic studies on various occupational groups using hand-held vibrating tools of the percussive, low-frequency type (less than about 40 Hz), there is evidence of an excess risk of premature osteoarthrosis of the elbow and the wrist. An excess risk for joint pathology has not been conclusively demonstrated to be caused by vibration exposure from tools with medium or high frequencies. An increased risk of osteoarthrosis also has been observed among workers with heavy manual tasks but no exposure to vibrating hand tools, for example, radiographically defined elbow osteoarthrosis among miners who had not drilled[1] and clinically defined distal interphalangeal osteoarthrosis (Heberden's nodes) among women with at least 10 years' exposure to work tasks with moderate or heavy physical demands.[55] A German study among 110 resin tappers reported an independent effect of years working as a resin tapper on the development of radiographically assessed elbow osteoarthrosis, whereas both age and length of time as resin tapper predicted wrist arthrosis.[56] The work of resin tappers is physically heavy and involves manual handling of heavy loads. In many studies, it has not been possible to differentiate between the effects of forceful hand exertions and low-frequency vibration, because they occur concomitantly.

Gemne and Saraste[27] suggest the following physical load factors to be etiologic for elbow and wrist osteoarthrosis: joint load associated with the manipulation of tools in manual work, repetitive movements possibly associated with minor traumatization, loading of the joint surfaces in extreme positions, and static work. With low-frequency vibrating tools, additional factors include shocks to the articular cartilage from the tool, additional articular load associated with a vibration-induced increase in the need for joint stabilization, the tonic vibration reflex (increasing muscle contraction), and a stronger grip on the tool handle induced when tactile sensibility is diminished by vibration.

Of the special types of pathology, pseudarthrosis of the scaphoid is considered to be the result of fracture. Microtraumatization has not been considered as an etiologic factor. The etiology of Kienböck's disease is not fully understood.[27] The relationship of bone cysts and vacuoles to physical work load factors has not been demonstrated.

Many of the studies with radiographic assessment of osteoarthrosis are old, and some of the exposures in these studies no longer exist in the industrialized countries.[57] In mining, the machinery is equipped with jack legs, and most miners are exposed to vibration for only occasional short periods. Similarly, the machinery used in road and house construction is now equipped with dampers.

Concerning the lower spine and the weightbearing joints, some epidemiologic and experimental studies have suggested that there is a range of optimal physical loading, below and above which the risk of structural changes increases.[58,59] A similar relationship between physical loading and the health of the joints of the upper limb might be likely. Whether this hypothesis is true will need to be investigated in future studies. The concepts of repetitive trauma and overloading have prevailed in occupational epidemiology and not much attention has been paid to underload or inactivity.

Most studies on radiographically detected osteoarthrosis have been cross-sectional and represent survivor populations. Therefore, it is likely that risk will be underestimated. Radiographic evaluation of the degenerative changes represents a valid and unbiased method of outcome assessment, provided that the assessors are blinded to the exposure of the subjects. The latency period after which the possible effects of physical work load factors may be seen on plain radiographs is probably some years. Therefore, it is preferable that these effects are evaluated against assessments of cumulative exposure. Modern imaging methods (eg, magnetic resonance imaging) might provide an assessment method for short- and long-term effects.

Compartment Syndrome

The muscles, nerves, and blood vessels in the forearm and hand are located in specific compartments defined by bones, membranes, and fasciae. Compartment syndrome denotes a condition in which the intracompartmental pressure is constantly or repeatedly increased to a level at which the compartmental structures may be injured. This may occur after trauma, such as fracture or crush injury to the arm. Compartment syndrome after strenuous exertion of the muscles is a well-known disease in the lower extremity. Some cases and case series of exertional compartment syndrome in the forearm and hand have also been described, although the occurrence of these conditions is not known,[60,61] nor have generally accepted diagnostic criteria nor indications for treatment been defined.[62]

There are two compartments in the forearm. The dorsal compartment includes the wrist and finger extensors, the supinator, and the radial nerve. The volar compartment includes the wrist and finger flexors, the pronator, and the median and ulnar nerves. There are five interosseous compartments in the hand. The compartment syndromes of the cases described thus far have been located in the volar and dorsal compartments of the forearm[61,62] as well as in the first dorsal interosseous compartment.[60] The afflicted workers have usually had hand-intensive work, although no epidemiologic studies on the association between work and these disorders have been published.

The symptoms of compartment syndrome include tenseness of the fascial boundaries of the compartment, pain during muscle contraction and later also during rest, and muscle weakness. In clinical examination, the compartment area is tender, there is pain on passive stretching, and there may be hypoesthesia in the distribution of the nerves running through the compartment.[63] Intracompartmental pressure measurements during rest, during activity, and after activity have been used to confirm the diagnosis, but full agreement on reference values does not exist.

The clinical picture of compartment syndrome is consistent with that of the cases sometimes seen by occupational health physicians. If valid diagnostic criteria could be determined for this disorder, some workers with previously poorly understood symptoms might be correctly diagnosed. Epidemiologists also would profit from diagnostic criteria, so that risk factors for this condition could be investigated.

Ulnar Artery Thrombosis (Hypothenar Hammer Syndrome)

The ulnar artery may be damaged and undergo subsequent thrombosis and vascular occlusion in the Guyon's canal on the ulnar aspect of the palm. A history of repeated trauma to the ulnar side of the palm (hypothenar eminence), such as intensive hammering or using the hypothenar eminence as a hammer, has often preceded the disease. In a group of 79 male employees in vehicle maintenance workshops who used the hand as hammer, the prevalence of this disorder was 14%. In a referent group of the same occupation not using the hand as hammer, the prevalence was 0%.[64] In a group of platers exposed to low-, medium-, and high-frequency vibration and pressure in the palm from tools as well as possible hammering with the hands, 37% had a positive response for Allen's test of the ulnar artery compared with 20% in the control group of office workers.[65] A positive result for Allen's test suggests impaired circulation in the ulnar artery.

Other Disorders

Ganglions in the Wrist and Hand

Ganglions are soft mucin-filled cysts that represent the majority of all soft-tissue tumors of the hand. The most typical location of the ganglion is the dorsoradial aspect of the wrist. The volar wrist ganglion, is typically located on the radial side of the flexor carpi radialis tendon. The third commonly occurring ganglion is located at the proximal pulley of the finger flexor tendon sheath at the level of the metacarpal heads. A volar wrist ganglion may cause entrapment of the median nerve in the carpal tunnel resulting in CTS. In rare cases, a ganglion may be located in Guyon's canal and cause entrapment of the ulnar nerve.

Ganglions are common, although the prevalence in populations is not well known. The prevalence of ganglions on clinical examination was 5% among 130 newspaper employees with at least moderately severe symptoms of work-related upper limb disorders, but only 1% among 99 nonsymptomatic controls.[46] In a clinical cross-sectional examination of 113 slaughterhouse workers (52 cutters, 38 butchers, and 23 meat by-product workers), five cases of painful carpal ganglia (four volar and one dorsal) were found.[6] All volar ganglia were found in cutters and all were in the dominant hand. Three were persistent after earlier surgery. Two workers had nocturnal paresthesiae of the median area and one also had a positive Tinel's sign and Phalen's test.

Controversy exists on the etiology of ganglia. Some consider them congenital and others believe that acute or repeated trauma plays a role in their development. Different opinions also exist on the pathogenesis of the ganglia.

The data presented above suggest that ganglia are a potentially significant work-related problem. Epidemiologic studies have suffered from difficulties in case definition because no valid objective method of assessment has been used to this point. Modern imaging methods, eg, ultrasound or magnetic resonance imaging, could be a feasible alternative for case ascertainment in etiologic studies on wrist and hand ganglia.

Olecranon Bursitis

Olecranon bursitis is an inflammation of the olecranon bursa on the dorsal side of the elbow. It may be caused by repeated mechanical trauma (traumatic, or "student's bursitis"). It also may be septic or associated with gout.

Dupuytren's Contracture

Dupuytren's contracture is a fibrosis of the palmar fascia of the hand leading to flexion contracture of the fingers. It is a familial disease transmitted by a single autosomal dominant gene. It is a common condition in people of North-European origin, affecting about 3% of the general population. The disease is twice as common among men as among women, and as many as 20% of males older than 60 years may have it. Dupuytren's contracture is associated with epilepsy, type 1 diabetes, alcohol consumption, and smoking.[66] The disease has been associated with trauma and heavy manual labor.[67] Few controlled studies have been carried out, however, and the role of occupational factors in the etiology of Dupuytren's contracture has not been generally accepted.[66,68]

Functional Impairment

Some of the upper limb disorders of workers can be classified into diagnostic entities. Because the number of individual diseases has often been small, many studies have suffered from low statistical power. Some investigators have chosen to measure various aspects of upper limb function and have used these measurements as the outcome instead of attempting to make a clinical diagnosis based on symptoms and signs (Table 1).[17] The assessment of function may offer more sensitive outcome measures. Not much is known, however, about the significance of slightly impaired function; eg, its predictive value.

A functional impairment score, composed of grip and pinch strength measurement, Semmes-Weinstein monofilament test, vibrometer, neurometer, and Tinel's and Phalen's sign, was constructed and used as one outcome in a study among meat-processing workers.[69] This was done in order to group the various pathologic conditions as one functional impairment entity. The results suggested lower scores for less repetitive jobs and for workers who rotated their jobs. Although this result was significant, even after adjustment for age and job seniority, gender was not taken into account in the analysis and remains a possible confounder.

Elbow, Forearm, Wrist, and Hand Pain

Some studies that have used subjective symptoms in the elbow, forearm, wrist, or hand as the outcome are listed in Table 5. These studies have been chosen on the basis that the localization of symptoms has been clearly indicated in the study and the symptoms have been judged moderate or severe, depending on their intensity or frequency. Subjective reporting of symptoms is liable to errors of recall. Whether a subject can remember lifetime sciatic pain has been shown to be dependent on occupation and age: those with physically less-demanding jobs have forgotten their symptoms more frequently than those with strenuous jobs, and young subjects have forgotten more frequently than the middle-aged subjects.[73] Studies on recall error of upper limb symptoms have not been reported, but one may expect the predictors for forgetting symptoms to be similar. The subjective assessment of physical work load factors in a cross-sectional study may be biased by the perception of symptoms and lead to spurious associations between exposure and symptoms.[74,75]

Many studies on upper limb symptoms have investigated the role of psychosocial factors at work. Some of these studies provide very little information on the physical work load factors,[71,76] or they report on populations in which there is little variation in physical work load.[76] Therefore, the relative

Table 5 Epidemiologic studies on elbow, wrist and hand symptoms

Study Population	Outcome	Exposure	Adjustment
162 female garment workers, 73 female hospital employees	Prevalence of persistent pain, numbness, or tingling in elbow, wrist, or hand (pain lasting for most days for 1 month or more within the past year), prevalence of CTS symptoms	See Table 1	None
652 industrial workers, 358 males and 294 females	symptoms of CTS (see Table 1)	4 exposure categories based on force and repetition (see Table 1)	None
102 male meatcutters, 107 female sausage makers, 118 female packers, and 141 men and 197 women in nonstrenuous tasks	Pain in the elbow during the preceding 7 days in three consecutive cross-sectional studies within a time period of 18 months	See Table 4	None, same gender and similar age structure between groups compared
50 supermarket checkers, 18 men and 32 women	sum score for wrist-hand symptoms, sum score for carpal tunnel symptoms	Individual indices of wrist flexion, wrist extension, forearm pronation, pinch grip, dragging, trunk flexion, based on observations and video recordings	None
973 newspaper employees, 577 men, 396 women	Prevalence of symptoms of hand/wrist disorders during the preceding year fulfilling the following criteria: no previous accident or nonwork-related injury, symptoms started since in current job, symptoms lasted for more than 1 week or occurred at least once a month	Hours worked per week, hours of VDT use per day, hours on telephone per day, number of brief breaks, number of long breaks, based on self-assessments	Demographic variables, work practices, job history, other work organizational factors, psychosocial factors
4,332 workers in various tasks in forestry industry, 3,205 men and 1,127 women	Case-referent study on incidence and persistence of severe forearm-hand pain (pain on 30 days or more during the preceding 12 months) during a follow-up of 1 year	Physical heaviness of work, postural factors of the trunk and extremities, repetitive movements of the wrist and fingers, risk of injury to the upper limb (questionnaire assessment)	Individual factors and psychosocial work characteristics

importance of physical versus psychosocial factors cannot be adequately evaluated in these studies.

There are associations between physical work load factors and distal upper limb symptoms in each of the studies listed in Table 5. These associations seem to be strong when the factors involved in physical work load have been evaluated objectively and in detail[13] or when the differences in work load between various occupations have been great.[54] Bernard and associates[71] found an exposure-effect relationship between subjectively reported hours of typing per day and symptoms of hand and wrist disorders. In a sample of symptomatic and nonsymptomatic workers, the subjective reports of this work load factor were validated against observations. Although the correlations of reported and observed durations were similar between symptomatic and nonsymptomatic subjects, both groups overestimated heavily the hours they spent typing. Thus, the results from studies based on self-assessments should be applied cautiously to preventive strategies in practice.

Exposed Prevalence or Incidence (%)	Referents' Prevalence or Incidence (%)	Risk (RR)	95% CI	Reference
Elbow 6.5	Elbow 2.8	2.4	1.2-4.2	Punnett et al 1985[12]
Wrist 16.8	Wrist 4.3	3.9	1.4-10.9	
Hand 27.3	Hand 10.3	2.7	1.3-5.2	
CTS symptoms 18.0	CTS symptoms 6.0	3.0	1.2-7.6	
HIF-HIR 10	LOF-LOR 1	unadj. RR:	0.3-8.5	Silverstein et al 1987[13]
LOF-HIR 3	LOF-LOR 1	1.6	0.4-11.3	
HIF-LOR 2	LOF-LOR 1	2.2	2.2-25.4	
		7.5		
Meatcutters 4	Nonstrenuous jobs, men 2	2.4	0.5-12.0	Viikari-Juntura et al 1991[54]
Sausage makers 12	Nonstrenuous jobs, women 4	3.3	1.2-9.2	
Packers 4	Nonstrenuous jobs, women 4	1.1	0.3-4.4	
Wrist flexion and extension associated with wrist-hand and carpal tunnel symptom score				Harber et al 1993[70]
		ORs for typing hours per day:		Bernard et al 1994[71]
		0 to 2 1.0	0.6-1.8	
		2 to 4 1.0	0.8-2.2	
		4 to 6 1.3	1.3-3.6	
		6 to 8 2.1	1.2-8.9	
		> 8 3.3		
Work with forward bent trunk more than 1 hour per day predicted incident severe pain, moderate to high risk of upper limb injury predicted persistent severe pain				Viikari-Juntura et al 1994[72]

In a small study among supermarket checkers,[70] wrist flexions and extensions showed a correlation with wrist/hand symptoms and carpal tunnel symptoms. The results of a small study of sign language interpreters showed that high frequency of wrist deviations, work envelop excursions, high pace of finger and hand movements, and low frequency of rest breaks were predictors of upper limb pain during work activities.[77]

Conclusion

There is substantial information on a variety of physical load factors as risk factors for CTS, tendon disorders, degenerative joint disorders, and vascular disorders. The role of physical factors in the etiology of nerve disorders other than CTS, epicondylitis, ganglions, and compartment syndrome has not been as adequately evaluated. In epidemiologic studies among working populations, the interest often has been restricted to repetitive and high physical loads, certain wrist and hand postures, and vibration associated with work tasks. Nonoccupational physical factors (eg, those associated with sports, and previous major traumas) are potential confounders that have not been thoroughly investigated. The effects of inactivity have not been addressed. Some older studies suggest unaccustomed work to be a major etiologic factor for tendon disorders, but the magnitude of this risk has not been evaluated in recent studies.

The recognition of physical load factors has remained mostly at a qualitative level with little information on exposure-effect relationships. More detailed information on physical exposure is needed for better elucidation of exposure-effect relationships. For conditions in which induction time is assumed to be short, emphasis should be on the exposure shortly before the disease onset, whereas for conditions in which induction time is long, it is important to measure cumulative exposure over months and years. Few methods have been described to assess cumulative physical exposure.

The studies that have put an emphasis on the assessment of physical work load often have not put much emphasis on psychosocial factors and vice versa. The result is that we do not know much about the role of physical versus psychosocial factors for different outcomes.

Work-related upper limb disorders represent a multitude of painful conditions. Epidemiologic studies have focused on diseases of nerves, tendons, muscle-tendon junctions, and muscle insertions. Some other studies have investigated localized pain with little attempt to elucidate the underlying pathology. It has been argued that painful conditions in the forearm are more common in the muscles than in the tendons or muscle-tendon junction.[78] High intracompartmental pressure might be a common denominator for some of these conditions as well as some poorly understood painful states. These disorders, however, lack validated diagnostic criteria.

Most studies had been limitations for investigating etiologic factors. A cross-sectional design has been often used in small samples of population, although most diseases, if verified by strict diagnostic criteria, are fairly rare among working populations. The studies have mostly been carried out among survivor populations with a possible selection bias. With few exceptions of studies on CTS, the case-control design has been little used. Prospective longitudinal studies are almost nonexistent. Nevertheless, epidemiologic studies that utilize recent advances in epidemiologic methods and results of past studies should be able to answer many of the remaining questions.

References

1. Lawrence JS: Rheumatism in coal miners: Part III. Occupational factors. *Br J Industr Med* 1955;12:249–261.
2. Obolenskaja AJ, Goljanitzki JA: Die seröse tendovaginitis in der klinik und im experiment. *Dtsch Z Chir* 1927;201:388–399.
3. Howard NJ: A new concept of tenosynovitis and the pathology of physiologic effort. *Am J Surg* 1938;42:723–730.
4. Corlett EN: Static muscle loading and the evaluation of posture, in Wilson JR, Corlett EN (eds): *Evaluation of Human Work: A Practical Ergonomics Methodology.* London, UK, Taylor & Francis, 1990, pp 542–570.
5. Waris P, Kuorinka I, Kurppa K, et al: Epidemiologic screening of occupational neck and upper limb disorders: Methods and criteria. *Scand J Work Environ Health* 1979;5(suppl 3):25–38.

6. Viikari-Juntura E: Neck and upper limb disorders among slaughterhouse workers: An epidemiologic and clinical study. *Scand J Work Environ Health* 1983;9:283–290.
7. Silverstein BA, Fine LJ, Armstrong TJ: Hand wrist cumulative trauma disorders in industry. *Br J Ind Med* 1986;43:779–84.
8. Golding DN, Rose DM, Selvarajah K: Clinical tests for carpal tunnel syndrome: An evaluation. *Br J Rheumatol* 1986;25:388–390.
9. Gellman H, Gelberman RH, Tan AM, et al: Carpal tunnel syndrome: An evaluation of the provocative diagnostic tests. *J Bone Joint Surg* 1986;68A:735–737.
10. deKrom MC, Knipschild PG, Kester AD, et al: Efficacy of provocative tests for diagnosis of carpal tunnel syndrome. *Lancet* 1990;335:393–395.
11. Hagberg M, Morgenstern H, Kelsh M: Impact of occupations and job tasks on the prevalence of carpal tunnel syndrome. *Scand J Work Environ Health* 1992;18:337–345.
12. Punnett L, Robins JM, Wegman DH, et al: Soft tissue disorders in the upper limbs of female garment workers. *Scand J Work Environ Health* 1985;11:417–425.
13. Silverstein BA, Fine LJ, Armstrong TJ: Occupational factors and carpal tunnel syndrome. *Am J Ind Med* 1987;11:343–358.
14. Nathan PA, Meadows KD, Doyle LS: Occupation as a risk factor for impaired sensory conduction of the median nerve at the carpal tunnel. *J Hand Surg* 1988:13B:167–170.
15. Barnhart S, Demers PA, Miller M, et al: Carpal tunnel syndrome among ski manufacturing workers. *Scand J Work Environ Health* 1991;17:46–52.
16. Chiang HC, Ko YC, Chen SS, et al: Prevalence of shoulder and upper-limb disorders among workers in the fish-processing industry. *Scand J Work Environ Health* 1993;19:126–131.
17. Stetson DS, Silverstein BA, Keyserling WM, et al: Median sensory distal amplitude and latency: Comparisons between nonexposed managerial/professional employees and industrial workers. *Am J Ind Med* 1993;24:175–189.
18. Armstrong TJ, Chaffin DB: Carpal tunnel syndrome and selected personal attributes. *J Occup Med* 1979;21:481–486.
19. Cannon LJ, Bernacki EJ, Walter SD: Personal and occupational factors associated with carpal tunnel syndrome. *J Occup Med* 1981;23:255–258.
20. Wieslander G, Norbäck D, Göthe C-J, et al: Carpal tunnel syndrome (CTS) and exposure to vibration, repetitive wrist movements, and heavy manual work: A case-referent study. *Br J Ind Med* 1989;46:43–47.
21. deKrom MC, Kester AD, Knipschild PG, et al: Risk factors for carpal tunnel syndrome. *Am J Epidemiol* 1990;132:1102–1110.
22. Stetson DS, Albers JW, Silverstein BA, et al: Effects of age, sex, and anthropometric factors on nerve conduction measures. *Muscle Nerve* 1992;15:1095–1104.
23. Rothman KJ: Types of epidemiologic study, in Rothman KJ (ed): *Modern Epidemiology*, ed 1. Boston, MA, Little Brown & Company, 1986, pp 51–76.
24. Armstrong TJ, Castelli WA, Evans FG, et al: Some histological changes in carpal tunnel contents and their biomechanical implications. *J Occup Med* 1984;26:197–201.
25. Smith EM, Sonstegard DA, Anderson WH Jr: Carpal tunnel syndrome: Contribution of flexor tendons. *Arch Phys Med Rehabil* 1977;58:379–385.
26. Radwin RG, Armstrong TJ, Chaffin DB: Power hand tool vibration effects on grip exertions. *Ergonomics* 1987;30:833–855.
27. Gemne G, Saraste H: Bone and joint pathology in workers using hand-held vibrating tools: An overview. *Scand J Work Environ Health* 1987;13:290–300.
28. Mathiassen SE, Winkel J: Quantifying variation in physical load using exposure vs time data. *Ergonomics* 1991;34:1455–1468.
29. Nathan PA, Keniston RC, Meadows KD, et al: Validation of occupational hand use categories. *J Occup Med* 1993;35:1034–1042.
30. Pearce N: Methodological problems of time-related variables in occupational cohort studies. *Rev Epidemiol Santé Publique* 1992;40(suppl 1):S43–S54.

31. Adams ML, Franklin GM, Barnhart S: Outcome of carpal tunnel surgery in Washington State workers' compensation. *Am J Ind Med* 1994;25:527–536.
32. Masear VR, Hayes JM, Hyde AG: An industrial cause of carpal tunnel syndrome. *J Hand Surg* 1986;11A:222–227.
33. Gartsman GM, Kovach JC, Crouch CC, et al: Carpal arch alteration after carpal tunnel release. *J Hand Surg* 1986;11A:372–374.
34. Harter BT Jr: Indications for surgery in work-related compression neuropathies of the upper extremity. *Occup Med* 1989;4:485–495.
35. Morris HH, Peters BH: Pronator syndrome: Clinical and electrophysiological features in seven cases. *J Neurol Neurosurg Psychiatry* 1976;39:461–464.
36. Werner C-O: Lateral elbow pain and posterior interosseous nerve entrapment. *Acta Orthop Scand* 1979;50(suppl 174):1–62.
37. Streib EW, Sun SF: Distal ulnar neuropathy in meat packers: An occupational disease? *J Occup Med* 1984;26:842–843.
38. Feldman RG, Goldman R, Keyserling WM: Classical syndromes in occupational medicine: Peripheral nerve entrapment syndromes and ergonomic factors. *Am J Ind Med* 1983;4:661–681.
39. Taylor-Jones THE: Tenosynovitis in untrained farm workers. *Br Med J* 1942;2:440.
40. Flowerdew RE, Bode OB: Tenosynovitis in untrained farm-workers. *Br Med J* 1942;2:367.
41. Luopajärvi T, Kuorinka I, Virolainen M, et al: Prevalence of tenosynovitis and other injuries of the upper extremities in repetitive work. *Scand J Work Environ Health* 1979;5(suppl 3):48–55.
42. Kuorinka I, Koskinen P: Occupational rheumatic diseases and upper limb strain in manual jobs in a light mechanical industry. *Scand J Work Environ Health* 1979;5(suppl 3):39–47.
43. Roto P, Kivi P: Prevalence of epicondylitis and tenosynovitis among meatcutters. *Scand J Work Environ Health* 1984;10:203–205.
44. Kurppa K, Viikari-Juntura E, Kuosma E, et al: Incidence of tenosynovitis or peritendinitis and epicondylitis in a meat-processing factory. *Scand J Work Environ Health* 1991;17:32–37.
45. Viikari-Juntura E: Interexaminer reliability of observations in physical examinations of the neck. *Phys Ther* 1987;67:1526–1532.
46. Bernard B, Sauter S, Petersen M, et al: Upper extremity musculoskeletal disorders among newspaper employees. *NIOSH Health Hazard Evaluation Report*. HETA 90-013-2277. Los Angeles, CA, U.S. Department of Health and Human Services, Centers for Disease Control and Prevention, National Institute for Occupational Safety and Health, January, 1993.
47. Mausner JS, Bahn AK: Measures of morbidity and mortality, in Mausner JS, Bahn AK (eds): *Epidemiology: An Introductory Text*. Philadelphia, PA, WB Saunders, 1974, pp 126–159.
48. Thompson AR, Plewes LW, Shaw EG: Peritendinitis crepitans and simple tenosynovitis: A clinical study of 544 cases in industry. *Br J Industr Med* 1951;8:150–158.
49. Goldstein SA, Armstrong TJ, Chaffin DB, et al: Analysis of cumulative strain in tendons and tendon sheaths. *J Biomech* 1987;20:1–6.
50. Moore JS: Function, structure, and responses of components of the muscle-tendon unit. *Occup Med* 1992;7:713–740.
51. Coppin EG, Livingstone SD, Kuehn LA: Effects on handgrip strength due to arm immersion in a 10 degree C water bath. *Aviat Space Environ Med* 1978;49:1322–1326.
52. Georgitis J: Extensor tenosynovitis of the hand from cold exposure. *J Maine Med Assoc* 1978;69:129–131.
53. Dimberg L: The prevalence and causation of tennis elbow (lateral humeral epicondylitis) in a population of workers in an engineering industry. *Ergonomics* 1987;30:573–579.

54. Viikari-Juntura E, Kurppa K, Kuosma E, et al: Prevalence of epicondylitis and elbow pain in the meat-processing industry. *Scand J Work Environ Health* 1991;17:38–45.
55. Bergenudd H, Lindgärde F, Nilsson B: Prevalence and coincidence of degenerative changes of the hands and feet in middle age and their relationship to occupational work load, intelligence, and social background. *Clin Orthop* 1989;239:306–310.
56. Jürgens WW, Ristow B, Pernack E-F: Zur Wirkung körperlicher Schwerarbeit auf das Bewegungssystem-Ergebnisse einer epidemiologischen Querschnittsstudie von Harzarbeitern. *Z Gesamte Hyg* 1990;36:155–158.
57. Starck J, Pyykkö I, Koskimies K, et al: Vibration exposure and prevention in Finland. *Nagoya J Med Sci* 1994;57(suppl):203–210.
58. Videman T: Connective tissue and immobilization: Key factors in musculoskeletal degeneration? *Clin Orthop* 1987;221:26–32.
59. Videman T, Nurminen M, Troup JD: 1990 Volvo Award in clinical sciences: Lumbar spinal pathology in cadaveric material in relation to history of back pain, occupation, and physical loading. *Spine* 1990;15:728–740.
60. Styf J, Forssblad P, Lundborg G: Chronic compartment syndrome in the first dorsal interosseous muscle. *J Hand Surg* 1987;12A:757–762.
61. Pedowitz RA, Toutounghi FM: Chronic exertional compartment syndrome of the forearm flexor muscles. *J Hand Surg* 1988;13A:694–696.
62. Rydholm U, Werner C-O, Ohlin P: Intracompartmental forearm pressure during rest and exercise. *Clin Orthop* 1983;175:213–215.
63. Matsen FA III, Winquist RA, Krugmire RB Jr: Diagnosis and management of compartmental syndromes. *J Bone Joint Surg* 1980;62A:286–291.
64. Little JM, Ferguson DA: The incidence of the hypothenar hammer syndrome. *Arch Surg* 1972;105:684–685.
65. Nilsson T, Burström L, Hagberg M: Risk assessment of vibration exposure and white fingers among platers. *Int Arch Occup Environ Health* 1989;61:473–481.
66. McFarlane RM: Dupuytren's disease: Relation to work and injury. *J Hand Surg* 1991;16A:775–779.
67. Bennett B: Dupuytren's contracture in manual workers. *Br J Ind Med* 1982;39:98–100.
68. Lugnegård H: The man behind the Dupuytren's contracture: The wild beast of the Seine. The most famous surgeon of his time. *Läkartidningen* 1983;80:5068–5069.
69. Higgs P, Young VL, Seaton M, et al: Upper extremity impairment in workers performing repetitive tasks. *Plast Reconstr Surg* 1992;90:614–620.
70. Harber P, Bloswick D, Beck J, et al: Supermarket checker motions and cumulative trauma risk. *J Occup Med* 1993;35:805–811.
71. Bernard B, Sauter S, Fine L, et al: Job task and psychosocial risk factors for work-related musculoskeletal disorders among newspaper employers. *Scand J Work Environ Health* 1994;20:417–426.
72. Viikari-Juntura E, Riihimäki H, Takala E-P, et al: Factors predicting pain in the neck, shoulders, and upper limbs in forestry work. *Työ Ja Ihminen* 1993;7:233–253.
73. Riihimäki H, Viikari-Juntura E, Moneta G, et al: Incidence of sciatic pain among men in machine operating, dynamic physical work, and sedentary work: A three-year follow-up. *Spine* 1994;19:138–142.
74. Wiktorin C, Karlqvist L, Winkel J, et al: Validity of self-reported exposures to work postures and manual materials handling. Stockholm MUSIC I Study Group. *Scand J Work Environ Health* 1993;19:208–214.
75. Viikari-Juntura E, Rauas S, Kuosma E, et al: Validity of self-reported physical work load in epidemiologic studies on musculoskeletal disorders. *Työ Ja Ihminen* 1993;7:288–298.
76. Hales TR, Sauter SR, Peterson MR, et al: Musculoskeletal disorders among visual display terminal (VDT) users in a telecommunications company. *Ergonomics* 1994;37:1603–1621.

77. Feuerstein M, Fitzgerald TE: Biomechanical factors affecting upper extremity cumulative trauma disorders in sign language interpreters. *J Occup Med* 1992;34:257–264.
78. Ranney DA, Wells RW, Moore A: Abstract: Forearm muscle strains: The forgotten work-related musculoskeletal disorder. International scientific conference on prevention of work-related musculoskeletal disorders. PREMUS, Sweden, May 12-14, 1992. *Arbete Och Hälsa* 1992;17:240–241.

Chapter 2
Epidemiology of Occupational Neck and Shoulder Disorders

Gunnar B. J. Andersson, MD, PhD

Introduction

Neck and shoulder disorders are combined in this review because symptoms from the neck and shoulder region are often poorly differentiated in epidemiologic surveys, and sometimes even purposely combined. Further, exposure factors for the shoulder muscles are difficult to separate from those affecting neck muscles because several muscles act on both the shoulder girdle and the upper spine.[1]

Clinical evaluations of reported complaints reveal that it is difficult to specifically attribute symptom reports obtained by an interview or questionnaire to specific neck and shoulder disorders.[2,3] Diagnoses are often approximate and based on exclusion of known causes of neck and shoulder pain. Most reported epidemiologic studies are cross-sectional and give prevalence rates only. Attempts at calculating prevalence odds ratios, etiologic fractions, and confidence intervals from these studies,[4] as well as performing meta-analysis[5] have generally supported a strong correlation between neck-shoulder complaints and certain types of work exposures. That relationship will be further explored in this review.

Although neck and shoulder disorders are difficult to separate, I have elected to divide the chapter into two segments: one on neck disorders and one on shoulder disorders. Unfortunately, overlap is unavoidable. Occupational neck and shoulder problems can be separated into three groups:[6] those that are relatively unique to industry, those that are not unique but occur regularly in certain types of work, and those that occur from external injury and have no special relationship to industry. This chapter will address the epidemiology of the first two groups but not the third.

Neck Disorders

A few studies have attempted to determine the prevalence of neck complaints, including pain, ache, stiffness, and discomfort, in general populations. Based on these studies, neck symptoms appear to affect 10% to 20% of the adult population annually. Westerling and Jonsson[7] analyzed a random sample of 2,537 18- to 65-year-old men and women in Stockholm, Sweden. Eighteen percent of the study population had neck-shoulder problems in the previous 12 months, 16% of the men and 20% of the women. The frequency of complaints increased with increasing age. Physically demanding jobs were associated with a significantly higher prevalence, but lifting per se was not. Takala and associates[8] reported similar data from a study consisting of a Finnish rural population of middle-aged women and men. The 1 year prevalence of pain, ache, or stiffness in the neck "occurring fairly often," was 18% in women and 16% in men. In another Finnish study of a general population sample (The Mini-Finland Study), four types of neck symptoms (or pathology) were examined: the tension neck syndrome, cervical spondylosis, cervical disk herniation, and myelopathy. At least one of these conditions was present in 14% of women and 9% of men who were 30 years of age and older.[9] In a comparable, large cross-sectional study of Swedish workers in different jobs, 12.3% said they experienced neck symptoms from the upper spine-neck area almost daily.[10] In another study of 2,500 workers "without special demands for neck and shoulder activity," Anderson[11] reported a prevalence of 15% over a 12-month period.

Cervical Herniated Disks

Kondo and associates[12] reviewed medical records in Rochester, Minnesota, from 1950 through 1974 to determine the incidence of cervical disk herniations. Protrusions and herniations were accepted into the study as long as they caused radicular symptoms. The annual incidence rates by gender were 6.5 per 100,000 for men and 4.6 for women, for a combined incidence of 5.5 per 100,000. The incidence for both sexes was highest among 45 to 54 year olds and slightly lower for 35 and 44 year olds. C5-6 was the disk most frequently affected, followed by C4-5 and C6-7.

Kelsey and associates[13] surveyed 20- to 64-year-old adults in New Haven and Hartford, Connecticut, who were identified as having a prolapsed cervical disk as determined by radiograph and myelography. Patients were divided into three groups: a surgical group, a probable group, and a possible group. These groups were compared to two control groups, one matched from the same medical services as the study patients and one obtained from a group of subjects who had cervical radiographs, but no prolapse. Subjects in the fourth decade of life were affected somewhat more often than individuals in other age groups. Men were affected 1.4 times more frequently than women. The C5-6 and C6-7 disks were involved in 75% of patients. Comparatively high odds ratios were calculated for frequent lifting, cigarette smoking, and frequent diving from a board (Table 1). Positive associations that were of borderline statistical significance or were not significant were operating vibrating equipment and driving or time spent in motor vehicles. Factors not associated with increased risk were participation in sports other than diving, number of pregnancies and live births, frequent twisting of the neck at work, sedentary work, wearing high heel shoes, and cigar or pipe smoking.

Prevalence of Occupational Neck Pain

Because classification and diagnostic criteria of neck pain vary greatly between reports in industry, it is difficult to compare studies. In a review of definition, cause, and pathogenesis of cervicobrachial syndromes, Waris[14] divided neck pain into cervical syndrome (CS) and tension neck syndrome (TNS). CS was defined as pain resulting from degenerative changes in the cervical spine causing pain radiating from the neck into the shoulder(s) and arm(s). TNS was defined as pain, fatigue, and stiffness in the neck muscles. Thoracic outlet syndrome (TOS) also was included as a syndrome of cervicobrachial pain, char-

Table 1 Odds ratios for association between several factors and a prolapsed cervical disk

Factor	Odds Ratio
Lifting	
0 times	1.0
<5	1.6
5 to 25	2.7
>25	0.9
Smoking (cigarettes)	1.7
Diving	
<10 times	1.0
10 to 25	2.3
>25	4.9
Golfing	2.0
Operating vibrating equipment	21.0

(Reproduced with permission from Kelsey JL, Githens PB, Walter SD, et al: An epidemiological study of acute prolapsed cervical intervertebral disc. *J Bone Joint Surg* 1984;66A:907–914.)

acterized by weakness and sensory disturbances in the arms. Modifications of the Waris classification have been used in the literature.

Hagberg and Wegman[4] reviewed the medical literature from 1966 to 1986 and calculated prevalence rates, odds ratios (OR) for occupational exposure, and etiologic fractions and their confidence intervals based on more than 200 reports. The etiologic fraction is an estimate of the impact of exposure; ie, the proportion of exposed cases attributable to the exposure. It is estimated by dividing the calculated odds ratio 1 (OR-1) by the odds ratio: (OR-1)/OR. Table 2 presents prevalence rates and odds ratios of radiographically verified cervical spondylosis (degenerative changes of the cervical spine). Odds ratios that significantly exceeded 1 were reported for meat carriers, dentists, miners, and heavy workers, while cotton workers were found to have fewer degenerative changes (both osteoarthritis [OA] and disk degeneration) than the general population. This would support the theory that high load on the cervical spine predisposes to degenerative changes. The point prevalences for cervical syndrome are listed in Table 3. Civil servants were found to have a prevalence odds ratio of 4.8 compared to iron foundry workers, with an etiologic fraction of 0.79. It has been hypothesized that the higher prevalence among civil servants is the result of a more static type of work among the civil servants, but a healthy worker effect cannot be excluded. Prevalence rates and odds ratios for thoracic outlet syndrome are given in Table 4. The rates vary considerably and none of the studies showed a significant odds ratio. Pooling the groups resulted in a significant standardized odds ratio (SOR) of 4.0, with an etiologic fraction of 0.75 for exposure to repetitive arm movements. Examples of such types of jobs would be cash register operators, light assembly line workers, and packers. It is hypothesized that this would occur because of the short cycle repetitive work occurring in those jobs.

TNS was found to have the highest prevalence rates of all shoulder-neck disorders studied (Table 5), and occurred more frequently in women than in men. Thus, female industrial workers in the United States had an odds ratio of 5.9

Table 2 Prevalence rates (number of cases per 100) and odds ratios of radiographically verified cervical spondylosis

Occupational Group	Gender	Prevalence Study Group	Prevalence Reference Group	Odds Ratio	Reference Number
Meat carrier	M	84	33	8.4	54
Dentists	M	42	14	5.3	55
Miners	M	76	51	4.5	18
Dentists	M	50	31	4.0	13
Miners	M	55	38	1.9	22
Heavy workers	M	55	42	1.7	19
Carriers	M	23	14	1.8	55
Manual workers	M	42	38	1.2	6
Miners	M	13	14	0.91	55
Cotton workers					
(OA)*	F	31	38	0.75	24
(DD)†	F	56	70	0.69	24
(OA)	M	41	53	0.61	24
(DD)	M	78	83	0.57	24

* OA, osteoarthritis
† DD, disk degeneration

(Reproduced with permission from Hagberg M, Wegman DH: Prevalence rates and odds ratios of shoulder-neck diseases in different occupational groups. *Br J Ind Med* 1987;44:602–610.)

Table 3 Prevalence rates (number of cases of 100) and odds ratios of cervical syndrome (cervical disk disease)

Occupational Group	Gender	Prevalence Study Group	Prevalence Reference Group	Odds Ratio	Reference Number
Slaughterhouse worker	M	5	1	8.5	35,9
Scissor makers	F	3	1	5.0	56,9
Civil servants	M	5	1	4.8	57,9
Data entry operators	F	1	2	0.54	48
Dockers	M	2	5	0.47	59
Assembly line packers	F	1	2	0.27	35
Iron foundry workers	M	1	5	0.07	57,59

(Reproduced with permission from Hagberg M, Wegman DH: Prevalence rates and odds ratios of shoulder-neck diseases in different occupational groups. *Br J Ind Med* 1987;44:602–610.)

compared with male industrial workers. When pooling the data entry operators, the standardized odds ratio was 3.0, with an etiologic fraction of 0.67. The hypothesized cause of TNS, exposure to static load on the shoulder-neck muscles, is to some degree supported by these data.

Although the review by Hagberg and Wegman[4] is exhaustive and helpful, they point out the difficulties in using published data. Confounding factors include poorly controlled studies, inadequate sample sizes, undetermined healthy worker effect, unquantified exposure, and unspecified effect (disease) criteria.

Table 4 Prevalence rates (number of cases per 100) and odds ratios of thoracic outlet syndrome

Occupational Group	Prevalence Study Group	Prevalence Reference Group	Odds Ratio	Reference Number
Assembly line packers	3	0	10.0	35
Asssembly line workers	14	0	9.6	41
Assembly line workers	44	14	3.9	41
Slaughterhouse workers	1	0	2.5	56,9
Cash register operators	32	17	1.7	41

(Reproduced with permission from Hagberg M, Wegman DH: Prevalence rates and odds ratios of shoulder-neck diseases in different occupational groups. *Br J Ind Med* 1987;44:602–610.)

Table 5 Prevalence rates and odds ratios for tension neck syndrome

Occupational Group	Gender	Prevalence Study Group	Prevalence Reference Group	Odds Ratio	Reference Number
Film rolling workers	F	100	65	118	60
Industrial workers	F	8	1	5.9	43
Lamp assemblers	F	91	65	5.1	60
Data entry operators		38	11	4.9	44
Typists	F	35	11	4.2	44
Scissor makers	F	61	28	4.1	35,56
Terminal operators	F	28	11	3.2	44
Data entry operators	F	47	28	2.3	58
Office workers	F	80	65	2.1	60
Assembly line packers	F	38	28	1.6	35
Slaughterhouse workers	M	5	28	0.15	35,9

(Reproduced with permission from Hagberg M, Wegman DH: Prevalence rates and odds ratios of shoulder-neck diseases in different occupational groups. *Br J Ind Med* 1987;44:602–610.)

In a subsequent analysis of the influence of work on cervical pain, Hagberg[10] concluded that although degenerative cervical spine changes were more common in some occupations, the increased risk is small and the relationship of degenerative changes and symptoms uncertain. Further, he concluded that no studies showed a true relationship between occupational stress and neck disease, or between thoracic outlet syndrome and occupational (physical and mental) stress. TNS, on the other hand, was thought to be more common in certain jobs with static demands on the neck and shoulder muscles.

Studies not reviewed in the Hagberg and Wegman study,[4] as well as studies after 1987 have sometimes reported conflicting results. Whitaker and associates[15] compared the prevalence of neck symptoms among 248 urologists and 113 general practitioners in Great Britain. Significantly more urologists than general practitioners had severe symptoms and frequent attacks, with a prevalence of 47.6% and 43.4%, respectively. The head position during uroscopy was believed to be at least in part responsible. Dimberg and associates[16] analyzed 2,814 industrial workers in a mechanical industry in Sweden. Neck symptoms were present in 293 workers, or 18% of the women and 9% of men.

Physical stress, the use of vibrating hand tools, and mental stress were associated with increased risk of neck symptoms.

Prevalence of Degenerative Changes in the Cervical Spine

Degenerative changes of the cervical spine include spondylarthrosis, disk degeneration, and apophyseal joint OA. Autopsy studies have indicated that degenerative changes are present in subjects as young as 30 years of age and in almost all individuals by age 70 years.[17] Nathan[18] actually found degenerative changes in the necks of all 40 year olds he examined.

Autopsy studies are less frequent than radiographic studies. Hult[19] found degenerative changes in from 61% to 100% of industrial workers and forest workers, the prevalence increasing with age (Table 6). Forest workers had significantly higher prevalence than industrial workers. The fifth cervical disk was the most frequently degenerated disk, followed by the fourth and the sixth disks. This supports reports by other investigators.[20,21] Hult[19] reported a strong correlation between cervicobrachial symptoms and increasing severity of degenerative changes. Lawrence and associates,[21] Kellgren and Lawrence,[22] and Friedenberg and Miller[20] found significant symptom-degeneration relationship when the degenerative changes were moderate and severe. Gore and associates[23] determined the prevalence of degenerative changes in 200 asymptomatic men and women. By age 60 to 65, 95% of the men and 70% of women had at least one identifiable degenerative change. Although gender was important, age was the main factor increasing prevalence and the C5-6 and C6-7 disks were those most often affected. The gender difference confirmed previous data by Kellgren and Lawrence[22] and Lawrence.[24] Hagberg and Wegman[4] found odds ratios for cervical spondylosis (radiographic degenerative changes) exceeding 1 for meat carriers, dentists, miners, and heavy workers. The highest etiologic fraction (0.88) was calculated for meat carriers.

Shoulder Disorders

Over the last two decades, occupational shoulder problems have increased in frequency to near epidemic proportions in Australia, Japan, Scandinavia, and the United States.[4,25-28] Surveys in Finland reveal that shoulder complaints actually exceed back complaints in many groups of workers, such as slaughterhouse workers[9] and drivers of large vehicles.[29] In Australia, shoulder pain is second to back pain in workers' compensation insurance costs.[25,30] In Sweden, occupational shoulder problems are second to back problems in the frequency of physician visits.[31]

Whether the increase in shoulder complaints is the result of ergonomic changes in industry brought about by automation and computerization, or

Table 6 Prevalence of radiographic changes of disk degeneration in cervical disks[19]

Age (Years)	Industrial Workers (%)	Forest Workers (%)
35 to 39	61	70
40 to 44	68	82
45 to 49	80	100

whether it is merely the result of increased awareness and recognition of an old problem is the subject of much study and debate. It is becoming increasingly apparent that both are true.

Prevalence of Occupational Cervicobrachial Disorders (OCD)

The term occupational cervicobrachial disorder (OCD) was first established by the Japan Association of Industrial Health in 1972.[32] It was used to describe a somewhat vague syndrome of pain about the shoulder posterior neck and parascapular musculature, the glenohumeral musculotendinous structures, and also pain radiating in the upper arm. In other words, it was not a pathologic or clinical diagnosis, but a symptom-based diagnosis. The same symptom complex is called repetitive stress injury (RSI) in Australia[25,30,33] and is considered one of the cumulative trauma disorders (CTDs) in the United States.[27]

OCD is especially common among keyboard operators and many types of light assembly workers.[25,27,34] Luopajärvi and associates[35] reported a prevalence among keypunch operators of 16% to 28%. By comparison, the incidence among cash register operators was 11% to 16%; typists, 13%; calculator operators, 10%; and light assembly line workers, 16%. A 1981 Australian survey of 122 data process workers showed that 78% had symptoms of OCD;[36] however, most symptoms were mild and only 26% of the whole group had obtained medical treatment. A later study included 52 additional process workers in the same office, with similar results.[37] The RSI epidemic in Australia is quite remarkable. The incidence of new reported cases rose from 2% in 1975 to 1976 to 21% in 1981 to 1982.[25] At Telecom Australia the rate of RSI began to rise in late 1983, peaked in 1984 (at a level about 30 times higher than in 1982), and began declining in 1985 to reach 1983 levels by 1987.[38] No specific work-related explanation was found.

O'Hara and associates[39] reviewed the Japanese literature on OCD, and found prevalence rates ranging from 2.4% to 28% for various kinds of employment. Only patients who needed medical care of had more severe symptoms were included. In their own study of 339 cash register operators, O'Hara and associates[39] found that 81% reported shoulder stiffness and 49%, right shoulder pain. Neck pain was reported by 31%; symptoms in the wrist, 13%; hand, 19%; and fingers, 13%. Other symptoms present in the cash register operators included general fatigue (82%), headaches (59%), insomnia (27%), and low back pain (42%). All of these symptoms were significantly more common in the study group than in office machine operators and other office workers.

General medical symptoms are common in patients with OCD. In a review article on clinical features, Miyake and associates[40] suggest that the initial symptoms of OCD involve the shoulder and neck, and that later various general symptoms follow as the condition progresses. Some investigators suggest that high levels of stress and subsequent muscle tension predispose to OCD.

Although light physical work seems to be associated with OCD symptoms, heavy physical work is not. In a cross-sectional study performed in Sweden, Westerling and Jonsson[7] actually found a negative correlation between heavy work and neck and shoulder problems. This should not be taken as an indication that heavy lifting prevents neck and shoulder problems, but it does support the fact that OCD is more prevalent among sedentary and light assembly workers. Westerling and Jonsson[7] also found that people with complaints from the neck and shoulder area had more sick leave for illnesses of all types than job-matched controls. Very few of the symptomatic individuals sought medical care for neck or shoulder pain. Within this group, women had a significantly higher number of absences due to sickness than men.

In another Swedish study, Sällström and Schmidt[41] compared the prevalence of OCD (including TOS) among cash register operators, office workers, and heavy industry workers. Forty-five percent of the workers reported symptoms (60% of the women and 34% of the men). Among female cash register operators, as many as 73% reported symptoms.

Punnett and associates[42] compared the incidence of persistent shoulder pain in female garment workers and hospital employees. Certain jobs among garment workers had higher prevalence of symptoms, such as "finishers" and "sewing machine operators." These jobs were characterized as posturally stressful, requiring repetitive movements of the fingers and wrists.

Stock[5] performed a meta-analysis of occupational musculoskeletal disorders of the neck and upper limbs. Only two studies involving the neck and shoulder met the inclusion criteria. One was a Finnish study of female food packers,[35] the other, a study from the United States of a mixed group of workers,[43] was found to have a higher validity. In the latter study, neck-shoulder disorders were a small part of a larger effort that included upper extremity trauma disorders in general. Luopajärvi and associates[35] reported an increased prevalence of shoulder disorders (mostly tendinitis) in the exposed group, with an odds ratio of 3.4. Silverstein[43] did not find a statistically significant increase in shoulder tendinitis in the highest exposure group, but found a significant increase in the high-force, low-repetition jobs (OR = 7.3).

Prevalent Shoulder Tendinitis and Rotator Cuff Tears

Herberts and associates[44] compared the prevalence of supraspinatus tendinitis in welders to that in office clerks. Shoulder pain was reported by 27% of the welders, compared to 2% of the clerks. On examination, 8% of the welders (ie, less than one third of those with shoulder complaints) were diagnosed as having supraspinatus tendinitis. Further investigation of the problem of rotator cuff tendinitis in shipyard workers by Herberts and associates[45] revealed that supraspinatus tendinitis was present in 18.3% of welders and 16.2% of plate workers studied. Both of these tasks involve heavy manual labor, but welding imposes a more static type of load on the shoulder. Hagberg and Wegman[4] pooled different studies and found that the odds ratio for occupational groups with work tasks at shoulder level was 11, with an etiologic fraction of 0.91 (Table 7). Thus, it appears that work at shoulder level, particularly work of a static nature, is associated with an increased risk of shoulder tendon disorders. Shoulder tendon disorders are common in certain types of repetitive work as well. The prevalence of rotator cuff tendinitis and biceps tendinitis in grocery store checkers has been reported at 15%, compared to 4% in noncheckers (OR 3.9).[46]

Prevalence of Degenerative Arthritis of the Shoulder

The relationship between OA of the shoulder and occupational factors other than direct trauma is unclear. A few studies lend support to the theory that specific occupations increase the risk of OA of the glenohumeral joint.

Kellgren and Lawrence[22] reported that the prevalence of degeneration of the glenohumeral joint in men was more common in physically heavy jobs. On the other hand, Petersson[47] not only did not find an occupational correlation, but found degeneration to be more prevalent in women. Cartilage degeneration and

Table 7 Prevalence rates (number of cases per 100) and odds ratios of rotator cuff tendinitis

Occupational Group	Prevalence Study Group	Prevalence Reference Group	Odds Ratio	Reference Number
Shipyard welders	18	2	13	44
Plate workers	16	2	11	45
Industrial workers (work at shoulder level)	69	17	11	61
Assembly line packers	9	4	2.6	35
Slaughterhouse workers	3	4	0.70	35,9
Scissor makers	2	4	0.56	35,56
Data entry operators	1	2	0.54	58

(Reproduced with permission from Hagberg M, Wegman DH: Prevalence rates and odds ratios of shoulder-neck diseases in different occupational groups. *Br J Ind Med* 1987;44:602–610.)

rotator cuff degeneration were found to occur at the same time in 76% of shoulders and were usually bilateral, making work factors less likely as causes. Not a single glenohumeral joint showed signs of degeneration before 60 years of age.

Katevuo and associates[48] compared the prevalence of OA in farmers and dentists in Finland. Of 40 dentists over the age of 49, 46% had radiographic evidence of OA, with 44% showing bilateral changes. In contrast, of 83 farmers studied, only 13% showed evidence of OA. The age-standardized odds ratio was 4.2 and the etiologic fraction was 0.76. Degenerative changes in the cervical and lumbar spine were also evaluated. Degenerative changes in the cervical spine were found in 52% of the dentists, compared with 19% of the farmers. In the lumbar spine, the findings were reversed. Spondylosis occurred in 22% of dentists and 43% of farmers. A dentist's work requires sustained static load on the shoulder and cervical spine with shoulders in moderate forward flexion and abduction. Moderate scapular elevation is also required, causing high sustained static loads on the glenohumeral joint. Bovenzi and associates[49] in Italy reported radiographic evidence of shoulder OA in 12% of shipping and grinding operators and 24% of heavy manual laborers. The average age in both groups was 39 years.

Acromioclavicular degenerative joint changes are more common than OA in the glenohumeral joint. DePalma[50] found changes in almost all subjects after age 50, and Petersson[51] frequently observed changes in 30- to 50-year-old individuals and regularly observed changes in people 60 years of age and older. Degeneration occurred as often in women as in men and was of the same severity in the left and right shoulders, making occupation an unlikely cause.

Sternoclavicular (SC) arthritis is not uncommon and is frequently asymptomatic.[52] Worcester and Green[53] found no relationship between SC osteoarthritis and occupation.

Discussion

Disorders of the neck and shoulder are common and often have similar symptoms. This makes it difficult to perform epidemiologic surveys using questionnaires, interviews, and pain drawings. In recent years, clinical classification has developed but is often based not only on history and physical examination but on imaging and other more elaborate techniques as well. Case definitions must be improved to allow further advances.

Exposure factors to the neck and shoulder are rarely, if ever, quantified. This makes it difficult to establish cause-and-effect relationships in the first place and exposure relationship subsequently. Techniques must be developed to allow quantification of level, duration, and variations of exposure.

Once better disease criteria and improved methods of measuring exposure are developed, the relationship between work, individual factors, and neck and shoulder disorders can be further clarified and intervention trials can be pursued.

Meanwhile, there is substantial evidence that certain types of physical activities are associated with an increased risk of neck and shoulder complaints. These include static work with the neck twisted, no flexion or extension, short cycle repetitive work, work with vibrating hand tools, work at or above shoulder level, and work with the shoulders abducted. These jobs can be addressed by a variety of generally applicable engineering and administrative controls while further evidence is gathered.

References

1. Winkel J, Westgaard R: Occupational and individual risk factors for shoulder-neck complaints: Part II. The scientific basis (literature review) for the guide. *Int J Industr Ergonomics* 1992;10:85–104.
2. Waris P, Kuorinka I, Kurppa K, et al: Epidemiologic screening of occupational neck and upper limb disorders: Methods and criteria. *Scand J Work Environ Health* 1979;5(suppl 3):25–38.
3. Kuorinka I, Viikari-Juntura E: Prevalence of neck and upper limb disorders (NLD) and work load in different occupational groups: Problems in classification and diagnosis. *J Hum Ergol* 1982;11:65–72.
4. Hagberg M, Wegman DH: Prevalence rates and odds ratios of shoulder-neck diseases in different occupational groups. *Br J Ind Med* 1987;44:602–610.
5. Stock SR: Workplace ergonomic factors and the development of musculoskeletal disorders of the neck and upper limbs: Meta-analysis. *Am J Ind Med* 1991;19:87–107.
6. Luck JV Jr, Andersson GBJ: Occupational shoulder disorders, in Rockwood CA Jr, Matsen FA III (eds): *The Shoulder.* Philadelphia, PA, WB Saunders, 1990, vol 2, pp 1088–1108.
7. Westerling D, Jonsson BG: Pain from the neck-shoulder region and sick leave. *Scand J Soc Med* 1980;8:131–136.
8. Takala J, Sievers K, Klaukka T: Rheumatic symptoms in the middle-aged population in southwestern Finland. *Scand J Rheumatol* 1982;47(suppl):15–29.
9. Viikari-Juntura E: Neck and upper limb disorders among slaughterhouse workers: An epidemiologic and clinical study. *Scand J Work Environ Health* 1983;9:283–290.
10. Hagberg M: *The Importance of the Work Environment to Symptoms from Neck and Shoulder.* Stockholm, Sweden, The Swedish Work Environment Fund, 1988, pp 1–141.
11. Anderson JA: Shoulder pain and tension neck and their relation to work. *Scand J Work Environ Health* 1984;10(spec no 6):435–442.
12. Kondo K, Molgaard CA, Kurland LT, et al: Protruded intervertebral cervical disk: Incidence and affected cervical level in Rochester, Minnesota, 1950 through 1974. *Minn Med* 1981;64:751–753.
13. Kelsey JL, Githens PB, Walter SD, et al: An epidemiological study of acute prolapsed cervical intervertebral disc. *J Bone Joint Surg* 1984;66A:907–914.
14. Waris P: Occupational cervicobrachial syndromes: A review. *Scand J Work Environ Health* 1979;5(suppl 3):3–14.

15. Whitaker RH, Green NA, Notley RG: Is cervical spondylosis an occupational hazard for urologists? *Br J Urology* 1983;55:585–587.
16. Dimberg L, Olafsson A, Stefansson E, et al: The correlation between work environment and the occurrence of cervicobrachial symptoms. *J Occup Med* 1989;31:447–453.
17. Heine J: Uber die arthritis deformans. *Virchows Arch Path Anat* 1926;260:521–663.
18. Nathan H: Osteophytes of the vertebral column: An anatomical study of their development according to age, race, and sex with considerations as to their etiology and significance. *J Bone Joint Surg* 1962;44A:243–268.
19. Hult L: Cervical, dorsal and lumbar spinal syndromes: A field investigation of a non-selected material of 1200 workers in different occupations with special reference to disc degeneration and so-called muscular rheumatism. *Acta Orthop Scand* 1954;17(suppl):7–102.
20. Friedenberg ZB, Miller WT: Degenerative disc disease of the cervical spine. *J Bone Joint Surg* 1963;45A:1171–1178.
21. Lawrence JS, Bremner JM, Bier F: Osteo-arthrosis: Prevalence in the population and relationship between symptoms and x-ray changes. *Ann Rheum Dis* 1966;25:1–24.
22. Kellgren JH, Lawrence JS: Rheumatism in miners: Part II. X-ray study. *Br J Industr Med* 1952;9:197–207.
23. Gore DR, Sepic SB, Gardner GM: Roentgenographic findings of the cervical spine in asymptomatic people. *Spine* 1986;11:521–524.
24. Lawrence JS: Rheumatism in cotton operatives. *Br J Industr Med* 1961;18:270–276.
25. McDermott FT: Repetition strain injury: A review of current understanding. *Med J Aust* 1986;144:196–200.
26. Aoyama H, O'Hara H, Oze Y, et al: Recent trends in research on occupational cervicobrachial disorder. *J Human Ergol* 1979;8:39–45.
27. Mallory M, Bradford H: An invisible workplace hazard gets harder to ignore. *Business Week* Janurary 30, 1989, pp 92–93.
28. Sommerich CM, McGlothlin JD, Marras WS: Occupational risk factors associated with soft tissue disorders of the shoulder: A review of recent investigations in the literature. *Ergonomics* 1993;36:697–717.
29. Backman AL: Health survey of professional drivers. *Scand J Work Environ Health* 1983;9:30–35.
30. Stone WE: Repetitive strain injuries. *Med J Aust* 1983;2:616–618.
31. Hammond G, Torgerson WR Jr, Dotter WE, et al: The painful shoulder, in MacAusland WR Jr (ed): *American Academy of Orthopaedic Surgeons Instructional Course Lectures*, XX. St. Louis, MO, CV Mosby, 1971, pp 83–90.
32. Keikenwan SI: Report of the Committee on Occupational Cervicobrachial Disorder of the Japan Association of Industrial Health. *Jap J Ind Health* 1973;15:304–311.
33. Browne CD, Nolan BM, Faithfull DK: Occupational repetition strain injuries: Guidelines for diagnosis and management. *Med J Aust* 1984;140:329–332.
34. Maeda K, Harada N, Takamatsu M: Factor analysis of complaints of occupational cervicobrachial disorder in assembly lines of a cigarette factory. *Kurume Med J* 1980;27:253–261.
35. Luopajärvi T, Kuorinka I, Virolainen M, et al: Prevalence of tenosynovitis and other injuries of the upper extremities in repetitive work. *Scand J Work Environ Health* 1979;5(suppl 3):48–55.
36. Taylor R, Pitcher M: Medical and ergonomic aspects of an industrial dispute concerning occupational-related conditions in data process operators. *Community Health Stud* 1984;8:172–180.
37. Ryan G, Mullerworth J, Pimble J: The prevalence of repetition injury in data process operators, in Adams AS, Stevenson MG (eds): *Ergonomics and Technological*

Change: Proceedings of the 21st Annual Conference of the Ergonomics Society of Australia and New Zealand. Parkville, Victoria, Ergonomics Society of Australia and New Zealand, 1984, pp 279–288.
38. Hocking B: Epidemiological aspects of "repetition strain injury" in Telecom Australia. *Med J Austr* 1987;147:218–222.
39. O'Hara H, Itani T, Aoyama H: Prevalence of occupational cervicobrachial disorder among different occupational groups in Japan. *J Hum Ergol* 1982;11:55–63.
40. Miyake S, Himeno J, Hosokawa M: Clinical features of occupational cervicobrachial disorder (OCD). *J Hum Ergol* 1982;11:109–117.
41. Sällström J, Schmidt H: Cervicobrachial disorders in certain occupations, with special reference to compression in the thoracic outlet. *Am J Ind Med* 1984;6:45–52.
42. Punnett L, Robins JM, Wegman DH, et al: Soft tissue disorders in the upper limbs of female garment workers. *Scand J Work Environ Health* 1985;11:417–425.
43. Silverstein BA: *The Prevalence of Upper Extremity Cumulative Trauma Disorders in Industry.* Ann Arbor, MI, University of Michigan, 1985. Thesis.
44. Herberts P, Kadefors R, Andersson G, et al: Shoulder pain in industry: An epidemiological study on welders. *Acta Orthop Scand* 1981;52:299–306.
45. Herberts P, Kadefors R, Hogfors C, et al: Shoulder pain and heavy manual labor. *Clin Orthop* 1984;191:166–178.
46. Baron S, Milliron M, Habes DJ: *Health Hazard Evaluation Report, HETA.* Cincinnati, OH, NIOSH, 1990, pp 88–344.
47. Petersson CJ: Degeneration of the gleno-humeral joint: An anatomical study. *Acta Orthop Scand* 1983;54:277–283.
48. Katevuo K, Aitasalo K, Lehtinen R, et al: Skeletal changes in dentists and farmers in Finland. *Commun Dent Oral Epidemiol* 1985;13:23–25.
49. Bovenzi M, Fiorito A, Volpe C: Bone and joint disorders in the upper extremities of chipping and grinding operators. *Int Arch Occup Environ Health* 1987;59:189–198.
50. DePalma AF (ed): *Degenerative Changes in the Sternoclavicular and Acromioclavicular Joints in Various Decades.* Springfield, IL, Charles C Thomas, 1957.
51. Petersson CJ: Degeneration of the acromioclavicular joint: A morphological study. *Acta Orthop Scand* 1983;54:434–438.
52. Yood RA, Goldenberg DL: Sternoclavicular joint arthritis. *Arthritis Rheum* 1980;23:232–239.
53. Worcester JN Jr, Green DP: Osteoarthritis of the acromio-clavicular joint. *Clin Orthop* 1968;58:69–73.
54. Schröter G, Rademacher W: Die Bedeutung von Belastung und aussergewöhnlicher Haltung für das Entstehen von Vershleiss-schäden der HWS dargestellt an einem Kollektiv von Fleischabträgern. *Z Gesamte Hyg* 1971;17:841–843.
55. Schröter G: Hat die berufliche Belastung Bedeutung für die Entstehung oder Verschlimmerung der Osteochondrose und Spondylose der Halswirbelsäule? *Deutsche Gesundheitswesen* 1959;14:174–177.
56. Kuorinka I, Koskinen P: Occupational rheumatic diseases and upper limb strain in manual jobs in a light mechanical industry. *Scand J Work Environ Health* 1979;5(suppl):3:39–47.
57. Partridge RE, Anderson JA, McCarthy MA, et al: Rheumatic complaints among workers in iron foundries. *Ann Rheum Dis* 1968;27:441–453.
58. Kukkonen R, Luopajärvi T, Riihimaki V: Prevention of fatigue amongst data entry operators, in Kvalseth TO (ed): *Ergonomics of Workstation Design.* London, UK, Butterworth-Heinemann, 1983, pp 28–34.
59. Partridge RE, Duthie JJ: Rheumatism in dockers and civil servants: A comparison of heavy manual and sedentary workers. *Ann Rheum Dis* 1968;27:559–568.
60. Onishi N, Nomura H, Sakai K, et al: Shoulder muscle tenderness and physical features of female industrial workers. *J Human Ergol* 1976;5:87–102.
61. Bjelle A, Hagberg M, Michaelsson G: Clinical and ergonomic factors in prolonged shoulder pain among industrial workers. *Scand J Work Environ Health* 1979;5:205–210.

Chapter 3
Work-Related Musculoskeletal Disorders in Computer Keyboard Operation

Laura Punnett, ScD

Introduction

Some of the same ergonomic stressors associated with soft-tissue disorders in industrial jobs also occur in the operation of video display units (VDUs), especially rapid and repetitive hand motion and awkward wrist and arm postures. Ohara and associates[1] noted that the mechanization of work, including that associated with data entry machines, has reduced the required force levels, but has made motion patterns more stereotyped and repetitive, increased the work pace, and produced localized stresses on body parts, such as the arms and shoulders. This parallels the development of manufacturing jobs over most of this century.

Both epidemiologic and laboratory studies provide evidence of biologic plausibility for an association between VDU and increased risk of musculoskeletal disorders. A literature review was conducted to determine the strength of the scientific evidence supporting the specific hypothesis that the occurrence of musculoskeletal and other soft-tissue disorders of the neck and upper extremity is elevated among operators of VDUs and related office keyboard machines. A further goal was to identify which, if any, specific features or physical demands of keyboard work might be associated with these disorders.

Methods

Various bibliographies and data bases were examined for pertinent references. Only epidemiologic studies were included, not laboratory experiments or studies of short-term effects of simulated exposures. Articles that did not define the population or methods sufficiently for evaluation or those that did not directly examine the relationship between job feature(s) and health endpoint(s) also were excluded.

Twenty articles were identified, primarily from the peer-reviewed scientific literature, plus a small number of conference proceedings and reports of Health Hazard Evaluations conducted by the United States National Institute of Occupational Safety and Health (NIOSH). These articles were reviewed according to standard epidemiologic criteria for evidence of casual association, particularly the absence of serious misclassification error, bias, or confounding; temporal sequence of cause and effect; and, if possible, exposure-response relationship.

In some cases, I carried out additional statistical analysis on the data provided in the article. For example, additional odds ratios were calculated for several papers. In addition, external comparisons could be made between some of the studies reviewed and an investigation that provided an estimate of disease frequency among industrial employees with low exposure both to forceful manual exertions and to repetitive manual work.[2,3] Three of the studies reviewed[4-6] used a case definition that was directly comparable, so that relative risks could be calculated for these groups of office workers in comparison to industrial workers in low ergonomic exposure jobs, after standardizing for gender.

Results

Twenty cross-sectional studies examined the risk of neck or upper extremity disorders in VDU or other keyboard work. On the basis of the information presented, seven studies[4-10] were found to have only very minor methodological flaws. Another four[11-14] had relatively minor weaknesses that might have affected only some of the findings or were otherwise not serious enough to invalidate the results. All of these 11 studies had relative risks that were significantly elevated for at least one aspect of keyboard or data entry work (Table 1). Overall, they showed evidence of increased risk of musculoskeletal disorders associated with VDU work per se, either dichotomized (yes/no) or in three or more levels of hours per week of keyboard operation.[4,5,7,8,10,11] Among these studies, the estimated relative risks (from both internal and external comparisons) for hand and wrist disorders, in relation to keyboard use of at least 4 hours per day, ranged from 0.7 to 7.9, with 13 of the 16 estimates greater than or equal to 2.0. A similar range of relative risks was found for neck, shoulder, arm, and elbow disorders, with nine of 16 estimates greater than or equal to 2.0. The magnitude of risk was correlated with cumulative exposure (in years) to keyboard work[4,5,12,13] and to the pace or intensity of the workload (eg, typing speed, data entry versus interactive tasks).[4-6] The use of non-neutral postures in keyboard operation was also a risk factor.[4,11] In a number of these investigations, exposure-response relationships were found for one or more of the risk factors studied.

In addition, VDU operators in three studies[4-6] had rates of hand/wrist disorders that were from about two to eight times higher than the expected rates in industrial jobs with low manual forces and low repetition rates, and comparable to or higher than the rates in highly repetitive, low-force industrial tasks (Tables 2 and 3).

Conclusions

The relative risks of shoulder, arm, and hand disorders were approximately 2.0 to 3.0 for keyboard work of at least 4 hours/day. (No evidence was found regarding the risk with fewer than 4 hours/day.) In comparisons among keyboard users, the relative risks were generally elevated for repetitive keyboard data entry work compared to non-keyboard clerical work, low-keyboard or interactive use. The relative risks were significantly higher than expected on the basis of low-force/low-repetition industrial work. The elevated relative risks persist after adjustment for gender (in about half the studies)[1-3,5,6] or in predominantly female study populations. The common set of implicated exposures demonstrates a consistency of findings that argues strongly for a causal relationship.

The excess risks observed in these studies may be due to a combination of factors. The first set of factors are inherent features of keyboard design, including

Table 1 Selected occupational risk factors for musculoskeletal disorders in 11 studies on ergonomic stressors in VDU and other keyboard operation

Ref	Neck/Shoulder	RR*	E-R†	Arm/Elbow	RR	E-R	Hand/Wrist	RR	E-R
4	Neck						Phase I		
	Low work variance	1.5					Hours typing/day (6 to 8 vs ≤ 2)	2.5	
	Hours on deadline/week (≥30 vs ≤ 10)	1.7					Hours on deadline/week (≤ 30 vs ≤ 10)	1.7	
	Hours on telephone/day (4 to 6 vs ≤ to 2)	1.4					Phase II Percent of day typing		+
	Shoulder						One-year increase in hours typing/day	9.1	
	Years employed		+						
	Job pressure	1.4							
	Low decision-making	1.6					One-year increase in overall workload	3.2	
5	Neck								
	Percent time typing		+	Reporter	2.5		Reporter	2.4	
	Years employed (reporter)		+	Percent time typing		+	Typing speed		+
	Years employed (other job)		+						
	Shoulder								
	Typing speed		+						
6	Neck/Shoulder			Surges in workload	1.2		Surges in workload		+
	Work pressure	1.2	+	Work pressure		+	Work pressure	1.3	+
	Variety of tasks	1.4		Overtime in past year		+	High information processing		+¶
	High information processing demands	1.3		Little decision-making	1.4	+	Little decision-making		+§
	Little decision-making	1.6							
11**	Neck/Shoulder	4.8		Data entry VDT work	8.0		Angle of wrist ulnar abduction (all operators)		+
	Data entry VDT work								
	Conversational VDT work	3.1		Conversational VDT work	2.8				
				Ulnar abduction > 20° (within data entry)	6.3				
				Ulnar abduction > 20° (within conversational)	8.8				

Table 1 Selected occupational risk factors for musculoskeletal disorders in 11 studies on ergonomic stressors in VDU and other keyboard operation (cont.)

Ref	Risk Factor							
	Neck/Shoulder	RR*	E-R†	Arm/Elbow	RR	E-R	Hand/Wrist	RR	E-R
12	Neck/Shoulder								
	Hours typing per day		+						
	Changes from sitting to standing per day		+						
13				Operators vs saleswomen	3.4		Operators vs saleswomen	2.0	
				Years employed (current job)		+			
8							Keyboard operator (> 4 hrs/day) administrative/clerical (< 4 hrs/day)		2.75¶
9	Neck						VDT use ≥ 4 vs 0 hrs/day (for numbness and tingling)	1.2	
	VDT ≥ 4 vs 0 hrs/day	4.5							
	Hours VDT work/day		+						
	Shoulder								
	VDT ≥ 4 vs 0 hrs/day	4.6							
	Hours VDT work/day		+						
10				Keyboard height		+			
				Document reach distance		+			
				Shoulder flexion		+			
				Wrist ulnar deviation		+			
14	Neck			Upper arm			VDT vs paper task	0.7	
	VDT vs paper task	2.0		VDT vs paper	1.1				
	Shoulder			Elbow					
	VDT vs paper task	1.6		VDT vs paper	0.8				

*RR, relative risk, generally estimated as prevalence odds ratio; estimates from multivariate analyses used when available

†E-R, exposure-response relationship; +, risk factor is found for 3 or more levels of exposure variable

¶For carpal tunnel syndrome only

§For all hand symptoms and for carpal tunnel syndrome

**Odds ratios calculated for tendon and muscle findings on physical examination

Table 2 Comparison of hand/wrist symptom and disorder prevalences among studies with comparable case definitions: Symptoms on interview alone

Ref		Prevalence of symptoms			Relative Risk		
		Male	Female	Both	Male	Female	Standardized
2[†]	LoF.LoR*	3%	16%	9%			
	LoF.HiR	12%	27%	22%			
4	Total (56% F)			22%			2.2
	Accounting/Finance	9%	25%		3.0	1.6	
	Circulation	16%	29%		5.3	1.8	
	Classified	8%	24%		2.7	1.5	
	Editorial	20%	39%		6.7	2.4	
5	Total (55% F)			23%			2.3

*LoF.LoR, low force, low repetition; LoF.HiR, low force, high repetition
[†]The prevalence of symptoms for a combined male-female population has been adjusted to the proportions of 55% female, 45% male to permit comparison with the results from references 4 and 5

Table 3 Comparison of hand/wrist symptom and disorder prevalences among studies with comparable case definitions: Symptoms plus findings on physical examination

Ref		Prevalence of disorders			Relative risk
		Male	Female	Both	Standardized
3[†]	LoF.LoR*	0%	3%	2%	
	LoF.HiR	2%	9%	7%	
6	Total (78% F)			12%	4.7

*LoF.LoR, low force, low repetition; LoF.HiR, low force, high repetition
[†]The prevalence of disorders for a combined male-female population has been adjusted to the proportions of 78% female, 22% male for comparison with reference 6

the repetitive finger motions involved in keying, the forces required to activate the keys, and the wrist postures that result from the (parallel-row) QWERTY keyboard layout. The second set includes factors extrinsic to the video display terminals themselves; ie, that result from the manner in which they are utilized (workstation dimensions, nature and content of the tasks performed, etc).

However, the effect of VDU work per se, whether measured in hours per week, intensity of keying, or duration of employment, does not appear to be entirely explained by the risk associated with the postures in which that work is performed. Where postural stresses were found to be significantly associated with musculoskeletal discomfort, these variables explained from about 15% to 40% of the variability. In contrast, the most consistent evidence for work-relatedness involved the intensity of and cumulative exposure to keyboard use.

References

1. Ohara H, Nakagiri S, Itani T, et al: Occupational health hazards resulting from elevated work rate situations. *J Human Ergol* 1976;5:173–182.
2. Silverstein BA: *The Prevalence of Upper Extremity Cumulative Trauma Disorders in Industry*. Ann Arbor, Michigan, University of Michigan, 1985. Thesis.

3. Silverstein BA, Fine LJ, Armstrong TJ: Hand wrist cumulative trauma disorders in industry. *Br J Industr Med* 1986;43:779–784.
4. Bernard B, Sauter S, Petersen M, et al: *Health Hazard Evaluation Report*. Los Angeles, CA, Los Angeles Times. National Institute of Occupational Safety and Health, HETA 90–013-2277, 1993.
5. Burt S, Hornung R, Fine LJ: *Health Hazard Evaluation Report*. Melville, NY, Newsday, Inc., National Institute of Occupational Safety and Health, HETA 89–250–2046, 1990.
6. Hales T, Sauter S, Petersen M, et al: *Health Hazard Evaluation Report*. Minneapolis, MN, U.S. West Communications, National Institute of Occupational Safety and Health, HETA 89–299–2230, 1992.
7. Knave BG, Wibom RI, Voss M, et al: Work with video display terminals among office employees: I. Subjective symptoms and discomfort. *Scand J Work Environ Health* 1985;11:457–466.
8. Nathan PA, Meadows KD, Doyle LS: Occupation as a risk factor for impaired sensory conduction of the median nerve at the carpal tunnel. *J Hand Surg* 1988;13B:167–170.
9. Rossignol AM, Morse EP, Summers VM, et al: Video display terminal use and reported health symptoms among Massachusetts clerical workers. *J Occup Med* 1987;29:112–118.
10. Sauter SL, Schleifer LM, Knutson SJ: Work posture, workstation design, and musculoskeletal discomfort in a VDT data entry task. *Human Factors* 1991;33:151–167.
11. Hünting W, Laubli T, Grandjean E: Postural and visual loads at VDT workplaces: I. Constrained postures. *Ergonomics* 1981;24:917–931.
12. Kamwendo K, Linton SJ, Moritz U: Neck and shoulder disorders in medical secretaries: Part I. Pain prevalence and risk factors. *Scand J Work Environ Health* 1985;11:457–466.
13. Maeda K, Hünting W, Grandjean E: Localized fatigue in accounting-machine operators. *J Occup Med* 1980;22:810–816.
14. Starr SJ, Thompson CR: Effects of video display terminals on telephone operators. *Human Factors* 1982;24:699–711.

Chapter 4
Perceived Exertion as a Function of Physical Effort

Vern Putz-Anderson, PhD
Katharyn A. Grant, PhD

Introduction

To what extent can a worker's perception of exertion be used to establish what is an acceptable level of work? There is an increasing body of knowledge that suggests that safe levels of work can be established using psychophysical and psycho-scaling tools to assess the worker's perception of exertion. The purpose of this chapter is to (1) review laboratory methods used to assess the perceived exertion of workers, (2) examine the role of task variables that affect perceived exertion (ie, force, work rate, and type of work—static versus dynamic) and (3) assess the potential of psychological methods for achieving the goal of establishing safe levels of work.

Numerous studies over the last 10 years have investigated the occupational causes of upper extremity musculoskeletal disorders. Armstrong and associates[1] recently reviewed a series of epidemiologic studies that linked various job or task attributes with disorders affecting the musculoskeletal system. To date, however, relatively few studies have been conducted that provide information which defines the limits of acceptable or safe manual work for the majority of healthy workers. One reason may be the manner in which human work capacity is assessed.

To assess work capacity and the potential for musculoskeletal injury, investigators rely on one or two approaches: If the work is heavy, but intermittent, biomechanical measures of strength may serve as indicators of work capacity. If the work is light, but continuous, physiological measures of endurance may be needed. Studies of muscle endurance, for example, provide useful information on the strength of an individual muscle or even a group of muscles. However, the problem is that even simple manual work activities can require the use of numerous muscles, joints, ligaments, and tendons in varying degrees.[2] Information on the functioning of one or more muscles cannot provide much predictive insight as to the level of exertion a worker is *willing* to experience to carry out the job safely.

The findings from a number of studies of muscle fatigue suggest that few muscle groups can maintain a static exertion or contractile force for more than a few minutes without the subject experiencing significant pain.[3] The actual duration of exertion depends on the load and the individual muscle group used. To measure the maximum duration of contraction, a load is selected that is some fraction of the individual's maximum voluntary contraction (MVC). The higher the level of MVC, the more rapid is the onset of fatigue and the shorter is the voluntary contraction duration. Rohmert[4] recognized this relationship as logarithmic. There is a logarithmic relationship between the holding time of a muscle group and the maximum force it is required to maintain; ie, as force increases, holding time decreases in a geometric progression.

The results of maximum-effort studies are useful in establishing the limiting endurance levels of physiologic fatigue for various exertions. The findings provide little guidance, however, in establishing submaximal or acceptable levels of effort for work performed over the course of an 8-hour day.

Ultimately, what work a person is willing to do each day depends on the level of fatigue experienced. When the discomfort from muscle fatigue exceeds a personal threshold, the worker seeks ways in which to reduce the aversive state. Depending on the job and supervision, a worker may conceal a rest break, change a work routine, or, at the extreme, stop working. If these recourses are prohibited and the worker is compelled to continue to work with increasing fatigue or pain and with reduced capacity, the safety of work is endangered and, over time, occupational impairments are likely.

Attempts at evaluating the effects of fatigue on worker behavior have been largely impeded by the lack of adequate methods of measurement. In the past researchers have tried to identify a single test to measure industrial fatigue.[5] Today, most industrial psychologists recognize that fatigue is more than a decline in muscle contraction, a fall in critical flicker fusion, or an increase in blood lactate concentration. Work fatigue can be regarded as a perceptual issue, an "experienced self-evaluation," integrating psychological (motivational) and sensory information.[6]

Although there are no single tests for isolating the experience of fatigue, psychophysical techniques have been used to research methods for quantifying the perception of physical events.[7] Psychophysics is concerned with the quantitative relationship between physical changes in stimulation and the subject's awareness of that stimulation. Some of the earliest psychophysical studies explored the perception of weight and force.[8,9] More recently, the variables of exertion, discomfort, and effort involved in work performance have been investigated.[10]

Perceived Exertion

Psychophysical studies of perceived exertion during work, for example, on a bicycle ergometer, indicate that perceived intensity increases with the physical work load according to a positively accelerating function, which can be described by a power function with an exponent of 1.6.[11] This relationship is consistent with Stevens's power model for subjective assessments.[12]

Stevens and Cain[13] expanded the research on the perception of muscular fatigue to include the role of duration. Recognizing that work is a function of force applied over time, Stevens and Cain identified a power function that describes the growth of perceived exertion (PE) with respect to load and duration of the exertion. Using data from hand grip contraction, the exponent for force was twice that for duration, as shown below. The relationship is expressed as $PE = k * Load^{1.7} * Duration^{0.7}$. The constant, k, defines individual strength differences.

The exponent for load indicates that the perception of exertion increases at a rapid rate relative to changes in the physical load, whereas the exponent for duration indicates a more gradual change in perceived exertion as duration increases. The exponents were derived from studies of highly repetitive work, such as bicycle pedaling. For static or eccentric work, the exponent would be larger. The implication is that with an equivalent load, perceived fatigue increases at a faster rate for static work than for dynamic work.[14,15] Regardless of the size of the exponent, it is apparent from the multiplicative relationship between load and duration (holding perceived effort constant) that variations in load will produce compensatory variations in duration. This reflects the everyday experience that heavy loads cannot be supported for as long as lighter loads.

Studies also indicate that individuals are capable of reliably estimating their endurance in a physical task and that there is a strong positive correlation between the objective and subjective aspects of a fatigue state.[16–18] Caldwell and Smith[19] and Park and Rodbard[20] suggested that the sensation of local muscle/joint pain is a reliable indicator of physiologic stress associated with physical work load. Moreover, Park and Rodbard noted that the subjective feelings associated with static loads increase consistently with the level of accumulated pain-inducing metabolites.

Further evidence of the close relationship between subjective and objective aspects of work endurance is reported by Tanii and associates.[21] In computing the endurance time course for different forces that loaded the arm, they found that the median time for onset of pain sensation occurs at between 30% and 40% of the maximum endurance time. For example, if the maximum endurance was 60 seconds for a given task, the subject would begin to experience pain between 18 and 24 seconds after the task began. Hence, the sensation of pain can be used as an early warning sign for overexertion that is time-locked to the course of maximum work endurance. Corlett and associates[22,23] also recognized that "acceptable discomfort" was a valid measure for evaluating how long a person could hold a work posture.

In addition to pain, several other studies in recent years have been conducted to evaluate the importance of physiological cues in the rating of exertion. Pandolf[24] concluded that two factors determine the level of perceived exertion: a local factor (ie, sensations or feelings of strain in the working muscles and/or joints) and a central factor (ie, sensations or feelings primarily associated with the cardiorespiratory system). Central factors contribute to the sensation of exertion when large muscle groups are involved and the work exceeds intensities of 50% aerobic power. Local factors contribute to the sensation of exertion for tasks in which static postures are maintained. For static postures, sensory cues are extracted primarily from muscle spindles, Golgi tendon organs, and various mechanoreceptors. As a result, joints such as the shoulder girdle with its rich supply of muscles and tendons are capable of responding to very distinct levels of static or repetitive loading.

Rating Scales

The two Borg scales provide a practical example of the application of psychophysical methods in the field of ergonomics.[25] In 1970, Borg[26] published the first of his scales, entitled the Rating of Perceived Exertion (RPE) scale (Table 1). The RPE scale consists of 15 numbers from 6 to 20, accompanied by nine descriptive labels that ranged from "no exertion" at one end to "maximum exertion" at the bottom of the scale. For practical purposes, he chose a simple category rating scale, in contrast to the ratio scaling methods used by Stevens and Cain.[13] The RPE scale was designed to grow linearly with exercise intensity and heart rate during work on a bicycle ergometer. Borg chose the numerical values on the RPE scale to correspond to one-tenth value of the heart rate. For example, a person performing a task in which a heart rate of 90 beats

Table 1 Borg 15-point rating of perceived exertion (RPE) scale*

Rating	Scale
6	No exertion at all
7	
8	Extremely light
9	Very light
10	
11	Light
12	
13	Somewhat hard
14	
15	Hard
16	
17	Very hard
18	
19	Extremely hard
20	Maximal exertion

* Scale of perceived whole-body exertion

per minute occurs would likely rate that task on the RPE scale as a 9 (very light). The RPE scale has proven useful in exercise physiology for the evaluation and monitoring of exercise intensities. In 1982, Borg[27] developed the second of his scales, which has become known as the CR-10 scale because it is based on category ratios of 0 to 10 (Table 2).[27] The CR-10 scale is widely used for assessing the level of muscular exertion during manual work, such as lifting or carrying. The numbers on the CR-10 scale are assigned expressions that are simple and understandable by most people. Exertions assigned a "10" are defined as "very, very strong" or "very, very heavy," usually the heaviest physical work perceived by the subject. Exertions rated as a "0.5" are considered "very, very weak" intensity or "very, very light" work. When using the scale, people are permitted to use decimals and to use values greater than 10.[25] Anchoring the highest number in a very well-defined maximum effort or exertion provides a point of reference for individuals, which aids in defining "same-

Table 2 Borg CR-10 Discomfort Rating Scale*

Rating	Scale
0	No discomfort at all
0.5	Very, very weak
1	Very weak
2	Weak
3	Moderate
4	Somewhat strong
5	Strong
6	
7	Very strong
8	
9	
10	Very, very strong (maximal)

* Scale of perceived muscular exertion

ness" for different individuals. The concept of the level of effort required to assign a value of 10 on the Borg CR-10 scale has become a public unit for comparisons between noise, vibration, pain, and exertion.

Because the Borg CR-10 scale is conceptually very simple and easy to administer, the rating procedure can be carried out at almost any stage during a work task. Typically, a subject provides a response by verbally indicating the numerical point on the scale that best represents his or her degree of exertion. An alternate procedure is to use one or more points on the scale as a criterion or target value for adjusting work load.

Yonda[28] and Deeb and associates[29] tested the hypothesis that the values on the Borg CR-10 scale, when multiplied by 10, are roughly equal to the percentage of maximum muscle strength (% MVC) that a given effort requires. For example, if an individual exerts a force and rates it as a "6" on the CR-10 scale, then that person is using roughly 60% of his or her maximum strength. This relationship is not perfectly linear; studies have shown that subjects consistently overestimate their efforts at lower forces and underestimate their efforts at high forces, with nearly perfect estimation occurring near 55% of MVC.[29,30] Deeb and associates[29] demonstrated that the RPE for a specific level of effort tends to increase with age, which is consistent with what is understood about the effect of aging on strength. To account for this age effect, psychophysical recommendations for working limits may need to be based on workers representing the spectrum of the working population.

Hogan and Fleishman[31] conducted a series of psychoscaling studies to assess the reliability and validity of subjective methods for measuring perceived physical effort (PPE). They developed a PPE index, which was a condensed version of the Borg 15-point RPE scale (Table 1). The PPE index consisted of a 7-point scale with the same labels as the Borg RPE scale with the numerical intervals reduced by half, beginning with "1" instead of "6." They found that relatively inexperienced participants could accurately and reliably characterize the physical effort of various common tasks using the PPE index. The tasks included activities such as sawing wood, carrying trays, operating a crane, and stocking shelves. The actual task ratings provided by the inexperienced participants were highly correlated (r = .88) with actual metabolic costs and measures of biomechanical or ergonomic demands. The authors concluded that the PPE index, even in the hands of inexperienced individuals, would be very useful as a job analysis method for physically demanding work.[32]

Acceptability Scaling

Much of the original psychophysical research into manual work has focused on ratings of maximum acceptable loads (RALs), ie, the individual's assessment of the maximal work load that can be tolerated without feeling overexertion or fatigue.[33] Measures of maximum acceptable frequency for a task are labeled as MAFs and, similarly, measures of maximum acceptable torque are labeled as MATs. The rationale for "acceptability scaling" is based on the view that the worker can best determine an appropriate individual work load based on his or her own interpretation of physical sensations resulting from the task. Psychophysical test protocols are usually designed to give the subject control over one task variable, such as load or frequency of exertion. The subject, based on perceived sensations of fatigue or exertion, adjusts the variable so that the subject can perform the task without experiencing excessive strain or fatigue.

Psychophysical methods including the use of both RPEs and RALs have proved valuable in the assessment of the individual's working capacity in manual material handling tasks. Chaffin and Andersson[34] concluded that until comprehensive dynamic testing methods and biomechanical models are developed, psychophysical limits, based on simulations of specific tasks of interest, may be the most accurate means of determining a person's acceptable performance limit for a given task. Poulton[35,36] also concluded that subjective rating techniques represent a valid procedure for assessing the subject's response to physical stimuli, reasoning that subjective assessment is the individual's "own perception" of a stimulus and, as such, provides a unique and valid response measure that no "objective measure" can replace.

Applications to Upper Extremity Work Activities

Despite widespread use in manual materials handling research, the application of psychophysical methods to the study of upper extremity work activities has only recently been explored. Interest in psychophysical techniques emanates from industry demands for guidelines or limits designed to prevent cumulative trauma disorders, combined with the difficulties inherent in assessing upper extremity work using more objective approaches. These difficulties with more objective work were demonstrated by Snook and Irvine[37,38] and Garg and Saxena,[39] who showed that physiologic measures of metabolic energy expenditure or heart rate criteria have little meaning in the study of upper extremity work. Similarly, although electromyography (EMG) can be helpful for quantifying muscular activity and fatigue, it requires expensive instrumentation, careful calibration, and an experimental design that preserves characteristic relationships between EMG and muscle. An advantage of psychophysical measures is that (unlike EMG) they are applicable to highly dynamic tasks, intermittent tasks, or exertions that involve combinations of several different muscles. Furthermore, psychophysical methods are less invasive in the workplace, require no expensive instrumentation or painstaking calibration to implement, and provide data that are readily interpretable.

Recent laboratory studies using psychophysical techniques to examine the effects of different variables on perceived exertion are described below (Table 3). These studies have also served to identify appropriate tool, task, and workstation designs for various manual activities. Much of this research yields insight into the reliability and reproducibility of psychophysically derived limits and the relationship between psychophysical measures and other measures of upper extremity exertion.

Variables Affecting Psychophysically Perceived Exertion

The results of psychophysical studies of upper extremity work are generally consistent with the results of biomechanical and epidemiologic studies; ie, conditions that impose biomechanical loads on the body and are associated with increased risk of musculoskeletal injury are also perceived as more stressful and less "acceptable" to workers than conditions that do not.

Force

Several studies clearly demonstrate that force of movement has a powerful effect on perceived exertion and the acceptability of manual work activities. As manual effort increases (often because the weight of a tool or object increases), the RPE increases.[40–47] Furthermore, increased manual force requirements generally have significant deleterious effects on the length of time sub-

Table 3 Psychophysical studies of upper extremity work

Reference	Task	Independent Variable(s)	Dependent Variable(s)	Psychophysical Method(s)	Results/Recommendations
Snook and Irvine[37,38]	Lifting boxes using arms	Box weight Lift height	MAF* of lift Heart rate	MAF determined using method of adjustment over 1 hour	MAF decreased with height and weight of lift. No difference in heart rate between conditions.
Garg and Saxena[39]	One-handed lifting in the horizontal plane	Load Reach distance	MAF of lift Heart rate RPE[†]	MAF determined using method of adjustment over 40-minute period Borg RPE scale	Increasing the load weight and lifting distance reduced MAF. At MAF, subjects rated exertion as fairly light to somewhat hard. No heart rate variation.
Hammarskjöld et al[60]	Sawing, nailing, and screwing (carpentry work)	Task type Day Time of day	RPE EMG[¶] Force exerted Motions Work time	Borg RPE scale	Screwing consistently rated as hard or very hard, sawing as somewhat hard, and nailing as fairly light.
Armstrong et al[52]	Powered hand tool use (assembly work)	Tool weight Tool handle diameter Vertical work distance Horizontal work distance Gender, stature, hand size	Rating of weight, handle size, grip force, and comfort of tools used	Attribute rated using a continuous scale (0–10), anchored at 0, 5, and 10	Weight and grip force assessments correlated with tool mass. Perceived handle size related to handle circumference. Discomfort increased with horizontal and vertical work distance.
Garg and Beller[61]	One-handed handle pulling	Speed of pull Vertical height of handle Angle of pull	RPE for elbow, shoulder, and back Comfort Pulling strength	Borg RPE scale	RPE and strength decreased, comfort increased with increased pulling speed. Pull height and angle had little effect on RPE.
Genaidy et al[40]	Holding weights and moving the	Task type (static, dynamic, and	RPE Heart rate Blood pressure	Borg RPE scale	RPE increased, endurance time decreased with weight. Static task

Table 3 Psychophysical studies of upper extremity work (cont.)

Reference	Task	Independent Variable(s)	Dependent Variable(s)	Psychophysical Method(s)	Results/Recommendations
	lower arm about the elbow.	combination) Weight Lift frequency	Time until exhaustion		associated with greatest RPE and blood pressure, shortest endurance time. Lift frequency had no effects.
Park et al[62]	Carpet trimming (3 studies)	Carpet type Type and direction of cut Knife temperature Blade angle	RPE, EMG Wrist deviation Grip force Length of cut	Borg CR-10 scale	RPE affected by carpet type and blade angle (straight blade associated with lowest RPE).
Snook et al[49,56]	Wrist motion against resistance (2 studies)	Wrist motion and grip type Repetition rate Days of exposure (2 vs 5 days/week)	MAT[§] Isometric wrist strength Tactile sensitivity Symptoms Errors Duration of force	MAT determined using method of adjustment (averaged and recorded each minute for 7 hours) Discomfort recorded on series of graded scales (0 to 3)	MAT decreased with repetition and hour of day; greater for wrist flexion than extension. No MAT difference between days. Increase in weekly work load (from 2 to 5 days) produced 36.3% decrease in MAT.
Ulin et al[45,50,53,54]	Driving screws (4 studies)	Vertical and horizontal work location Tool type Tool mass Work rate	RPE Discomfort rating	Borg CR-10 scale Body part discomfort survey	RPE increased with tool mass, vertical and horizontal work distance, and work pace.
Marley and Fernandez[41] Kim and Fernandez[42] Dahalan and Fernandez[43]	1. Drilling holes in sheet metal 2. Wire crimping (All simulated tasks)	1. Force, wrist flexion 2. Grip force as a % of MVC,** grip duration	MAF RPE Blood pressure EMG No discomfort measure	MAF determined using method of adjustment over a 20-minute period RPE-Borg scale	MAF decreased, RPE increased with increasing force, duration, and wrist flexion. RPE and MAF (–) correlated. RPE, HR[††], EMG, and blood pressure (+) correlated.
Krawczyk[44]	3 studies: 1. Moving plastic bottles	1. Bottle weight, frequency and distance of	1. RPE, discomfort 2. PW,** RPE,	RPE—10 cm visual analog scale (anchored at ends) Discomfort of 11 body parts	RPE increased with weight and frequency but not distance of transfer. For combination task, RPE

56 Epidemiologic and Psychologic Laboratory Studies

Perceived Exertion as a Function of Physical Effort   57

Table 3 Psychophysical studies of upper extremity work (cont.)

Reference	Task	Independent Variable(s)	Dependent Variable(s)	Psychophysical Method(s)	Results/Recommendations
	2. Moving containers (combination task)	movement, time 2. Frequency and distance of movement, time 3. % time spent on each task	discomfort 3. RPE, discomfort	(ranked) PW determined using method of adjustment over 8-hour period	and discomfort were minimized when time was evenly split between tasks. PW decreased with increased frequency and distance of movement. RPE and PW stable during workday; discomfort increased.
Putz-Anderson and Galinsky[48]	Lifting and lowering a tool handle (4 studies)	1. Discomfort level, force as a % of MVC 2. Repetition rate, force 3. Repetition rate, tool weight 4. Repetition rate, reach height	Work duration (time until onset of a specified level of fatigue)	Borg CR-10 scale used to designate fatigue/discomfort criterion	Work duration increased with fatigue criterion; decreased with increased force, tool weight, reach, and repetition. Increases in force or repetition attenuated the other's effect. No change in average work time through workday. Limiting fatigue maintained rest effectiveness.
Harber et al[47]	Repetitive grasping motions	Wrist position Force Repetition rate Grip type	RPE Comfort (overall and wrist)	Borg CR-10 scale (RPE) Discomfort scale (1–8, anchored at 4 points)	RPE and discomfort affected by grip type, force, wrist position, and rapid repetition.
Grant et al[46]	Grasping and moving tool handles (3 studies)	Handle shape/diameter Tool weight	RPE Grip force Forearm EMG	RPE measured using Borg CR-10 scale	RPE increased with weight, not affected by handle shape or diameter. RPE correlated with grip force, EMG.

* MAF, maximum acceptable frequency
† RPE, rating of perceived exertion
¶ EMG, electromyography
§ MAT, maximum acceptable torque
** PW, preferred container weight; MVC, maximum voluntary contraction
†† HR, heart rate

jects can work without becoming excessively fatigued and the rate of work subjects find acceptable for an 8-hour period.[37,39,41–43,48]

Repetition

Likewise, researchers are in nearly universal agreement that the repetitiveness of manual work (ie, the work rate) has a direct impact on the RPE and RAL.[44,47–50] All agree that increasing the rate of task repetition increases the level of perceived stress associated with the task. Furthermore, as the rate of repetition increases, the length of time workers are able to work without fatigue decreases and the acceptable force of exertion required by the task is reduced.[44,48,49] There is also evidence that as repetition rates continue to increase, compensatory mechanisms for reducing the stress associated with manual work become less effective. For example, Putz-Anderson and Galinsky[48] found that at extremely high rates of repetition, reducing the force required to perform the task was relatively ineffective in forestalling shoulder fatigue and discomfort. Similarly, Snook and associates[49] found that even though subjects were encouraged to adjust force requirements to avoid discomfort, and subjects actually did reduce force levels as repetition rates increased, subjects reported more discomfort throughout the workday when repetition rates were high. Although these findings do not invalidate studies that suggest that trade-offs are possible to achieve acceptable work loads, they do challenge the assumptions and recommendations of many ergonomists—namely, that high rates of repetition are permissible if awkward postures or manual forces associated with manual work can be reduced.

Posture

Awkward working postures frequently result from the faulty layout and design of workstations and tools.[51] It has been suggested that psychophysical measures represent a direct method for evaluating the interface between tools, tasks, and workers for the purpose of establishing design criteria for tools and workstations.

To evaluate this hypothesis, Armstrong and associates[52] asked workers in an automotive assembly plant to rate the handle size, grip comfort, and posture comfort of tools used during their work activities. Objective measures of handle circumference and the horizontal and vertical location of the tool relative to the body were collected, along with data on worker gender, stature, hand breadth, and hand length. The results indicated that workers' subjective assessments strongly correlated with tool, task, and worker attributes (Table 3). While acknowledging a need for further studies, Armstrong and associates argued that psychophysical ratings could be used to target and prioritize areas for ergonomic interventions.

In an extension of this work, Ulin and associates[45,50,53,54] conducted a series of laboratory studies to examine the effect of work location/orientation on the RPE in manual assembly operations. Subjects rated the exertion associated with driving screws into perforated sheet metal at different horizontal and vertical work locations with different pneumatic screwdrivers using the Borg CR-10 scale. The results agreed favorably with predictions based on anthropometric and biomechanics data, indicating that exertion is minimized when tools and workstations allow workers to maintain neutral wrist and shoulder postures during their work activities. As a result, specific design guidelines for minimizing perceived exertion were offered.

Other studies tend to confirm that worker tolerance for various work conditions is increased when extreme joint deviations are avoided. Garg and Saxena[39] and Krawczyk[44] found that doubling the reach distance in a manual transfer task reduced the maximum acceptable frequency of transfer by about 18% and the preferred weight of transfer by 37%. Marley and Fernandez[41] and Kim and Fernandez[42] found that the MAF of work in a drilling task was optimized when workers were allowed to perform the task with a neutral wrist posture. As angle of wrist flexion increased, the MAF decreased and RPE increased.

Job Content

Rotating workers between dissimilar jobs or giving workers responsibility for a larger number of work tasks is frequently proposed as an administrative means of controlling musculoskeletal stress. The goal of these strategies is to reduce the load on any one muscle group by breaking up long periods of static muscle contraction and by spreading the work load over additional body parts.

Recognizing that the mechanisms of injury associated with static and dynamic exertions are different, and that many jobs have both static and dynamic activities, Genaidy and associates[40] undertook a study to examine the effects of static and dynamic arm tasks on RPEs, endurance time, blood pressure, and the heart rate. Subjects performed three tasks: (1) a static task in which subjects held equal loads in both hands with the upper arms freely hanging at the sides and the elbows flexed at 90°; (2) a dynamic task in which subjects lifted loads in both hands by repetitively flexing and extending the elbow; and (3) a combination task in which the subject held a load in the left hand as described in (1) and lifted an equal load in the right hand as described in (2). The RPE and blood pressure measures indicated that the static arm task was the most stressful, followed by the combination task and the dynamic task. This agrees with findings by Stevens and Krimsley[14] and deVries[15] that perceived fatigue increases at a faster rate for static work than for dynamic work, if load is held constant. Genaidy and associates[40] also noted that static effort induces the blood vessels in the working muscle to compress; therefore, the muscle does not receive sufficient nutrients from the blood and waste products rapidly accumulate. Although energy expenditure and heart rate measurements are usually insensitive to disturbances in small muscle groups, Genaidy and associates demonstrated that psychophysical measures provide a valid indicator of these effects during manual work tasks.

The effect of varying job content on psychophysical stress was also examined by Krawczyk.[44] Workers either transferred objects along a conveyor with the left hand or drove screws with a pneumatic screwdriver using the right hand. Various amounts of time were recorded for each task. The results indicated that perceived exertion and body part discomfort were minimized when the workers' time was evenly divided between the two tasks. Krawczyk noted that not only did the evidence indicate the positive effects of work enlargement but also that this evidence would have been more difficult to obtain using more objective means.

Potential of Psychophysical Methods for Establishing Safe Levels of Work

Reliability Reliability refers to the consistency or stability of measures of a variable over time or across representative samples.[55] Researchers have repeatedly examined the reliability of psychophysically derived limits for upper extremity work by replicating trials under similar task conditions. Garg and Saxena[39] reported no significant differences in RPEs or in the maximum frequency of lift selected by subjects in two replications of a one-handed lifting task conducted using six weight-distance combinations. In two studies to identify MATs for various patterns and frequencies of wrist motion, Snook and associates[49,56] reported no significant differences in MATs from day to day during either experiment. Similarly, Putz-Anderson and Galinsky[48] compared work trial durations resulting from three replications of various repetitive arm tasks. In each trial, subjects were instructed to initiate a rest pause each time sensations in the shoulder exceeded a prespecified threshold of discomfort. The researchers reported no significant differences in average work trial duration between replications of the same task. This finding was interpreted as demonstrating that subjects were able to reliably monitor their own feelings of discomfort, and that providing appropriate rest breaks was an effective method of preventing overaccumulation of fatigue. Finally, Marley and Fernandez[41] and Kim and Fernandez[42] both reported that subjects were consistent in their selection of acceptable work rates for three experimental replications of a hand-held pneumatic drilling task.

Validity Measurement techniques are considered valid if they measure what they purport to measure. As previously discussed, evidence for the validity of RPEs and RALs is provided by several studies that demonstrate strong correlations with objective measures of muscular exertion. More recent studies of upper extremity work tasks tend to corroborate the reports of earlier researchers. In experiments in which subjects were required to repeatedly grasp and move various tool handles, Grant and associates[46] found that the RPE was significantly correlated with both the grip force exerted during the task (measured using a strain gauge embedded in the handle) and with the amplitude of EMG signals measured in the forearm. Marley and Fernandez,[41] Kim and Fernandez,[42] and Dahalan and Fernandez[43] also found that the RPE was strongly correlated with the pulse rate, systolic blood pressure, and forearm EMG amplitudes during drilling and gripping tasks.

With reference to laboratory experiments, results are also considered valid to the extent to which the findings can be generalized to nonlaboratory situations.[57] The validity of applying limits derived from laboratory studies to industrial settings has only recently been addressed. One issue relates to the selection of subjects for psychophysical studies of manual work. There is evidence from manual material handling research to indicate that subjects who are inexperienced or are not sufficiently trained (usually college students) tend to overestimate their capacity to work for an 8-hour period. This source of bias is easily avoided by limiting study participation to experienced industrial workers and by providing training at the beginning of the experiment.

There is also a concern that certain psychosocial processes, such as high arousal, that can occur at a specific workplace may not be present in a laboratory setting where psychophysical data usually are collected. High arousal can temporarily lower or elevate the threshold for experiencing a sensation of discomfort from the locomotor system. This effect could reduce the generalizability of laboratory-based psychophysical data for use at the work site.[58] For example, an individual experiencing extremely high levels of arousal, such as from fast-paced, high-demand work conditions, could fail to notice the onset of local muscle discomfort until many minutes after the incident occurred.

Another concern relates to the validity of generalizing from laboratory data that are collected on subjects during psychophysical tests which are considerably shorter in duration than the 8-hour typical work duration experienced by most workers. Are workers able to accurately judge from a 20-minute or even a 2-hour test what their capacity for work is over an 8-hour day? Because increasing trial duration can considerably increase the cost of experimentation, some researchers have attempted to examine and characterize the bias introduced by limited trial durations. Krawczyk[44] compared preferred weights and RPEs gathered at intermediate points during a manual transfer experiment (ie, after 1 or 2 hours) with results gathered at the end of an 8-hour work period. The difference between weights and RPEs selected in the first 2 hours and the last 2 hours of work averaged only 5% and 8%, respectively.

Slightly different findings were reported in two experiments by Snook and associates.[49,56] In two experiments, Snook and associates found that although MAT tended to decrease during the course of an 8-hour workday, the difference between forces selected after the first hour of work and the fifth hour of work was generally less than 10%, and forces did not decline significantly after the fifth hour. However, Snook also found that the duration of the workweek had a significant effect on the acceptability of manual forces. Comparing results from study I (in which subjects worked 2 days per week for 10 weeks) with results gathered in study II (in which subjects worked 5 days per week for 4 weeks—a work schedule more typical of industrial operations), the average force that workers found acceptable was 36.3% lower in study II, if all other task-related factors are held constant. Because the difference in work schedule was the only explanation that was provided for the dramatic difference in the results of these two experiments, a need for additional research on this topic is suggested.

Perhaps the ultimate test of the validity of psychophysical measures is their ability to separate safe work conditions from those that cause injury. Some of the most compelling evidence for the validity of psychophysical methods in establishing safe levels of manual lifting, pushing, and pulling has been reported by Snook and associates, noted above. In a report in which they compared three approaches to the prevention of low back injuries, they concluded that designing jobs with maximum weight limits that are acceptable to 75% of the population will reduce back injuries by 33%.[59] To date, however, there are limited work site data to demonstrate that designing tasks in accordance with psychophysically derived limits will reduce the morbidity associated with forceful and repetitive manual tasks. One main explanation is that psychophysical methods have been used only recently to derive recommendations for preventing upper extremity disorders. Field studies are needed to relate the incidence and severity of upper extremity injuries to the extent to which manual demands are judged acceptable by experienced workers.

Summary

There is growing evidence that, when carefully applied, psychophysical methods provide a practical means for achieving the goal of establishing safe levels of work. To date, laboratory results indicate that psychophysically derived limits are consistent and reproducible. Psychophysical measures of effort also appear to correlate with other physiologic measures of effort, as well as predictions based on anthropometric and biomechanical analyses. Additional evidence is needed to demonstrate that designing work in accordance with psychophysically derived limits will eliminate or reduce the rate of musculoskeletal injury associated with manual work.

References

1. Armstrong TJ, Buckle P, Fine LJ, et al: A conceptual model for work-related neck and upper-limb musculoskeletal disorders. *Scand J Work Environ Health* 1993; 19:73–84.
2. Engin, AE. On the biomechanics of the shoulder complex. *J Biomech* 1980;13:570–590.
3. Chaffin DB: Localized muscle fatigue: Definition and measurement. *J Occup Med* 1973;15:346–354.
4. Rohmert W: Problems in determining rest allowances: Part 1. Use of modern methods to evaluate stress and strain in static muscular work. *Appl Ergonomics* 1973;4:91–95.
5. Broadbent DE: Is a fatigue test now possible? *Ergonomics* 1979;22:1277–1290.
6. Bartley SH: *Fatigue: Mechanism and Management*. Springfield, IL, Charles C Thomas, 1965.
7. Stevens SS, Galanter EH: Ratio scales and category scales for a dozen perceptual continua. *J Exp Psychol* 1957;54:377–411.
8. Stevens JC, Mack JD: Scales of apparent force. *J Exp Psychol* 1959;58:405–413.
9. Eisler H: Subjective scale of force for a large muscle group. *J Exp Psychol* 1962;64: 253–257.
10. Jones LA: Perception of force and weight: Theory and research. *Psychol Bull* 1986; 100:29–42.
11. Borg G: Simple rating methods for estimation of perceived exertion, in Borg G (ed): *Physical Work and Effort*. Oxford, UK, Pergamon Press, 1977, pp 39–47.
12. Stevens SS: On the psychophysical law. *Psychol Rev* 1957;64:153–181.
13. Stevens JC, Cain WS: Effort in isometric muscular contractions related to force level and duration. *Perception and Psychophysics* 1970;8:240–244.
14. Stevens JC, Krimsley AS: Build up of fatigue in static work: Role of blood flow, in Borg G (ed): *Physical Work and Effort*. Oxford, UK, Pergamon Press, 1977, pp 145–155.
15. deVries HA: Method for evaluation of muscle fatigue and endurance from electromyographic fatigue curves. *Am J Phys Med* 1968;47:125–135.
16. Hosman J: Adaptation to muscular effort. Stockholm, Sweden, University of Stockholm, 1967.
17. Eason RG: Electromyographic study of local and generalized muscular impairment. *J Appl Physiol* 1960;15:479–482.
18. Lloyd AJ, Voor JH, Thieman TJ: Subjective and electromyographic assessment of isometric muscle contractions. *Ergonomics* 1970;13:685–691.
19. Caldwell LS, Smith RP: Pain and endurance of isometric muscle contractions. *J Eng Physiol* 1966;5:25–32.
20. Park SR, Rodbard S: Effects of load and duration of tension on pain induced by muscular contraction. *Am J Physiol* 1962;203:735–738.
21. Tanii K, Sadoyama T, Sanjo Y, et al: Appearance of effort-depending changes in static local fatigue. *J Hum Ergol* 1973;2:31–45.
22. Corlett EN, Bishop RP: A technique for assessing postural discomfort. *Ergonomics* 1976;19:175–182.
23. Corlett EN, Manenica I: The effects and measurement of working postures. *Appl Ergonomics* 1980;11:7–16.
24. Pandolf KB: Influence of local and central factors in dominating rated perceived exertion during physical work. *Percept Mot Skills* 1978;46:683–698.
25. Borg GA: Psychophysical bases of perceived exertion. *Med Sci Sports Exerc* 1982; 14:377–381.
26. Borg G: Perceived exertion as an indicator of somatic stress. *Scand J Rehabil Med* 1970;2:92–98.

27. Borg G: Psychophysical scaling with applications in physical work and the perception of exertion. *Scand J Work Environ Health* 1990:16 (suppl 1):55–58.
28. Yonda RA: An investigation of the human ability to replicate task-produced forces on a load cell: A method for determining the magnitude of forces exerted by workers engaged in manual materials handling activities. Buffalo, NY, State University of New York at Buffalo, 1986. Unpublished thesis.
29. Deeb JM, Drury CG, Pendergast DR: An exponential model of isometric muscular fatigue as a function of age and muscle groups. *Ergonomics* 1992;35:899–918.
30. Jones LA, Hunter IW: The relation of muscle force and EMG to perceived force in human finger flexors. *Eur J Appl Physiol* 1982;50:125–131.
31. Hogan JC, Fleishman EA: An index of physical effort required in human task performance. *J Appl Psychol* 1979;64:197–204.
32. Hogan JC, Ogden GD, Gebhardt DL, et al: Reliability and validity of methods for evaluating perceived physical effort. *J Appl Psychol* 1980;65:672–679.
33. Snook SH, Irvine CH, Bass SF: Maximum weights and work loads acceptable to male industrial workers: A study of lifting, lowering, pushing, pulling and walking tasks. *Am Ind Hyg Assoc J* 1970 31:579–586.
34. Chaffin DB, Andersson GBJ: *Occupational Biomechanics*. New York, NY, Wiley & Sons, 1991.
35. Poulton EC: Bias in ergonomic experiments. *Appl Erg* 1973;4:17–18.
36. Poulton EC: Qualitative subjective assessments are almost always biased, sometimes completely misleading. *Br J Psychol* 1977;68:409–425.
37. Snook SH, Irvine CH: Maximum frequency of lift acceptable to male industrial workers. *Am Ind Hyg Assoc J* 1968;29:531–536.
38. Snook SH, Irvine CH: Psychophysical studies of physiological fatigue criteria. *Hum Factors* 1969;11:291–300.
39. Garg A, Saxena U: Maximum frequency acceptable to female workers for one-handed lifts in the horizontal plane. *Ergonomics* 1982;25:839–853.
40. Genaidy AM, Houshyar A, Asfour SS: Physiological and psychophysical responses to static, dynamic and combined arm tasks. *Appl Ergonomics* 1990;2:63–67.
41. Marley RJ, Fernandez JE: Psychophysical frequency and sustained exertion at varying wrist posture for a drilling task. *Ergonomics* 1995;38:303–325.
42. Kim CH, Fernandez JE: Psychophysical frequency for a drilling task. *Int J Indust Ergonomics* 1993;12:209–218.
43. Dahalan JB, Fernandez JE: Psychophysical frequency for a gripping task. *Int J Indust Ergonomics* 1993;12:219–230.
44. Krawczyk S: Psychophysical determination of work design guidelines for repetitive upper extremity transfer tasks over an eight hour workday. Ann Arbor, MI, University of Michigan, 1993. Unpublished dissertation.
45. Ulin SS, Armstrong TJ, Snook SH, et al: Examination of the effect of tool mass and work postures on perceived exertion for a screw driving task. *Int J Indust Ergonomics* 1993;12:105–116.
46. Grant KA, Habes DJ, Putz-Anderson V: Psychophysical and EMG correlates of force exertion in manual work. *Int J Indust Ergonomics* 1994;13:31–39.
47. Harber P, Hsu P, Pena L: Subject-based rating of hand-wrist stressors. *J Med* 1994;36:84–89.
48. Putz-Anderson V, Galinsky T: Psychophysically determined work durations for limiting shoulder girdle fatigue from elevated manual work. *Int J Indust Ergonomics* 1993;11:19–28.
49. Snook SH, Vaillancourt DR, Ciriello VM, et al: Psychophysical studies of repetitive wrist motion: Part I: Two day per week exposure. *Ergonomics*, in press.
50. Ulin SS, Armstrong TJ, Snook SH, et al: Perceived exertion and discomfort associated with driving screws at various work locations and at different work frequencies. *Ergonomics* 1993;36:833–846.
51. Putz-Anderson V: *Cumulative Trauma Disorders: A Manual for Musculoskeletal Disorders of the Upper Limbs*. London, UK, Taylor and Francis, 1988, pp 61–64.
52. Armstrong TJ, Punnett L, Ketner P: Subjective worker assessments of hand tools used in automobile assembly. *Am Ind Hyg Assoc J* 1989;50:639–645.

53. Ulin SS, Snook SH, Armstrong TJ, et al: Preferred tool shapes for various horizontal and vertical work locations. *Appl Occup Environ Hyg* 1992;7:327–337.
54. Ulin SS, Armstrong TJ, Snook SH, et al: Effect of tool shape and work location on perceived exertion for work on horizontal surfaces. *Am Ind Hyg Assoc J* 1993;54:383–391.
55. Sanders MS, McCormick EJ (eds): *Human Factors in Engineering and Design.* New York, NY, McGraw-Hill, 1987.
56. Snook SH, Vaillancourt DR, Ciriello VM, et al: Psychophysical studies of repetitive wrist motion: Part II. Five day per week exposure. *Ergonomics,* in press.
57. Dember WN, Jenkins JJ, Teyler TJ: *General Psychology,* ed 2. Hillsdale, NJ, L Erlbaum Associates, 1984.
58. Theorell T, Harms-Ringdahl K, Ahlberg-Hulten G, et al: Psychomotor job factors and symptoms from the locomotor system: A multicausal analysis. *Scand J Rehabil Med* 1991;23:165–173.
59. Snook SH, Campanelli RA, Hart JW: A study of three preventive approaches to low back injury. *JOM* 1978;20:478–481.
60. Hammarskjöld E, Harms-Ringdahl K, Ekholm J: Shoulder-arm muscular activity and reproducibility in carpenters' work. *Clin Biomech* 1990;5:81–87.
61. Garg A, Beller D: One-handed hynamic pulling strength with special reference to speed, handle height and angles of pulling. *Int J Indust Ergonomics* 1990;6:231–240.
62. Park D, Yun MH, Freivalds A: Knife replacement studies at an automobile carpet manufacturing plant. Proceedings of the Human Factors Society 35th Annual Meeting, San Francisco, CA, 1991, pp 848–852.

Chapter 5
The Relationship Between Workplace Psychosocial Factors and Musculoskeletal Disorders in Office Work: Suggested Mechanisms and Evidence

Steven L. Sauter, PhD
Naomi G. Swanson, PhD

Introduction

There are increasing indications that workplace psychosocial factors are somehow involved in the etiology of work-related musculoskeletal disorders. For example, an extensive review of the epidemiologic literature on this subject by Bongers and de Winter[1] concluded that monotonous work, perceived high workload and time pressure, and low control and social support were all related to musculoskeletal symptoms among workers.

The International Labor Office (ILO) has defined workplace psychosocial factors in very broad terms, synonymous with conditions that give rise to job stress.[2] These conditions include not only aspects of work, ranging from the nature of tasks to relationships at work to management practices (often grouped loosely under the rubric "work organization"), but also psychological attributes of workers (needs and expectations, personality, culture, etc).

In this chapter we will attempt to elucidate the potential causal mechanisms and pathways linking workplace psychosocial factors and musculoskeletal disorders in video display terminal (VDT) work. The intent is not to diminish the importance of ergonomic factors or biomechanical mechanisms in the etiology of work-related musculoskeletal disorders, but rather to suggest a more holistic explanatory framework that incorporates psychosocial factors as well as physical environmental or ergonomic factors. Research supporting this framework is presented.

In this discussion, we adopt a vernacular that is generally consistent with the ILO concept of psychosocial factors. Specifically, the expression "psychosocial factors" is used to refer to attributes of both jobs and the individual, including the individual's extra-work environment, which contribute to job stress. The expression "work organization" is used very broadly in reference to any work-related risk factor for job stress, in contrast to "individual factors," which interact with working conditions in the development of job stress.

Musculoskeletal Disorders and Psychosocial Mechanisms

Three types of explanations for the association between work-related psychosocial factors and musculoskeletal disorders seem especially plausible and have been described by several authors.[1,3-6] In a report on VDT work and musculoskeletal disorders among newspaper editors, NIOSH[7] suggested three possible explanations for this association: (1) psychosocial demands and job stress may produce increased muscle tension and exacerbate task-related biomechanical strain, (2) psychosocial demands may affect awareness and reporting of musculoskeletal symptoms or affect perceptions of their cause, or (3) a causal or correlational relationship exists between psychosocial and physical workload demands. These types of mechanisms have been suggested previously by several investigators.[1,3-6]

The present paper incorporates all of these pathways into a formal causal model, which builds on earlier efforts by the authors to model the relationship between psychosocial factors and musculoskeletal disorders.[5]

According to this model, shown in Figure 1, musculoskeletal disorders can be traced ultimately to the nature of work technology, which includes the nature of both tools and of work systems. In the case of office or VDT work, the chief tool is the VDT and computer and the nature of work can be defined as mechanized or automated information. As shown in the model, there is a direct pathway from VDT or office technology to physical demands (as defined by workstation ergonomics) and a direct pathway from office technology to work organization. (The influence of industrialization and mechanization on the specialization of work, recognized since Adam Smith,[8] is an example of the latter pathway.) The pathway from work organization to physical demands suggests that the physical demands of work are exacerbated by organizational demands, for example, increased specialization leads to increased repetition.

The model shows a direct pathway between work organization and psychological strain (stress) which, in turn, influences musculoskeletal outcomes through two routes. First, psychological strain is hypothesized to increase muscle tension, and possibly other autonomic effects, which compound biomechanical strain induced by physical demands of the task. This effect is depicted by the arrow between psychological strain and biomechanical strain in

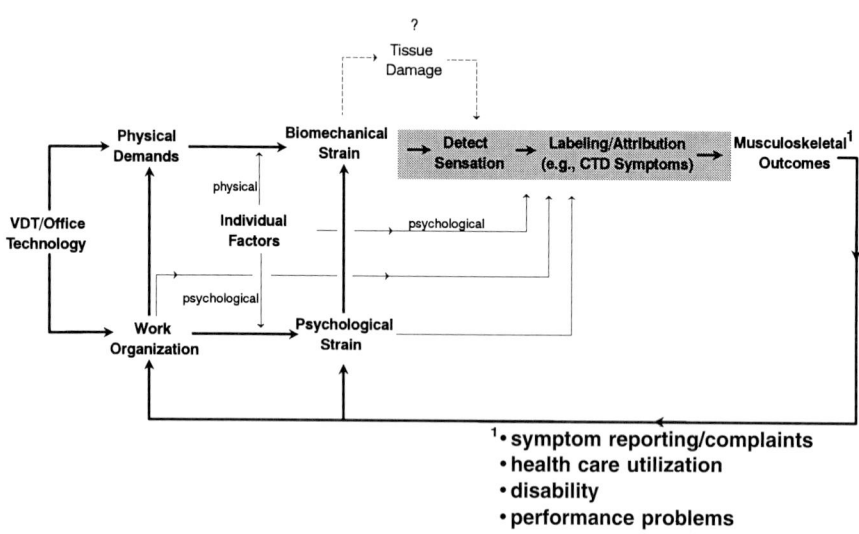

Fig. 1 An ecological model of musculoskeletal disorders in VDT work.

Figure 1. Second, psychological strain is hypothesized to moderate the relationship between biomechanical strain and the appearance of symptoms. (Moderating effects are denoted by the thin arrows in Figure 1.)

The model depicted in Figure 1 suggests that the relationship between biomechanical strains (ie, internal physiologic events) and the development of musculoskeletal symptoms is mediated by a complex of psychological processes (denoted by the shaded area in Figure 1), which involves the detection and labeling or attribution of somatic information (ie, symptoms). As discussed by Cioffi,[9] development of symptoms is not a direct or predetermined response to some internal physical event, rather, it is a highly plastic interpretive process subject to influence by contextual factors. Unfortunately, however, the rather extensive psychological literature on the perception and attribution of symptoms (reviewed by Cioffi[9]) has received little or no attention in ergonomics and occupational health.

With regard to the perception of symptoms, Figure 1 shows that the connection between biomechanical strain and musculoskeletal outcomes is influenced not only by psychological strain, but also by individual and work organization factors apart from the possible contribution of these factors to psychological strain. Factors such as organizational safety climate, for example, may have a direct influence on how workers detect, interpret, and respond to symptom information, regardless of whether safety climate results in stress.

For ease of presentation, multiple effects are combined in Figure 1 under "musculoskeletal outcomes." Space permitting, it would be more appropriate to describe these effects in terms of a continuum of events involving first the development of symptoms, then symptom reporting and health care utilization, then sick leave utilization and disability, and so on. It can be postulated that psychological factors as discussed above are instrumental in the evolution of each stage.

Figure 1 also shows a pathway from biomechanical strain to tissue damage to somatic interpretation. The broken lines comprising this pathway indicate that physical damage or disease is not necessarily integral to the model, ie, all that is essential are conditions that give rise to musculoskeletal symptoms.

Finally, the model suggests that the experience of musculoskeletal disorders feeds back to influence stress at work and it is likely that these disorders also prompt work redesign. It is because of these closed-system properties, as well the fact that the model incorporates input from both the physical and psychosocial work environment, that we refer to the model as an "ecological" model of musculoskeletal disorders.

Recently, researchers from the TNO Institute of Preventive Health Care in the Netherlands have described a generic model of workplace psychosocial factors and musculoskeletal disease with pathways similar to those depicted in Figure 1.[1,4] It should be noted, however, that the authors were reluctant to represent this model as an "explanatory" model. Rather they describe it as a vehicle for their extensive review of studies exploring associations between psychosocial factors and musculoskeletal disorders. However, an important distinguishing feature of the present model is the attention to cognitive processes that mediate between biomechanical strain and the development of musculoskeletal disorders.

The Evidence

There are insufficient data to fully substantiate the pathways between work organization and musculoskeletal disorders illustrated in Figure 1. Key problems in the extant literature, as pointed out by Bongers and de Winter,[1] include inadequate exposure assessment for the physical or work organization factors and failure to effectively disentangle the effects of these two sets of variables on musculoskeletal outcomes. Further, although many studies link work organization and musculoskeletal outcomes, the effect size is often quite small. Also few studies establish intermediary effects, which is essential to identifying specific pathways. In addition, most of the pertinent studies have cross-sectional designs, which limit casual inferences, including direction of causation, between psychosocial and musculoskeletal measures. These deficiencies notwithstanding, we believe that select studies offer circumstantial support for several of the pathways in Figure 1. These supportive studies are discussed below, with the emphasis on investigations of musculoskeletal disorders in office and VDT workers.

The Pathway From Office Technology to Work Organization

The mechanization of office work, which was associated with the introduction of the typewriter at the turn of the century, produced changes in the organization of office work not unlike the effects of mechanization in manufacturing processes. Guiliano[10] suggested that the mechanized or "industrial" office resulted in the standardization of office jobs and fragmentation of tasks and responsibilities that are characteristic of assembly line work. Video display terminal (computer) technology offers promise for reversal of these effects through enlargement of tasks and skills in office work.[11] However, the indication is that some types of VDT work are still stuck in the industrial age or may even exacerbate the adverse organizational aspects of office mechanization.[12] For example, in a 1981 NIOSH investigation[13] comparing clerical workers who used VDTs with those who did not, VDT users were reported to have significantly less autonomy and role clarity and greater work pressure and management control over work processes. Identical findings were obtained in a subsequent NIOSH investigation of VDT users and nonusers in Wisconsin.[5,14] A much larger study at Columbia University in 1987[12] compared all-day VDT users with part-time users and several groups of typists and clerical workers. In contrast to all other study participants, the all-day VDT users reported significantly higher levels of workload demand and repetition and lower levels of decision latitude, ability to learn new things on the job, and understanding of the overall work process.

Additional studies have investigated organizational aspects of VDT work, but strict comparisons with noncomputerized workplaces have been difficult in recent years because VDTs have become ubiquitous and, thus, suitable comparison groups are unavailable. Still, review of this work suggests a pattern of effects consistent with the reduction of tasks, skills, and autonomy, etc, as discussed above.[15]

Pathways From Work Organization to Musculoskeletal Outcomes

An impressive number of studies in the last decade have linked work organizational factors to upper extremity musculoskeletal signs and symptoms among VDT/keyboard users.[3,14,16–28] Factors predictive of musculoskeletal outcomes in these studies included limited rest pauses, routine tasks, uncertain job future, highly variable workload, time pressure and heavy workload demands, high mental workload, low co-worker and supervisory support, low worker autonomy, and low work group cohesion. Several of these factors (eg, heavy workload demand, low autonomy, low supervisory support, and low [peer] group cohesion) were predictive of musculoskeletal problems in multiple studies.

Figure 1 shows two principal pathways (thick, or "bold" arrows) from work organization factors to musculoskeletal disease; one mediated by psychological strain and one mediated by increased physical demand. With regard to the latter, it is evident that the VDT itself imposes musculoskeletal demands relating to the posture required to do the work (ie, to view the display and operate the keyboard). However, it is intuitive that the extent of exposure to these demands as well as the exposure to other generic risk factors such as repetitive motion (eg, excessive keying) are influenced by work organization factors such as workload demands and the complexity of tasks (which would affect cycle time). At least two studies have shown a relationship between organizational and physical stressors in VDT work,[5,12] with correlations as high as 0.38 reported between these two classes of variables.[5] Although a purely correlational relationship (resulting from the effect of technology on both work organization and physical demands) cannot be ruled out, data by Lim and Carayon[22] argue for a direct causal link between organizational demands and physical demands. Using path analysis to explore the relationship between organizational factors, ergonomic demands, and psychological stress, Lim and Carayon reported a significant pathway from organizational factors to physical ergonomic demands.

Research is available also in support of linkages in the pathway between work organization and musculoskeletal disorders which is mediated by psychological strain. Using structural analysis methods, Sauter and associates[5] found that factors such as job future uncertainty, social support, and workload demands influenced somatic symptoms in VDT users by way of an intermediary effect on mood disturbances. A study of keyboard operators performing postal letter sorting tasks[17] linked every element in the pathway mediated by psychological strain in Figure 1. Specifically, tasks involving increased visual search and memory demand were associated with reports of increased mental strain, spectral changes in the forearm electromyogram (EMG) and increased forearm tremor, and increased musculoskeletal discomfort. Similar multilink associations were reported by investigators from the Karolinska Institute,[29] although the study population did not include office workers. Increased psychological demands at work were associated with increased worry, fatigue, and sleep problems which, in turn, were associated with behavioral indicators of muscle tension, which were associated with increased back, neck, and shoulder discomfort.

Other studies address specific links within the psychologically mediated pathway. Lim and Carayon[22] and Bergqvist and associates[16] reported associations between indicators of psychological strain (fatigue and stomach reactions, respectively) and upper extremity musculoskeletal symptoms[16,22] and diagnosed disorders of the upper extremities.[16]

As early as 1951, Lundervold[30] demonstrated effects of psychological demands on muscle tension in keyboard operators, supporting the link between psychological strain and biomechanical strain in the present model. More recently, Westgaard and Bjorklund[31] and Waersted and associates[32] investigated static muscle loading as a possible mechanism linking work organization, psychological strain, and musculoskeletal disorders among VDT users. Consistent with extensive prior research showing effects of psychological demands on muscle tension (as reviewed by Ursin and associates[6] and Waersted and associates[32]), increases in low level muscle tension in the trapezius were induced by increasing the complexity and attentional demands of VDT tasks. Although the overall group effects were modest, averaging about 0.5% to 1.0% of maximum voluntary contraction (MVC), considerable interindividual variability was seen, with some subjects producing sustained loads up to 6.0% MVC. The latter level is within the range thought by Jonsson[33] to pose risk for musculoskeletal disease with chronic exposure. In this regard, it is notable that Kogi[34] reported Japanese research showing sustained loads in the range of 10% to 30% MVC in the forearm extensors among office machine operators (although a linkage to psychosocial demands was not suggested).

It is plausible that the direct, neurogenic effects of psychological demand on muscle tension and biomechanical strain are complemented by stress-related endocrine effects on neuromuscular function.[22,29] However, there has been little empirical study of such mechanisms.

Despite the evidence supporting the pathway in Figure 1 from organizational factors to musculoskeletal outcomes via psychological strain, it is difficult to rule out a competing pathway involving direct effects of organizational factors or psychological strain on the perception and attribution of symptoms, ie, the pathway denoted by the thin arrows from work organization and psychological strain in Figure 1. (This effect is examined in the discussion of somatic interpretation below.) But a more fundamental issue is whether effects attributed to the pathways from work organization to psychological strain or symptom perception are possibly confounded by physical effects related to (1) the path from work organization through physical demands, or (2) the covariation of physical and organizational demands resulting from the effects of technology on both of these classes of variables.

Two lines of evidence can be raised against the confounding hypothesis. First, for several types of variables found to predict musculoskeletal outcomes among VDT users, a significant effect on physical demand would seem unlikely. Examples of these types of variables include low group cohesion, work clarity, and staff support, which were predictive of repetition strain injury (RSI) cases in the study of Ryan and Bampton[26] or uncertainty regarding job future and reduced supervisory support, which were predictive of musculoskeletal symptoms in a NIOSH study of telecommunications workers.[24] Unlike organizational variables such as time pressure or repetitive work, it is difficult to see how changes in these conditions could elicit changes in physical workload demands (ie, the pathway to physical demands would not seem to be operative).

More compelling are the results of studies that statistically separated effects relating to physical and organizational factors and, thus, are able to demonstrate effects unique to the psychological pathway. This counterargument to the confounding hypothesis, however, rests on the adequacy of the exposure assessment for physical demands (and also psychosocial factors), which has been a difficult issue and may be problematic in many studies. Using multiple regression methods, Sauter and associates[5,14] reported a significant association between worker autonomy and musculoskeletal symptoms in VDT users after adjusting for a wide variety of variables denoting physical stressors. Similarly, NIOSH[3] found an association between supervisory support and hand/wrist symptoms in news editors after adjusting for the amount of time spent typing. Additionally, Bergqvist and associates,[16] Lim and Carayon,[22] and Ryan and Bampton[26] all were able to separate to some extent the effects of physical and organizational factors in predicting musculoskeletal problems in VDT users.

Similar evidence of effects uniquely attributable to psychosocial variables comes from Arndt,[35] Linton,[36] and Theorell and associates,[29] although none of these studies employed VDT users. The Arndt[35] and Theorell and associates[29] studies are of particular interest. Arndt found increased EMG activity in assembly line workers who were asked to speed up, but who were unable to respond with increased work speed (virtually eliminating any possibility of a confound with a physical influence on the muscle response observed). Like several VDT studies, Theorell and associates[29] found effects of psychological demands on back, neck, and shoulder symptoms after adjusting for physical demands (lifting demands, awkward postures). Like Gomer and associates,[17] however, he was also able to demonstrate intermediate linkages of psychosocial demands to psychological strain, self-reported muscle tension, and, ultimately, musculoskeletal discomfort.

Finally, inherent limitations of cross-sectional studies (the predominant methodology in VDT health research) pose a potential problem. The cited associations between organizational factors and musculoskeletal disorders might result from an influence of symptoms on job perceptions, not the reverse. Two studies, however, tend to discount this possibility. Hopkins[21] studied the organizational environment in workplaces with high and low prevalences of RSI. Ratings of organizational factors, however, were obtained from asymptomatic workers only (thereby eliminating the possibility of a symptom influence on job perceptions). Almost without exception, ratings of organizational factors were more negative in the high (RSI) prevalence workplaces. Similar findings are reported by Hales and associates,[20] who observed an association between fear of job loss and neck, shoulder, and elbow symptoms in directory assistance operators. Fear of job loss ratings within job sites were rescored based on ratings obtained from asymptomatic workers, and then associations with musculoskeletal symptoms were re-examined. Reanalysis showed that symptom levels were still positively associated with fear ratings; ie, higher in units with higher fear ratings.

Psychological Mediation of the Pathway From Biomechanical Strain to Musculoskeletal Outcomes

Thus far, it has been suggested that psychosocial factors might contribute to musculoskeletal disorders via two pathways: one involving effects on physical workplace demands and a second involving stress-related effects on muscle function. A third possible mechanism bears some similarity to what has been referred to as an "iatrogenic" process.

The iatrogenic hypothesis has been heavily promoted as an explanation for the surge in upper extremity musculoskeletal disorders witnessed internationally in the last decade. According to this hypothesis, musculoskeletal discomfort and fatigue are endemic to VDT work. Environmental forces, including not only medical practitioners, but also social and cultural factors, legal/compensation systems, and workplace industrial relations then encourage the interpretation of discomfort as signals of underlying injury and promote the development of sick roles and disability.[37-40] Although the iatrogenic hypothesis has not been tested empirically in the context of VDT work, this type of explanation finds support in the medical anthropologic and sociologic literature that identifies significant cultural variations in response to somatic symptoms.[41,42]

The iatrogenic hypothesis converges with an extensive area of investigation in psychology, which may offer a theoretically broader and richer formulation for explaining iatrogenic-like effects on musculoskeletal disorders. Extensive research in social and cognitive psychology in the last two decades has tried to explain how people interpret internal somatic information such as sensations associated with emotional response or illness. Space does not permit more than the briefest summary of this work[9,43] but the theory and findings suggest that response to somatic signals involves a multistage perceptual and attributional process that is governed by cognitive and environmental factors.

First, as in the perception of any stimulus, whether or not a somatic stimulus is even noticed depends on factors such as the degree of arousal of the individual and the salience of competing stimuli (which could mask the somatic stimulus). Second, once detected, explanations for the somatic sensation are sought, which involves labeling the sensation and then deducing its cause. Social psychological research has shown that this inferential process is highly influenced by situational factors. In the classic studies in this area, subjects were injected with epinephrine to induce psychological and physiological arousal, but were uninformed about the effects. It was then demonstrated that self-labeling of the resulting arousal state as euphoria or anger could be readily manipulated by exposure of the subjects to euphoric or angry confederates.[44] Importantly, this attributional process is understood to be a natural, probably hard-wired, and lawful process that has survival value for the organism;[9,43] ie, it is normal to seek causal explanations for events in and around us and to rely on contextual cues when the stimuli are ambiguous, which is often the case with somatic sensations.

In the current model of musculoskeletal disorders, it is suggested that somatic interpretation processes as discussed here (shaded area in Figure 1) mediate between biomechanical strain and musculoskeletal outcomes, and that these processes are influenced by various psychosocial factors (thin parallel inputs to the shaded processes). Within this framework, several effects of stress and psychosocial factors on musculoskeletal disorders seem plausible, although studies to confirm these effects have not been undertaken.

With regard to the detection of symptoms, it is possible that stress-related arousal may sharpen sensitivity to otherwise subthreshold musculoskeletal stimuli. Similarly, work organization might influence the relative salience of musculoskeletal signals. For example, competition for attention to musculoskeletal stimuli may be considerably reduced in dull routine tasks in comparison to more varied, challenging tasks that provide richer environmental stimulation. This may help to explain, for example, why clerical-level VDT jobs are associated with increased musculoskeletal symptoms[13,16,18] or why monotonous work was associated with neck symptoms in a Swedish working population.[36] Ironically, as discussed by Pennebaker,[43] this mechanism might also increase the health risk for workers in more challenging, engrossing tasks by reducing their relative awareness to somatic danger signals. Could this suppression phenomenon partially explain, for example, the reportedly high prevalence of musculoskeletal disorders among news editors?[7,45]

It is also possible to suggest ways in which psychosocial conditions might influence the labeling and attribution of musculoskeletal sensations. Assuming that people hold implicit hypotheses that stress promotes disease, it is predictable that musculoskeletal sensations arising in the context of stressful working conditions might be interpreted as signals of injury or disease. Further, attribution of these symptoms to the job might seem natural in the presence of adverse organizational conditions such as a negative safety climate. NIOSH[7] found, for example, that perceived lack of management support for ergonomic programs nearly doubled the odds for neck symptoms among news editors.

Effects of personality or dispositional factors on musculoskeletal disorders in office work[16,27] and in other occupations[6,46] might also be explained within the somatic interpretation framework. It is possible, for example, that negative affectivity, referring to a state (or trait) characterized by undifferentiated subjective distress,[47] colors the labeling of sensations in negative (disease) terms. In this regard, Bergqvist and associates[16] found that negative affectivity predicted both neck and shoulder discomfort among VDT users. (Self-reports of working conditions might be similarly [ie, adversely] affected, tending to inflate associations of organizational factors and musculoskeletal outcomes.) Although negative affectivity is commonly discussed as an individual or personality characteristic,[47] it is plausible that, like job attitudes such as job dissatisfaction, negative affectivity could be shaped by chronic exposure to stressful working conditions. These two perspectives would have different implications (ie, in terms of focusing on the person or the job) in attributing the cause of health outcomes associated with negative affectivity and in the design of interventions.

Although the current model highlights somatic interpretations, it is important to emphasize that this process has not been investigated in the context of work-related musculoskeletal disorders, and thus the significance of this mechanism in comparison with other mechanisms suggested in the current model is unknown. It is very doubtful that this mechanism alone could fully explain the relationship between psychosocial factors and musculoskeletal disorders seen in the extant literature. Several studies have demonstrated significant associations between workplace psychosocial factors and more objective indices of musculoskeletal disorders involving clinical evaluation of subjects.[16,20,24,26,47,48] Use of more objective methods for assessing musculoskeletal disorders obviates, to a considerable extent, the influence of cognitive and inferential effects integral to the somatic interpretation mechanism.

Feedback Effects

Finally, the current model shows reciprocal effects of musculoskeletal disorders on work organization and psychological strain. This pathway is highly intuitive. For example, adjustments in job tasks such as assignment to "light duty" or other forms of work redesign are commonly made for injured or symptomatic workers. Regarding effects on psychological strain, Ghiringhelli[49] reported fear of health impairment to be an important source of stress among VDT users. Data supporting such effects are very limited, however. Sauter and associates[5] conducted a series of analyses showing reciprocal prediction of illness symptoms and mood states in a sample of office workers, including VDT users. One other study, with a longitudinal design permitting stronger causal inference, reported this type of effect in a sample of office and production workers. Leino[48] found that 1973 to 1978 stress symptom scores predicted rheumatic symptoms and clinically defined musculoskeletal disorders upon follow-up in 1983. Among male workers, however, rheumatic symptoms and musculoskeletal disorders from 1973 to 1978 also predicted stress symptoms in 1983.

Summary and Direction

A theoretical model suggesting multiple causal linkages between workplace psychosocial factors and musculoskeletal disorders in VDT work is presented. This model does not diminish the importance of physical environmental/ergonomic factors in the etiology of musculoskeletal disorders in VDT work that is supported in prior research.[50,51] Rather, psychosocial effects are depicted as complementary to and interactive with effects of physical workplace demands. Furthermore, the psychological mechanisms linking or mediating psychosocial factors and musculoskeletal disorders are discussed as normal psychological processes, in contrast to clinical or abnormalistic characterizations by others.[52,53]

Evidence presented in support of the psychosocial pathways suggested in these models is neither perfect nor complete. More powerful study methods employing longitudinal designs, improved exposure (to both psychosocial and ergonomic demands) and health assessment, and improved analytical schemes, such as structural analysis, would be useful in substantiating and isolating the effects of psychosocial factors. Further research is needed to evaluate the strength of specific pathways postulated in the model. For example, to our knowledge, studies have not investigated the magnitude of static muscle loads during actual workplace exposure to known psychosocial stressors (eg, deadline work, electronic monitoring, etc) in the office workplace. Thus, the need for further analytic study is evident.

From a prevention imperative, an additional course of investigation is worth consideration. Specifically, case studies of organizational interventions to prevent musculoskeletal disorders in VDT work suggest rather powerful effects of psychosocial factors. According to Westin,[54] for example, the Federal Express Corporation has been able to maintain high levels of productivity with minimal experience of musculoskeletal disorders among VDT users by adopting a "people-technology" philosophy that gives priority to improving job design to minimize monotony, by adoption of participative management practices, and by improved employee education, among other measures.

Intervention studies often do not permit the type of control or manipulation needed to define specific mechanisms or pathways of effect. Furthermore, naturalistic interventions are not always pure enough to isolate specific causal factors. Indeed, the people-technology philosophy at Federal Express also included a commitment to improve ergonomics. Still, these types of studies have a high degree of ecological validity and can be much more powerful motivators of preventive action than the more molecular investigations that have been examined in this paper.

References

1. Bongers PM, de Winter CR: *Psychosocial Factors and Musculoskeletal Disease: A Review of the Literature.* Leiden, The Netherlands, TNO Gezondheidsonderzoek, 1992, NIPG Report 92.028.
2. The Joint ILO/WHO Committee on Occupational Health: *Psychosocial Factors at Work: Recognition and Control.* Geneva, Switzerland, International Labour Office, 1986.
3. Bergqvist UO: Video display terminals and health: A technical and medical appraisal of the state of the art. *Scand J Work Environ Health* 1984;10(suppl 2):1–87.
4. Bongers PM, de Winter CR, Kompier MA, et al: Psychosocial factors at work and musculoskeletal disease. *Scand J Work Environ Health* 1993;19:297–312.
5. Sauter SL, Gottlieb MS, Rohrer KM, et al: *The Well-Being of Video Display Terminal Users: An Exploratory Study.* Madison, WI, University of Wisconsin, 1983.
6. Ursin H, Endresen IM, Ursin G: Psychological factors and self-reports of muscle pain. *Eur J Appl Physiol Occup Physiol* 1988;57:282–290.
7. National Institute for Occupational Safety and Health: Health Hazard Evaluation Report, in *Los Angeles Times.* Los Angeles, CA, January 1993, HETA 90–013–2277.

8. Smith A: *An Inquiry Into the Nature and Causes of the Wealth of Nations.* Chicago, IL, University of Chicago Press, 1977.
9. Cioffi D: Beyond attentional strategies: A cognitive-perceptual model of somatic interpretation. *Psychol Bull* 1991;109:25–41.
10. Guiliano VE: The mechanization of office work. *Sci Am* 1982;247:149–164.
11. Johansson G, Aronsson G: Stress reactions in computerized administrative work. *J Occup Behav* 1984;5:159–181.
12. Stellman JM, Klitzman S, Gordon GC, et al: Work environment and the well-being of clerical and VDT workers. *J Occup Behav* 1987;8:95–114.
13. Smith MJ, Cohen BG, Stammerjohn LW Jr: An investigation of health complaints and job stress in video display operations. *Hum Factors* 1981;23:387–400.
14. Sauter SL, Gottlieb MS, Jones KC, et al: Job and health implications of VDT use: Initial results of the Wisconsin-NIOSH study. *Commun Assoc Comput Mach* 1983;26:284–294.
15. Report on a World Health Organization Meeting: Working with visual display terminals. Psychosocial aspects and health. *J Occup Med* 1989;31:957–968.
16. Bergqvist U, Wolgast E, Nilsson B, et al: Musculoskeletal disorders among visual display terminal workers: Individual, ergonomic and work organizational factors. *Ergonomics*, in press
17. Gomer FE, Silverstein LD, Berg WK, et al: Changes in electromyographic activity associated with occupational stress and poor performance in the workplace. *Hum Factors* 1987;29:131–143.
18. CLC Labour Education and Studies Centre: *Towards a More Humanized Technology: Exploring the Impact of Video Display Terminals on the Health and Working Conditions of Canadian Office Workers.* Ottawa, Ontario, CLC Labour Education and Studies Centre, December, 1982.
19. Green R, Briggs C: Prevalence of overuse injury among keyboard operators: Characteristics of the job, the operator and the work environment. *J Occup Health Safety* 1990;6:109–118.
20. Hales TR, Sauter SL, Peterson MR, et al: Musculoskeletal disorders among visual display terminal (VDT) users in a telecommunications company. *Ergonomics* 1994;37:1603–1621.
21. Hopkins A: Stress, the quality of work, and repetition strain injury in Australia. *Work Stress* 1990;4:129–138.
22. Lim SY, Carayon P: An integrated approach to cumulative trauma disorders in computerized offices: The role of psychosocial work factors, psychological stress and ergonomic risk factors, in Smith MJ, Salvendy G (eds): *Human Computer Interaction: Applications and Case Studies.* Amsterdam, The Netherlands, Elsevier Science Publishers, 1993, pp 880–885.
23. Linton SJ, Kamwendo K: Risk factors in the psychosocial work environment for neck and shoulder pain in secretaries. *J Occup Med* 1989;31:609–613.
24. National Institute for Occupational Safety and Health: *Health Hazard Evaluation Report.* Cincinnati, OH, U.S. West Communications, HETA Report 89–299–2230.
25. Pot F, Padmos P, Brouwers A: Determinants of the VDU operator's well-being, in Knave B, Wildeback PG (eds): *Work With Display Units.* Amsterdam, The Netherlands, 1987, pp 16–25.
26. Ryan GA, Bampton M: Comparison of data process operators with and without upper limb symptoms. *Comm Health Studies* 1988;12:63–68.
27. Spillane RM, Deves LA: Psychosocial correlates of RSI reporting. *J Occup Health Safety* 1988;4:21–27.
28. Westgaard RH, Jensen C, Hansen K: Individual and work-related risk factors associated with symptoms of musculoskeletal complaints. *Int Arch Occup Environ Health* 1993;64:405–413.
29. Theorell T, Harms-Ringdahl K, Ahlberg-Hulten G, et al: Psychosocial job factors and symptoms from the locomotor system: A multicausal analysis. *Scand J Rehabil Med* 1991;23:165–173.

30. Lundervold AJS: Electromyographic investigations of position and manner of working in typewriting. *ACTA Physiol Scand* 1951;84(suppl):1–171.
31. Westgaard RH, Bjorklund R: Generation of muscle tension additional to postural muscle load. *Ergonomics* 1987;30:911–923.
32. Waersted M, Bjorklund RA, Westgaard RH: Shoulder muscle tension induced by two VDU-based tasks of different complexity. *Ergonomics* 1991;34:137–150.
33. Jonsson B: Kinesiology with special reference to electromyographic kinesiology. *Electroencephalogr Clin Neurophysiol* 1978;34(suppl):417–428.
34. Kogi K: Finding appropriate work-rest rhythm for occupational strain on the basis of electromyographic and behavioural changes. *Electroencephalogr Clin Neurophysiol* 1982;36(suppl):738–749.
35. Arndt R: Work pace, stress, and cumulative trauma disorders. *J Hand Surg* 1987;12A:866–869.
36. Linton SJ: Risk factors for neck and back pain in a working population in Sweden. *Work Stress* 1990;4:41–49.
37. Bell DS: "Repetition strain injury": An iatrogenic epidemic of simulated injury. *Med J Aust* 1989;151:280–284.
38. Cleland LG: "RSI": A model of social iatrogenesis. *Med J Aust* 1987;147:236;238–239.
39. Hadler NM: Industrial rheumatology: The Australian and New Zealand experiences with arm pain and backache in the workplace. *Med J Aust* 1986;144:191–195.
40. Hadler NM: Cumulative trauma disorders: An iatrogenic concept. *J Occup Med* 1990;32:38–41.
41. Hocking B: Anthropologic aspects of occupational illness epidemics. *J Occup Med* 1987;29:526–530.
42. Mechanic D: Social psychologic factors affecting the presentation of bodily complaints. *N Engl J Med* 1972;286:1132–1139.
43. Pennebaker JW (ed): *The Psychology of Physical Symptoms*. New York, NY, Springer-Verlag, 1982.
44. Schachter S, Singer JE: Cognitive, social, and physiological determinants of emotional state. *Psychol Rev* 1962;69:379–399.
45. National Institute for Occupational Safety and Health: *Health Hazard Evaluation Report*. Melville, NY, Newsday, Inc, 1990, HETA 89–250–2046.
46. Bigos SJ, Battie MC, Spengler DM, et al: A prospective study of work perceptions and psychosocial factors affecting the report of back injury. *Spine* 1991;16:1–16.
47. Toomingas A, Theorell T, Michelsen H, et al: Associations between perceived psychosocial job factors and prevalence of musculoskeletal disorders in the neck and shoulder regions. *Arbete och Hälsa* 1992;17:289–290.
48. Leino P: Symptoms of stress predict musculoskeletal disorders. *J Epidemiol Commun Health* 1989;43:293–300.
49. Ghiringhelli L: Collection of subjective opinions on use of VDUs, in Grandjean E, Vigliani E (eds): *Ergonomic Aspects of Visual Display Terminals*. London, UK, Taylor & Francis, 1982, pp 227–231.
50. Hunting W, Laubli T, Grandjean E: Postural and visual loads at VDT workplaces: I. Constrained postures. *Ergonomics* 1981;24:917–931.
51. Sauter SL, Schleifer LM, Knutson SJ: Work posture, workstation design, and musculoskeletal discomfort in a VDT data entry task. *Hum Factors* 1991;33:151–167.
52. Lucire Y: Neurosis in the workplace. *Med J Aust* 1986;145:323–327.
53. Spillane RM, Deves LA: RSI: Pain, pretence or patienthood? *J Indust Rel* 1987;19:41–48.
54. Westin AF: Organizational culture and VDT policies: A case study of the Federal Express Corporation, in Sauter SL, Dainoff MJ, Smith MJ (eds): *Promoting Health and Productivity in the Computerized Office: Models of Successful Ergonomic Interventions*. London, UK, Taylor & Francis, 1990, pp 147–168.

Directions for Future Research

Epidemiologic studies of work-related upper limb disorders have contributed to our knowledge about the occupational causes of these disorders. Despite the progress of the last 30 years, there are still important gaps in our knowledge. The following recommendations involve both methods to improve future studies and interesting hypotheses that need further investigation. Progress in these areas would enhance our knowledge and promote the development of more effective prevention strategies. The discussion by the participants in this section focused more on the identification of predictors and causes of these disorders rather than on the equally important question of what is the most effective treatment of these disorders or how to prevent their progression to disability. The recommendations for future research begin with a discussion of improvements in surveillance for these disorders because surveillance data have provided the impetus for initiation of epidemiologic studies and is critical in determining whether efforts to prevent these disorders have been successful.

Develop a more effective surveillance system for work-related upper limb disorders.

Work-related upper limb disorders are a common problem in working populations. Official statistics show an increase in incidence of these disorders in many countries during the past decade. The increase is possibly related to many factors, including changes in working conditions, in diagnostic criteria or patterns of medical care, in the awareness of the disorders among workers and health care providers, increased job insecurity, and legislation. A national surveillance system that provides more uniform information on specific disorders and associated occupational exposure conditions would be helpful in identifying the possible causes for the observed increased incidence and in the future for evaluating the impact of prevention activities.

There is a need to develop standard classification for the disorders and standard definitions for risk exposure factors. These methods, if internationally accepted, would allow comparisons between nations. Currently, there is no national reporting system in the United States that collects information on all occupations and industries (much less specific relevant risk factors). The development of an improved national surveillance system requires multidisciplinary scientific agreement concerning how to collect information on disorders and exposures. Additionally, there would need to be agreement between different federal and state agencies, resulting in changes in reporting mechanisms in the United States.

Develop exposure assessment methods for epidemiologic studies.

Most epidemiologic studies of work-related upper limb disorders suffer from inadequate exposure measures, thus, limiting both the strength of associations that can be demonstrated and the ability to generalize results. The lack of standardized, readily applicable methods for measuring occupational exposures remains a major impediment to etiologic studies. Simple, noninvasive, inexpensive accurate exposure assessment methods are needed, as are methods that can be used in diverse workplaces and exposures. It is necessary to develop a clearer idea of which combination of exposure conditions are most hazardous in order to develop better measurement tools for exposure.

Current exposure assessment methods represent a continuum between more expensive and accurate methods to less expensive and accurate methods. The most accurate direct measurement methods, such as electronic goniometers, may be useful for stereotypic jobs. This approach is costly for studies of nonstereotypic work or where only a few workers are performing each specific job. In these latter situations, investigators usually rely on a less accurate method, such as recording work exposures by observers in the workplace or the review of video recording of work. Another common method used when many workers are studied is the questionnaire. However, while workers can accurately describe whether they have or have not been "exposed," their ability to quantify the level of exposure is more limited. None of these methods address the problem that measurements of current working conditions may not accurately describe past working conditions, particularly if there have been changes. In some situations, the past exposure may be a more important causal factor than the current exposure. A better understanding of the precision and accuracy of the current available methods is needed from the most complex and expensive to the least complex and expensive. There is also a need for exposure assessment strategies that consider whether within-worker variability or between-worker variability represent the greatest source of exposure misclassification. It is likely that no single method will be the best for all studies. Simple methods for assessing exposures may not only assist research studies but also may have great utility in improving the assessment of exposure by occupational health professionals, supervisors, and workers engaged in ongoing efforts to reduce existing levels of exposure to recognized hazards.

Develop diagnostic tools for soft-tissue disorders of the upper limb.

As is often true in low back pain, the nature of tissue pathology in workers with upper limb pain commonly remains unknown. This is specifically true with regard to pain assumed to originate from muscles or tendons. The diagnosis of these disorders is often based on the symptom of local pain and on the ability of the health care provider to provoke pain by applying pressure to tissue or stretching the tissues. Some of the common physical findings have limited repeatability and perhaps validity. The validation has been difficult without a diagnostic gold standard and with an inadequate understanding of the underlying pathology. The pathophysiology and diagnosis of carpal tunnel syndrome are substantially clearer than many other work-related upper limit disorders.

Use of modern imaging methods, such as magnetic resonance imaging or ultrasound, may allow the pathology in typical clinical cases to be seen in the acute stage. Disorders under study should first be tendon-related, such as epicondylitis or peritendinitis. Cases could be compared to age- and gender-matched asymptomatic controls stratified perhaps on broad occupational categories, such as construction or office workers. Overstratification would reduce the study's ability to examine the role of occupational factors. Imaging could be used as the gold standard for investigating the validity of simpler and less expensive clinical tests for use in epidemiologic studies and medical surveillance activities. Different gold standards may be applicable for epidemiologic and clinical studies because epidemiologic studies of active workers will generally study less severe disorders.

Develop a prognosis for forearm signs and symptoms.

Although a number of soft-tissue disorders have been characterized (eg, epicondylitis, carpal tunnel syndrome), the prognosis of other work-related upper limb disorders have not. Many nonspecific symptoms are localized in the forearm. Some authors have emphasized the common nature of signs and symptoms in the forearm muscles and the lack of information on their natural course. In some cases, the symptoms are similar to those of a chronic compartment syndrome. If the prognosis for these forearm signs and for symptoms is substantial impairment of health, then additional research and prevention activities should focus on them.

Follow-up studies of cases should be conducted and grouped according to the nature and severity of symptoms and signs. The employment status and exposure of the cases should be ascertained throughout the follow-up. Change in levels of exposure as well as absence from work are potential factors in determining the natural history of these signs and symptoms.

Develop a standard nomenclature and assessment method for "work organization" factors and "psychosocial stressors," which can be integrated into epidemiologic studies.

There have been a number of studies associating both physical and work organizational factors to work-related upper limb disorders; however, it has been difficult to disentangle the exposures. "Monotonous" work, for example, may or may not be "repetitive" (eg, watching a monitor all day to detect errors versus watching a monitor and keying intensively on a keyboard). Because most studies that attempt to look at both psychosocial and physical stressors are cross-sectional, the direction of the association is not always clear. The extent to which work organization factors contributes to the development of musculoskeletal disorders has a direct bearing on prevention strategies in the workplace.

Longitudinal studies that measure the psychosocial and physical stressors (either retrospectively or prospectively) in large populations are required. The development, if feasible, of assessment methods for psychosocial occupational exposures that are more objective than the currently used method of worker questionnaire would be useful. Without these more objective methods, studies that compared the perceptions about the nature of occupational exposure of workers with symptoms to those without symptoms would be useful in determining whether workers with symptoms can objectively describe their psychosocial work environment. Each group of workers should have similar work environments.

Organizational intervention studies are necessary but difficult to conduct. They require sustained organizational support, which may be difficult to maintain, particularly in the context of external dynamic economic changes.

Evaluate the relationship among cognitive/attention demands, muscle activity, and pathophysiology in patients and controls with disorders associated with repetitive motion.

Laboratory studies have demonstrated an increase in static muscle loads with increases in attentional work demands. This has led to the hypothesis that mental tasks can increase muscle activity in the upper limb. These demands and their effects may be even more pronounced in the actual work environment than in the laboratory environment.

Although prospective studies are appealing, it may be more efficient to compare cognitive/attentional demands in case-control studies. Studies that measure the magnitude of, for example, trapezius muscle loads during exposure to known psychosocial stressors (eg, deadline work) would begin to test the pathways postulated by Sauter and Swanson in this section. Physical loads of the work would be an important confounder or effect modifier in these studies.

Evaluate the relationship between localized fatigue, discomfort, perceived exertion, and musculoskeletal disorders.

Despite widespread use in manual handling research, psychophysical methods of studying upper limb activities have only recently been explored. If these methods are useful predictors, guidelines for safe levels of exposure could be set, which would prevent development of upper limb disorders. If valid predictors, psychophysical methods may be useful because they may require fewer resources than epidemiologic studies with their extensive assessment of exposures and health outcomes.

Although laboratory studies indicate that psychophysically derived limits are consistent and reproducible, they have not been used extensively in field studies as predictors of adverse health outcomes. A comparison of different exposure assessments methods (psychophysical, biomechanical, physiological) in epidemiologic studies will shed light on the utility of this method of exposure assessment. Psychophysical methods in particular may underestimate the effects of infrequent high-peak demand activities that have been associated with upper extremity tendon disorders in some epidemiologic studies. A less ambitious approach would consist of smaller worksite studies in which job changes, based on psychophysical limits, would be evaluated with simple outcome measures such as body part discomfort and perceived exertion scores. The problem with this approach is that both exposure limits and response measures are based on subjective perceptions.

Overall, there are many opportunities to improve the ability of epidemiologic studies to contribute knowledge that can be used to design effective preventive strategies.

Section 2

Pathophysiology: Biomechanical Loads

Section Editor:
Kai-Nan An, PhD

Kai-Nan An, PhD
Thomas J. Armstrong, PhD
Louis U. Bigliani, MD
William P. Cooney III, MD
Evan L. Flatow, MD
Benjamin M. Hillberry, PhD
Peter J. Keir, BSc
Rajeev Kelkar, MS
Wendi A. Latko, ME

Anne E. Moore, MSc, PEng
Bernard F. Morrey, MD
Van C. Mow, PhD
Roger G. Pollock, MD
David Rempel, MD
Richard P. Wells, MEng, PhD
Savio L-Y Woo, PhD
John W. Xerogeanes, MD

Overview

Activity-related musculoskeletal disorders have complex multifactorial etiology, including not only the physical aspects of activity that people perform but also the psychosocial factors. These disorders may involve muscular, tendinous, ligamentous, and nervous tissues and onset may be either acute (overexertion) or chronic (overuse). The focus of this section is to document the models of the musculoskeletal system, the loads tissues bear during function compared to tissue tolerance or failure data, and the use of these models to help document the exposure of people to physical stressors during work, leisure, sports, and the activities of daily living. Figure 1 illustrates the presumed relationship between activity and potential musculoskeletal disorders. These relationships have been most studied in work and sport settings; however, activities of daily living have received some attention.

Activity-related musculoskeletal disorders represent a significant burden to the individuals concerned and to health care and workers' compensation schemes. In jurisdictions in North America "sprains and strains" are typically the largest category of claims in workers' compensation schemes, representing over half of claims and dollar costs. Disorders of the upper limb and low back disorders are usually both well represented in this total.

A number of sources of information, ranging from biomechanics, epidemiology, and clinical case series, have identified a number of major extrinsic (external) risk factors associated with the development of musculoskeletal disorders. These include forcefulness, adverse posture, repetition or continuous activity, and duration of exposure. In addition, there are a number of potentiating factors that are commonly mentioned, including cold, vibration, and use of gloves.

For work exposures there are ample and consistent findings that a variety of localized musculoskeletal symptoms and clinically identifiable conditions are associated with work. Force, whether recorded as a hand grip force or as a muscle activation relative to a maximal effort, has been found to be related to musculoskeletal disorders. Repetitiveness is a commonly identified risk factor but one that is frequently poorly defined; qualitatively, it has connotations of

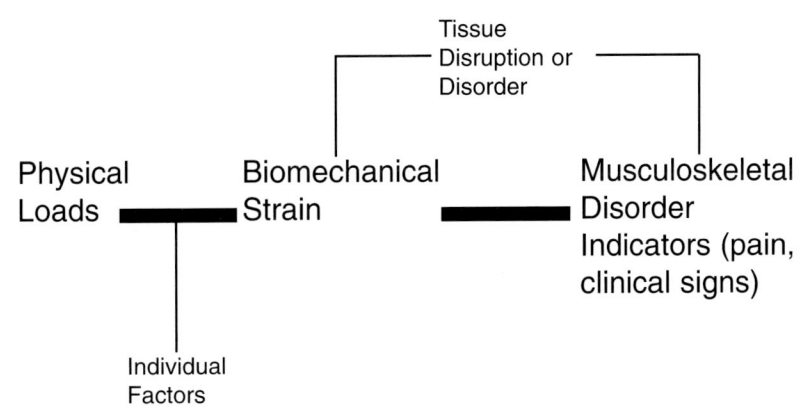

Fig. 1 Presumed relationship between activity and potential musculoskeletal disorders.

the same work elements repeated many times. Despite this imprecision, repetition has been found to be related to the development of musculoskeletal disorders. Posture has been found to be a consistently strong risk factor for injury in the upper limb, especially for the shoulder.

Biomechanical models, in the context of this section, have been used to describe the motions of, and forces acting on, the limb segments, including joint motion during function using rigid body models. For example, through the use of external forces and limb accelerations, moments of force at the elbow during pitching can be predicted. In addition, through the incorporation of the biologic materials properties, the response of the tissue to load can be grossly predicted. The models available to study activity-related musculoskeletal disorders are in preliminary stages of development; we are not sure of the mechanisms of injury. This is complicated by a lack of a good animal model of these disorders and the delicate balance of physical strain and restorative responses. Models are only as good as their parameters; we are developing a better database of quantitative anatomy (shapes of joint surfaces, sizes of muscles, geometry of the carpal canal) as well as properties of the various tissues. These data are frequently collected in the laboratory under conditions not representative of sport or work (eg, low strain rate, acute [minutes or hours] exposures). The biofidelity of the models available, therefore, remains to be shown for the study of activity-related musculoskeletal disorders. An example from the spine modeling area is instructive. Until recently, the estimates of the compression forces on the disks of the lower back during strenuous tasks routinely exceeded the measured compression strength of lumbar motion segments (disk plus vertebrae). Efforts to better capture the complex functional anatomy of the lumbar spine coupled with measures of maximum strength of lumbar motion segments under physiologic conditions have reduced or eliminated this uncomfortable state of affairs. The upper limb is certainly as complex a problem and points to the highest possible attention being paid to modeling efforts.

Modeling is not the only approach to investigate these phenomena. It may be possible to directly measure potentially injurious responses under field conditions. Carpal tunnel pressure measured via an implanted flexible catheter is one such variable that shows promise for a class of nerve compression disorders at the wrist; elevated pressure has been shown to lead to nerve disorders. Alternatively, a technique directly utilizing the perceptions of people (psychophysics) may be used. This technique is widely used in psychology and has seen some success in mapping the perceptions of people to manual materials handling as well as proposing limits for industrial tasks. This approach is currently being expanded to the upper limb.

Biomechanical models of the upper limb can provide the link between the physical activities that people do and the disorders they acquire. Because the upper limb is a multi-link chain with a very large number of degrees of freedom, without a conceptual model to provide guidance, it becomes difficult to relate a description of the activity to musculoskeletal disorders. For example, in the depiction of manual material handling tasks to elucidate the link between work and low back pain, one could describe the load lifted by a person and the distance away from the body of this mass. It has been found more useful to compute the joint moment (the product of the force and the distance). This is done based on a biomechanical model, which demonstrates that tissue loads are better reflected by moment than either load or posture separately.

In a similar manner, finger force exerted on a piano keyboard along with the position of the fingers can be used to estimate finger joint loading and thus preferred positions. Alternatively, quantitative modeling of the acromion/

supraspinatus interaction can help explain the epidemiologically documented link between shoulder posture and shoulder disorders.

Although modeling is not the only method by which the relationships between activity and musculoskeletal disorders can be studied, modeling appears to possess a number of strengths to recommend it. Models help us understand the many simultaneous and interacting physical stressors that act on the upper limb during activity. If based on sound anatomy and solid pathophysiology, such models may form a bridge between the performance of work and sport and the cellular or other descriptions of the degenerative/inflammatory processes involved in activity-related musculoskeletal disorders.

Chapter 6

Physical Stressors: Their Characterization, Assessment, and Relationship With Physical Work Requirements

Thomas J. Armstrong, PhD
Wendi A. Latko, ME

Introduction

Work-related musculoskeletal disorders are a major cause of worker impairment, disability, and compensation in many hand-intensive occupations. The pathogenesis of these disorders is not fully understood, but it appears to involve exposure to certain external physical stressors, such as repetitive exertions and awkward postures. It has been proposed that these external stressors produce a series of internal biomechanical and physiologic disturbances (Fig. 1).[1] Physical stressors are related to work requirements, such as production standards and work equipment, and to individual factors, such as body size and capacity. Physical stressors, their measurement and their relationship with work requirements, will be presented in this chapter. Although work requirements may have physical and psychological components, this chapter focuses only on their physical aspects.

Measurement of Physical Stressors

Physical stressors include repetitive and sustained exertions, forces, posture stresses, work duration, contact stresses, vibration, and low temperatures. Methods for measuring physical stressors have not yet been standardized; however, they draw on several standard methods, including observation, direct measurement, calculation, electromyography (EMG), goniometry, and psychophysics. The stressors, measurement techniques, and causal factors are listed in Table 1. The suitability of each method depends on the stressor and work situation under consideration, the desired accuracy and precision, and the available resources.

Repetition

Repetition refers to the temporal aspect of work. Some investigators have characterized repetition in terms of the number of exertions per unit time or frequency.[2-6] An exertion is defined as the contraction of a muscle to produce force or movement.

Other investigators have characterized repetition as the number of parts produced per unit time or cycle time.[7-13] A cycle is defined as a sequence of ex-

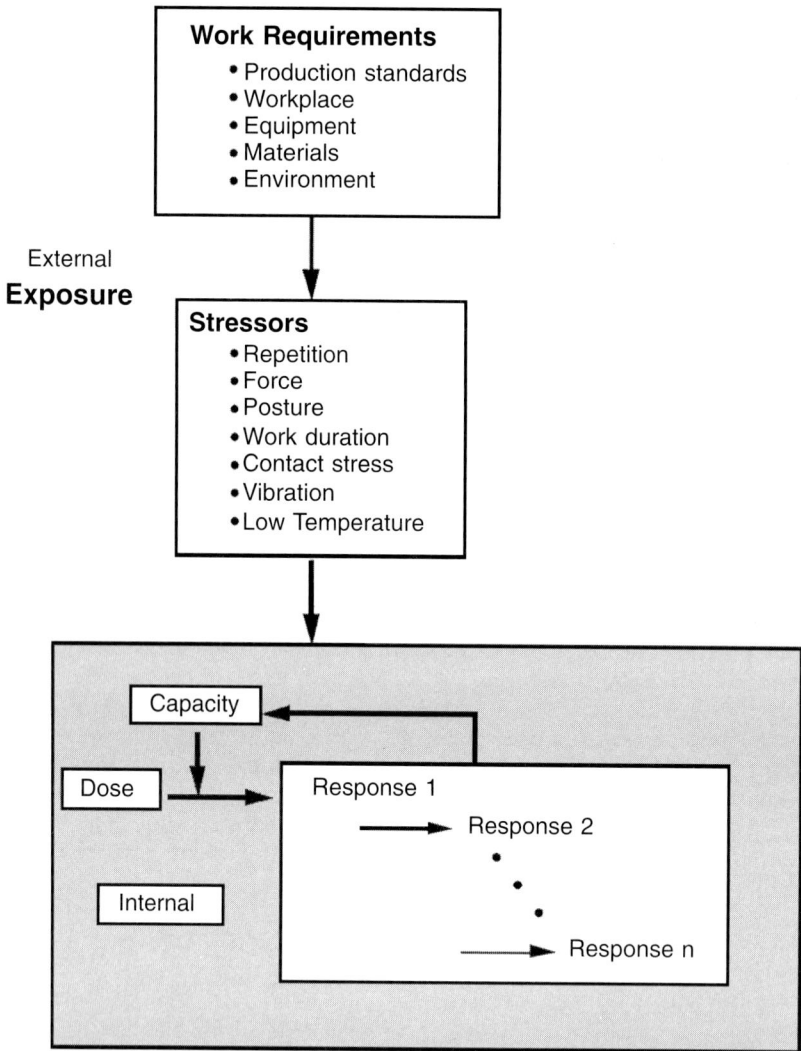

Fig. 1 Work requirements expose workers to physical stressors that lead to a series of cascading dose-response events. (Adapted with permission from Armstrong TJ, Buckle P, Fine LJ, et al: A conceptual model for work-related neck and upper-limb musculoskeletal disorders. *Scand J Work Environ Health* 1993;19:73–84.)

ertions or movements. One or more cycles is typically required to complete work on a part. Thus, for repetitive jobs, the number of exertions per unit time, the cycle time and the parts per unit time are all related. In some cases, they may be the same.

Exertions per unit time, work quantities per unit time, and cycle times may or may not be directly comparable. For example, 12,000 keystrokes/h (33.3 words/min) is considerably higher than 1,200 keystrokes/h (3.3 words/min). If the operators can remove their hands from the keyboard and relax when not

Table 1 Key attributes, methods of assessment, and causal factors of specific physical stressors

Stressor and Attributes	Assessment Methods	Factors
Repetition		
Exertion frequency	Observations	Production standard
Recovery time	Time study	Pacing
Percent recovery	Work sampling	Incentives
Cycle time	Interviews (workers, supervisors)	Work quantities per unit time
Velocity & acceleration	Rankings/ratings	Methods
Force	EMG	Work incentives
Posture	Force measurements	Worker rotation
	Goniometers	Manufacturing process
	Accelerometers	Mechanical aids
	Keystroke counts	Quality control
Duration		
Hours	Interviews (workers, supervisors)	Work schedules
Days	Time cards	Work standards
Percent time	Production records	Incentives
Force		
Peak	Observations	Friction
Average	Interviews (workers, supervisors)	Weight of work objects
Amplitude probability	Rankings/ratings	Balance
distribution	EMG	Reaction forces/torques
	Force transducers	Drag forces
		Mechanical aids
		Gloves
		Handles
		Quality control
Posture		
Range of motion	Observations	Work location
Average	Interviews (workers, supervisors)	Work orientation
Time position	Rankings/ratings	Work object shape
	Goniometers	
	Work equipment specifications	
Contact stress		
Force	Observations	Force factors
Area	Interviews (workers, supervisors)	Area of contact
Location	Rankings/ratings	Location of contact
Duration	Force measurements	Gloves
	Work equipment specifications	
Vibration		
Frequency	Observations	Tool drive train
Displacement	Interviews (workers, supervisors)	Bit condition
Velocity	Rankings/ratings	Abrasive
Acceleration	Work equipment specifications	Isolation/dampening
Duration		Gloves
Low Temperature		
Temperature	Observations	Temperature of air
Conductivity	Interviews (workers, supervisors)	Work objects
Duration	Rankings/ratings	Air exhaust
	Thermometers	Gloves

keying, then 1,200 keys/min would be much less stressful than 12,000 keys/min. If the operators must keep their hands positioned over the keys while waiting for information or for the computer to respond, then there may not be recovery between successive keystrokes and a lower keystroke rate may be as stressful as a higher rate.

Characterization of repetition in terms of exertion frequency is also affected by the kind of work under consideration. For example, keyboard work entails brief exertions of the fingers to activate the keys, whereas manufacturing work involves longer exertions of the hands and wrists to transfer and assemble parts. Manufacturing work may involve further differences, depending on the sizes and locations of the work objects. Work measurement procedures utilize performance ratings to characterize these differences.[14,15] The rating is based on the speed of the movements, the frequency and duration of voluntary pauses, and standardized performance norms.

Force

Assessment of repetition requires information about force. When investigators count exertions or cycle times, there is an assumption that they are separated by a rest pause. In some cases this pause can be seen; for example, a worker may put a part in a machine, activate the controls, and then wait for the machine to cycle. In other cases, the pause is not so obvious; for example, a worker drives screws in parts on a passing assembly line and waits for the next part, but holds the tool while waiting.

In some cases, the magnitude of the force can be estimated from the weight and friction of the work object.[16] The hand must apply enough contact force to produce enough friction to overcome gravity, drag, or reaction forces on the work object. In the case of holding a suitcase, the required finger force will be equal to the weight of the suitcase. In the case of holding a file folder against gravity, the required force can be computed as the weight divided by two times the coefficient of friction.[17] For other tasks, such as swinging a hammer or picking up an irregularly shaped part, there may not be a straightforward way of computing the force. In practice, most workers usually exert more than the minimum required force. Johansson and Westling[18] refer to this as the "safety margin."

Another way of assessing exertions is with recordings of muscle electric patterns, or electromyograms (EMGs).[19] Lundervold[20] used EMGs to examine the relationship between forearm, arm, shoulder, and trunk muscle contractions in typing. This work led to important conclusions about how the work load in keyboard tasks is affected by worker, work station, task, and environmental parameters. Armstrong and associates[21] described a system for recording work, postures, and EMGs using motion pictures. This system was later used to assess force patterns in sewing and meat processing jobs.[4,22] Radwin and associates[23] used surface EMG recordings to study muscle responses to torque reaction forces of power tools used to drive threaded fasteners.

Jonsson[24] proposed a technique for characterizing task force requirements using amplitude probability distributions of the surface EMGs. He proposed normalizing EMGs as a fraction of maximum and then summarizing the recordings from a given worker performing a given task as a cumulative frequency histogram. The fraction of time an individual muscle group is working above a given relative force then could be determined. A limitation of amplitude probability distributions is that they do not indicate the duration of exertions; that is, it is not possible to distinguish between a work regime in which a worker alternates between 1-second work and 1-second recovery or one that entails 1-minute work and 1-minute recovery. For example, a keyboard task that entails one 0.3-sec exertion to press a key every second could have an amplitude frequency distribution which is similar to that for a packing task which requires one 3-second exertion every 10 seconds. Linderhed[25] proposed adding the duration of exertion to the amplitude probability distribution. It then would be possible to determine whether exertions at a given level are short enough to avoid excessive physiological or biomechanical disturbances or whether periods between exertions are long enough for recovery. Linderhed's method could be expanded to include other stressors, such as contact stresses, posture, vibration, and low temperature, in addition to force and frequency. Although it is not yet possible to determine risk based on force and frequency profiles, these are important tools for characterizing exposure in epidemiological studies.

Armstrong and associates[26] used psychophysics to assess the force required to use hand tools in automobile assembly. Subjects were asked to rate force on a scale of zero to ten, where zero was "too light," five was "just right," and ten was "too heavy." There was a clear demarcation between tools with a mass of less than 1.5 kg, which were generally "just right," and tools with a mass greater than 2.5 kg, which were generally "too heavy." Additional studies are needed to calibrate measures of perceived exertion and their association with injury risk.

In some cases, forces can be measured directly or indirectly with force gauges. Armstrong and associates[27] used force gauges to measure keyboard reaction forces in keyboard work. This arrangement was satisfactory for comparing keyboards with different key activation forces, but could not be used for high-fidelity dynamic finger force measurements. Flexibility of the keyboard causes high-frequency force components to be attenuated and low-frequency components to be amplified. Rempel and associates[28] overcame this problem by placing strain gauges in the caps of the keys. Other investigators have attempted to mount force gauges on the tips of the fingers.[29] It appears that these devices may be used where the finger is exerted against a flat surface, but problems may be encountered in manipulating of objects of different sizes and shapes. Also, placement of materials such as gloves between the finger and work objects is likely to affect the force exerted by the worker.[30]

Direct force, EMG, and psychophysical measurements only provide information about the level of muscle activity. Studies of fatigue suggest that muscle movement also is an important exertion stress parameter (See Chapter 20 by Fridén and Lieber). Exertions are classified as static, concentric (shortening), or eccentric (lengthening). Static exertions are required to maintain body position and to hold tools and work objects. Concentric exertions are required when the hand moves or closes against an external load; examples are lifting, cutting, and squeezing. Eccentric exertions are required when the body resists movement of an external load; examples are lowering work objects and resisting the torque reactions of power tools as they start and stop. Antagonistic muscle groups may alternate between eccentric and concentric work; examples can be seen in the finger flexor and extensor muscles in keyboard work.

Several systems have been proposed for characterizing repetition in terms of movements. Drury[31] proposed a system in which repetition was characterized by counting wrist excursions from neutral. Wrist postures were determined from videotapes of workers performing their jobs. A similar technique was adopted by Higgs and associates[6] to characterize repetition in a study of upper extremity impairment. Marras and Schoenmarklin[32] characterized repetition strictly in terms of the velocity and acceleration of wrist movements. Wrist movements were recorded from an electromechanical goniometer attached to workers' wrists while they performed their jobs. They concluded that wrist acceleration was the most important factor in Occupational Safety and Health Administration (OSHA) reportable cumulative trauma disorders, but acknowledged that acceleration was a factor of force.

Posture Stresses

In addition to velocity and acceleration, posture is an important problem in its own right. As early as 1713, Ramazzini[33] talked about "unnatural posture" and "perpetual movement of the hand in the same manner." Gray[34] referred to "close ringing" motions. Performing detailed observations in a case-controlled study of 90 workers using keyboards, Duncan and Ferguson[35] found that shoulder depression, shoulder flexion, shoulder abduction, ulnar wrist deviation and wrist extension were related to occupational myalgia. Corlett and associates[36] proposed a method for characterizing posture in which the joint ranges of motion were divided into zones. The average zone of each joint could then be estimated from observations of a worker performing a given task. Building on the work of Bishop and associates, Armstrong and associates[21] proposed estimating shoulder elbow and wrist angles from successive frames of motion pictures made of workers as they performed their jobs. Overall hand posture was characterized by indicating the fingers involved in a pinch, press, or power grip.[4,37] Armstrong[38] used plots of these data to characterize upper limb postures and to identify stressful postures of poultry processors, which was useful during the redesign of their knives.

A number of investigators have proposed using electromechanical goniometers for real time posture recordings.[39–43] Theoretically, an electrogoniometer enables investigators to identify stressful postures and provides several options for characterizing static and dynamic posture attributes. Radwin and Lin[44] proposed using a power spectral analysis to characterize posture. They found that peak spectral magnitudes and frequency components corresponded closely with joint displacement amplitudes and repetition rates. Although investigators have considered the theoretical bases of how goniometers work, there are no published studies demonstrating the accuracy and precision of these devices with respect to known postures or other measurement devices. Preliminary investigations suggest that accuracy may be degraded for some upper limb positions and that there may be interference between channels when movement occurs about various joint axes. Further studies are necessary to determine the operating limitations of these systems.

Armstrong and associates[26] utilized psychophysics to assess postures associated with using hand tools. Workers were simply asked to rate the posture on a scale of zero to ten, where 0 was easiest imaginable and ten was hardest imaginable. Ulin and associates[45] compared visual analog scales with the 10-point Borg scale to assess postures of persons driving threaded fasteners at heights ranging from 40 cm to 190 cm. Although no practical differences were found between the scales, under laboratory conditions, subjects seemed to prefer the Borg scale.

Work Duration and Contact Stress

Work duration can be expressed in terms of hours per day or in some cases percent of shift devoted to a particular task.[8,46–49] Information about work duration can be obtained from production records and interviews with workers and supervisors.

Contact stress is defined as force divided by area of contact or as a pressure. In some cases contact stress can be calculated from force and area measurements. In a recent laboratory study of pain-pressure thresholds of all areas of the hand, Fransson-Hall and Kilbom[50] calculated pressures using force measurements and knowledge of the area of contact. Lundborg and associates[51] investigated the relationship between pressure on the palmar side of the wrist and intracarpal canal pressure. Pressure was measured inside the wrist with a catheter and pressure transducer; pressure on base of the palm was measured simply as the force applied to a known area. Once the relationship between palmar wrist pressure and intracarpal canal pressure was determined, force was applied to the base of the palm to study the effect of intracarpal pressures on median nerve function. Quantitative contact stress measurements are seldom possible in most field settings. Contact stress is usually characterized as a yes or no categorical variable. In some cases it is characterized in terms of worker comfort patterns.[52,53] Workers are asked to point at areas of discomfort on their hands or to shade in areas of discomfort on a drawing of a hand.

Vibration and Low Temperatures

Environmental stressors include vibration and low temperatures. Vibration may act directly on tissues to produce injury or it may affect the force and posture used to handle work objects.[13,54–56] Vibration is a vector quantity with properties of frequency, displacement, velocity, and acceleration. Quantitative vibration measurements require tri-axial accelerometers, amplifiers, and frequency analyzers. As a practical matter, such measurements are not feasible and vibration may be indicated categorically as yes or no or as hours of exposure.[13,57,58]

It is not known whether low temperature affects tissue tolerance to mechanical stressors, but it does affect sensory and motor performance.[59–65] Temperature exposure measurements are assessed from the temperature of ambient air and from the temperature of work objects. The measurements may be influenced by the insulative value of clothing, thermal conductivity of work objects, and air exhaust from hand tools.

Physical Stressors and Work Requirements

Exposure to physical stressors—repetitive exertions, forces, posture stresses, work duration, contact stresses, vibration, and low temperatures—are related to work requirements, individual factors, and environmental factors (Table 1). Work requirements include work standards, work processes, workplace layout, tools, equipment, and materials. Individual factors include the worker's abilities, skills, size, and fitness. Environmental factors include vibration and ambient air temperatures.

Work requirements specify the quantity and quality of work to be performed in a given period of time.[15] They also specify the method, tools, and workstation that are to be used to attain the standard. Consequently, the standard is an important determinant of how many exertions a worker will perform in a given amount of time; how much recovery time will be available; how much force a worker will have to exert to hold and use work objects; where a worker will have to reach; how long a worker will hold a vibrating tool, control, or work object; how long a worker will hold a cold object; and how long a worker will spend in a cold environment.

The standard may include work incentives that reward workers for exceeding the production standards. Rewards may be given to individuals or to groups of workers or teams. In the latter case, individuals are subjected to group pressures as well as individual financial pressures to attain high production rates and repetition. Incentives also encourage workers to handle larger loads than they might without the incentive. Finally, incentives may discourage workers from taking the time to properly adjust and maintain their work stations and equipment.

The load pattern on a given joint and muscle group will vary from one job to another. Many employers now routinely rotate workers between different jobs to avoid exceeding the capacity of any one joint or muscle group.[24] Rotations require additional worker training and may expose additional workers to excessive stressors. Additional research is required to determine optimal rotation schedules.

Seven- to 8-hour work shifts and 5-day work weeks are normal in the United States; however, 10- and 12-hour work shifts and 6-day work weeks are not unusual. Long shifts and long work weeks increase worker exposures to physical stressors. They also reduce the amount of recovery time between shifts. Work schedules are generally driven by production demands and the cost of hiring additional workers versus the cost of overtime by existing workers. Additional data are needed so that employers can include the human cost of overtime in such decisions.

Some work processes and employers permit workers to work ahead of schedule and to achieve their work standard before the end of the shift. Working ahead may increase the frequency of exertion and reduce recovery time between exertions. In addition, workers may exert additional force to handle larger quantities of materials at a time. They may also assume more stressful postures to reach ahead of the production line. Additional research is needed to determine whether the possible adverse effects of increased repetition are offset by the shortened shift.

Work methods are affected by manufacturing processes and product designs. For example, attaching parts with adhesive requires fewer exertions than would be required for threaded fasteners. Consequently, a part could be attached with adhesives with less repetition than if it were attached with screws. Also, the use of adhesives would eliminate exposure to posture and vibration stresses from the power tool. Process modifications that reduce required exertions sometimes increase the production standard so that there is no net reduction of repetition. Manufacturing processes also affect exposure to other stressors.

The quality of work materials affects how many exertions are required to meet the standard. In a finishing operation, parts that do not meet quality specifications may require additional exertions to inspect and remove the excess material. Additional force may be required to cut or file away excess material. In an assembly operation, substandard parts may not fit properly and may require additional motions to reject or additional force to make them fit.

Repetition and force are also affected by maintenance of equipment. Dull cutters will require more force and motions than sharp cutters. Similarly, worn bits will require more force to engage a fastener than a well-maintained bit.[66]

The specification of work equipment and the work station determines worker posture. For example, assembly of a part on the underside of a suspended vehicle overhead will require that the hands remain above the worker's head. If the vehicle is positioned on its side, the worker can face the vehicle and work with the elbows at the sides of the body. The posture may also be affected by worker size.[67] A short worker will have to reach higher than a tall worker for a work object at a fixed location; however, if the work object is held in one hand while it is worked on with the other hand, posture will not be affected. Employers can exercise some control over posture by making work locations adjustable and providing workers with adjustable seating.

Physical stressors can be increased or decreased in some cases by worker behavior. Worker skill affects how many exertions are required to complete some jobs. It may also influence force of exertion and posture. Skills training may help to reduce exposure to these stressors in certain tasks, such as typing. Methods such as biofeedback may be helpful in some aspects of worker training. Workers can be taught how to arrange their work and adjust their work station to minimize posture stresses and needless exertion of force. They also can be trained in how to select the best tools and how to use them most efficiently.

Summary

Exposure to certain physical stressors, such as repetitive and forceful exertions, posture stresses, contact stresses, vibration, and low temperature appear to be related to the development of work-related musculoskeletal disorders. These physical stressors are directly related to the physical work requirements of the job. Physical work requirements of a job include work rate, methods, equipment, and work objects, and thus specify what workers do and how they do it. In specifying these aspects of a worker's job, physical work requirements in part determine the level at which the worker is exposed to the above physical stressors.

Although methods for quantifying exposure to physical stressors have not been standardized, many useful methods have been adapted from existing methods of job analysis and physiologic measurement. Observation, direct measurement, calculation, EMG, goniometry, and psychophysics are all used to quantify exposure to the various stressors. The choice of which method to apply in a given situation depends on the particular characteristics of the workplace and job under consideration, the available resources, and the level of precision required.

Further research is needed to develop standard methods of quantifying exposure that can be applied in a wide variety of industries and occupations. In addition, although the above physical stressors appear to be related to the pathogenesis of these disorders, more epidemiologic studies are necessary to establish a dose-response relationship between the physical stressors and medical outcomes that can be used to specify acceptable work designs.

References

1. Armstrong TJ, Buckle P, Fine LJ, et al: A conceptual model for work-related neck and upper-limb musculoskeletal disorders. *Scand J Work Environ Health* 1993;19: 73–84.
2. Obolenskaja AJ, Goljanitzki JA: Die seröse tendovaginitis in der klinik und im experiment. *Dtsch z Chir* 1927;201:388–399.
3. Hammer AW: Tenosynovitis. *Med Record* 1934;140:353–355.
4. Armstrong TJ, Foulke JA, Joseph BS, et al: Investigation of cumulative trauma disorders in a poultry processing plant. *Am Indust Hygiene Assoc J* 1982;43:103–116.

5. Barnhart S, Demers PA, Miller M, et al: Carpal tunnel syndrome among ski manufacturing workers. *Scand J Work Environ Health* 1991;17:46–52.
6. Higgs P, Young VL, Seaton M, et al: Upper extremity impairment in workers performing repetitive tasks. *Plast Reconstr Surg* 1992;90:614–620.
7. Kuorinka I, Koskinen P: Occupational rheumatic diseases and upper limb strain in manual jobs in a light mechanical industry. *Scand J Work Environ Health* 1979;5(suppl 3):39–47.
8. Hunting W, Grandjean E, Maeda K: Constrained postures in accounting machine operators. *Appl Ergonomics* 1980;11:145–149.
9. Luopajarvi T, Kuorinka I, Virolainen M, et al: Prevalence of tenosynovitis and other injuries of the upper extremities in repetitive work. *Scand J Work Environ Health* 1979;5(suppl 3):48–55.
10. Punnett L, Keyserling WM: Exposure to ergonomic stressors in the garment industry: Application and critique of job-site work analysis methods. *Ergonomics* 1987;30:1099–1116.
11. Silverstein BA, Fine LJ, Armstrong TJ: Occupational factors and carpal tunnel syndrome. *Am J Indust Med* 1987;11:343–358.
12. Armstrong TJ, Fine LJ, Goldstein SA, et al: Ergonomics considerations in hand and wrist tendinitis. *J Hand Surg* 1987;12A:830–837.
13. Armstrong TJ, Fine LJ, Radwin RG, et al: Ergonomics and the effects of vibration in hand-intensive work. *Scand J Work Environ Health* 1987;13:286–289.
14. Barnes RM (ed): *Motion and Time Study: Design and Measurement of Work*, ed 7. New York, NY, John Wiley & Sons, 1980.
15. Niebel BW: *Motion and Time Study*, ed 8. Homewood, IL, RD Irwin Publishers, 1988.
16. Armstrong TJ: Mechanical considerations of skin in work. *Am J Indust Med* 1985;8:463–472.
17. Buchholz B, Frederick LJ, Armstrong TJ: An investigation of human palmar skin friction and the effects of materials, pinch force and moisture. *Ergonomics* 1988;31:317–325.
18. Johansson RS, Westling G: Roles of glabrous skin receptors and sensorimotor memory in automatic control of precision grip when lifting rougher or more slippery objects. *Exper Brain Res* 1984;56:550–564.
19. Basmajian JV, De Luca CJ (eds): *Muscles Alive: Their Functions Revealed by Electromyography*, ed 5. Baltimore, MD, Williams & Wilkins, 1985.
20. Lundervold A: Electromyographic investigations during typewriting. *Ergonomics* 1958;1:226–233.
21. Armstrong TJ, Chaffin DB, Foulke JA: A methodology for documenting hand positions and forces during manual work. *J Biomech* 1979;12:131–133.
22. Armstrong TJ, Chaffin DB: Carpal tunnel syndrome and selected personal attributes. *J Occup Med* 1979;21:481–486.
23. Radwin RG, Armstrong TJ, Vanbergeijk E: Vibration exposure for selected power hand tools used in automobile assembly. *Am Indust Hygiene Assoc J* 1990;51:510–518.
24. Jonsson B: The static load component in muscle work. *Eur J Appl Physiol* 1988;57:305–310.
25. Linderhed H: A new dimension to amplitude analysis of EMG. *Int J Indust Ergon* 1993;11:243–247.
26. Armstrong TJ, Punnett L, Ketner P: Subjective worker assessments of hand tools used in automobile assembly. *Am Indust Hygiene Assoc J* 1989;50:639–645.
27. Armstrong TJ, Foulke JA, Martin BJ, et al: Investigation of applied forces in alphanumeric keyboard Work. *Am Ind Hyg Assoc J* 1994;55:30–35.
28. Rempel D, Klinenberg E, Serina E, et al: Finger force during computer keyboard work: Part II. Relation of keyswitch make force to applied force and surface EMG. *Proceedings of the 12th Triennial Congress of the International Ergonomics Association*. Toronto, Canada, Human Factors Association of Canada, 1994, vol 2, pp 201–203.

29. Dario P, De Rossi D: Tactile sensors and the gripping challenge. *IEEE Spectrum* 1985;Aug:46–52.
30. Hertzberg HTE: Some contributions of applied physical anthropology to human engineering. *Ann NY Acad Sci* 1955;63:616–636.
31. Drury CG: A biomechanical evaluation of the repetitive motion injury potential of industrial jobs. *Seminars in Occupational Medicine* 1987;2:41–49.
32. Marras WS, Schoenmarklin RW: Wrist motions in industry. *Ergonomics* 1993;36:341–351.
33. Ramazzini B: *De Morbis Artificum Bernardini Ramazzini Dietriba*. Chicago, Illinois, The University of Chicago Press, 1940.
34. Gray H: *Anatomy, Descriptive and Surgical*, ed 13. Philadelphia, PA, Lea Brothers & Co, 1893.
35. Duncan J, Ferguson D: Keyboard operating posture and symptoms in operating. *Ergonomics* 1974;17:651–662.
36. Corlett EN, Madeley SJ, Manenica I: Posture targeting: A technique for recording working posture. *Ergonomics* 1979;22:357–366.
37. Chao EY, Opgrande JD, Axmear FE: Three-dimensional force analysis of finger joints in selected isometric hand functions. *J Biomech* 1976;9:387–396.
38. Armstrong TJ: Development of a biomechanical hand model for study of manual activities, in Easterby R, Kroemer KHE, Chaffin DB (eds): *Anthropometry and Biomechanics: Theory and Application*. New York, NY, Plenum Press, 1982, pp 183–192.
39. Chao EY, An KN, Askew LJ, et al: Electrogoniometer for the measurement of human elbow joint rotation. *J Biomech Eng* 1980;102:301–310.
40. Chao EYS: Justification of triaxial goniometer for the measurement of joint rotation. *J Biomech* 1980;13:989–1006.
41. Palmer AK, Werner FW, Murphy D, et al: Functional wrist motion: A biomechanical study. *J Hand Surg* 1985;10A:39–46.
42. Ojima H, Miyake S, Kumashiro M, et al: Dynamic analysis of wrist circumduction: A new application of the biaxial flexible electrogoniometer. *Clin Biomech* 1991;6:221–229.
43. Moore A, Wells R, Ranney D: Quantifying exposure in occupational manual tasks with cumulative trauma disorder potential. *Ergonomics* 1991;34:1433–1453.
44. Radwin RG, Lin ML: An analytical method for characterizing repetitive motion and postural stress using spectral analysis. *Ergonomics* 1993;36:379–389.
45. Ulin SS, Ways CM, Armstrong TJ, et al: Perceived exertion and discomfort versus work height with a pistol-shaped screwdriver. *Am Indust Hyg Assoc J* 1990;51:588–594.
46. Oxenburgh M: Musculoskeletal injuries occurring in word processor operators, in Adams AS, Stevenson MG: *Ergonomics and Technological Change: Proceedings of the 21st Annual Conference of the Ergonomics Society of Australia and New Zealand*. Parkville, Victoria, Ergonomics Society of Australia and New Zealand, 1984, pp 137–143.
47. Margolis W, Kraus JF: The prevalence of carpal tunnel syndrome symptoms in female supermarket checkers. *J Occup Med* 1987;29:953–956.
48. MacDonald G, Robertson M, Erickson J: Carpal tunnel syndrome among California dental hygienists. *Dental Hyg* 1988;62:322–327.
49. Waersted M, Westgaard RH: Working hours as a risk factor in the development of musculoskeletal complaints. *Ergonomics* 1991;34:265–276.
50. Fransson-Hall C, Kilbom A: Sensitivity of the hand to surface pressure. *Applied Ergonomics* 1993;24:181–189.
51. Lundborg G, Gelberman RH, Minteer-Convery M, et al: Median nerve compression in the carpal tunnel: Functional response to experimentally induced controlled pressure. *J Hand Surg* 1982;7A:252–259.
52. Karlqvist L, Bjorksten MG: Design for prevention of work-related musculoskeletal disorders, in Bullock MI (ed): *Ergonomics: The Physiotherapist in the Workplace*. Edinburgh, Scotland, Churchill Livingstone, 1990, pp 149–181.

53. Tannen KJ, Stetson DS, Silverstein BA, et al: An evaluation of scissors for control of upper extremity disorders in an automobile upholstery plant, in Karwowski W (ed): *Trends in Ergonomics/Human Factors III*. Amsterdam, The Netherlands, North Holland Publishers, 1986, pp 631–639.
54. Brammer AJ, Pyykko I: Vibration-induced neuropathy: Detection by nerve conduction measurements. *Scand J Work Environ Health* 1987;13:317–322.
55. Lundborg G, Dahlin LB, Danielsen N, et al: Intraneural edema following exposure to vibration. *Scand J Work Environ Health* 1987;13:326–329.
56. Radwin RG, Armstrong TJ, Chaffin DB: Power hand tool vibration effects on grip exertions. *Ergonomics* 1987;30:833–855.
57. Rothfleisch S, Sherman D: Carpal tunnel syndrome: Biomechanical aspects of occupational occurrence and implications regarding surgical management. *Orthop Rev* 1978;7:107–109.
58. Cannon LJ, Bernacki EJ, Walter SD: Personal and occupational factors associated with carpal tunnel syndrome. *J Occup Med* 1981;23:255–258.
59. Provins KA, Morton R: Tactile discrimination and skin temperature. *J Appl Physiol* 1960;15:155–160.
60. Green BG: The effect of skin temperature on vibrotactile sensitivity. *Percept Psychophys* 1977;21:243–248.
61. Dusek R: Effect of temperature on manual performance, in FR Fischer (ed): *Protection and Functioning of the Hands in Cold Climates*. Washington, DC, National Research Council, 1957, pp 63–76.
62. Gaydos HF, Dusek ER: Effects of localized hand cooling versus total body cooling on manual performance. *J Appl Physiol* 1958;12:377–380.
63. Lockhart JM: Effects of body and hand cooling on complex manual performance. *J Appl Physiol* 1966;50:57–59.
64. Bensel CK, Lockhart JM: Cold-induced vasodilatation onset and manual performance in the cold. *Ergonomics* 1974;17:717–730.
65. Lockhart JM, Kiess HO, Clegg TJ: Effect of rate and level of lowered finger surface temperature on manual performance. *J Appl Physiol* 1975;60:106–113.
66. Nenzen B: Aching arms? Aching shoulders? Worn tools: Another cause of injury. *Working Environment* (Sweden) 1987, pp 22–23.
67. Ulin SS, Ways CM, Armstrong TJ, et al: Perceived exertion and discomfort versus work height with a pistol-shaped screwdriver. *Am Indust Hyg Assoc J* 1990;51:588–594.

Chapter 7

Dynamic Effects of Work on Musculoskeletal Loading

Benjamin M. Hillberry, PhD

Introduction

Repetitive motion disorders of the upper extremity are usually associated with work-related biomechanical stresses caused by routine repeated movements. This is particularly true for activities involving the hand that lead to carpal tunnel syndrome (CTS). Garment workers, meat cutters, grocery checkers, electronic assembly workers, typists, musicians, packers, and carpenters are at increased risk due to grasping, pinching, awkward positions of the hand and wrist, and use of vibrating tools. The risk is enhanced by highly repetitive movements associated with the task.[1] Manifestations of CTS include pain, numbness, and weakness in the median nerve distribution. These conditions are believed to be caused by compression or irritation of the median nerve within the carpal tunnel region of the hand.[1-3]

The carpal tunnel is an area in the palm of the hand that is bounded by the carpal bones and a firm, transverse ligament across the palmar side of the wrist.[3] The median nerve and the nine flexor tendons pass through this region. Enlargement of the tissue within the tunnel can result in increased pressure, causing nerve compression. A higher pressure has been observed in the carpal tunnel of CTS patients versus controls.[4,5] The maximum pressure was found to occur in the distal third of the tunnel, showing a direct correlation with the conduction impairment in the median nerve for CTS patients.[4,6] When pressure in the carpal tunnel is released by cutting the transverse carpal ligament, pain and numbness tend to subside, further indicating a correlation between carpal tunnel pressure and CTS.[3] Carpal tunnel pressure also is significantly higher in CTS patients whose ligament was cut than in controls. The pressure also increases proportionately with flexion or extension of the wrist for both subjects with and without CTS.[5] Magnetic resonance imaging (MRI) of the carpal tunnel in subjects with CTS revealed swelling of the median nerve, flattening of the median nerve, tendon sheath edema in traumatic tenosynovitis, excessive fat within the carpal tunnel, and a large abductor pollicis muscle.[7] This further substantiates the role of pressure on CTS. Schuind and associates[8] hypothesized that CTS results from a vicious cycle: "After an initial episode of mechanical stress, synovium swelling, occurring in a restrictive anatomical space, enhances friction and thus increases further swelling and fibrous hyperplasia."

The work-related symptoms that develop, along with the above hypothesis by Schuind and associates, suggest that biomechanical stresses may be the driving force in the development of CTS. Understanding the forces in the tendons and muscles of the hand for those tasks that lead to CTS can provide a better

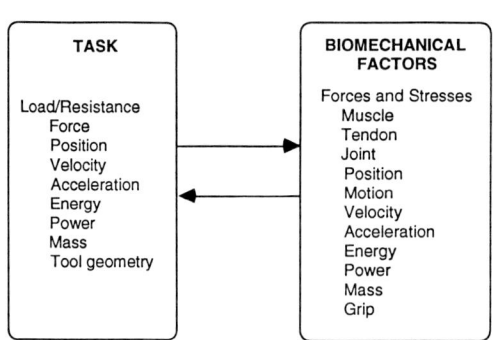

Fig. 1 Parameters describing the task and the biomechanical forces and stresses.

understanding of the factors that initiate the process. Furthermore, the workload and its duration could be determining factors in an overuse condition. Physiologic conditions also are important factors, but the driving forces that create the conditions for CTS are directly related to the biomechanical stresses caused by the forces and by the repetitions that are necessary to perform the tasks. Understanding the biomechanical loading can help in identifying those conditions of the task that predispose to repetitive motion disorders. Techniques for performing the task can be altered and tools can be improved to reduce the tendency for repetitive motion injury.

Determining the mechanical factors required to perform the task and the biomechanical factors at work as the subject adapts to the task can provide quantitative measure of the demands on the subject and can indicate methods for evaluating changes in the task. Computer models of the task interfaced with computer models of the hand can assist in developing quantitative biomechanical conditions that may be determining factors in the development of cumulative motion disorders. Both the task and the hand require dynamic models that account for position, velocity, and accelerations involved in the activity. Dynamic measurements of these parameters and the forces are necessary to quantify the models.

The task provides the load or resistance in terms of forces and displacements necessary to perform the activity. The body, or segment(s) thereof, provide the necessary input to overcome this resistance (Fig. 1). Studies of piano playing and video display terminal (VTD) entry (typing) have used these concepts to determine biomechanical factors in the fingers and hand.[9,10] The models and the results are described below. A method for synthesizing improved finger position for piano playing is also discussed.[11]

Finger Model

Several static mathematical models for the finger have been developed to describe the tendon and joint forces.[9,11–17] An and associates[13] established average locations for the tendon paths using cadaver studies. Chao and An[14,15] developed a three-dimensional finger model. Because of the large number of unknown quantities in the model, an optimal criterion was required to find a solution. Weightman and Amis[16] developed a two-dimensional static model to study pinching activities. They found that using only the two-dimensional sagittal plane coordinates for the tendon paths established by An and associ-

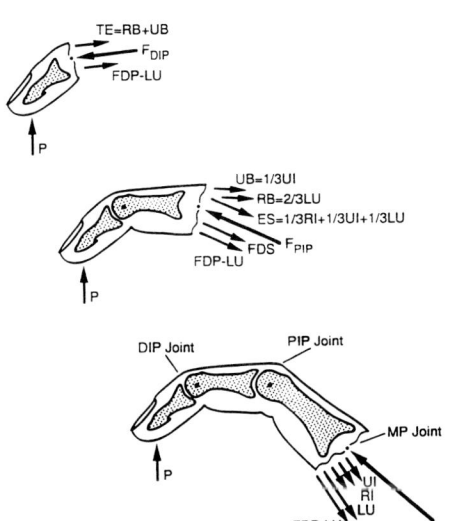

Fig. 2 Free body diagrams of the finger segments illustrating the tendon and joint forces required to provide equilibrium conditions with the applied fingertip force, P.[15,16] TE, terminal extensor; FDP, flexor digitorum profundus; UB, ulnar band; RB, radial band; ES, extensor slip; FDS, flexor digitorum; UI ulnar interosseous, RI radial interosseous; LU, lumbrical; F_{DIP}, DIP joint force; F_{PIP}, PIP joint force; F_{MP}, MP joint force. INT = UI + RI + LU. (Adapted with permission from Weightman B, Amis AA: Finger joint force predictions related to design of joint replacements. J Biomed Eng 1982;4:197–205.)

ates,[13] introduced a maximum tendon tension error of only 1%. Weightman and Amis assumed that the intrinsic muscle tension (INT) could be represented as one variable, INT, which is made up of the radial interosseous (RI), ulnar interosseous (UI), and lumbrical (LU) muscles (Fig. 2), each proportioned according to their physiologic cross-sectional area (PSCA).[18]

Harding and associates[9,11] developed a two-dimensional finger model very similar to that of Weightman and Amis[16] for studying finger forces during piano playing. As with other models, Harding's model assumes that friction in the finger is negligible, only flexor tendons are loaded during the keystrike, and damping in the fingertip pulp is negligible.

Harding and associates[9,11] used a commercial motion measurement system (WATTSMART) to measure position, velocity, and acceleration of the finger segments during rapid trill keystrike. This system computes the positions of light-emitting diodes attached to the fingers. The maximum inertia force due to finger mass was only 2.6% of the keystrike force and, therefore, a static finger model could be used. Because only flexion is considered, the model is deterministic.

The finger model was derived from free body analyses for each of the finger segments as illustrated in Figure 2. For fixed finger size, the joint and tendon forces depend on the fingertip force and the angular position of the finger (Fig. 3). Using measured values for these parameters at peak load, the model can be used to determine the maximum values of the joint and tendon forces.

Characterization of the Task

The task can be described in terms of the required force, displacement, velocity, acceleration, and energy loss for the system. Mathematical models and direct measurements can aid in characterizing the load. The measurements must be made over the range of physiologic velocities used during the task, and care must be taken to avoid artifacts in the data. Frequently, the measurement method can change the load due to transducer location or mass.

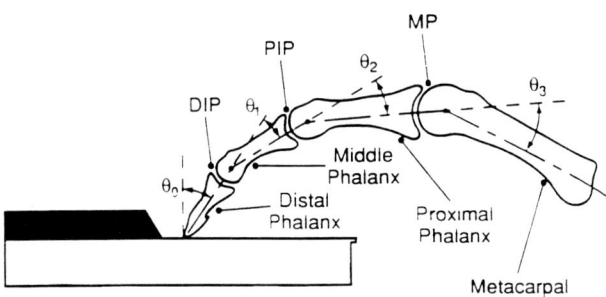

Fig. 3 Angular finger posture described by the four joint angles, θ_0, θ_1, θ_2, θ_3. MP, metaphalangeal joint; DIP, distal metatarsophalangeal joint; PIP, proximal interphalangeal joint. (Reproduced with permission from Wolf FG, Keane MS, Brandt KD, et al: An investigation of finger joint and tendon forces in experienced pianists. *Med Probl Perform Artists* 1993;8:84–95.)

Piano Key

As the fingertip strikes the piano key, a force is imparted, causing the key to accelerate. The required fingertip force is determined by the key mass and its acceleration. This force increases the velocity as the key is depressed and, just prior to the end of the stroke, the hammer leaves the key to strike the wire. It is the velocity of the hammer that determines the sound volume.

Keystrike force versus time was measured using a small load cell placed on the key.[17] Two randomly selected legato keystrikes compared in Figure 4 illustrate the force during key depression (shaded region) and the bottoming out force (peak) for keystrikes of the same accoustic volume. Figure 4, *top*, shows a smoother keystrike, a lower peak force, and a lower bottoming out force. This illustrates how technique can reduce the loading. Force versus displacement curves also can be used to determine the required energy and to evaluate keystrike efficiencies.

Before the finger model could be evaluated during piano playing, it was necessary to develop a method of measuring the fingertip force for each keystrike. Because the fingertip force accelerates the key, key velocity was found to correlate with the applied force. An electronic piano with weighted keys (to give the same feel as a conventional piano) was used. With the electronic piano, the velocity of the key is measured just prior to bottoming out. This velocity measure is used in the electronic piano to control the acoustic volume. A musical instrument digital interface (MIDI) standard is used in electronic musical instruments to interface with other instruments and with computers. The velocity parameter corresponding to the volume is readily available at the computer interface. The piano keystrike force is measured with a load cell and calibrated to this MIDI key velocity parameter. The correlation is shown in Figure 5. This calibration curve permits a direct measurement of keystrike force for each key during piano performance.

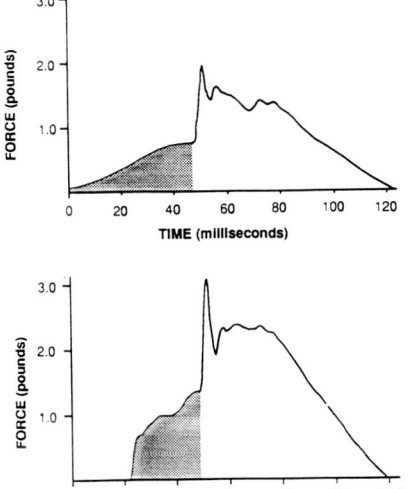

Fig. 4 Force versus time for two randomly selected legato keystrikes with identical acoustic volume and sound. (Reproduced with permission from Harding DC, Brandt KD, Hillberry BM: Minimization of finger joint forces and tendon tensions in pianists. *Med Probl Perform Artists* 1989;4:103–108.)

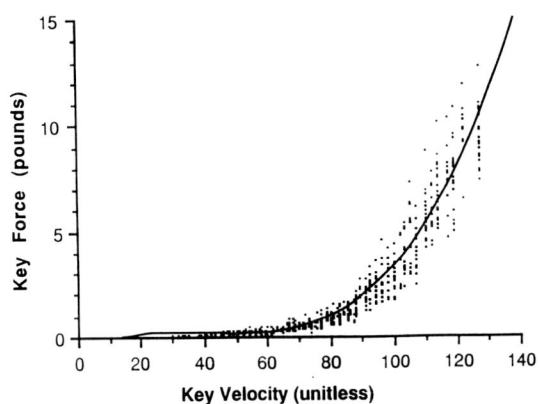

Fig. 5 Fingertip keystrike force versus MIDI key velocity calibration data for all keystrikes from several subjects. (Reproduced with permission from Harding DC, Brandt KD, Hillberry BM: Minimization of finger joint forces and tendon tensions in pianists. *Med Probl Perform Artists* 1989;4:103–108.)

Computer Keyboard

For a given computer keyboard, the mechanical resistance of a key could be modeled by accounting for the mass, spring rate, and damping of the key mechanism. This would require modeling each different keyboard, however.

Alternatively, the keystrike force can be measured. In one method, miniature strain gauges are attached to individual keys, but this requires instrumenting all of the keys. In another method, the reaction forces are measured using a dynamometer created by placing load cells under the keyboard. This method has been used in my laboratory to compare finger forces during computer entry for CTS and control subjects.[10]

To obtain accurate dynamic measurements of the fingertip force, the resonant frequency of the dynamometer must be large compared to the frequency content of the keystrike. This requires a very stiff support for the keyboard and a very stiff load path through the load cells and their support. The schematic shown in Figure 6 illustrates the load cell-support combination for the dynamometer. This system has three load cells to support the keyboard, providing a high stiffness and a high natural frequency of 190 Hz. The system has been shown to provide very accurate measurements of the fingertip forces at regular typing speeds.

Biomechanical Forces in the Fingers During Piano Performance

Methods

The finger tendon and joint forces were determined for eight professional pianists ranging in years of experience from 12 to 59 years.[19] Each subject had 1 week to practice a passage from Mendelssohn's *Song Without Words (op. 19, No. 2)*. During recording, a vertically positioned video camera provided an aerial view of the fingers to assure sagittal plane motion. A horizontally positioned camera recorded the sagittal plane motion of the finger. Using a single frame display on the video, the angular position of the finger was measured at the position of maximum key travel.

The fingertip force was determined from the MIDI software using the calibration curve (Fig. 5). Keystrikes by the forefinger were selected from the music passage for analysis with the computer finger model. Only keystrikes were analyzed for which all pianists approached the key with the same three keystrikes prior to the keystrike selected. Ten notes in the passage were selected for analysis.

The joint and tendon forces in the finger were determined by the computer model as values normalized for a unit fingertip force. These values, called force coefficients, described the effect of finger posture (angular position) on the joint and tendon force. These coefficients, when multiplied by the fingertip force, give the actual joint and tendon forces. Finger segment lengths were loaded

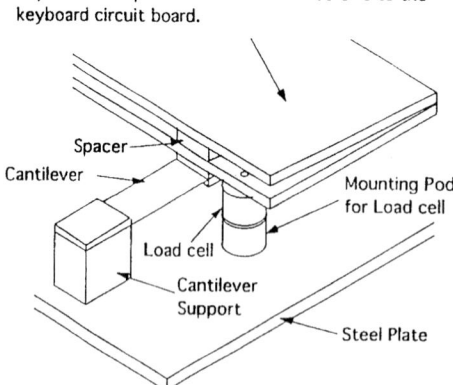

Fig. 6 Schematic of keyboard dynamometer for measuring computer keystrike force.

into the computer for each subject. The model determined the joint and tendon forces for hand size, finger posture, and fingertip force.

Results and Discussion

The effect of finger posture is clearly illustrated in Figure 7. The DIP joint force for a curved finger posture is less than half that for a straighter finger posture. The wide variation in joint and tendon forces is illustrated in Figure 8 for five different finger postures.

The results from the tests of the eight professional pianists show that for the ten notes analyzed, the average keystrike force for each subject varied from 2.0 N to 5.6 N. The pianist with the fewest years of experience struck the keys with significantly greater force than the more experienced subjects. This is perhaps expected because greater proficiency should lead to more effortless and efficient keystrikes. This confirms the hypothesis that the efficiency of performing a task is improved with experience. This has been shown quantitatively among athletes.[20] In repetitive tasks, studies of experienced workers can illustrate techniques for training new workers that will avoid high initial biomechanical stresses during the training period.

Comparison of the biomechanical parameters, joint and tendon forces, for the eight professional pianists showed a wide variation in both finger posture and keystrike force. The effect of finger posture is illustrated by comparing the normalized tendon and joint force coefficients for each subject as they strike the same note in the passage (Table 1). These results indicate a wide variation in finger posture or technique, suggesting that each individual will develop a preferred technique. Finger posture also varied significantly from note to note for the same subject, creating large variations in joint and tendon forces. The finger posture for the lowest and the highest DIP joint force for subject 4 are compared in Figure 9. The effect of finger posture is given by the normalized force coefficient for the DIP joint force, which in this case is 2.3 times higher for the straighter finger (note 2) posture. Interestingly, the keystrike force was 5.6 times higher for note 2, which resulted in a 12.7 times higher actual joint force. Similar results were observed for the other joint and tendon forces and other subjects.

The pianist's musical expression for the dynamic levels within the musical passage resulted in very large variability in the magnitude of the keystrike force. Table 2 gives the keystrike force and the resulting tendon and joint forces for

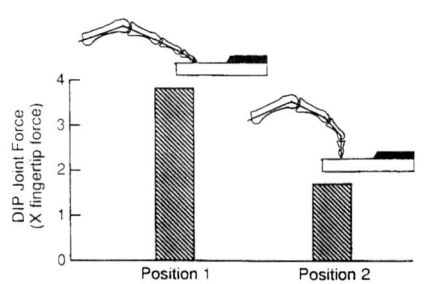

Fig. 7 Comparison of distal interphalangeal (DIP) joint force for two different finger postures with unit finger tip force. (Reproduced with permission from Harding DC, Brandt KD, Hillberry BM: Minimization of finger joint forces and tendon tensions in pianists. *Med Probl Perform Artists* 1989;4:103–108.)

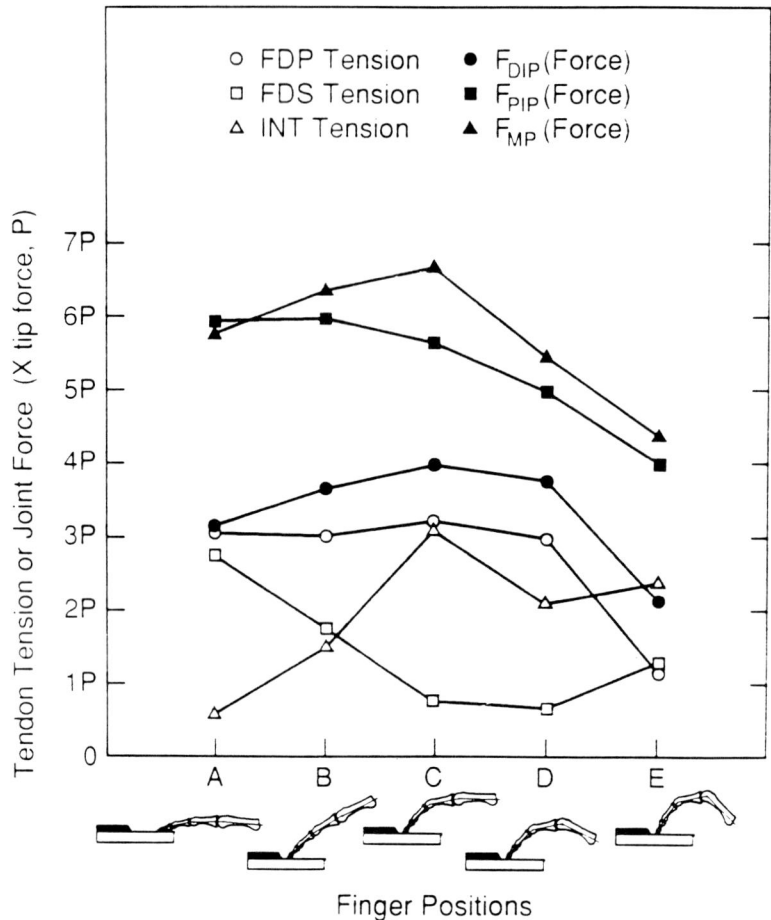

Fig. 8 Tendon and joint forces for five different finger postures with unit fingertip force. FDP, flexor digitorum profundus; FDS, flexor digitorum superficialis; INT, ulnar interosseous + radial interosseous + lumbrical; DIP, distal interphalangeal joint; PIP, proximal interphalangeal joint; MP, metaphalangeal joint.

each subject playing note 1. The wide variation observed between subjects is the result of the artistic expression of the musical performance. This type of variation may not occur in work-related tasks.

Joint and tendon stresses can be readily determined by dividing the corresponding forces by the respective cross-sectional areas. Hand size can become a significant factor. Provided that the keystrike force is the same as in a subject with larger hands, a subject with smaller hands will have smaller joint areas and, therefore, higher joint stresses.

These results show the importance of technique to the biomechanical forces and stresses in the fingers. These methods are directly applicable to work-related tasks and can be used to compare techniques between subject groups. (Typists with and without CTS are compared below.) The models can provide

Table 1 Tendon and joint force coefficients (unity finger tip force) for all subjects striking the note 1*

Joint or tendon	Subject							
	1	2	3	4	5	6	7	8
DIP	2.66	2.70	1.74	1.71	2.46	2.80	2.51	2.32
PIP	4.57	3.88	3.88	4.22	5.18	4.39	4.37	4.17
MP	4.92	3.79	4.31	4.69	6.92	5.33	4.66	4.50
FDP	1.84	1.86	0.71	0.70	1.31	1.78	1.58	1.38
FDS	1.47	0.99	1.63	2.08	1.38	0.68	1.44	1.37
INT	2.01	0.72	2.29	2.13	4.69	3.29	1.64	2.11

* DIP, distal interphalangeal joint; PIP, proximal interphalangeal joint; MP, metaphalangeal joint; FDP, flexor digitorum profundus; FDS, flexor digitorum superficialis; INT, sum of the radial and ulnar interossei, and lumbrical intrinsic muscle tendon forces. The variations in these values are due to finger posture only.

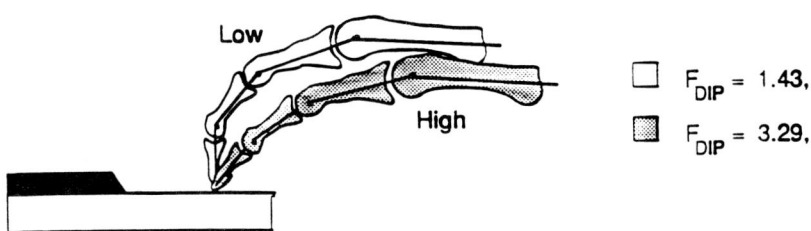

Fig. 9 Finger postures for the lowest and highest distal interphalangeal (DIP) joint force coefficients for subject 4.

a basis for creating techniques that will reduce biomechanical loads and stresses, and thereby improve performance efficiency.

Biomechanical Forces in the Fingers of Computer Users With and Without CTS

The similarity in finger motion between computer VDT usage and piano playing has prompted me to use the above methods to study the biomechanical forces in the fingers of subjects with and without CTS.

Methods

Fifteen subjects whose primary job function is typing on a computer keyboard were selected for the study. Eight subjects had a previous history of CTS injury and seven control subjects had no previous CTS injury. The dynameter (described above) was used to measure the keystrike forces. A WATTSMART notion analysis system was used to measure the motion of the forefinger and middle fingers of the right hand, synchronous with the keystrike force. All subjects used the same keyboard, typed the same passage, and followed the same test protocol.

Table 2 Keystrike force and joint and tendon forces for all subjects striking note 1*

Joint or tendon	Subject							
	1	2	3	4	5	6	7	8
DIP	7.23	7.33	1.32	1.21	6.67	9.60	25.31	9.81
PIP	12.39	10.52	2.93	3.01	14.05	15.03	44.16	17.63
MP	13.34	10.28	3.26	3.34	18.79	18.25	47.08	19.00
FDP	5.01	5.05	0.54	0.50	3.56	6.08	15.97	5.85
FDS	3.98	2.68	1.23	1.48	3.74	2.34	14.56	5.78
INT	5.45	1.95	1.73	1.52	12.72	11.27	16.60	8.93
Keystrike Force	2.71	2.71	0.76	0.71	2.71	3.43	10.10	4.23

* The joint and tendon forces are obtained by multiplying the force coefficients of Table 1 by the keystrike force. (Force measured in Newtons.)

The keystrike force and finger posture were input to Harding's finger model to determine the tendon and joint forces. The t-test was used to compare the statistical difference in the mean values between subjects with and without CTS.

Results and Discussion

Numerous statistical comparisons have been studied. The primary observations are presented below.

Subjects with CTS applied different middle finger forces from those without CTS ($0.05 < \alpha < 0.1$) with the mean keystrike force 30% higher for the subjects with CTS. There were no statistically significant differences in the finger and hand angular positions between the two groups. Subjects with CTS held the wrist straight or slightly drooped versus slightly raised for the subjects without CTS. The mean wrist angles were statistically different between the two groups. The keystrikes with a more curved finger had lower force coefficient values. Subjects without CTS had larger FDP tendon displacements ($0.05 < \alpha < 0.1$), whereas subjects with CTS had larger FDS tendon displacements.

These preliminary results demonstrate that the biomechanical factors, tendon and joint forces, can be determined from these models. In addition, the models can be used to determine posture or techniques to reduce the loading conditions. These forces and the tendon displacements under load may contribute to the development of CTS in the hands.

Minimization of Finger and Tendon Joint Forces

Harding and associates[11] developed a minimization algorithm for determining the finger posture that would reduce the joint or tendon force. Use of the algorithm showed that a more-curved finger posture results in lower forces, which substantiates the methods generally taught by piano teachers. The combination of such methods with the boundary limits of acceptable or possible techniques can contribute to the development of methods to reduce the biomechanical loading.

Summary

Quantitative evaluation of the task provides the input parameters for models that describe the internal biomechanical forces, stresses, and displacements of the body segments. These biomechanical stresses could be the driving force for repetitive motion injury. The model provides not only quantitative evaluation of the activity but also a tool for synthesizing alternate techniques of reducing those parameters that may increase the risk of injury. The models also can be used to evaluate energy expenditure. Experience and practice have been shown to lead to more efficient performance techniques.[20] Assessing these techniques can provide information for improving training methods.

References

1. Baker EL, Ehrenberg RL: Preventing the work-related carpal tunnel syndrome: Physician reporting and diagnostic criteria. *Ann Intern Med* 1990;112:317–319.
2. Centers for Disease Control: Occupational disease surveillance: Carpal tunnel syndrome. *JAMA* 1989;262:886–889.
3. Schenck RR: Carpal tunnel syndrome: The new "industrial epidemic". *AAOHN J* 1989;37:226–231.
4. Luchetti R, Schoenhuber R, Alfarano M, et al: Carpal tunnel syndrome: Correlations between pressure measurement and intraoperative electrophysiological nerve study. *Muscle Nerve* 1990;13:1164–1168.
5. Rojviroj S, Sirichativapee W, Kowsuwon W, et al: Pressures in the carpal tunnel: A comparison between patients with carpal tunnel syndrome and normal subjects. *J Bone Joint Surg* 1990;72B:516–518.
6. Nathan PA, Srinivasan H, Doyle LS, et al: Location of impaired sensory conduction of the median nerve in carpal tunnel syndrome. *J Bone Joint Surg* 1990; 15B:89–92.
7. Mesgarzadeh M, Schneck CD, Bonakdarpour A, et al: Carpal tunnel: MR imaging, part II. Carpal tunnel syndrome. *Radiology* 1989;171:749–754.
8. Schuind F, Ventura M, Pasteels JL: Idiopathic carpal tunnel syndrome: Histologic study of flexor tendon synovium. *J Hand Surg* 1990;15A:497–503.
9. Harding DC, Brandt KD, Hillberry BM: Minimization of finger joint forces and tendon tensions in pianists. *Med Probl Perform Artists* 1989;4:103–108.
10. Keane MS: *Biomechanical Study of Hand Usage in Video Display Terminal Operators*. Lafayette, Indiana, Purdue University, 1993. Thesis.
11. Harding DC, Brandt KD, Hillberry BM: Finger joint force minimization in pianists: Using optimization techniques. *J Biomech* 1993;26:1403–1412.
12. Smith EM, Juvinall RC, Bender LF, et al: Role of the finger flexors in rheumatoid deformities of the metacarpophalangeal joints. *Arthritis Rheum* 1964;7:467–480.
13. An KN, Chao EY, Cooney WP III, et al: Normative model of human hand for biomechanical analysis. *J Biomech* 1979;12:775–788.
14. Chao EY, An KN: Determination of internal forces in human hand. *J Eng Mech Div* 1978;104:255–272.
15. Chao EY, An KN: Graphical interpretation of the solution to the redundant problem in biomechanics. *J Biomed Eng* 1978;100:159–167.
16. Weightman B, Amis AA: Finger joint force predictions related to design of joint replacements. *J Biomed Eng* 1982;4:197–205.
17. Harding DC: *Minimization of Finger Joint Reaction Forces and Tendon Tensions in Pianists*. Lafayette, Indiana, Purdue University, 1989. Thesis.
18. Amis AA, Dowson D, Wright V: Muscle strengths and musculo-skeletal geometry of the upper limb. *Eng Med* 1979;8:41–48.
19. Wolf FG, Keane MS, Brandt KD, et al: An investigation of finger joint and tendon forces in experienced pianists. *Med Probl Perform Artists* 1993;8:84–95.
20. Cavanagh PR, Kram R: Mechanical and muscular factors affecting the efficiency of human movement. *Med Sci Sports Exerc* 1985;17: 326–331.

Chapter 8

Applications of Biomechanical Hand and Wrist Models to Work-Related Musculoskeletal Disorders of the Upper Extremity

Richard P. Wells, MEng, PhD
Peter J. Keir, BSc
Anne E. Moore, MSc, PEng

Work-related musculoskeletal disorders (WMSDs) have complex multifactorial etiologies, including the physical aspects and psychosocial factors of the workplace. Models are necessary to help determine and explain the effects of the many interacting physical stressors that affect the hand, wrist, and forearm during work. For example, biomechanical models of the hand and wrist can demonstrate the connection between the physical aspects of work done by individuals and the resultant disorders that develop in tissues.[1]

The need for more representative measurements of exposure in epidemiological studies of WMSDs has been recognized.[2] In addition, models may help in determining the mechanisms of injury. Biomechanical modeling offers the possibility of synthesizing variables that are probably related to the pathophysiology of injury, but which cannot be measured directly, for example, calculating low back compression in the study of manual materials handling tasks.

Moore and associates[3] developed a comprehensive approach that integrated the classic risk factors of force, posture, repetitiveness, and duration and produced a profile of biomechanical risk factors for use in industrial settings. These risk factors reflected the loading caused by different static postures, repeated extreme postures, and dynamic movements. Table 1 shows the biomechanical risk factors proposed. Most of the proposed mechanisms of injury combine more than one of the classic risk factors.

Figure 1 illustrates the submodels that link the external exposure variables. Input to the model includes continuously monitored hand and wrist postures and forces and muscle activation (electromyographic [EMG] signals) over the duration of the task in the arms and shoulders. The submodels are based on the best available anatomic and pathophysiologic data. For example, the tendon loads can be predicted from optimization models[4] combined with empiric data of passive muscle forces.[5] Further processing estimates the risk to particular tissues.

In a laboratory simulation, many of the proposed biomechanical risk factors responded to task changes in a manner predictive of the injury potential

Table 1 WMSD injury mechanisms and related modeled risk factors

Disorder	Proposed Pathophysiology	Modeled Biomechanical Risk Factor
Carpal tunnel syndrome*†	Force of tendons on median nerve	Peak normal pressure Cumulative pressure against flexor retinaculum
Tenosynovitis	"Bearing loads" on sheath	Peak normal pressure Cumulative normal pressure
	Movement of tendon with respect to the sheath	Cumulative tendon excursion
	Friction between tendon and tendon sheath	Frictional work
Tendinitis	Strain and cumulative strain in tendon	Peak tendon tension Impulse of tendon force
Muscle pain and disorders	Static or uninterrupted activation	"Static" muscle load (10th percentile APDF‡) EMG "gaps" EVA§
	Dynamic muscle use	EMG (50th and 90th percentiles APDF) EVA

*Carpal tunnel syndrome may also be secondary to tenosynovitis and other causes
†Elevated intra carpal tunnel pressure is a strong risk factor but comprehensive models are not yet available
‡APDF, amplitude probability distribution function
§EVA, Exposure variability assessment

of the tasks.[3] In an initial study of 153 workers with physical examinations,[1] several of the measures, including tendon excursion and static muscle contraction, have been found to be significantly related to injury.[6,7]

Nonmodeling Approaches to Predicting Disorders in the Hand and Wrist

In addition to modeling, another method for studying the relationships between work and musculoskeletal disorders is by using external measures of physical exposure, such as job classification, expert evaluation of the "heaviness" of a job or measures of force exerted, wrist posture, grip type, or frequency of movement (repetitiveness).

Ample and consistent findings show that a variety of localized musculoskeletal symptoms and clinically identifiable conditions are associated with work-related risk factors determined using observational or video-aided techniques.[8] Force, whether recorded as a hand grip force or as a muscle activation related to a maximal effort, has been found to be related to WMSDs. Repetitiveness is a commonly identified risk factor, but one that frequently is poorly defined. Qualitatively, it has connotations of the same work elements repeated many times. Despite this, repetition has been associated with WMSDs. Posture has been found to be a consistently strong risk factor for injury in the upper limb, especially for the shoulder.

Posture probably has been used widely in the field as a risk factor because it can be determined relatively easily and acts as a surrogate for many other risk

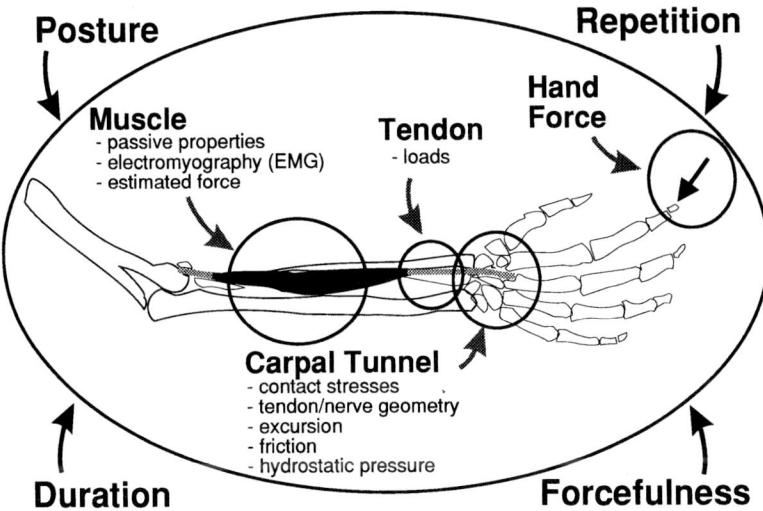

Fig. 1 Schematic diagram illustrating the measured (external) risk factors and the modeled biomechanical risk factors.

factors. Postures deviating from neutral frequently are predictive of the moment at a joint, and thus tissue load, because of both tension in passive tissues and moments to support the body parts against gravity. Changes in the musculoskeletal geometry that may modify the pressure in a compartment or alter contact stresses (and thus frictional loads) on tendons may also be captured by observing posture. In addition, postural changes can be used to determine repetitiveness. More recently, measurements of wrist angular acceleration have been found to be important in distinguishing between jobs with high and low reported rates of carpal tunnel disorders.[9]

Modeling Approaches to Predicting Disorders in Tendons of the Hand and Wrist

One suggested mechanism for tenosynovitis is reduced lubrication between tendons and tendon sheaths caused by excess relative movement.[10] High peak loads and cumulative strain have been suggested as a mechanism for tendinitis.[11] A model for assessing tenosynovitis was proposed by Wells and associates[12] and was recently put into effect.[3] In this model, the frictional work done by the tendon sliding through its sheath is calculated. One type of frictional work is the result of a "belt-pulley" interaction when the wrist deviates from a straight position.[13] Besides this type of frictional work, it is suggested that a non-negligible resistance to movement must be present to move the tendons through the carpal tunnel, even in the straight position. Estimates extrapolated from the work of Goldstein[14] put this resistance at around 5 N in the neutral position. However, in humans, values of the order 0.5 N have been measured (Paul Smutz, PhD, personal communication). Therefore, excursion of the tendons at the wrist (caused by finger and wrist movement) in both deviated and straight postures will create an energy input, possibly beyond the

114 Pathophysiology: Biomechanical Loads

ability of the tissue to recover. Thus, high tendon excursion has both a biologic and epidemiologic link to WMSDs and tenosynovitis.[6]

Nerve Disorders in the Hand and Wrist

Insult to the median nerve, whether from increased hydrostatic pressures in the carpal canal[15] or from mechanical insult (contact stresses) upon the nerve by overlying tendon(s)[13] has been often suggested as a likely mechanism of work-related carpal tunnel syndrome.

Mechanical stress to the median nerve can be predicted by modified belt-pulley models of the wrist, which are an output of our biomechanical model. Magnetic resonance imaging performed on living subjects exerting known forces in a variety of functional postures enabled estimates of the radius of curvature of the extrinsic flexor tendon. Thus, estimates of the load exerted on the supporting structures within the carpal canal during gripping tasks could be assessed.[16] Using mathematical differentiation, the instantaneous radii of curvature were calculated throughout the length of the carpal tunnel. The vectors shown in Figure 2 were produced using the radius of curvature in the radioulnar and dorsopalmar directions. (Note: Figure 2 is a schematic and not meant to represent actual tendon locations.) The direction of the force vectors in Figure 2 are consistent with the suggested movement of the median nerve through the tendons while moving from flexion to extension.[17] The direction of the forces from the tendons would appear to permit such movement. Although the MRI data do not conclusively demonstrate median nerve movement, the forces acting on the tendons support the movement hypothesis. With movement of the median nerve through the flexor tendons or movement of the tendons around

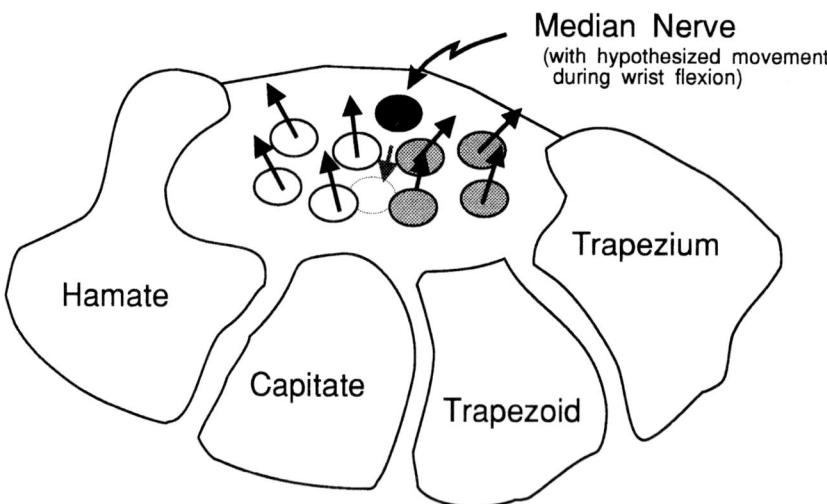

Fig. 2 Schematic of the loads exerted on the supporting structures in the carpal tunnel. A two-finger pinch with the wrist in 20° of flexion is illustrated. Only tendons of the flexor profundus and flexor superficialis are shown. Loaded tendons are shaded. The median nerve is black. (Reproduced with permission from Keir PJ, Wells R: Normal forces on wrist structures transmitted by the flexor tendon. *Proceedings of the 2nd North American Congress of Biomechanics.* Ann Arbor, MI, University of Michigan, 1992, pp 35–36.)

the median nerve, increased frictional forces and damage on the tendon synovium might be expected.[18] The magnitude of the transmitted (normal) tendon forces depends on the tendon axial load and the radius of curvature.

Hydrostatic pressures, on the other hand, are only measurable using invasive techniques. Models of the carpal tunnel may soon allow intracarpal pressure estimates based on such data as posture and force.

Muscle Disorders in the Hand and Wrist

Muscular loading during upper limb intensive work has been linked to the development of chronic muscular problems in the shoulder and neck.[2,19] Recent clinical findings have also suggested that forearm muscular pain may be an overlooked problem in studying work-related chronic musculoskeletal injuries.[1] Although work-related muscular pain is well accepted in the shoulder, pain in the forearm is usually attributed to tendinitis or epicondylitis.

One suggested mechanism for muscle pain is fatigue-induced hypoxia leading to metabolic changes resulting from low-level continuous activation. Another possible mechanism is increased intracompartmental pressure and physical disruption of the muscle with high force contractions.

The major approach to determining potential for development of muscle work-related disorders, especially to the trapezius and other shoulder and neck musculature, has been electromyography (EMG). Appropriate processing of the EMG signal can establish the association between the work performed and the muscle usage required. Jonsson[20] described a technique in which the frequency of occurrence of any particular level of EMG is calculated. An amplitude probability distribution function (APDF) curve is developed based on this calculation. The static level of this curve describes the ability of the muscle to rest at least 10% of the time during the performance of a task and appears important in the development of chronic work-related muscle problems. If the value is greater than zero, the muscle is not given the chance to completely rest at least 10% of the time during a task. Although this is a useful method of quantifying muscle use throughout the duration of a task, it gives no indication of the duration of each rest pause (ie, whether the rests come as numerous pauses or as one big pause). Veiersted and associates[21] addressed this by using a gaps analysis, which determines the number of times the muscle is turned off (less than 0.5% MVC). It appears that people with pain have fewer gaps. More recently, Mathiassen and Winkel[22] have proposed a measure, exposure variability assessment (EVA), which combines elements of both these approaches.

Our recent study of 153 women 28 to 50 years of age from six industries (automotive trim, food retail, packaging, clothing, electronics, and metal parts assembly) examined the relationship between muscle activation and WMSD in highly repetitive tasks.[7] EMG of the forearm flexors (midpoint of a line between the medial epicondyle and radial styloid) and extensors (over the extensor muscle mass just distal to the lateral epicondyle) was monitored bilaterally while the workers were videotaped performing their normal tasks at their workstations. Physical signs of specific injury to muscles, tendons, and nerves in the upper limb, neck, and shoulder were assessed.[1] Specific to forearm muscles, the lateral and medial epicondyles, and the flexor and extensor muscles were all palpated separately. Each muscle was activated individually. Forearm muscle disorders were diagnosed based on: (1) findings of pain and/or tenderness correctly located to the structure being stressed and (2) complaints of work-induced pain at the same site. Pain or tenderness was classified as (1) muscle-related if it occurred in the proximal half of the forearm, more than a thumb width distal to the epicondyle; (2) epicondylitis if it occurred directly on the epicondyle; and (3) tendinitis if it occurred on the intervening tendon of origin. After drop out and exclusion due to previous injury or language and technical problems, 111 right limbs and 110 left limbs of the remaining patient population were used in the analysis.

Muscle pain without pain in the tendon of origin was established in 12% of the arms of the subjects examined. Separate variance-independent t tests were used to examine the relationship between each specific injury site and the appropriate EMG site. The strongest relationship ($p < .05$) occurred on the left side between static extensor EMG and pain or tenderness isolated to the extensor muscle belly (Fig. 3).

Uses of Modeling in the Work-Related Musculoskeletal Disorders of Video Display Operators

The medical problems associated with keyboard use for activities such as typing and data entry have promoted increased research in these areas. Rose[23] investigated the postures assumed during typing and data entry and found that certain postures elicited high forearm extensor activation levels. We have used a planar model of the index finger[24] combined with empirical data of the passive properties of the extrinsic hand and wrist musculature[25] to predict the loads on the wrist extensor musculature during static typing postures.[26]

Wrist extensor load increased with increasing wrist extension to balance the flexor moments caused by gravity and flexor muscle forces (Fig. 4). Positioning of the wrist in neutral required 12.7% of the available extensor moment, whereas a posture of 30° of wrist extension required a minimum of 30% of the available moment. It is interesting to note that although the gravitational moment due to the weight of the hand decreases as the wrist becomes more extended, the passive moment caused by the flexors increases, dramatically increasing the effort required by the extensor. The contribution of the wrist flex-

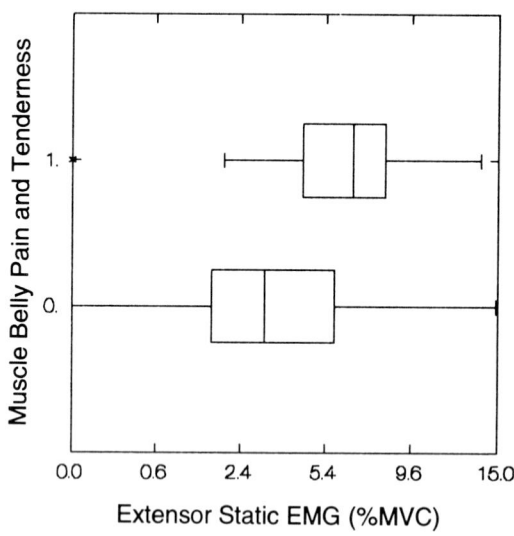

Fig. 3 Relationship between extensor muscle pain and static extensor muscle activation. (Reproduced with permission from Moore A, Wells R, Ranney D: The relationship between pain and tenderness and electromyographic measures in the forearms of workers performing repetitive manual tasks, in *Proceedings of the International Society of Biomechanics Congress.* Paris, France, International Society of Biomechanics, 1993, pp 898–899.)

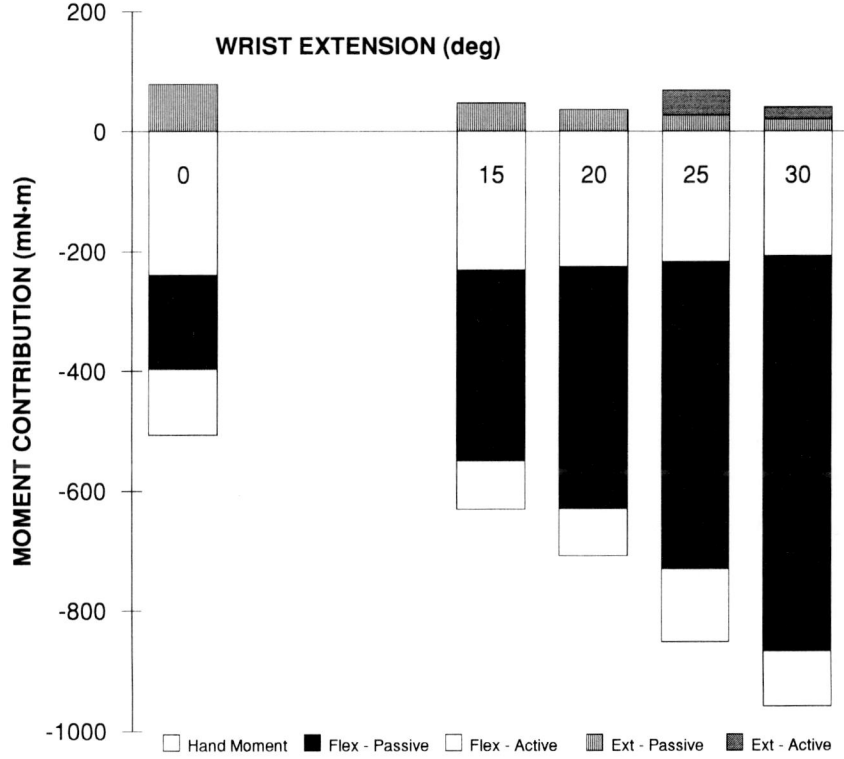

Fig. 4 Relationship between wrist extension angle and wrist flexor moment sources during VDT work. Moments include passive and active contributions from the wrist and finger flexors as well as the flexor moment induced by gravity. A wrist extensor moment is required to balance these moments. (Reproduced with permission from Keir P, Wells R: The effect of typing posture on wrist extensor loading, in *Proceedings of the Biannual Conference of the Canadian Society for Biomechanics.* Kingston, ON, Queens University, 1994.)

ors (flexores carpi radialis and ulnaris and palmaris longus) provides most of the passive flexor moments. This proportion increased with increasing wrist extension angle. These data parallel the findings of Rose,[23] whose protocol altered the finger posture as well as the height of the keyboard relative to the forearm. The 30% extensor activation level noted in his EMG evaluation of typing postures was associated with numeric entry. Because typing postures require ulnar deviation of approximately 15°,[27] one might expect greater activity or loading of the extensor carpi ulnaris.

A field study of ten operators of video display terminals (VDT) who also handled written materials lends some support to the theory that forearm extensor loading may be an important risk factor for this task.[28] EMG signals from the forearm flexors, forearm extensors, and upper fibers of the trapezius were monitored bilaterally while the workers performed their normal tasks at their workstations. The APDF and EMG gaps were computed for each EMG signal. The only static load noted in the combined APDF curves was for the right extensor muscle, although dynamic and peak levels were higher for the trapezius EMG. It should be noted that individually, several operators had static load levels greater than zero with their extensor and trapezius muscles (the ratio of arms with static load to total arms assessed was 9/19 for the extensors and 9/19 for the trapezius); however, very few had static levels greater than zero with the flexor muscles (2/19). Of the three muscle groups studied, the forearm extensors had the fewest gaps.

All of the operators tested had adjustable chairs; however, few had any form of wrist support. Most operators had adjusted their chairs so their elbows were comfortable at their side or their arms rested on surrounding furniture. In many cases, however, the wrists had to be maintained in extension against gravity in order to keep the fingers above the keyboard.

The results show that muscles in the forearm, especially on the extensor side, are subjected to low level continuous or repeated loading while performing this task. Recent evidence that even moderate deviations from a neutral typing posture can significantly elevate intracarpal pressures[15] supports the control of extended and deviated postures in the prevention of work-related musculoskeletal disorders to both the nerve and muscle tissues of keyboard operators.

A Modeling Approach to Assessing the Effectiveness of Job Rotation in Highly Repetitive Tasks

Job rotation is an organizational strategy that has been advocated to prevent the development of work-related musculoskeletal injuries after engineering controls have failed to reduce musculoskeletal stress. One recommendation on job rotation is that the jobs be dissimilar. The goal is to "dilute" the exposure of the worker to potentially injurious stressors of particular tissues. Thus, it would be beneficial to have multiple indices to describe the musculoskeletal loading of different parts of the body for jobs used in job rotation programs.

We have used the modeling approach described above to assess quantitatively the utility of existing rotation schemes.[28] Details of the equipment and procedures used are described in the preceding section. In addition, a lightweight wrist transducer and glove recorded the postures of the wrist, proximal interphalangeal joint, and metacarpophalangeal joint of the fingers. Six factors related to injury mechanisms in the carpal tunnel were calculated from an analytical model of the hand and forearm.[3] The variables described tendon loading and movement (tendon force, tendon excursion, tendon excursion velocity, tendon normal pressure impulse) and work factor or the frictional work done on the tendon sheaths (Table 1).

The study investigated two existing job rotation schemes at two different companies. The first rotation was at an electronics assembly facility and included four jobs: two loading operations (A and B), a screwrunning task (C), and an inspection task (D). The second rotation was at an automotive trim plant and included three jobs in rotation: glue application using a spray gun (E), and two jobs involving vacuum forming, edge turning, and stapling operations that differed by the use of either an overhead conveyor (F) or a belt conveyor (G). Only demands on the right side are described.

Differences in jobs A, B, and D of the electronics plant and jobs E, F, and G of the trim plant were small (Table 2). The static level of the trapezius for job C was much higher (10.9%) than any other job of the electronics rotation, differing by 75%. This job would benefit from rotation. The factors that describe forearm loading illustrate that the jobs within the rotation schemes have different demands. In electronics assembly, job C showed highest demand upon the finger flexors and extensors due to high handgrip forces maintained over a large part of the cycle.

In the automotive trim task rotation, job E was characterized by long duration gripping with the wrist in flexion. This is seen in the static level of the flexors as well as the high cumulative pressure in the flexor direction, which indicates sustained load on the median nerve in the carpal tunnel. Jobs F and G were characterized by pinch grips in a flexed posture with high peak loads, as seen in the tendon loads and normal (flexor) pressure impulse. This is mirrored in the high median load in all muscle groups, especially job F.

The seated electronics assembly was characterized by relatively lighter demands on the hand and wrist with higher shoulder loads and fixed postures of the shoulder girdle. On the other hand, the standing automotive trim tasks were characterized by high loads on the hand and wrist with lower shoulder loads. In neither case was the rotation scheme particularly beneficial, based on the profile of risk factors.

Summary

While modeling is not the only method by which the relationships between work and musculoskeletal disorders can be studied, we believe it has a num-

Table 2 Biomechanical risk factors in two rotation schemes

Musculoskeletal Load Factor		Electronics Assembly (n=6)				Automotive Trim (n=2)		
		A	B	C	D	E	F	G
Peak tendon force (N)		57.8	95	112.6	99.6	94.8	146.4	194.0
Cumulative tendon force Impulse (Ns/hr) (× 10³)		19.1	22.6	64.8	31.2	61.7	101.4	87.9
Cumulative excursion (cm²/hr) (× 10³)		3.6	4.2	4.5	4.9	6.4	6.6	5.7
Peak excursion velocity (cm/sec)		18	17	33	44	20	14	16
Cumulative normal pressure impulse (Flexion) (Ns/cm²/hr)		203	139	146	254	5254	1609	1886
Cumulative work factor (J/cm²/hr)		0.31	0.66	0.48	0.19	0.42	0.63	0.33
APDF* of finger flexors (%MVC)	Static	0.7	1.1	0.8	0.1	1.3	0.4	0.5
	Median	3.4	3.1	5.7	2.8	8.5	14.2	9.1
	Peak	8.7	12.8	16.9	11.1	22.2	35.5	32.3
APDF of finger extensors (%MVC)	Static	1.4	3.1	3.1	0.4	0.8	0.3	0
	Median	5.6	5.2	8.9	4.4	12.9	18.8	12.4
	Peak	13.4	14.2	20.1	16.8	36.3	47.4	37.7
APDF of trapezius (%MVC)	Static	3.3	3.7	10.9	4.8	0	0.8	1.5
	Median	12.1	14.3	20.3	11.7	4.9	14.1	8.2
	Peak	22.1	24.1	31.8	24.6	29.7	31.0	25.2

* APDF, Amplitude probability distribution function
(Reproduced with permission from Wells RW, Orr SE, Moore AE: Selection of jobs for a job rotation program, in Hagberg M, Kilbom A (eds): *Proceedings of the International Scientific Conference on Prevention of Work-Related Musculoskeletal Disorders (PREMUS)*. Stockholm, Sweden, National Institute of Occupational Health, 1992, pp 327–329.)

ber of strengths to recommend it. Models help explain the many simultaneous and interacting physical stressors that act on the hand, wrist, and forearm during work. If based on sound anatomy and solid pathophysiologic findings, such models may be suitable for measuring exposure in epidemiologic studies as well as studying mechanisms of injury.

Acknowledgments

The authors would like to thank the Ontario Workplace Health and Safety Agency, the Ministry of Labour, and the NSERC for support of parts of this research.

References

1. Ranney D, Wells R, Moore A: Upper limb musculoskeletal disorders in highly repetitive industries: Precise anatomical physical findings. *Ergonomics*, in press.
2. Hagberg M: Occupational musculoskeletal stress and disorders of the neck and shoulder: A review of possible pathophysiology. *Int Arch Occup Environ Health* 1984;53:269–278.
3. Moore A, Wells R, Ranney D: Quantifying exposure in occupational manual tasks with cumulative trauma disorder potential. *Ergonomics* 1991;34:1433–1453.
4. An K-N, Chao EY, Cooney WP, et al: Forces in the normal and abnormal hand. *J Orthop Res* 1985;3:202–211.
5. Wells R, Ranney D, Keir P: Passive force length properties of cadaveric human forearm musculature, in Schuind F, An K-N, Cooney WP III, et al (eds): *Advances in the Biomechanics of the Hand and Wrist*. New York, NY, Plenum Press, 1994, pp 31–40.
6. Wells R, Ranney D, Moore A, et al: Relationship between chronic musculoskeletal disorders and work exposures: Results from repetitive manual task, in Hagberg M, Kilbom A (eds): *International Scientific Conference on Prevention of Work-Related Musculoskeletal Disorders (PREMUS)*. Stockholm, Sweden, National Institute of Occupational Health, 1992, pp 324–326.
7. Moore A, Wells R, Ranney D: The relationship between pain and tenderness and electromyographic measures in the forearms of workers performing repetitive maunal tasks, in *Proceeding of the International Society of Biomechanics Congress*. Paris, France, International Society of Biomechanics, 1993, pp 898–899.
8. Hagberg M (ed): *Work-related Musculoskeletal Disorders (WMSD): A Handbook on Prevention*. London, UK, Taylor and Francis, 1994.
9. Marras WS, Schoenmarklin RW: Wrist motions in industry. *Ergonomics* 1993;36:341–351.
10. Rowe ML: The diagnosis of tendon and tendon sheath injuries. *Sem Occup Med* 1987;2:1–6.
11. Goldstein SA, Armstrong TJ, Chaffin DB, et al: Analysis of cumulative strain in tendons and tendon sheaths. *J Biomech* 1987;20:1–6.
12. Wells RP, Moore A, Ranney D: Evaluation of hand intensive tasks using biomechanical load factors, in Haselgrave CM (ed): *Work Design in Practice*. London, UK, Taylor and Francis, 1990.
13. Armstrong TJ, Chaffin DB: Some biomechanical aspects of the carpal tunnel. *J Biomech* 1979;12:567–570.
14. Goldstein SA: *Biomechanical Aspects of Cumulative Trauma to Tendons and Tendon Sheaths*. Ann Arbor, MI, University of Michigan, 1981. Thesis.
15. Rempel D, Bloom T, Tal R, et al: A method of measuring intracarpal pressure and elementary hand manoeuvres, in Hagberg M, Kilbom A (eds): *Proceedings of the International Scientific Conference on Prevention of Work-Related Musculoskeletal Disorders (PREMUS)*. Stockholm, Sweden, National Institute of Occupational Health, 1992, pp 249–251.

16. Keir PJ, Wells R: Normal forces on wrist structures transmitted by the flexor tendon. *Proceedings of the 2nd North American Congress of Biomechanics.* Ann Arbor, MI, University of Michigan, 1992, pp 35–36.
17. Armstrong TJ, Castelli WA, Evans FG, et al: Some histological changes in carpal tunnel contents and their biomechanical implications. *J Occup Med* 1984;26:197–201.
18. Skie M, Zeiss J, Ebraheim NA, et al: Carpal tunnel changes and median nerve compression during wrist flexion and extension seen by magnetic resonance imaging. *J Hand Surg* 1990;15A:934–939.
19. Aaras A: Postural load and the development of musculo-skeletal illness. *Scand J Rehabil Med* 1987;18(suppl):5–35.
20. Jonsson B: Measurement and evaluation of local muscular strain in the shoulder during constrained work. *J Human Ergol* 1982;11:73–88.
21. Veiersted KB, Westgaard RH, Anderson P: Pattern of muscle activity during sterotyped work and its relation to muscle pain. *Int Arch Occup Environ Health* 1990;62:31–41.
22. Mathiassen SE, Winkel J: Quantifying variation in physical load using exposure-vs-time data. *Ergonomics* 1991;34:1455–1468.
23. Rose MJ: Keyboard operating posture and actuation force: Implications for muscle over-use. *Applied Ergonomics* 1991;22:198–203.
24. Wells RP, Ranney DA, Keeler A: The interaction of muscular and passive elastic forces during unloaded finger movements: A computer graphics model, in Perren SM, Schneider E (eds): *Biomechanics: Current Interdisciplinary Research.* Dordrecht, The Netherlands, Martinus Nijhoff Publishers, 1985, pp 743–748.
25. Keir P, Wells R: The effect of typing posture on wrist extensor loading: *Proceedings of the Biannual Conference of the Canadian Society for Biomechanics.* Kingston, ON, Queen's University, 1994.
26. Serina E, Tal R, Rempel D: Wrist and arm angles during typing. *Proceedings of the Marconi Keyboard Research Conference.* Ann Arbor, MI, University of Michigan, 1994.
27. Wells R, Ranney DA, Moore A: Relationship between forearm muscle pain/tenderness and work exposures: Results from repetitive manual tasks, in *Occupational Disorders of the Upper Extremities, Proceedings of a Conference Held at the University of Michigan.* Ann Arbor, MI, University of Michigan, 1992.
28. Wells RW, Orr SE, Moore AE: Selection of jobs for a job rotation program, in Hagberg M, Kilbom A (eds): *Proceedings of the International Scientific Conference on Prevention of Work-Related Musculoskeletal Disorders (PREMUS).* Stockholm, Sweden, National Institute of Occupational Health, 1992, pp 327–329.

Chapter 9
Musculoskeletal Loading and Carpal Tunnel Pressure

David Rempel, MD

In the 1950s, Tanzer[1] used a mercury-filled bag to measure fluid pressure within the carpal tunnels of live subjects. Since then, the measurement technique has been refined through use of the wick catheter,[2] a pressure transducer tipped catheter, and, most recently, a multi-perforated, saline-filled catheter.[3] Although studies have elucidated parts of the relationship between carpal tunnel pressure (CTP) and carpal tunnel syndrome (CTS), the role of elevated CTP in the pathophysiology of CTS is still somewhat speculative.[4-9] The hypothesis underlying the material presented in this chapter is that an adequate dose of prolonged and elevated CTP from repeated hand activities can initiate the cascade of events leading to nerve entrapment.

Role of CTP in Disease

CTS is an entrapment of the median nerve within the carpal tunnel at the wrist. This small tunnel is tightly occupied by the median nerve and by nine tendons, each in a gelatinous sheath. CTS is associated with factors, such as space-occupying lesions (eg, anomalous muscle, tumor), or conditions associated with tissue swelling (eg, pregnancy, myxedema, congestive heart failure, tenosynovitis), that increase the pressure inside the tunnel.

The precise pathophysiology linking repetitive hand activity to CTS is unknown, but a number of mechanisms have been proposed. Three possible mechanisms are: (1) friction associated with repetitive tendon motions leading to flexor tendon sheath irritation and swelling; (2) repeated direct mechanical trauma to the median nerve by structures within the carpal tunnel; and (3) prolonged elevated pressure within the carpal tunnel leading to ischemia, tissue swelling, and epineural fibrosis. An expanded explanation of the third mechanism is that the elevated pressures limit microvascular flow and lead to protein leakage, epineurial edema, and, eventually, epineurial fibrosis.[2] Evidence supporting this ischemic mechanism is indirect and is summarized in the following paragraphs.

First, carpal tunnel pressure is almost always higher in patients with CTS than in normal subjects (Table 1). It is only in patients with very severe cases of CTS that the pressure has been reported to be low.[9] These "end-stage" cases may have adapted to the prolonged elevations in pressure with a reduction of tissue volume or by some other mechanism not yet defined.

Second, parts of the ischemic mechanism are supported by surgical experience. In early CTS, the symptoms experienced by the patient may stem from

Table 1 Summary of studies comparing mean carpal tunnel pressure among healthy subjects to pressures in patients with carpal tunnel syndrome

Study	Carpal Tunnel Patients*				Control Subjects*			
	N†	Neutral	Flexion	Extension	N†	Neutral	Flexion	Extension
Gelberman, et al, 1981[2]	15	32	94	110	12	2.5	—	—
Werner, et al, 1983[27]	16	31	75	105	—	—	—	—
Szabo & Chidgey, 1988[9]	22	10	32	51	6	5	16	27
Okutsu, et al, 1989[31]	62	43	192	222	32	14	144	158
Luchetti, et al, 1989[4]	30	26	—	—	4	13	—	—
Rojviroj, et al, 1990[32]	61	12	27	33	32	4	9	13

*Mean pressures at different wrist postures are included when available
†Number of subjects studied
(Adapted with permission from Weiss N, Gordon L, Bloom T, et al: Wrist position of lowest carpal tunnel pressure: Implications for splint design. *J Bone Joint Surg*, in press.)

poor nutrition of the nerve fibers when circulation is initially impaired. At this point, effective treatment involves eliminating or reducing the pressure in the carpal tunnel.[5,8] Prolonged venous insufficiency leads to protein leakage and edema, which causes other structural changes associated with more severe sensory and motor deficits; but these changes are still reversible if circulation can be restored through decompression.[8,10] If the edema continues, however, fibroblast invasion and endoneurial fibrosis will result, and, once the nerve has been damaged, the return of full function is delayed or unlikely to occur even after carpal tunnel release.

Third, histologic studies of the flexor tendon sheaths biopsied during carpal tunnel release show edema and vascular changes consistent with long-standing ischemia.[11] Edema was observed in 85% and vascular sclerosis in 98% of 177 wrists with idiopathic CTS; both findings were significantly more frequent than in the control wrists.[12] Inflammation was an uncommon finding. Others have observed similar vascular thickening within the synovial sheath, suggesting an ischemic mechanism.[13]

Fourth, several animal studies have defined the effects of nerve compression. Short-term, low-pressure compression of a nerve will lead to decreased blood flow, tissue edema, and acute nerve dysfunction.[6] Compression of a rabbit tibia nerve to 30 mm Hg blocked epineurial venule blood flow and axonal transport, and increased vascular permeability.[14] Increasing compression to 50 mm Hg reduced endoneurial and arteriolar blood flow, 60 mm Hg caused complete ischemia in 60% of nerves, and 80 mm Hg blocked all blood flow. Acute increases in pressure led to changes in nerve function along with the vascular effects. In a canine model, nerve conduction velocity was significantly reduced at a tissue pressure of 30 mm Hg after 8 hours and 50 mm Hg caused complete nerve block.[15] Likewise, in a rat sciatic nerve model, a pressure of 30 mm Hg for 120 minutes led to a complete conduction block.[16] To differentiate the pathophysiologic role of cyclical loading versus sustained pressure, Szabo[17] tested the neurophysiologic effects on the rat tibia nerve of 20,000 cycles of loading at 1 Hz versus 5 hours of constant hydrostatic loading. The average applied hydrostatic pressure for both types of loading appeared to be the critical predictor of nerve damage, rather than the cyclical loading peak, minimum, or frequency.

Fifth, in humans, similar physiologic changes occur after acute elevation of CTP. A device that applied external pressure over the carpal tunnel was used to compress the median nerve at the wrist in 25 normal humans.[18] The device was adjusted to maintain a constant CTP. Every 10 minutes, nerve conduction, vibrometry, two-point discrimination, and Semmes-Weinstein monofilament tests were conducted. This study revealed a critical threshold of carpal tunnel pressure between 40 and 50 mm Hg for acute nerve dysfunction. The study also provided additional evidence that acute nerve dysfunction is an ischemic process: among nine hypertensive subjects, the critical threshold varied with blood pressure and was approximately 30 mm Hg below the diastolic pressure.

Sixth, crude, chronic nerve compression rat and rabbit models have demonstrated physiologic and histologic changes similar to those seen in human compressive neuropathies.[19] Five months after the loose banding of the rat sciatic nerve, slowing of nerve conduction velocity, perineural thickening, and segmental demyelination were observed.[20] In the rabbit, surgical reduction of the carpal tunnel volume led to edema, vascular proliferation, and fibrosis after 3 weeks.[21]

When taken together, these studies suggest that CTP plays an important role in the pathophysiology of CTS and possibly in finger flexor tenosynovitis. If this is the case, then understanding how musculoskeletal loading and hand postures influence CTP should explain how certain repeated hand activities lead to the development of CTS. In the next sections, the studies linking hand activities to predictable changes in CTP will be reviewed.

Wrist Posture and CTP

Minute to minute variations in CTP are strongly influenced by wrist angle. In 12 normal subjects, Gelberman and associates[2] observed that passive extension or flexion of the wrist caused the CTP to increase on average from 2.5 to 30 mm Hg.[2] A similar, but higher increase in CTP was observed at extremes of wrist extension and flexion in patients with CTS. These findings have been observed by others (Table 1). The differences in CTP levels in the various studies can be ascribed to differences in measurement and task technique (eg, anesthesia, use of patients with paraplegia, forearm in different positions, etc). In spite of these differences, certain patterns emerge. Among both CTS patients and normal subjects, CTP increases by a factor of two to ten with passive flexion or extension.

To extend these findings to typical hand activities, it would be of value to know whether CTP is similarly elevated during active wrist motion and what the relationship is between CTP and wrist angle. To this end, my coworkers and I[22] measured CTP in 20 healthy subjects using a multiperforated, saline-filled catheter, while simultaneously recording wrist posture with an electrogoniometer. The system is unique in that it allows complete freedom of hand movement while the carpal tunnel pressure and wrist angle are monitored continuously. Subjects were instructed to slowly move the wrist throughout the full range of extension and flexion and of ulnar and radial deviation. Data were sampled every 0.25 seconds. When subjects moved their wrists from neutral position to extension or flexion, or to ulnar, or radial deviation, the CTP increased dramatically and repeatably; in some cases up to 180 mm Hg. The average lowest CTP in this healthy population was 7 ± 5 mm Hg. The mean wrist position associated with the lowest pressure was 2° of flexion and 3° of ulnar deviation.

In all subjects, the relationship of carpal tunnel pressure to wrist angle was parabolic, increasing more with greater wrist extension or flexion (Fig. 1). A

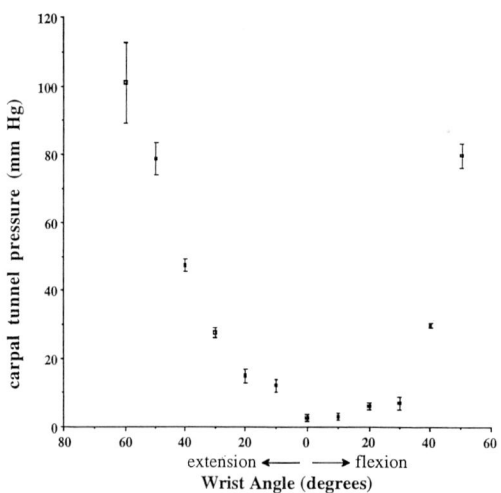

Fig. 1 Example of carpal tunnel pressure as a function of wrist extension-flexion in one healthy subject (error bars represent standard error). (Reproduced with permission from Weiss N, Gordon L, Bloom T, et al: Wrist position of lowest carpal tunnel pressure: Implications for splint design. *J Bone Joint Surg*, in press.)

similar parabolic relationship is observed for ulnar-radial deviation and an example is presented in Figure 2. The parabolic curves were offset up or down with changes in the metacarpophalangeal joint angles of the index and long fingers. Similar but elevated curves were observed in four patients with CTS. The pressures at extremes of wrist posture were consistent with those in the studies summarized in Table 1.

The findings presented in this section provide a potential pathophysiologic link with the epidemiologic studies that show an increased risk of CTS when working with the wrist in a non-neutral position.[23] However, wrist posture is

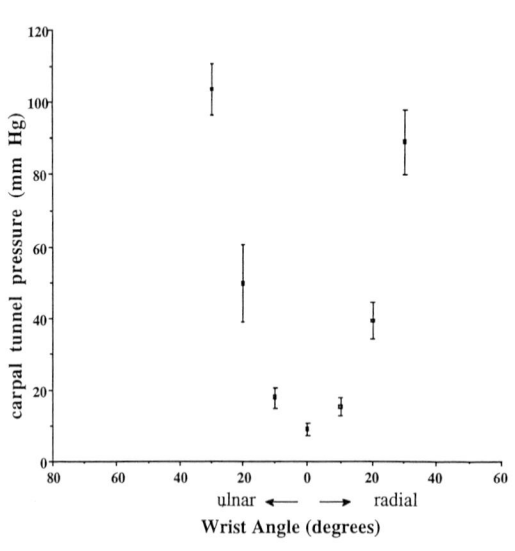

Fig. 2 Example of carpal tunnel pressure as a function of wrist ulnar-radial deviaton in one healthy subject (error bars represent standard error). (Reproduced with permission from Weiss N, Gordon L, Bloom T, et al: Wrist position of lowest carpal tunnel pressure: Implications for splint design. *J Bone Joint Surg*, in press.)

not the only determinant of carpal tunnel pressure. Fingertip and tendon loading also influence pressure.

Tendon Loading and CTP

Repeated grip force and pinch force have been identified as risk factors for activity-related CTS.[24] A possible mechanism linking loading of flexor tendons to damage to the median nerve involves elevations of CTP with fingertip loading. Smith and associates[25] demonstrated that CTP is increased with tendon loading in cadavers. They replaced the median nerve with a balloon pressure transducer and applied 5- and 10-lb static loads to the finger flexor tendons. This loading resulted in elevated pressures of between 30 and 90 mm Hg in the region of the median nerve.

A similar increase in CTP occurs in healthy, live subjects. CTP was measured in 14 subjects while each of them pressed on a load cell with the index finger.[26] The load cell was mounted on a test fixture that allowed for fixed adjustments of the subject's wrist in flexion and extension. The subject was instructed to press down (toward the palm) on the pinch meter with the tip of the index finger to 0, 6, 9, and 12 N force. The other fingers were not loaded. The task was repeated with the wrist in three angles of extension.

With the wrist in 15° of extension, active increase of fingertip loading led to an increase in CTP (Fig. 3). The CTP versus load curves were offset up by constant amounts with increasing wrist deviation from neutral. Elevation of pressure may be due to regional pressure changes in the carpal tunnel due to flexor

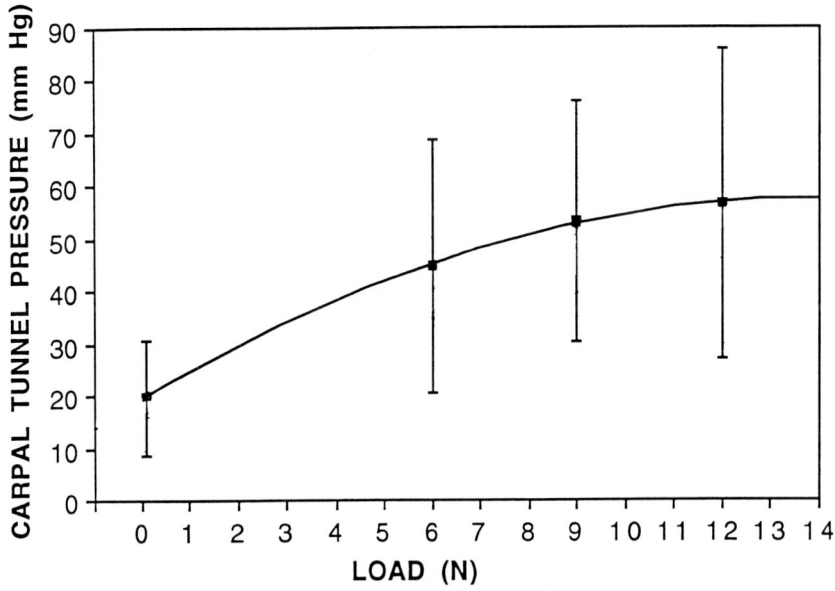

Fig. 3 Relationship of carpal tunnel pressure versus fingertip loading in 14 subjects. The wrist is in the neutral position. Error bars are standard deviation. (Reproduced with permission from Rempel D, Smutz WP, So Y, et al: Effect of fingertip loading on carpal tunnel pressure. *Trans Orthop Res Soc* 1994;19:698.)

tendon loading or changes in the effective volume of the carpal tunnel due to changes of structures, such as the lumbrical muscles, within the carpal tunnel.

Repetitive Hand Activity and CTP

Finally, CTP is elevated and fluctuates dramatically in subjects performing repetitive hand activities. Werner and associates[27] observed that in subjects with CTS, active motion of the wrist and fingers increased CTP more than passive motion. Szabo and Chidgey[9] confirmed that in CTS patients, CTP increases more in response to repetitive passive motion than in normal subjects.

Dynamic changes in CTP occur in normal subjects performing typical repetitive hand tasks. Nineteen subjects were instructed to move 1-lb cans in and out of a box, at the rate of one can every 3 seconds, while CTP and wrist position were monitored in real time.[3] Figure 4 illustrates the fluctuation of CTP in one subject performing this task. The resting baseline pressure of 5 mm Hg rose to a mean of 27 mm Hg during the repetitive task. The mean CTP for the 19 subjects rose from a resting value of 8 mm Hg to a value of 18 mm Hg during the task; this was a significant difference ($p = 0.0003$). In several subjects, the mean pressure during material handling was greater than 30 mm Hg.

A similar rise in CTP has been observed in subjects performing a typing task. The CTP and wrist angles from one subject typing for 2 minutes is shown in Figure 5.[28] The upper curve is the CTP during typing; the lower two curves are wrist posture as tracked by an electrogoniometer. The CTP at rest was near 12 mm Hg but rose to 40 mm Hg during typing. As in the material-handling task, the pressure dropped to its original baseline within seconds of concluding the task.

Although the act of typing, by itself, increases CTP, the mean CTP during typing was strongly influenced by wrist angle. During the experiment, the key-

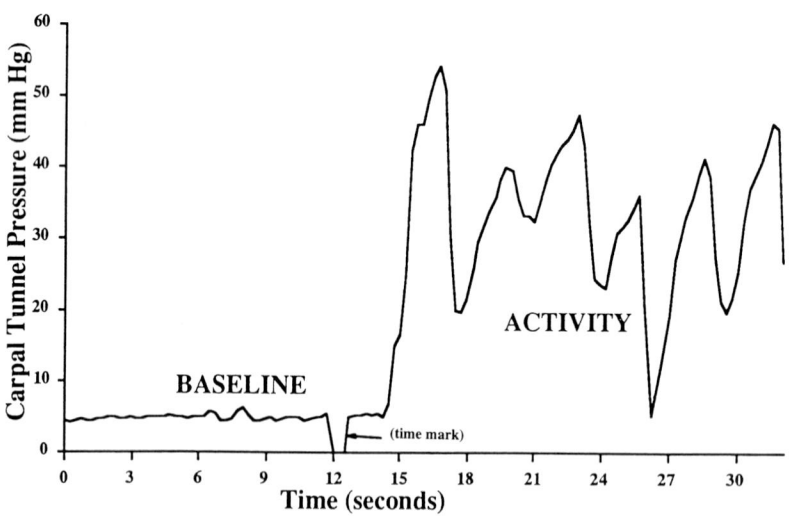

Fig. 4 Carpal tunnel pressure changes in one subject moving 1-lb cans in and out of a box at the rate of one can every 3 seconds. (Reproduced with permission from Rempel D, Manojlovic R, Levinsohn D, et al: The effect of wearing a flexible wrist splint on carpal tunnel pressure during repetitive hand activity. J Hand Surg 1994;19A:106–110.)

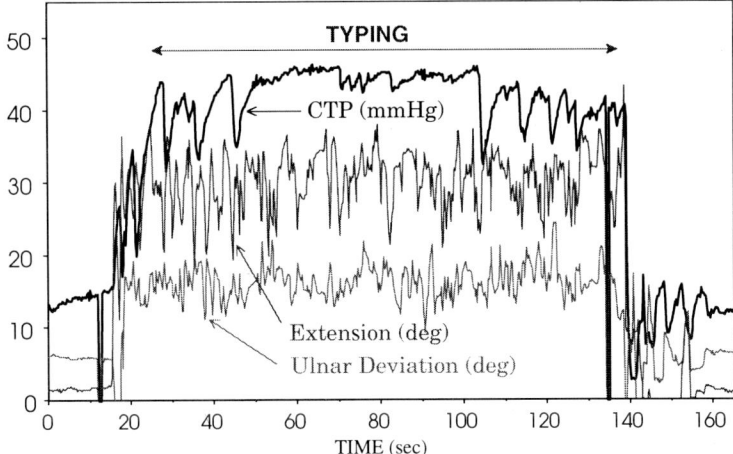

Fig. 5 Carpal tunnel pressure and wrist posture in one subject during typing for a 2-minute period. The upper line is carpal tunnel pressure. The lowest line is wrist extension-flexion angle, the middle line is wrist ulnar/radial deviation as tracked by an electrogoniometer.

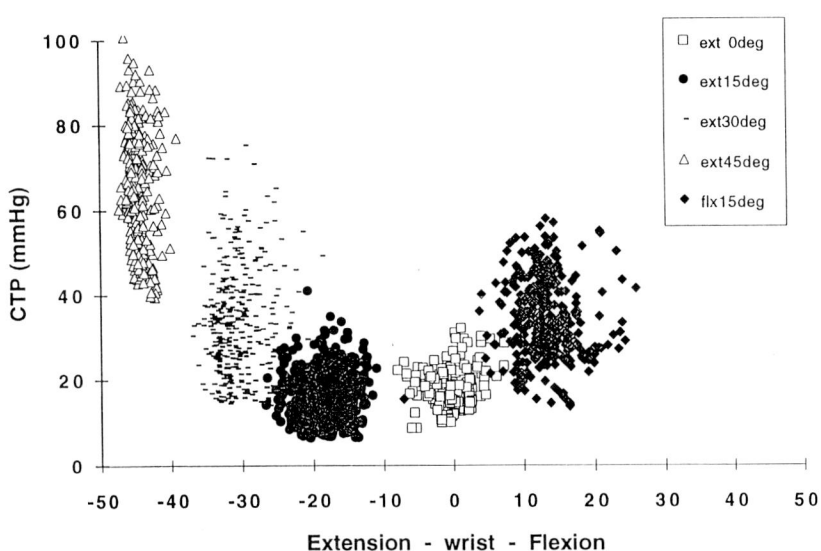

Fig. 6 Carpal tunnel pressure versus wrist angle in one subject during typing. The subject typed with the keyboard adjusted so that the wrist was in five different angles of wrist extension and flexion. Each data "cloud" represents 5 minutes of typing on one keyboard configuration.

board was tilted so that the subject's wrist extension angle was changed. Six subjects typed for 5 minutes each with their wrists at 45°, 30°, 15°, and 0° of extension and 15° of flexion. As shown in Figure 6, the mean pressure for one subject during typing increased dramatically with increasing wrist deviaton from neutral. Each cloud contains the pressure versus wrist angle points sampled during a 5-minute period of typing on one keyboard configuration. In this subject, the mean CTP, when typing with the wrist at 45° of extension, is 60 mm Hg. Figure 7 demonstrates similar findings among the five other subjects studied. The lowest CTP occurred at mean wrist angles of 0° or 15° extension. Many computer operators actually maintain wrist extension angles of 25° to 60° when typing at their workstations.[29]

Conclusion

The median nerve and flexor tendon synovium are exposed to elevated fluid pressure within the carpal tunnel during repetitive hand activities. Among normal subjects the resting CTP is low, and even when the pressure is elevated during hand activity it returns rapidly to a low level after task completion.[2,30] On the other hand, after CTS patients complete a similar task, the CTP returns to its elevated "resting" pressure more slowly.[9] The changes in tissue structure and function leading to this difference in the handling of tissue pressure and fluid movement may involve an ischemic process.

The pressure increase to which the median nerve is exposed during activity, although it is of a low level, is great enough to reduce the flow of blood in the epineurial venules.[7,10,14] Prolonged disturbances of venule microcirculation can produce retrograde effects on the capillary circulation, resulting in anoxic injury to endothelial cells, subsequent increase in vascular permeability, and endoneurial and synovial edema. Because there are no lymphatics within the median nerve through which this fluid can drain, the excess fluid in the endoneurium or the tendon synovium is not easily dissipated and may ultimately affect fiber function.

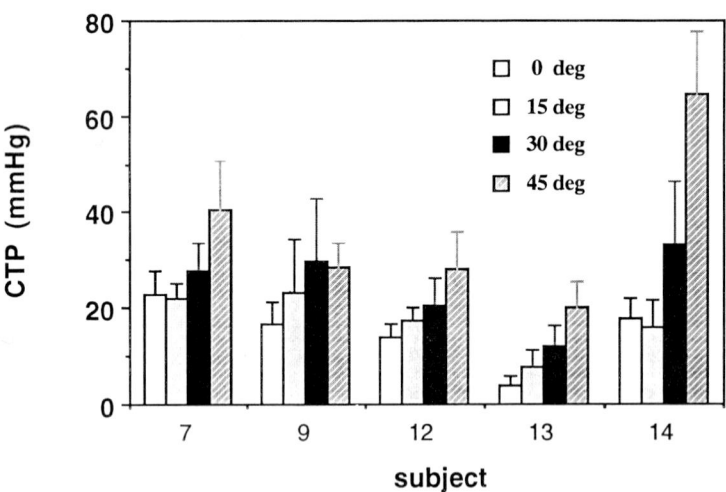

Fig. 7 Carpal tunnel pressure versus wrist angle for five subjects in a study. Each column represents mean pressure during a 5-minute typing task at that wrist angle.

The rate of this process would be controlled by the duration and degree of ischemia, the sensitivity of the tissues to ischemia, and the rate of transfer of tissue fluids. Any factors (eg, activity, anatomic, fluid retention) that prevent the usual return of CTP to a low level during the course of the day may prolong disturbances of microcirculation and lead to epineurial edema. Tasks that require the wrist to be in an extreme position for long periods of time maintain CTP at a high level and may produce this effect.

Animal and human data suggest that repeated and prolonged elevations of CTP may play a role in the pathophysiology of CTS, although a direct link has not been proven. A dose-response, parabolic relationship exists between CTP and wrist angle; the greater the wrist deviation from neutral, the greater the CTP. In addition, a dose-response relationship between CTP and fingertip loading has been demonstrated. Finally, repetitive hand and finger activities can lead to a rise in CTP, and this relationship is strongly influenced by mean wrist angle.

Acknowledgments

Some of the work presented was supported by CDC-NIOSH grant no. K01OH00121-01.

References

1. Tanzer RC: The carpal-tunnel syndrome: A clinical and anatomical study. *J Bone Joint Surg* 1959;41A:626–634.
2. Gelberman RH, Hergenroeder PT, Hargens AR, et al: The carpal tunnel syndrome: A study of carpal canal pressures. *J Bone Joint Surg* 1981;63A:380–383.
3. Rempel D, Manojlovic R, Levinsohn D, et al: The effect of wearing a flexible wrist splint on carpal tunnel pressure during repetitive hand activity. *J Hand Surg* 1994;19A:106–110.
4. Luchetti R, Schoenhuber R, De Cicco G, et al: Carpal-tunnel pressure. *Acta Orthop Scand* 1989;60:397–399.
5. Lundborg G: The intrinsic vascularization of human peripheral nerves: Structure and functional aspects. *J Hand Surg* 1979;4A:34–41.
6. Lundborg G, Gelberman RH, Minteer-Convery M, et al: Median nerve compression in the carpal tunnel: Functional response to experimentally induced controlled pressure. *J Hand Surg* 1982;7A: 252–259.
7. Rydevik B, Lundborg G, Bagge U: Effects of graded compression on intraneural blood flow: An in vivo study on rabbit tibial nerve. *J Hand Surg* 1981;6A:3–12.
8. Sunderland S: The nerve lesion in the carpal tunnel syndrome. *J Neurol Neurosurg Psych* 1976;39:615–626.
9. Szabo RM, Chidgey LK: Stress carpal tunnel pressures in patients with carpal tunnel syndrome and normal patients. *J Hand Surg* 1989;14A:624–627.
10. Gelberman RH, Rydevik BL, Pess GM, et al: Carpal tunnel syndrome: A scientific basis for clinical care. *Orthop Clin North Am* 1988;19:115–124.
11. Yamaguchi DM, Lipscomb PR, Soule EH: Carpal tunnel syndrome. *Minn Med* 1965;48:22–33.
12. Fuchs PC, Nathan PA, Myers LD: Synovial histology in carpal tunnel syndrome. *J Hand Surg* 1991;16A:753–758.
13. Scelsi R, Zanlungo M, Tenti P: Carpal tunnel syndrome: Anatomical and clinical correlations and morphological and ultrastructural aspects of the tenosynovial sheath. *Ital J Orthop Traumatol* 1989;15:75–80.
14. Dahlin LB, Nordborg C, Lundborg G: Morphologic changes in nerve cell bodies induced by experimental graded nerve compression. *Exper Neurol* 1987;95:611–621.

15. Hargens AR, Akeson WH, Mubarak SJ, et al: Fluid balance within the canine anterolateral compartment and its realtionship to compartment syndromes. *J Bone Joint Surg* 1978;60A:499–505.
16. Szabo RM, Sharkey NA, Foerster BV: Effects of acute nerve compression evaluated in a rat tibial nerve model. *Trans Orthop Res Soc* 1991;16:683.
17. Szabo RM: Pathophysiologic and clinical factors in cumulative trauma of the upper extremity. Presented at the 61st Annual Meeting of the American Academy of Orthopaedic Surgeons, New Orleans, Louisiana, February 24, 1994.
18. Gelberman RH, Szabo RM, Williamson RV, et al: Tissue pressure threshold for peripheral nerve viability. *Clin Orthop* 1983;178:285–291.
19. Mackinnon SE, Dellon AL, Hudson AR, et al: Chronic human nerve compression: A histological assessment. *Neuropath Appl Neurobiol* 1986;12:547–565.
20. O'Brien JP, Mackinnon SE, MacLean AR, et al: A model of chronic nerve compression in the rat. *Ann Plastic Surg* 1987;19:430–435.
21. Lluch AL: Thickening of the synovium of the digital flexor tendons: Cause or consequence of the carpal tunnel syndrome? *J Hand Surg* 1992;17B:209–212.
22. Weiss N, Gordon L, Bloom T, et al: Wrist postion of lowest carpal tunnel pressure: Implications for splint design. *J Bone Joint Surg*, in press.
23. de Krom MC, Kester AD, Knipschild PG, et al: Risk factors for carpal tunnel syndrome. *Am J Epidemiol* 1990;132:1102–1110.
24. Silverstein BA, Fine LJ, Armstrong TJ: Occupational factors and carpal tunnel syndrome. *Am J Ind Med* 1987;11:343–358.
25. Smith EM, Sonstegard DA, Anderson WH Jr: Carpal tunnel syndrome: Contribution of flexor tendons. *Arch Phys Med Rehabil* 1977;58:379–385.
26. Rempel D, Smutz WP, So Y, et al: Effect of fingertip loading on carpal tunnel pressure. *Trans Orthop Res Soc* 1994;19:698.
27. Werner CO, Elmqvist D, Ohlin P: Pressure and nerve lesion in the carpal tunnel. *Acta Orthop Scand* 1983;54:312–316.
28. Rempel D, Horie S: Effect of wrist posture during typing on carpal tunnel pressure, in Grieco A, Molteni G, Occhipinti E, et al (eds): *Proceedings of Work with Display Units: Fourth International Scientific Conference*. Milan, Italy, 1994, pp 27–28.
29. Sauter SL, Schleifer LM, Knutson SJ: Work posture, workstation design, and musculoskeletal discomfort in a VDT data entry task. *Human Factors* 1991;33:151–167.
30. Graham B, Adkins P, Kutz JE: Dynamic carpal tunnel pressures in actively exercising workers. *Proc Am Soc Surg Hand* 1991;16:3–4.
31. Okutsu I, Ninomiya S, Hamanaka I, et al: Measurement of pressure in the carpal canal before and after endoscopic management of carpal tunnel syndrome. *J Bone Joint Surg* 1989;71A:679–683.
32. Rojviroj S, Sirichativapee W, Kowsuwon W, et al: Pressures in the carpal tunnel: A comparison between patients with carpal tunnel syndrome and normal subjects. *J Bone Joint Surg* 1990;72B:516–518.

Chapter 10
The Relationship Between Upper Limb Load Posture and Tissue Loads at the Elbow

Kai-Nan An, PhD
William P. Cooney III, MD
Bernard F. Morrey, MD

Introduction

Throughout the literature, repetitive motion disorders have been defined imprecisely and identified under a variety of names, such as repetitive stress syndrome, overuse syndrome, repetitive strain injury, and cumulative trauma disorder. This diversity of terminology suggests that the pathology underlying the condition is, at best, poorly understood. Specific disorders, however, are generally believed to arise from a summation of mechanical loads applied beyond the tolerance of the biologic tissues. Repetitive motion disorders are most prominent among performers and athletes whose professions demand exceptionally long and vigorous practices for them to achieve a high level of performance.

In the elbow joint, such painful disorders appear in all tissue types[1] (Table 1). This chapter reviews the mechanical loads associated with these disorders. In general, the loads across the elbow joint consist of muscle and joint forces encountered in normal activities, valgus and varus stresses, axial compressive forces, as well as wrist and forearm muscles loads.

Table 1 Repetitive motion disorders in the elbow joint

Tissue Type	Disorder Manifestation
Osseous	Angular change; hypertrophy
Articular	Degenerative arthrosis; loose body; spur; osteophyte in the olecranon; osteochondritis dissecans
Synovial	Reactive synovitis and effusion
Ligamentous	Collateral ligament tear; stretch; calcification
Tendon	Epicondylitis; distal biceps and triceps rupture
Muscular	Myofascitis and hypertrophy; compartment syndrome in anconeus
Bursae	Radiobicipital and olecranon inflammation
Nerve	Cubital tunnel entrapment

Anatomy

A brief review of elbow anatomy[2] is useful for the discussion of the associated repetitive motion disorders. The distal humerus comprises two condyles, which form the articular surfaces of the trochlea and capitellum, that articulate with the proximal ulna and radius at the elbow joint (Fig. 1). Proximal to the trochlea, the prominent medial epicondyle serves as a source of attachment for the ulnar collateral ligament as well as the hand flexor and forearm pronator muscle groups. The lateral epicondyle serves as the attachment for the lateral collateral ligaments as well as the hand extensor and forearm supinator muscle group (Fig. 2).

The proximal radius consists of the radial head, with a depression in the mid portion, which articulates with the capitellum. The radial tuberosity, located distally to the head and neck of the radius, is the source of attachment of the biceps tendon. Anterior and covering the attachment is the bicipitoradial bursa, which protects the tendon during full pronation.

The proximal ulna provides the primary articulation and stability of the elbow. The sigmoid notch articulates with the trochlea of the humerus. The anterior and distal aspect of the notch is composed of the coronoid process, which provides the anterior articulating surface of the humeroulnar joint and is the insertion site of the brachialis muscle. The olecranon, comprising the proximal aspect of the notch, provides the posterior articulation of the humeroulnar joint and is the site of the triceps tendon. The most proximal tip is protected from the tendon by the subtendinous bursa (Fig. 3).

On the anterior aspect of the distal humerus, the radial fossa and coronoid fossa accommodate the radial head and coronoid process during full elbow flexion. Posteriorly, the olecranon fossa receives the olecranon during full extension of the elbow joint.

The three major flexors of the elbow are the biceps, brachialis, and brachioradialis. The biceps is the major flexor with a large physiologic cross-sectional area (4.6 cm^2) and a moderated mechanical advantage (20 mm to 40 mm).[3] The brachialis muscle has the largest physiologic cross-sectional area (7.0 cm^2)

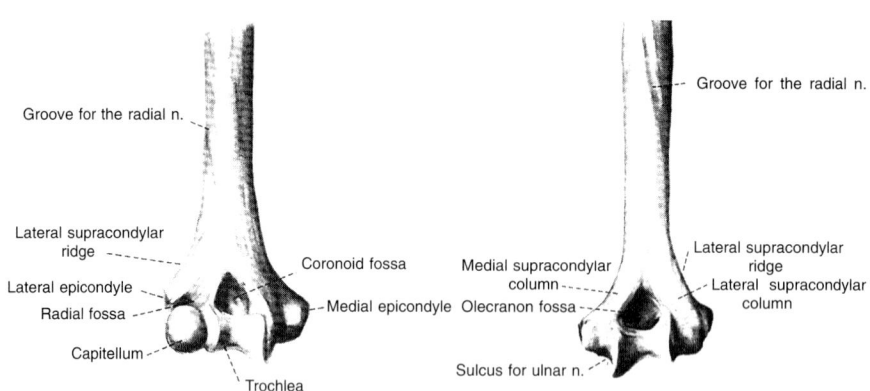

Fig. 1 Left, The bony landmarks of the anterior aspect of the distal humerus. **Right,** The prominent medial and lateral supracondylar bony columns as well as other landmarks of the posterior aspect of the distal humerus. (Reproduced with permission from Morrey BF: Anatomy of the elbow joint, in Morrey BF (ed): *The Elbow and Its Disorders*, ed 2. Philadelphia, PA, WB Saunders, 1993, pp 16–52).

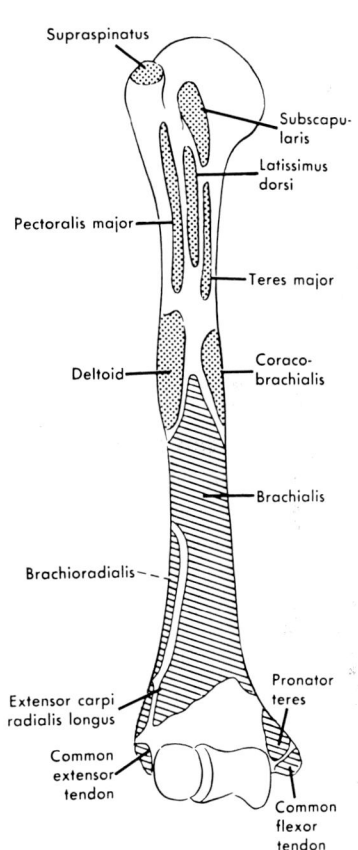

Fig. 2 Anterior humeral origin and insertion of muscles that control the elbow joint. (Reproduced with permission from Morrey BF: Anatomy of the elbow joint, in Morrey BF (ed): *The Elbow and Its Disorders*, ed 2. Philadelphia, PA, WB Saunders, 1993, pp 16–52).

but a poor mechanical advantage (15 mm to 33 mm). The brachioradialis is the minor flexor, which has the least physiologic cross-sectional area (1.5 cm^2). The triceps brachii and anconeus are the two major extensors of the elbow. The physiologic cross-sectional area of the three heads of the triceps combined is relatively large (19 cm^2). In addition to these major elbow flexors and extensors, the wrist and hand muscles that cross the elbow joint also provide flexion (flexor carpi radialis and ulnaris) and extension (extensor carpi radialis and ulnaris, and flexor digitorum superficialis).

Muscle and Joint Forces in Elbow Function

Studying the force across the elbow joint is a difficult task. Several analyses of varying degrees of sophistication have been performed.[4–9] In sagittal plane motion, the elbow joint is assumed to be a hinge joint. Forces and moments at the joint, which result from the loads applied at the hand or distal forearm, are balanced by the muscles, tendons, ligaments, and contact forces on the articular surfaces (Fig. 4). Based on a free body analysis, equilibrium equations have been developed for such force calculation. For static balance of weight in the hand or at the distal forearm, the muscle and joint forces have been estimated

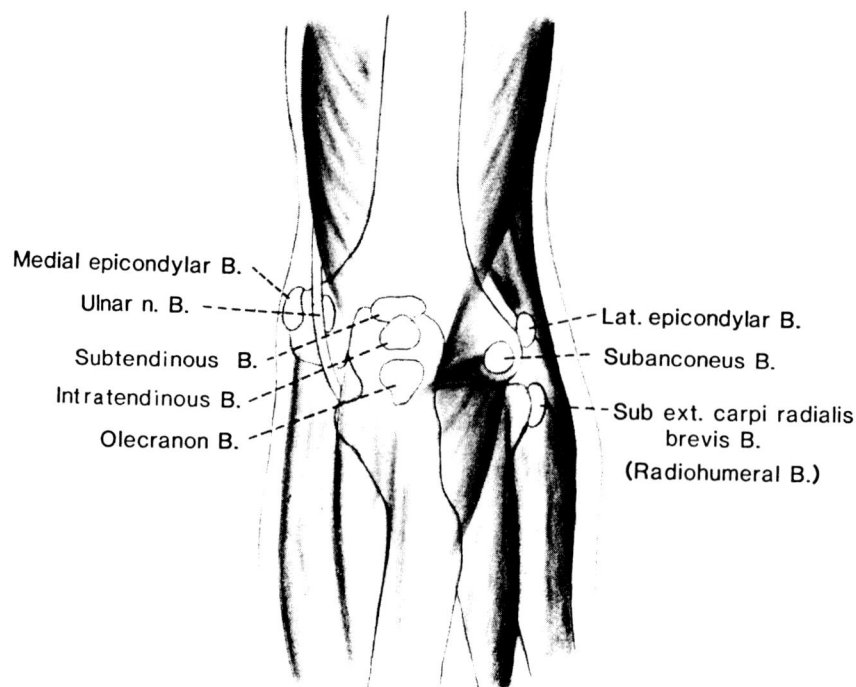

Fig. 3 Posterior view of the elbow demonstrating the superficial and deep bursae that are present about this joint. (Reproduced with permission from Morrey BF: Anatomy of the elbow joint, in Morrey BF (ed): *The Elbow and Its Disorders*, ed 2. Philadelphia, PA, WB Saunders, 1993, pp 16–52).

in the unit of the weight (Table 2). When lifting a 10 N weight in the hand, 20-, 40-, and 8-N forces are expected in the biceps, brachialis, and brachioradialis, respectively. The corresponding joint force could be in the range of 60 N. In laboratory tests, the maximum flexion strengths of the elbow with the weight at the wrist level are in the range of 90 to 150 N at 0° flexion, 110 to 190 N at 30° of flexion, 220 to 383 N at 90° of flexion, and 178 to 307 N at 120° of flexion. Under these strenuous lifting conditions, muscle forces as high as two times the body weight, and joint forces up to four times the body weight, are expected.[9]

Under high-speed forearm movement, inertial loads are generated at the elbow joint. In laboratory tests, the maximal speed of flexion and extension of the forearm throughout the full range of movement was analyzed.[5] For movements lasting 0.25 seconds, angular velocity of 18 radians/s and angular accelerations of 570 radians/s² were observed. During an experiment testing abrupt arrest, deceleration could occur in the range of 1,100 radians/s². However, analysis of the joint forces during these actions suggested that the articulations were not subjected to forces beyond those seen during maximal isometric efforts.

Valgus-Varus Stress

Given its anatomic design, the elbow joint allows only flexion-extension and forearm pronation-supination motion. Rotation in the frontal plane for valgus or varus motion is not possible for a normal intact elbow. The passive struc-

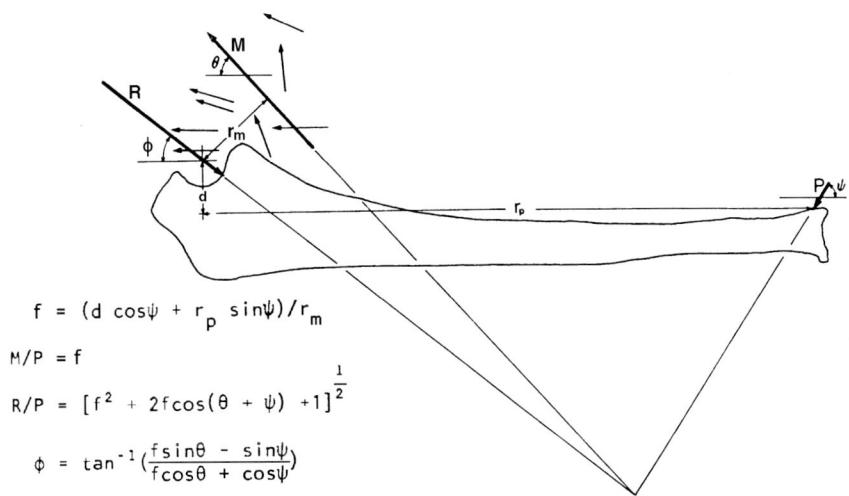

Fig. 4 Free-body diagram of isolated forearm. External force P applied at r_p from the joint center with an angle of y to the ulnar axis. Combined muscle force M has moment arm r_m and is oriented with the ulnar axis. The resultant force R is oriented with the ulnar axis by an angle. All forces applied to the ulna are under equilibrium conditions. (Reproduced with permission from An KN, Morrey BF: Biomechanics of the elbow, in Morrey BF (ed): *The Elbow and Its Disorders*, ed 2. Philadelphia, PA, WB Saunders, 1993, pp 53–72.)

$$f = (d\cos\psi + r_p \sin\psi)/r_m$$

$$M/P = f$$

$$R/P = [f^2 + 2f\cos(\theta + \psi) + 1]^{\frac{1}{2}}$$

$$\phi = \tan^{-1}\left(\frac{f\sin\theta - \sin\psi}{f\cos\theta + \cos\psi}\right)$$

tures responsible for resisting valgus-varus stress have been extensively examined. For resisting the valgus stress, the medial collateral ligament (MCL) is the primary stabilizer and the radial head is the secondary stabilizer. The anterior band of the MCL stabilizes the joint throughout nearly the entire range of elbow flexion. The posterior band is usually less important at the range of full extension. The anterior capsule, although quite thin, provides resistance to valgus and varus stress at full extension of the elbow joint.[9]

The lateral radial collateral ligament is generally responsible for resisting varus stress. More recently, the importance of the lateral ulnar collateral ligament in preventing posterolateral instability has been recognized. The contribution of articular geometry to elbow stability has also been examined. With the elbow in extended position, or at 90° of flexion, valgus stress was resisted

Table 2 Muscle and joint force in resisting load on the distal forearm

Joint Flexion (°)	Muscles (in the unit of external applied forces)			Joint Forces
	Biceps	Brachialis	Brachioradialis	
0°	0.12	0.19	0.04	1.17
30°	1.43	2.18	0.47	3.89
60°	2.35	3.58	0.77	5.89
90°	2.65	4.03	0.86	6.31
120°	2.23	3.39	0.73	5.10
150°	1.22	1.85	0.40	2.60

primarily (75% to 85%) by the proximal half of the sigmoid notch; whereas, the varus stress was resisted primarily by the distal half or the coronoid portion of the articulation.[10]

The valgus-varus moment could not be generated actively by the major elbow flexors and extensors as confirmed by strength and electromyographic measurements.[11] With the elbow at 90° of flexion, the internal and external shoulder rotations generated corresponding 25- and 17-N•m adduction and abduction moments at the elbow. Under such strenuous valgus and varus stresses, the electromyographic signals of the major elbow muscles are relatively quiet, with the exception of the anconeus muscle.[11] However, oppositional force due to normal muscle contraction may help the congruent elbow joint resist any passive valgus and varus moment at the joint during upper extremity movements.[10]

Athletes participating in overhead or throwing sports place repetitious high valgus stress on the medial aspect of the elbow joint.[12–15] During throwing motion, the acceleration phase of the arm begins with the elbow in a flexed position between 90° and 120°, followed by rapid extension to 25° of flexion as the ball is released. This event usually takes place over 30 to 40 milliseconds.[13] The average angular velocity over this arc of motion has been estimated to exceed 5,000°/s, with peak angular acceleration of 500,000°/s^2.[14] An average of 100 to 120 N•m of varus torque is needed to prevent the forearm from rotating in the valgus direction at the point of maximum shoulder external rotation.[15,16] A peak valgus torque, preventing rotation in the varus direction, occurs shortly after the ball is released.[15]

Can this excessive amount of valgus stress be resisted by the passive capsuloligamentous structures in conjunction with the congruent joint articulating surfaces? In the previous study, the failure loads of the anterior and posterior bands of the MCL were found to be 260 N and 159 N, respectively.[17] This ligament failure strength implies that a maximum valgus stress at the elbow joint should be in the range of 28 N•m. In a recent study, the ultimate torque to failure of the elbow under valgus stress was found to average 33 N•m (WP Smutz, EP France, SP Kupferman, et al, personal communication, 1994). If the estimated valgus stress in baseball pitching is correct, the strength of the static structure could resist only one third to one fourth of the valgus stress across the joint. Therefore, the contribution of the congruent joint surface under the compressive force of muscle contraction must likely play an important role as demonstrated by the electromyographic activities of the triceps, wrist flexor-pronator, and anconeus muscles.[15,18] In general, it is believed that the valgus stress during overhead throwing should at least produce microscopic tears within the ligaments. Continuous throwing can lead to attenuation or rupture of the weakened ligament.[12]

Repetitive valgus stress could also result in compression injury to the articular surface.[19] Osseous manifestations of repetitive elbow stress consist of bony hypertrophy, loose bodies, osteophytes, traction spur formation, and osteochondral defects.[20] Impingement of the medial tip of the olecranon on the medial wall of the olecranon fossa may result in synovitis, osteophytes, and loose bodies.[19]

Load Induced by Wrist and Hand Muscles

Several flexors and extensors of the wrist and hand originate from the distal humerus. The force generated on these muscles and tendons, therefore, may cause disorder at the elbow joint. Lateral epicondylitis, or tennis elbow, is the most common elbow affliction in adults. The precise pathology of the condition is debated, with as many as 14 pathologic features reported in the literature (W Regan, LE Wold, JR Coonrad, et al, unpublished data, 1989). In general, the lateral tendinitis primarily involves the origin and the muscle-tendon junction of the extensor carpi radialis brevis. Occasionally, the anterior edges of the extensor digitorum communis and the underside of the extensor carpi radialis longus are also involved, and the origin of the extensor carpi ulnaris is rarely involved.[21]

The tension in the extensor carpi radialis brevis muscle generates either wrist extension or resists wrist flexion torque. Based on a biomechanical model, it has been shown that grasping and pinching always cause a flexion moment at the wrist joint. To avoid flexion, there must be equilibrium of moments, which is attained by activity of the extensor muscles.[22] In grasp and pinch, the extensor carpi radialis brevis and longus and extensor digitorum communis are all active. The effect of preimpact hand forces and impact location on the postimpact force loading on the hand in the tennis forehand drive was examined by using force sensing resistor and strain gauges.[23]

The forces on the base of the index finger and on the lower hypothenar eminence show a consistent inverse relationship. About 50 milliseconds prior to impact the hypothenar force increased in preparation for ball impact. Postimpact (40 to 50 milliseconds after impact) peak forces on the base of the index finger were variable but recorded up to 214 N. The hand grip strength has been found to be a function of the object size as well as the posture of the wrist joint. For a given size of object, there is an optimal wrist position for maximum grip strength (Fig. 5).[24] In general, the larger the handle of the device, the better the leverage for controlling the torsion of the racket. However, for better grip, the proper circumference for the handle has been found to be the distance from the mid palmar crease to the distal ring finger (Fig. 6).[25]

The backhand stroke, which results in a tremendous wrist flexion moment, most commonly is associated with tennis elbow. A late backhand stroke and off-center racquet contact are the two basic stresses leading to tennis elbow.[26]

The tensile strengths of the bone-tendon unit of the common extensor and flexor tendons have recently been measured to average 1,000 and 1,920 N, respectively (JS Han, J Ryu, personal communication, 1994). These data, combined with the load data, could provide information in regards to potential microscopic tissue damage.

Axial Loading

With the elbow extended and axially loaded, the distribution of the stress across the joint has been calculated to be approximately 40% across the ulnohumeral joint and 60% across the radiohumeral articulation.[27,28] In addition, contraction of the biceps creates great axial force on the radial head, especially at the extended elbow.[29] The greatest force transmitted to the radial head occurs with the forearm in pronation when the interosseous membrane is relatively lax. However, in this position, the maximum possible force transmitted to the radiohumeral joint was measured as approximately 0.9 times body weight.[29]

In a military push-up, peak forces exerted on the elbow joint along the forearm axis averaged 45% of the body weight when the hands were placed directly under the shoulder. Axial forces were significantly decreased when the hands were positioned either apart from or superior to the normal position.[30] During swing-through axillary crutch gait, moments and axial forces at the elbow joint were found to be significant.[31] Changing gait speed significantly af-

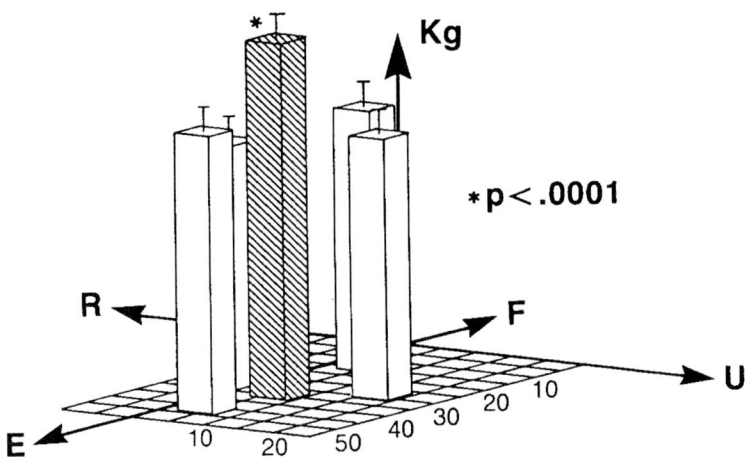

Fig. 5 Mean (± SE) grip strengths in self-selected positions (hatched bar) and positions of deviation (shown in °) into flexion (F), extension (E), and radial (R) and ulnar (U) deviation. Grip strengths were significantly lower in each of the deviated positions than in the self-selected position. (Reproduced with permission from O'Driscoll SW, Horii E, Ness R, et al: The relationship between wrist position, grasp size, and grip strength. J Hand Surg 1992;17:169–177.)

fected the load transmission at the hand and elbow. Changing handle position significantly affected the moment at the elbow. Increasing the elbow flexion angle by raising the crutch handle resulted in a significant increase in elbow flexion moment as well.[31] Video and force plate analysis of young female gymnasts showed that the elbow joint flexed during the double-arm support phase of the back handspring and the reaction forces at the hand produced a large compressive force that averaged 2.37 times body weight and sizeable valgus moments at the elbow joint that averaged 0.03 times body weight times height.[32] The combination of compressive forces and total number of repetitions resulted in lateral compressive injuries, such as osteochondritis dissecans of the capitellum. The etiology of the bone lesion is believed to be vascular insufficiency.[33,34] One interesting suggestion is that compressive forces at the radiocapitellar joint produce focal arterial injury and subsequent bone death.[19] In gymnastics, the upper extremities are used as weightbearing limbs, and the repetitive, high-impact loads on the elbow and wrist provide more opportunity for chronic injuries.[35]

Tendon Loading and Biologic Response

Various types of pathologies and disorders often develop as a result of cumulative loading and repetitive motion. In general, muscles, tendons, and ligaments provide and transmit tensile forces. However, transverse compressive and frictional forces on the surfaces of these tissues are encountered as the paths of these tissues (tendons, muscles, and ligaments) change direction when wrapping around bony structure or a pulley. The magnitudes of these forces are influenced significantly by the magnitude and direction of external loading and

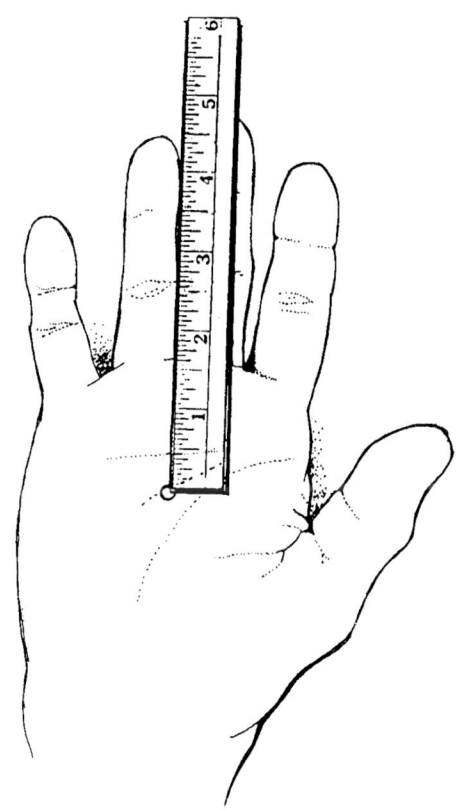

Fig. 6 Author's method of determining proper racket grip size. (Reproduced with permission from Nirschl RP: Sports and overuse injuries to the elbow, in Morrey BF (ed): *The Elbow and Its Disorders*, ed 2. Philadelphia, PA, WB Saunders, 1993, pp 537–552.)

joint posture. The relationship of these forces to the potential development of soft-tissue disorders has been postulated.

Due to the relative short lever arms of the muscles and tendons as compared to that of external loading on the upper limb, the forces required to balance the joint are in the range of two to five times that of the external loadings. For example, during strenuous tip pinch the tension in the flexor tendons can range from 100 to 250 N.[36] This amount of tension represents only 10% to 20% of the ultimate strength of the associated tendon,[37] which can be considered to be relatively safe from possible gross rupture. However, this amount of tension could put the tendon at the end of the toe region and at the beginning of the linear region on the force-elongation curve. Micro damage of the collagen bundles, or even of the interwoven links, could be possible. Such accumulated trauma could evoke biologic and inflammatory responses, leading to disorders such as tendinitis.

As the tendon changes its path, transverse compressive forces develop between the tendon and the surrounding tissues. The amount of compressive force is approximately equal to twice the tension in the tendon multiplied by the sine of half the angle of the changing tendon direction. When the tendon is running straight, the angle is zero and the transverse force on the tendon is equal to zero. In the case where the tendon is bent 90° during finger joint flexion, the transverse force could be as high as 1.732 times the tendon tension. Stress analysis of tendons under such loading has shown that the hydrostatic compressive stress and distortional strain in the region correlate to the formation of cartilaginous and fibrous matrix.[38] The fibrocartilaginous zone developed in the tendon may represent the functional adaption to the compressive load.[39] Such fibrocartilaginous transformation might also be the trigger leading to the calcifying tendinitis of the rotator cuff tendon in the shoulder.[40]

When the tendon glides through the pulley, friction is encountered at the interface. This friction between the pulley and tendon has been postulated to be related to cumulative trauma disorders.[41,42] Again, the magnitude of friction was found to be proportional to the magnitude of the tendon tension and the angle of contact between the tendon and pulley.[43] With increasing joint angles during flexion or extension, the angle of the tendon path increased, as did the friction force. In addition, repetitive motion would further cause irritation at the interface due to friction. Such irritation, again, could evoke a series of biologic responses of the tendon sheath and surrounding synovial tissue and eventually lead to soft-tissue disorders such as tenosynovitis.

Summary

In general, the load environment experienced by the soft tissues in the upper extremity can be complex and is significantly influenced by the external loading and joint configuration. Biologic reaction in response to each of the specific types of loadings could lead to certain pathologies of repetitive motion syndromes.

References

1. Berger RA: Overuse syndrome of the elbow, in Morrey BF (ed): *The Elbow and Its Disorders*, ed 2. Philadelphia, PA, WB Saunders, 1993, pp 604–609.
2. Morrey BF: Anatomy of the elbow joint, in Morrey BF (ed): *The Elbow and Its Disorders*, ed 2. Philadelphia, PA, WB Saunders, 1993, pp 16–52.
3. An KN, Hui FC, Morrey BF, et al: Muscles across the elbow joint: A biomechanical analysis. *J Biomech* 1981;14:659–669.
4. Amis AA, Dowson D, Wright V: Elbow joint force predictions for some strenuous isometric actions. *J Biomech* 1980;13:765–775.
5. Amis AA, Dowson D, Wright V: Analysis of elbow forces due to high-speed forearm movements. *J Biomech* 1980;13:825–831.
6. An KN, Kwak BM, Chao EY, et al: Determination of muscle and joint forces: A new technique to solve the indeterminate problem. *J Biomech Eng* 1984;106: 364–367.
7. An KN, Kaufman KR, Chao EY: Physiological considerations of muscle force through the elbow joint. *J Biomech* 1989;22:1249–1256.
8. An KN, Himeno S, Tsumura H, et al: Pressure distribution on articular surfaces: Application to joint stability evaluation. *J Biomech* 1990;23:1013–1020.
9. An KN, Morrey BF: Biomechanics of the elbow, in Morrey BF (ed): *The Elbow And Its Disorders*, ed 2. Philadelphia, PA, WB Saunders, 1993, pp 53–72.
10. An KN, Morrey BF, Chao EY: The effect of partial removal of proximal ulna on elbow constraint. *Clin Orthop* 1986;209:270–279.
11. Funk DA, An KN, Morrey BF, et al: Electromyographic analysis of muscle across the elbow joint. *J Orthop Res* 1987;5:529–538.
12. Jobe FW, Stark H, Lombardo SJ: Reconstruction of the ulnar collateral ligament in athletes. *J Bone Joint Surg* 1986;68A:1158–1163.
13. Jobe FW, Elattrache NS: Diagnosis and treatment of ulnar collateral ligament injuries in athletes, in Morrey BF (ed): *The Elbow and Its Disorders*, ed 2. Philadelphia, PA, WB Saunders, 1993, pp 566–570.
14. Pappas AM, Zawacki RM, Sullivan TJ: Biomechanics of baseball pitching: A preliminary report. *Am J Sports Med* 1985;13:216–222.

15. Werner SL, Fleisig GS, Dillman CJ, et al: Biomechanics of the elbow during baseball pitching. *J Orthop Sports Phys Ther* 1993;17:274–278.
16. Feltner M, Dapena J: Dynamics of the shoulder and elbow joints of the throwing arm during a baseball pitch. *Int J Sport Biomechanics* 1986;2:235–259.
17. Regan WD, Korinek SL, Morrey BF, et al: Biomechanical study of ligaments around the elbow joint. *Clin Orthop* 1991;271:170–179.
18. DiGiovine NM, Jobe FW, Pink M, et al: An electromyographic analysis of the upper extremity in pitching. *J Shoulder Elbow Surg* 1992;1:15–25.
19. Bennett JB: Articular injuries in the athlete, in Morrey BF (ed): *The Elbow And Its Disorders*, ed 2. Philadelphia, PA, WB Saunders, 1993, pp 581–595.
20. Gore RM, Rogers LF, Bowerman J, et al: Osseous manifestations of elbow stress associated with sports activities. *AJR* 1980;134,971–977.
21. Nirschl RP: Muscle and tendon trauma: Tennis elbow, in Morrey BF (ed): *The Elbow and Its Disorders*, ed 2. Philadelphia, PA, WB Saunders, 1993, pp 537–552.
22. Snijders CJ, Volkers AC, Mechelse K, et al: Provocation of epicondylalgia lateralis (tennis elbow) by power grip or pinching. *Med Sci Sports Exerc* 1987;19:518–523.
23. Knudson DV: Factors affecting force loading on the hand in the tennis forehand. *J Sports Med Phys Fitness* 1991;31:527–531.
24. O'Driscoll SW, Horii E, Ness R, et al: The relationship between wrist position, grasp size, and grip strength. *J Hand Surg* 1992;17A:169–177.
25. Nirschl RP: Tennis elbow. *Orthop Clin North Am* 1973;4:787–800.
26. Schnatz P, Steiner C: Tennis elbow: A biomechanical and therapeutic approach. *J Am Osteopath Assoc* 1993;93:778–788.
27. Halls AA, Travill A: Transmission of pressures across the elbow joint. *Anat Rec* 1964;150:243–247.
28. Walker PS (ed): Laxity, flexibility and stability, in *Human Joints and Their Artificial Replacements*. Springfield IL, Charles C. Thomas, 1977, pp 167–210.
29. Morrey BF, An KN, Stormont TJ: Force transmission through the radial head. *J Bone Joint Surg* 1988;70A:250–256.
30. Donkers MJ, An KN, Chao EY, et al: Hand position affects elbow joint load during push-up exercise. *J Biomech* 1993;26:625–632.
31. Reisman M, Burdett RG, Simon SR, et al: Elbow moment and forces at the hands during swing-through axillary crutch gait. *Phys Ther* 1985;65:601–605.
32. Koh TJ, Grabiner MD, Weiker GG: Technique and ground reaction forces in the back handspring. *Am J Sports Med* 1992;20:61–66.
33. Panner HJ: A peculiar affection of the capitulum humeri, resembling Calvé-Perthes' disease of the hip. *Acta Radiol* 1929;10:234–242.
34. Woodward AH, Bianco AJ Jr: Osteochondritis dissecans of the elbow. *Clin Orthop* 1975;110:35–41.
35. Meeusen R, Borms J: Gymnastic injuries. *Sports Med* 1992;13:337–356.
36. An KN, Chao EY, Cooney WP, et al: Forces in the normal and abnormal hand. *J Orthop Res* 1985;3:202–211.
37. Pring DJ, Amis AA, Coombs RR: The mechanical properties of human flexor tendons in relation to artificial tendons. *J Hand Surg* 1985;10B:331–336.
38. Giori NJ, Beaupre GS, Carter DR: Cellular shape and pressure may mediate mechanical control of tissue composition in tendons. *J Orthop Res* 1993;11:581–591.
39. Okuda Y, Gorski JP, An KN, et al: Biochemical, histological, and biomechanical analyses of canine tendon. *J Orthop Res* 1987;5:60–68.
40. Sarkar K, Uhthoff HK: Ultrastructural localization of calcium in calcifying tendinitis. *Arch Path Lab Med* 1978;102:266–269.
41. Armstrong TJ, Chaffin DB: Some biomechanical aspects of the carpal tunnel. *J Biomech* 1979;12:567–570.
42. Moore A, Wells R, Ranney D: Quantifying exposure in occupational manual tasks with cumulative trauma disorder potential. *Ergonomics* 1991;34:1433–1453.
43. Uchiyama S, Coert JH, Berglund L, et al: Method for the measurement of friction between tendon and pulley. *J Orthop Res* 1995;13:83–89.

Chapter 11
Shoulder Biomechanics and Repetitive Motion

Roger G. Pollock, MD
Evan L. Flatow, MD
Louis U. Bigliani, MD
Rajeev Kelkar, MS
Van C. Mow, PhD

Introduction

The shoulder is characterized foremost by its great mobility, which facilitates prehensile activities of the upper extremity in multiple planes. The glenohumeral joint is notable anatomically for its relative lack of bony constraint and its heavy reliance on the surrounding soft tissues for both static and dynamic stabilization. These tissues include the musculotendinous structures, particularly the rotator cuff, that provide dynamic stabilization and the capsuloligamentous tissues, particularly the glenohumeral ligaments and labrum, that provide static support. Activities requiring repetitive motion, particularly overhead activities, appear to be involved in the pathogenesis of several clinical shoulder syndromes, including rotator cuff disease, glenohumeral instability, and osteoarthritis of the glenohumeral joint. These activities may contribute to alterations in the structure or material properties of the surrounding soft tissues, leading to shoulder impairment, which is manifested clinically by pain and limitations in motion and function. Specific anatomic factors that are native to certain individuals, such as a particular acromial morphology, increased ligamentous laxity, or decreased articular congruence, may contribute to an environment in which the repetitive activities have a deleterious effect on shoulder function. This chapter will focus on the anatomic and biomechanical factors that may be involved with the pathogenesis of repetitive motion disorders of the shoulder.

Anatomic Factors

Glenohumeral Articular Anatomy

The glenohumeral joint is characterized by relatively little bony constraint. Two factors have been cited historically to explain the reduced contribution of articular geometry to shoulder stability: the smaller surface area of the glenoid relative to the humeral head[1] and the supposed relative shallowness of the glenoid articular surface compared with that of the humeral head.[2] More recently, an optical technique, stereophotogrammetry, has been used for the precise determination of surface topology, surface areas, and cartilage thickness in several diarthrodial joints.[3-6] This technique has demonstrated that the geometry of normal glenohumeral joint articular surfaces may be described by portions of spheres with deviations from sphericity of less than 1% of the radii (Fig. 1).[6] The ratio of the radii of curvature of the articular surface of the matching humeral head as compared to the glenoid surface ranged from 0.89 to 1.09 and averaged 0.99 ± 0.05 standard deviation (SD). The radii of corresponding humeral heads and glenoid were not statistically different, and the absolute difference of the radii was less than 2.0 mm in 88% of matched pairs and less than 3.0 mm in all pairs (Table 1). These data show that the glenoid is not flat, as is suggested by plain radiographs, which image only the bony contours and not the articular surfaces. In these studies, the cartilage of the glenoid was found to be thicker at the periphery than in the center. The articular cartilage contributes to the contour and, thus, to the stability of the glenohumeral articulation. However, the ratio of the surface area of the humeral head to the glenoid was almost 3:1. The small surface area of the glenoid, which does not enclose the humeral head (such as is the case in the hip joint, another ball-and-socket joint), allows great mobility of the shoulder, but at the price of less bony stability.

Capsuloligamentous Stabilizers

Because the bony glenohumeral articulation provides limited stability, the soft tissues surrounding the joint play an important role in joint stabilization. Much has been written about the importance of the chief static glenohumeral stabilizers, the glenohumeral ligaments and the labrum. Bankart[7] reported that the detachment of the labrum from the anterior glenoid rim was "the essential lesion" for recurrent anterior dislocation. Bost and Inman[8] expanded the emphasis on the labrum, describing it as a ring of dense fibrocartilaginous tissue

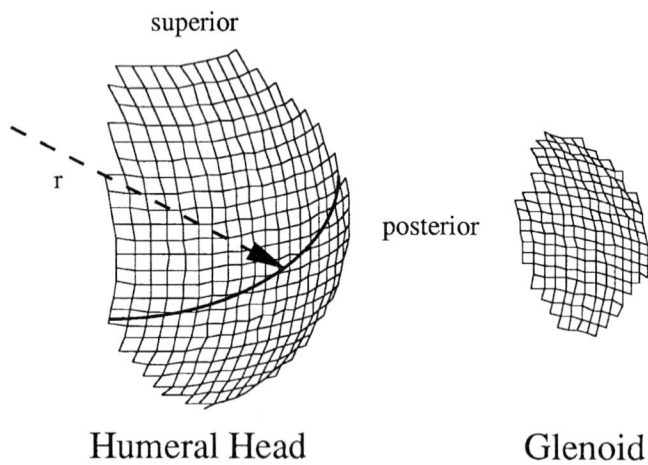

Fig. 1 Three-dimensional computer graphics representations of the cartilage surface of the humeral head and glenoid obtained using stereophotogrammetry. (Reproduced with permission from Soslowsky LJ, Flatow EL, Bigliani LU, et al: Articular geometry of the glenohumeral joint. *Clin Orthop Rel Res* 1992;285:181–190.)

Table 1 Radius of curvature*

Specimen	Cartilage (mm)		Bone (mm)	
	Male	Female	Male	Female
Humeral head	26.85±1.40	23.27±1.69	26.10±1.41	23.15±2.09
Glenoid	26.37±2.42	23.62±1.56	34.56±1.74	30.28±3.16

*Data reported as means ± standard deviations.
(Reproduced with permission from Soslowsky LJ, Flatow, EL, Bigliani LU, et al: Articular geometry of the glenohumeral joint. *Clin Orthop* 1992;285:181–190.)

that deepens the glenoid and enhances stability. Moseley and Overgaard[9] reported in a histologic study that the labrum was not a fibrocartilaginous disc like the meniscus of the knee; rather, it consisted of a redundant fold of fibrous capsular tissue with very little fibrocartilage. More recently, Cooper and associates[10] have clarified the structure of the labrum with further anatomic, histologic, and vascular studies. They found that the morphology of the labrum varies regionally around the rim of the glenoid. More superiorly, the labrum is meniscal in appearance and is more loosely attached and mobile. Anteroinferiorly and posteroinferiorly, the labrum is firmly attached to the glenoid rim and appears as a fibrous extension of the glenoid. Thus, the labrum appears to serve both as an attachment site for the glenohumeral ligaments[11] and, perhaps, as a stabilizer by increasing the constraining wall height of the small glenoid surface,[12] thereby adding to the curvature initially created by the glenoid articular cartilage.

The glenohumeral ligaments have been recognized to play a role in stabilization of the shoulder, especially at extremes of the range of motion. Townley[13] introduced the concept of a capsular mechanism, in which the entire anterior capsule acts to stabilize the glenohumeral joint against anterior dislocations. Turkel and associates[14] demonstrated in a series of radiographic and ligament-sectioning studies using cadavers that the position and tightness or laxity of the anterior structures (subscapularis muscle, middle glenohumeral ligament [MGHL], and inferior glenohumeral ligaments [IGHL]) vary with different positions of abduction and external rotation. These studies showed that no single structure stabilized the glenohumeral joint in all positions. As abduction and external rotation increase, the static stabilizing function shifts from the superior to the inferior structures. In the clinical position of anterior instability, namely 90° of abduction and full external rotation, the IGHL was the crucial static restraint. Further biomechanical studies of anterior instability in cadavers have verified these findings.[15–17]

Until recent years, few reports had focused on the intrinsic mechanical and structural properties of these static stabilizers. Reeves[18] determined the tensile strength of the labrum, the anteroinferior capsule, and the subscapularis tendon in cadavers from various age groups. He observed that in younger specimens, the glenoid attachment is the weakest point; whereas, in the older cadavers, the capsule and subscapularis were weaker and failed before the labral attachment. Kaltsas[19] tested the anterior capsule as a whole, with the shoulder positioned in 90° of abduction, and demonstrated that the anteroinferior capsule usually ruptured first at a force of 2,000 N. More recently, structural and mechanical properties of a single important stabilizer, the IGHL, have been determined.[20–22] In these experiments, the IGHL was divided into its three anatomic regions, as previously described by Turkel and associates:[14] a superior band, an anterior axillary pouch, and a posterior axillary pouch (Fig. 2). Structurally, the superior band was consistently the thickest region, averaging 2.79 mm, with the ligament thickness decreasing from anterosuperiorly to posteroinferiorly. The resting lengths of all three anatomic regions did not differ significantly.[20]

With respect to tensile properties of the IGHL, regional variations in strain to failure were seen. At slow testing rates (0.004 or 0.04 mm/s), the anterior axillary pouch failed at a higher strain (34%) than either of the other two regions ($p < 0.001$). This was true for both bone-ligament-bone and midsubstance ligament measurements. Average midsubstance failure strains represented only 35% to 45% of the total specimen strain at failure, indicating strain variations along the course of the ligament, with the greatest strain existing near the ligament insertions. Failure stresses (average, 5.5 MPa) did not differ significantly among the three regions of the IGHL at the slow strain rates.[21] At the fast rate (4.0 mm/s), the anterior axillary pouch again had the highest strain at failure. In this case, however, significant differences in tensile failure stress were found, with the superior band and anterior axillary pouch failing

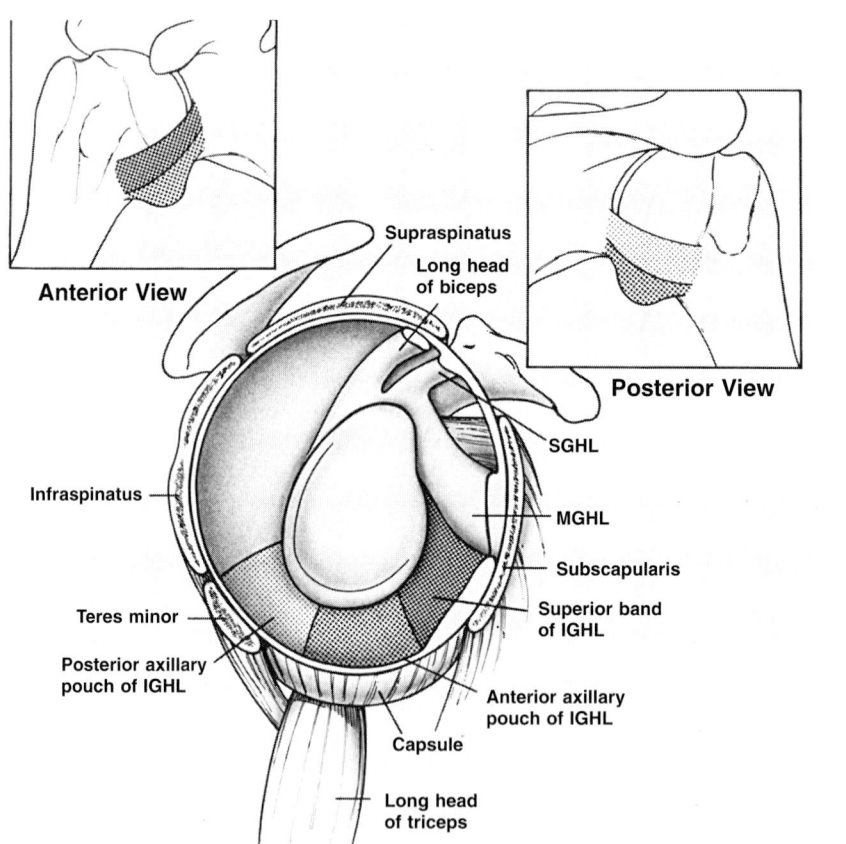

Fig. 2 Anatomic drawings of the three regions of the inferior glenohumeral ligament (IGHL) from both infrascapular and extrascapular views. (SGHL, superior glenohumeral ligament; MGHL, middle glenohumeral ligament.)

at significantly higher stress than the posterior axillary pouch region.[22] In the comparison of the fast and slow strain rate data, the superior band demonstrated the greatest strain rate dependency (failure stress increased 62% at the higher rate), followed closely by the anterior axillary pouch (+ 42%).

Biochemical and histologic studies of the IGHL have also been undertaken recently. O'Brien and associates[23] reported that three well defined layers of collagen fibers make up this ligament. The fibers of the inner and outer layers extend in a coronal axis from the glenoid to the humerus, wheras those of the middle layer are oriented perpendicularly to these layers. Biochemical analysis has shown a higher proteoglycan content in the superior band than in the other regions of the IGHL, although no regional differences in water, collagen, or hydroxypyridinium cross-links were found.[24] The higher proteoglycan content of the superior band may explain, in part, the more viscoelastic behavior of this region and would support the hypothesis that the viscoelastic stiffening effect is caused by the flow of interstitial fluid, which, in turn, is due to compaction of the proteoglycan molecules as the collagen fibers are straightened (uncrimped) during tensile loading.

Musculotendinous Stabilizers

The musculotendinous tissues, chiefly the rotator cuff muscles, serve to provide both mobility and dynamic stability for the shoulder. Inman and associates[25] first demonstrated in electromyographic (EMG) analyses of the shoulder that the rotator cuff muscles are active continuously during abduction and flexion and play a role in depressing the humeral head as well as in compressing it against the glenoid. In this manner, the rotator cuff stabilizes the joint against the vertical (shearing) component of force exerted by the deltoid. More recent EMG studies performed on the shoulders of throwing athletes have demonstrated decreased activity of the subscapularis muscle as well as of the scapular protractors in throwers with instability, suggesting a role for subtle differences in neuromuscular control in anterior instability.[26] These studies emphasize the role of the scapular stabilizers in providing dynamic stability for the shoulder. Using a biomechanical model, Cain and associates[27] have demonstrated that the posterior rotator cuff can reduce strain in the anterior capsular structures by pulling the humeral head posteriorly during external rotation of the shoulder. Clark and associates[28] also have suggested that the rotator cuff muscles and capsular ligaments may interact functionally because the cuff tendons blend tightly with the capsule at their humeral insertion. Contraction of the rotator cuff then may create tension in the ligaments, thus dynamizing the ligaments. Warner and associates[29] have further studied the interrelationship between the glenohumeral ligaments during simulated rotator cuff contraction and have documented reciprocal length changes in the ligaments with varying arm positions.

Repetitive Activity and Rotator Cuff Disease

As discussed above, the rotator cuff muscles center the humeral head in the glenoid and serve as dynamic stabilizers for the glenohumeral joint. These tendons pass under the relatively rigid coracoacromial arch, which consists of the acromion, acromioclavicular joint, coracoacromial ligament, and coracoid, before they insert into the proximal humerus. An interposed subacromial bursa promotes smooth gliding of these structures. However, bursitis, tendinitis, and failure of the tendon fibers resulting in tears of the rotator cuff are quite common clinical disorders of the shoulder. Activities requiring repetitive motion, particularly overhead activities, appear to be involved in the pathogenesis of rotator cuff disease. The underlying causes of rotator cuff disease appear to be multifactorial, with intrinsic tendon factors interacting with extrinsic structural factors and patterns of repetitive use to produce these tendon tears.

Clinical and pathologic studies have found a consistent pattern of tendon failure, with tears initiating uniformly at the supraspinatus insertion, usually on the inferior or articular surface. These partial thickness tears progress to full thickness supraspinatus tears and then progress to involve adjacent tendons.[30–32] Historically, there have been many theories about how and why these tears occur. Codman[30] reported that most of these tears resulted from trauma, although others have pointed out that many patients with rotator cuff tears present either without any history of trauma or after a trivial injury.[31,32] Experimental efforts to reproduce rotator cuff tears in cadavers by forcefully disrupting the scapula-supraspinatus muscle-tendon-humerus complex have resulted in failure of the complex anywhere but at the tendon insertion, further suggesting that trauma alone usually is not the mechanism of clinical tendon failure.[33]

Hypovascularity of the supraspinatus tendon insertion has also been implicated in tendon failures. Microinjection studies have demonstrated decreased blood flow to the region of the supraspinatus insertion,[34,35] particularly on the deep (articular) surface of the tendon.[34] However, more recent microvascular studies using Doppler flowmetry have demonstrated that there is, in fact, hypervascularity in the supraspinatus tendon insertion,[36] thus questioning the role of blood supply as a factor in the initiation of rotator cuff degeneration. Degenerative changes associated with aging, such as thinning of fiber fascicles, fibrillation, and fiber failures, have been described.[37,38] These observations have led Ogata and Uhthoff[39] to refer to disease of the rotator cuff as a "primary tendinopathy." However, if this process is an intrinsic tendon disorder, it remains unclear why it occurs first almost exclusively in one region, the supraspinatus insertion.

Mechanical factors have long been implicated in the pathogenesis of rotator cuff disease. Meyer[40] implicated mechanical wearing under the acromion as an important contributing factor in rotator cuff degeneration and biceps tendon ruptures. He suggested that it was the repetitive use of the shoulder that led to degenerative changes in the tissues. Neer[41] demonstrated that spurs and excrescences are found on the undersurface of the anterior aspect of the acromion, and he believed that this region of the acromion (not the lateral region, as had previously been implicated) was responsible for mechanical impingement on the supraspinatus tendon. Neer[42] related this process of mechanical impingement to the entire spectrum of rotator cuff disease, which he divided into three stages. More recently, Bigliani and associates[43] have classified the shape of the acromion into three categories: type I, flat; type II, curved; and type III, hooked. Moreover, they have correlated acromial morphology with the incidence of rotator cuff tears in cadavers, showing that those acromions that were curved or hooked and thus projected downward onto the tendon were associated with a higher incidence of rotator cuff tears.[44] These clinical and anatomic studies suggest that certain morphologies or alterations with aging in the anatomy of the coracoacromial arch cause compression of the underlying rotator cuff tendon and act as the primary extrinsic factor responsible for tendon damage and rotator cuff tears.

Basic research studies have also demonstrated a correlation between subacromial contact and regions of tendon damage. Nasca and associates[45] employed a dye technique to show that subacromial contact increases between 45° and 90° of abduction and that the regions of contact correlate with the usual site of tendon pathology. Pressure sensitive film has also been used to demonstrate that the highest subacromial pressures develop with the arm in 90° of abduction.[46] More recently, stereophotogrammetry has been used in a cadaver study to quantitate contact of the acromion on the rotator cuff in varying degrees of abduction in the scapular plane[47] (Fig. 3). This study showed that the supraspinatus tendon and the undersurface of the acromion are in closest proximity between 60° and 120° of humeral elevation. As the arm is raised, contact shifts from the anterolateral edge of the acromion to more medial regions. On the humeral side, contact is located proximally on the supraspinatus tendon at 0° of elevation and shifts distally so that, in the range from 60° to 120°, contact is greatest at the supraspinatus tendon insertion, correlating with the region of clinical tendon damage. Moreover, contact was more pronounced for shoulders with Type III (hooked) acromial morphology.[47]

Other biomechanical factors besides compression of the tendon on the undersurface of the acromion may contribute to rotator cuff damage. Lindblom[48] observed that, with the arm in abduction, the inferior (articular surface) fascicles of the supraspinatus tendon were in tension while the superior (bursal surface) fibers remained lax. By applying load to the tendon with the arm in abduction, he produced ruptures first in the inferior fibers of the tendon. Thus, differential fiber length and inhomogeneous tensile stress and strains within the tendon may play a role in fiber failure as well as mechanical compression. Recently, Jobe (C Jobe, personal communication) has suggested that the undersurface of the rotator cuff may abut on the glenoid, leading to isolated undersurface tearing, particularly in high demand overhead athletes. Several biomechanical factors, thus, may contribute to failure of the rotator cuff.

Rotator cuff failure appears to be related to multiple factors, some intrinsic to the aging tendon and others related to the extrinsic mechanical environment. The greater frequency of rotator cuff pathology in the dominant versus the nondominant shoulder, in paraplegic patients who subject the shoulder to frequent high loading, and the earlier age of presentation in overhead competitive athletes all point to a role for repetitive use in rotator cuff disease. However, much remains unproven about the exact mechanisms of rotator cuff degeneration, and much remains to be learned about the biomechanical and biochemical properties of these tissues.

Repetitive Microtrauma and Glenohumeral Instability

High demand repetitive use of the shoulder has also been implicated in the etiology of glenohumeral instability in a subset of patients. Historically, since the time of Hippocrates, shoulder dislocations had been classified as either "traumatic" or "atraumatic." Shoulders were thought to become unstable either on the basis of a major traumatic injury or congenital laxity of the glenohumeral ligaments. Neer pointed out that there was a subset of patients who had "acquired" instability as a result of repeated minor injuries to the glenohumeral joint capsule.[49,50] These patients typically are involved with high demand sports activities that require repetitive overhead motion, such as throwing, swimming (especially the butterfly and backstroke), and weightlifting. These patients tend to have inherent joint laxity, although they have less than those in the atraumatic group. The pathology encountered in these shoulders is an acquired enlargement of the glenohumeral joint volume.[50] Splitting and partial

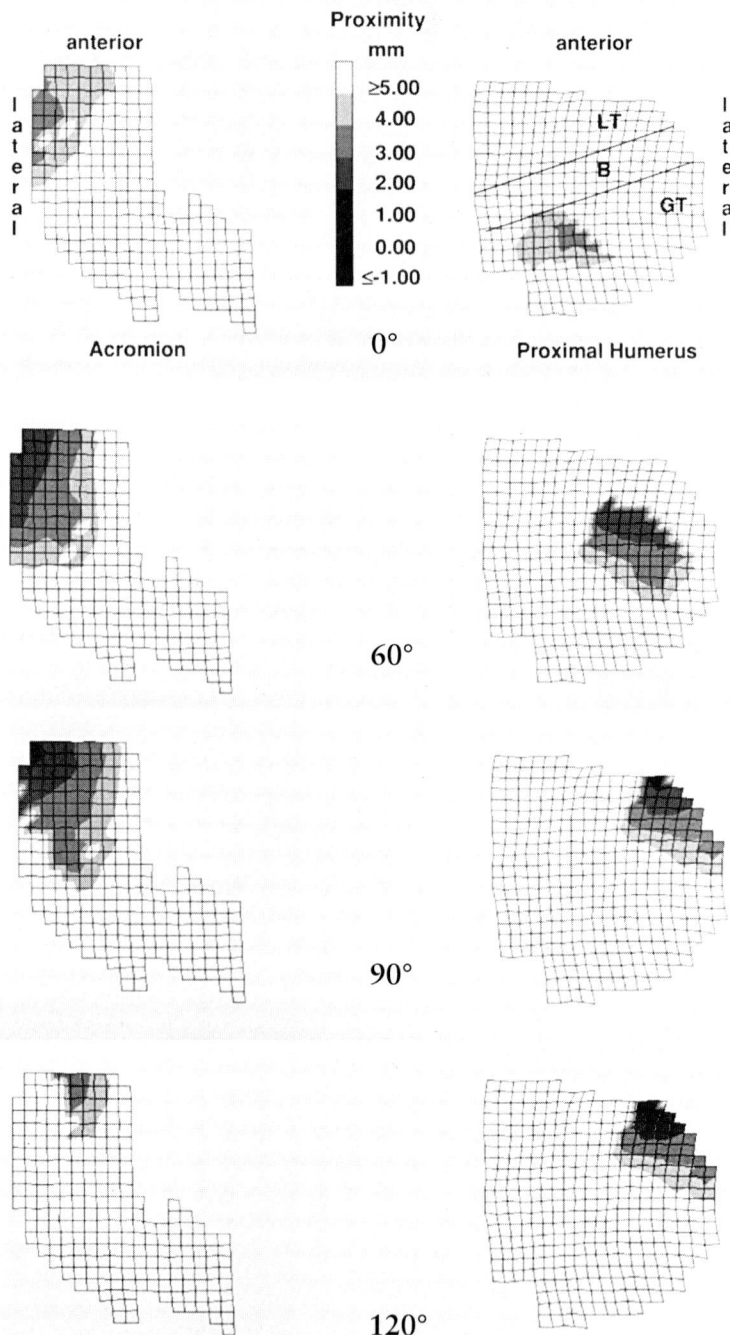

Fig. 3 Subacromial contact patterns for a right shoulder at 0° (**top**), 60°, 90°, and 120° of arm elevation in the scapular plane in the external starting rotation. B, biceps region; GT, greater tuberosity; LT, lesser tuberosity. Gray levels represent proximity of one surface to the other. (Reproduced with permission from Soslowsky LJ: *Studies on Diarthrodial Joint Biomechanics With Special Reference to the Shoulder.* New York, NY, Columbia University, 1991. Thesis.)

detachment of the labrum is frequently seen, although complete detachment (a Bankart lesion) is less common in this group.

In Neer's series,[49,50] the acquired instability group was the largest subset of patients. The significance of this type of instability is that these shoulders frequently have capsular ligament damage that allows instability in more than one direction. In addition to anterior dislocation or subluxation, there may be instability in inferior and/or posterior directions. Neer[49] described multidirectional instability as occurring in three directions, but the frequent presence of bidirectional instability (anteroinferior or posteroinferior) is increasingly cited, particularly in the overhead athletic population with shoulder instability.[51–53] Neer[49] pointed out that an attempt to repair a multidirectional instability with a standard unidirectional repair will often fail; usually, it leaves the inferior instability unaddressed. In the case of a tight unidirectional repair performed on a multidirectionally unstable shoulder, it may even cause a fixed subluxation in the opposite direction. Persistent instability or the development of glenohumeral arthritis may occur in this setting.[49] The inferior capsular shift procedure was designed to address these additional elements of instability by reducing the volume of the glenohumeral joint capsule on all three sides when necessary.[49]

This procedure as well as other capsulolabral procedures on the middle and medial capsule, which balance the static stabilizers and address multiple components of instability when these are present, have produced a high rate of success in the treatment of glenohumeral instability.[51–54] Prevention of further episodes of instability and return to full function, including participation in high demand overhead sports, have been achieved with these repairs in a high percentage of patients with acquired shoulder instability.

Although repetitive microtrauma has been implicated as an etiology of instability in the shoulders of overhead athletes, few scientific data exist concerning this mechanism. Jobe and associates[55] have suggested that sports requiring overhead use may stress the tissues to near their physiologic limits. If these stresses are applied at a rate that is greater than the rate of tissue repair, these repetitive insults can produce damage to the tissues. It is well-accepted that if a material is subjected to a large number of loading cycles, it will fail at a stress lower than its ultimate tensile stress. It is quite possible that the repetitive high velocity motions of the shoulder during certain sports activities cause fatigue failure to the fibers of the glenohumeral ligaments because the endurance limit is exceeded during these motions.[56] It has been shown that the IGHL undergoes significant stretching before ultimate failure when it is tested in uniaxial tension.[20–22] To date, plastic deformation of this ligament during cyclic testing using subfailure stresses has not been demonstrated. It is suspected that the high demand repetitive loading of certain shoulders may lead to fatigue failure of the IGHL fibers, resulting in stretching of the ligament and impairment of the proprioceptive function of the capsule. Indeed, axonal fibers of different diameters have been identified in the glenohumeral ligaments, suggesting a proprioceptive role for these ligaments.[57] Moreover, differences have been demonstrated in shoulder proprioception between stable shoulders and unstable shoulders before and after repair.[58]

All throwing athletes do not develop instability. Thus, deficits in neuromuscular facilitation may underlie the development of damage to the capsular structures by inadequately shielding these structures from excessively high stresses. Capsular damage may lead to further proprioceptive deficiency. The role of tissue repair in this scenario of capsular damage from repetitive stresses is also poorly understood and will require future investigation. The hypothesis remains unproven that damage to the glenohumeral ligaments from repetitive microtrauma leads to compromise of their structural load support and proprioceptive functions. However, the greater frequency of symptomatic laxity in the dominant versus the nondominant arms of overhead athletes and the greater laxity in the dominant shoulders of throwing athletes suggest a role for repetitive high demand use in the development of glenohumeral instability in the "at risk" shoulder.

Repetitive Loading and Glenohumeral Arthritis

Osteoarthritis of the glenohumeral joint is certainly less common than that of the hip and knee, although it has long been recognized as a clinical entity. DePalma and associates[59,60] noted cartilage lesions in cadaver shoulders similar to those seen in the major weightbearing joints of the lower extremities. Similar findings were reported by Neer[61] and Petersson,[62] who found focal articular lesions in 10% to 23% of all cadaveric shoulders. DePalma and associates[60] noted that the changes in the glenoid surface were seen first, and that they occurred as early as the second decade. These changes consisted of softening, furrowing, and fibrillation in the superficial layers of the central glenoid region. Later, irregular scalloped and ulcerated areas were seen in the cartilage, and the adjacent bone became dense and hypertrophied. These investigators hypothesized that the degenerative changes must be due to high contact stresses acting on the relatively small glenoid during normal repetitive shoulder activities. Degenerative changes on the humeral head, especially at the periphery, were also documented although these were less severe than the corresponding glenoid changes. This discrepancy was attributed to the assumption that the contact areas of the smaller glenoid are subjected to more frequent wear and tear. Neer[61] specified that the focal areas of wear develop at the point of maximum joint reaction force when the arm is elevated between 60° and 100°, which is the frequent shoulder position for function. As these degenerative changes progress, the glenoid becomes smooth and eburnated but develops more bone loss posteriorly. This sloping glenoid may then allow the humeral head to become posteriorly subluxed. These earlier studies, thus, documented the anatomic changes and their progression and attributed these changes to repetitive mechanical loading, although the precise contact areas and stresses were not quantified.

Secondary osteoarthritis of the glenohumeral joint has been reported as a sequela of both traumatic dislocations and the surgical treatment of shoulder instability.[63] Neer and associates[49,50,64] postulated that the etiologic mechanism for the development of osteoarthritis after an instability repair (referred to by Neer as "arthritis of dislocation") is the performance of a standard unidirectional instability repair on a shoulder that is multidirectionally loose. Unidirectional tightening in this setting displaces the humeral head away from the side of the repair, causing a shift in normal joint contact and accentuating stresses in the new region of contact (ie, posteriorly on the glenoid after a tight anterior repair). Samilson and Prieto[63] correlated the limitation of external rotation after surgery with the severity of degenerative changes. More recently, Hawkins and Angelo[65] reported on the development of osteoarthritis in shoulders after a Putti-Platt capsulorrhaphy. They suggested that this repair can act as a restrictive anterior tether, leading to alterations in joint biomechanics and generating abnormal compressive and shear forces at the articular surfaces when the shoulder is used.

Biomechanical studies performed in recent years have begun to shed light on the kinematics and contact pattern of the glenohumeral joint, both before and after surgical procedures on the joint. Harryman and associates[66] demonstrated that with passive manipulation significant glenohumeral translations occur at the extremes of motion: anteriorly with flexion and posteriorly with extension. Surgical tightening of the posterior capsule increased the anterior translation in flexion and adduction.[66] Janevic and associates[67] studied glenohumeral joint contact in cadavers before and after performing a Bankart repair or a capsular shift on these shoulders. They found that overtightening the capsule resulted in shifting the humeral head and the joint contact posteriorly during loading in abduction, extension, and external rotation. Recent work in which stereophotogrammetry was used to study glenohumeral translations and contact patterns in cadavers during abduction in the scapular plane by simulated muscle forces has provided precise quantitative information.[68,69] Observation of minimal joint translations in all three planes correlates well with earlier findings that the articular surfaces are close-fitting spheres.[6,68] Moreover, in more congruent joints, the humeral head remains almost perfectly centered on the glenoid (range of posteroanterior translation = 1.5 mm), whereas in relatively less congruent joints there is increased translation through the range of motion (range of posteroanterior translation = 3.6 mm).[68] In these studies, glenohumeral contact areas were found to be greatest at more functional arm positions than at the extremes of elevation. In general, as the humerus is elevated, humeral contact migrates from an inferior region to a superior region while glenoid contact shifts posteriorly.[69] Additionally, after anterior capsular tightening, humeral head translation increases significantly in a posterior direction (0.63 ± 0.24 mm).[70] Relatively incongruent joints (mismatch of radii of curvature greater than 2.5 mm) demonstrate a trend for increased posterior translation, and articular contact on the glenoid demonstrates a similar posterior shift and a reduction in contact area[70] (Fig. 4).

Repetitive loading may interact with inherent anatomic and tissue factors to produce glenohumeral arthritis. Due to the large differences in surface area between the glenoid and the humeral head, there is asymmetry in the duration of load support (ie, the duty cycle), with glenoid cartilage loading being more frequent and longer. With repetitive activities involving the shoulder, the number of cycles of stress on the glenoid cartilage will be greater than the number on the humeral head. Intrinsic differences in the mechanical properties of the glenoid articular cartilage versus those of the humeral articular cartilage may also contribute to this unfavorable mechanical situation. Ebara and associates[71] have recently shown that bovine glenoid articular cartilage is less stiff than humeral head cartilage in tension, although similar work has not yet been reported on human glenohumeral cartilage. If such intrinsic differences exist in human glenohumeral cartilage, they might further predispose the less-stiff glenoid cartilage to earlier degenerative changes, as has been observed clinically. However, other factors must also exist for the development of glenohumeral osteoarthritis. All shoulders have a great discrepancy in surface area between the humeral head and the glenoid, and many are subject to frequent repetitive activities, yet only a small percentage (10% to 20%) develop osteoarthritic changes. In some cases, soft-tissue imbalances created through excessively tight instability repairs have been implicated because they produce abnormal joint contact and stress distributions. Perhaps other factors, such as relatively increased retroversion of the glenoid and relatively decreased congruence of the articulating surfaces of the glenohumeral joint, may account for development of degenerative changes in certain shoulders. Much of this re-

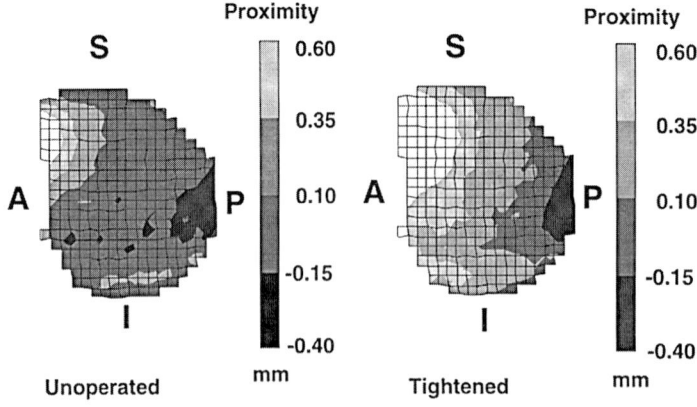

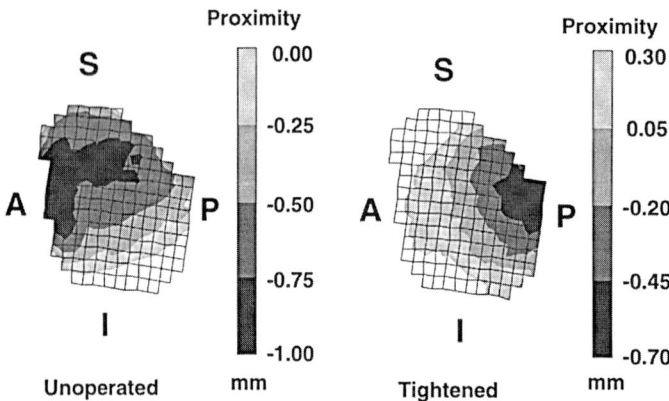

Fig. 4 Patterns of glenoid contact for congruent (**top**) and incongruent (**bottom**) glenohumeral joints in the unoperated and anteriorly tightened states at 130° of arm elevation in the scapular plane. Gray levels represent proximity of one surface to the other. S, superior; P, posterior; I, inferior; A, anterior.

mains speculative. Further investigation is required on the properties of these tissues and on their interaction with the mechanical forces placed on the glenohumeral joint with repetitive use of the extremity.

Conclusion

Repetitive loading appears to be a factor in the development of several major pathologic conditions affecting the shoulder, including rotator cuff disease, glenohumeral instability, and osteoarthritis of the glenohumeral joint. It is not repetitive use alone that results in these pathologic entities. Many shoulders are subjected to these repetitive stresses, but only a relatively small percentage develop one or more of these clinical syndromes. Rather, it appears that a specific anatomic or mechanical milieu is necessary for the repetitive loading to exert a deleterious effect. Thus, for example, the shoulder with a hooked acromial morphology may be at higher risk for developing rotator cuff disease than one with a flat acromion. Similarly, if a throwing athlete's shoulder has poor neuromuscular protective mechanisms or impaired proprioception, it may be at a higher risk for developing acquired glenohumeral instability. An anatomic factor, such as a relatively small incongruence between the humeral head and glenoid articular surfaces, may lead to significant differences in joint contact and kinematics, perhaps predisposing the joint to degenerative changes. In the last decade, we have seen dramatic advances in our understanding of glenohumeral anatomy and biomechanics. Scientific explanations for many of the astute clinical observations of the preceding decades have been advanced. However, our understanding of the mechanisms of these shoulder disorders is far from complete. The task remains to define more clearly and completely what the underlying anatomic, mechanical, and biologic factors are and how they interrelate to produce these clinical shoulder syndromes.

References

1. Saha AK: *Theory of the Shoulder Mechanism: Descriptive and Applied*. Springfield, IL, Charles C Thomas, 1961.
2. O'Brien SJ, Arnoczky SP, Warren RF, et al: Developmental anatomy of the shoulder and anatomy of the glenohumeral joint, in Rockwood CA Jr, Matsen FA III (eds): *The Shoulder*. Philadelphia, PA, WB Saunders, 1990, vol 1, pp 1–33.
3. Soslowsky LJ, Ateshian GA, Pollock RG, et al: An in situ method to determine diarthrodial joint contact areas using stereophotogrammetry. *Adv Bioengineering* 1989;15:129–130.
4. Ateshian GA, Soslowsky LJ, Mow VC: Quantitation of articular surface topography and cartilage thickness in knee joints using stereophotogrammetry. *J Biomech* 1991;24:761–776.
5. Huiskes R, Kremers J, de Lange A, et al: Analytical stereophotogrammetric determination of three-dimensional knee-joint geometry. *J Biomech* 1985;18:559–570.
6. Soslowsky LJ, Flatow EL, Bigliani LU, et al: Articular geometry of the glenohumeral joint. *Clin Orthop* 1992;285:181–190.
7. Bankart ASB: Recurrent or habitual dislocation of the shoulder-joint. *Br Med J* 1923;2:1132–1133.
8. Bost FC, Inman VT: The pathological changes in recurrent dislocation of the shoulder: A report of Bankart's operative procedure. *J Bone Joint Surg* 1942;24A:595–613.
9. Moseley HF, Overgaard B: The anterior capsular mechanism in recurrent anterior dislocation of the shoulder: Morphological and clinical studies with special reference to the glenoid labrum and the gleno-humeral ligaments. *J Bone Joint Surg* 1962;44B:913–927.
10. Cooper DE, Arnoczky SP, O'Brien SJ, et al: Anatomy, histology, and vascularity of the glenoid labrum: An anatomical study. *J Bone Joint Surg* 1992;74A:46–52.
11. McLaughlin HL: Recurrent anterior dislocation of the shoulder: I. Morbid anatomy. *Am J Surg* 1960;99:628–632.
12. Fukuda K, Chen CM, Cofield RH, et al: Biomechanical analysis of stability and fixation strength of total shoulder prostheses. *Orthopedics* 1988;11:141–149.
13. Townley CO: The capsular mechanism in recurrent dislocation of the shoulder. *J Bone Joint Surg* 1950;32A:370–380.
14. Turkel SJ, Panio MW, Marshall JL, et al: Stabilizing mechanisms preventing anterior dislocation of the glenohumeral joint. *J Bone Joint Surg* 1981;63A:1208–1217.

15. Ovesen J, Nielsen S: Stability of the shoulder joint: Cadaver study of stabilizing structures. *Acta Orthop Scand* 1985;56:149–151.
16. O'Connell PW, Nuber GW, Mileski RA, et al: The contribution of the glenohumeral ligaments to anterior stability of the shoulder joint. *Am J Sports Med* 1990;18:579–584.
17. Terry GC, Hammon D, France P, et al: The stabilizing function of passive shoulder restraints. *Am J Sports Med* 1991;19:26–34.
18. Reeves B: Experiments on the tensile strength of the anterior capsular structures of the shoulder in man. *J Bone Joint Surg* 1968;50B:858–865.
19. Kaltsas DS: Comparative study of the properties of the shoulder joint capsule with those of other joint capsules. *Clin Orthop* 1983;173:20–26.
20. Pollock RG, Soslowsky LJ, Bigliani LU, et al: The mechanical properties of the inferior glenohumeral ligament. *Trans Orthop Res Soc* 1990;15:510.
21. Bigliani LU, Pollock RG, Soslowsky LJ, et al: Tensile properties of the inferior glenohumeral ligament. *J Orthop Res* 1992;10:187–197.
22. Ticker JB, Bigliani LU, Soslowsky LJ, et al: Viscoelastic and geometric properties of the inferior glenohumeral ligament. *Orthop Trans* 1992;16:304–305.
23. O'Brien SJ, Neves MC, Arnoczky SP, et al: The anatomy and histology of the inferior glenohumeral ligament complex of the shoulder. *Am J Sports Med* 1990;18:449–456.
24. Ticker JB, Flatow EL, Pawluk RJ, et al: The inferior glenohumeral ligament: A correlative biomechanical, biochemical, and histological investigation. *Trans Orthop Res Soc* 1993;18:313.
25. Inman VT, Saunders JB, Abbott LC: Observations on the function of the shoulder joint. *J Bone Joint Surg* 1944;26A:1–30.
26. Glousman R, Jobe F, Tibone J, et al: Dynamic electromyographic analysis of the throwing shoulder with glenohumeral instability. *J Bone Joint Surg* 1988;70A:220–226.
27. Cain PR, Mutschler TA, Fu FH, et al: Anterior stability of the glenohumeral joint: A dynamic model. *Am J Sports Med* 1987:15:144–148.
28. Clark J, Sidles JA, Matsen FA: The relationship of the glenohumeral joint capsule to the rotator cuff. *Clin Orthop* 1990;254:29–34.
29. Warner JJP, Caborn DNM, Berger R, et al: Dynamic capsuloligamentous anatomy of the glenohumeral joint. *J Shoulder Elbow Surg* 1993;2:115–133.
30. Codman EA (ed): *The Shoulder: Rupture of the Supraspinatus Tendon and Other Lesions In or About the Subacromial Bursa.* Boston, MA, Thomas Todd, 1934.
31. Cofield RH: Rotator cuff disease of the shoulder. *J Bone Joint Surg* 1985;67A:974–979.
32. Cuff tears, biceps lesions, and impingement, in Neer CS II (ed): *Shoulder Reconstruction.* Philadelphia, PA, WB Saunders, 1990, pp 41–42.
33. Wilson CL, Duff GL: Pathologic study of degeneration and rupture of the supraspinatus tendon. *Arch Surg* 1943;47:121–135.
34. Lohr JF, Uhthoff HK: The microvascular pattern of the supraspinatus tendon. *Clin Orthop* 1990;254:35–38.
35. Rathbun JB, Macnab I: The microvascular pattern of the rotator cuff. *J Bone Joint Surg* 1970;52B:540–553.
36. Swiontkowski MF, Iannotti JP, Boulas HJ, et al: Intraoperative assessment of rotator cuff vascularity using laser Doppler flowmetry, in Post M, Morrey BF, Hawkins RJ (eds): *Surgery of the Shoulder.* St. Louis, MO, Mosby Year Book, 1990, pp 208–212.
37. Brewer BJ: Aging of the rotator cuff. *Am J Sports Med* 1979;7:102–110.
38. Uhthoff HK, Sarkar K: Pathology of rotator cuff tendons, in Watson MS (ed): *Surgical Disorders of the Shoulder.* Edinburgh, Churchill Livingstone, 1991, pp 259–270.
39. Ogata S, Uhthoff HK: Acromial enthesopathy and rotator cuff tear: A radiologic and histologic postmortem investigation of the coracoacromial arch. *Clin Orthop* 1990;254:39–48.

40. Meyer AW: Chronic functional lesions of the shoulder. *Arch Surg* 1937;35:646–674.
41. Neer CS II: Anterior acromioplasty for the chronic impingement syndrome in the shoulder: A preliminary report. *J Bone Joint Surg* 1972;54A:41–50.
42. Neer CS II: Impingement lesions. *Clin Orthop* 1983;173:70–77.
43. Bigliani LU, Morrison DS, April EW: The morphology of the acromion and its relationship to rotator cuff tears. *Orthop Trans* 1986;10:228.
44. Morrison DS, Bigliani LU: The clinical significance of variations in acromial morphology. *Orthop Trans* 1987;11:234.
45. Nasca RJ, Salter EG, Weil CE: Contact areas of the "subacromial" joint, in Bateman JE, Welsh RP (eds): *Surgery of the Shoulder*. Philadelphia, PA, BC Decker Inc, 1984, pp 134–139.
46. Jerosch J, Castro WH, Sons HU, et al: Etiology of sub-acromial impingement syndrome: A biomechanical study. *Beitr Orthop Traumatol* 1989;36:411–418.
47. Soslowsky LJ, Flatow EL, Pawluk RJ, et al: Subacromial contact (impingement) on the rotator cuff in the shoulder. *Trans Orthop Res Soc* 1992;17:424.
48. Lindblom K: On pathogenesis of ruptures of the tendon aponeurosis of the shoulder joint. *Acta Radiol* 1939;20:563–577.
49. Neer CS II, Foster CR: Inferior capsular shift for involuntary inferior and multidirectional instability of the shoulder: A preliminary report. *J Bone Joint Surg* 1980; 62A:897–908.
50. Neer CS II (ed): *Shoulder Reconstruction*. Philadelphia, PA, WB Saunders, 1990, pp 273–362.
51. Bigliani LU, Kurzweil PR, Schwartzbach CC, et al: Inferior capsular shift procedure for anterior-inferior shoulder instability in athletes. *Orthop Trans* 1989;13: 560.
52. Altchek DW, Warren RF, Skyhar MD, et al: T-plasty modification of the Bankart procedure for multidirectional instability of the anterior and inferior types. *J Bone Joint Surg* 1991;73A:105–112.
53. Pollock RG, Owens JM, Nicholson GP, et al: Anterior inferior capsular shift procedure for anterior glenohumeral instability: Long-term results. Presented at the 60th Annual Meeting of the American Academy of Orthopaedic Surgeons, San Francisco, CA, Feb. 1993.
54. Jobe FW, Giangarra CE, Kvitne RS, et al: Anterior capsulolabral reconstruction of the shoulder in athletes in overhand sports. *Am J Sports Med* 1991;19:428–434.
55. Jobe FW, Tibone JE, Jobe CM, et al: The shoulder in sports, in Rockwood CA Jr, Matsen FA III (eds): *The Shoulder*. Philadelphia, PA, WB Saunders, 1990, vol 2, pp 961–990.
56. Mow VC, Flatow EL, Foster RJ: Biomechanics, in Simon SR (ed): *Orthopaedic Basic Science*. Rosemont, IL, American Academy of Orthopaedic Surgeons, 1994, pp 397–446.
57. Jerosch J, Clahsen H, Grosse-Hackmann A, et al: Effects of proprioceptive fibers in the capsule tissue in stabilizing the glenohumeral joint. *Orthop Trans* 1993; 16:773.
58. Lephart SM, Warner JJP, Borsa PA, et al: Proprioception of the shoulder joint in healthy, unstable, and surgically repaired shoulders. *J Shoulder Elbow Surg* 1994;3:371–380.
59. DePalma AF, Callery G, Bennett GA: Variational anatomy and degenerative lesions of the shoulder joint, in Blount WP, Banks SW (eds): *American Academy of Orthopaedic Surgeons Instructional Course Lectures VI*. Ann Arbor, MI, JW Edwards, 1949, pp 255–281.
60. DePalma AF, White JB, Callery G: Degenerative lesions of the shoulder joint at various age groups which are compatible with good function, in Pease CN, Banks SW (eds): *American Academy of Orthopaedic Surgeons Instructional Course Lectures VII*. Ann Arbor, MI, JW Edwards, 1950, pp 168–180.
61. Neer CS II: Degenerative lesions of the proximal humeral articular surface. *Clin Orthop* 1961;20:116–125.

62. Petersson CJ: Degeneration of the gleno-humeral joint: An anatomical study. *Acta Orthop Scand* 1983;54:277–283.
63. Samilson RL, Prieto V: Dislocation arthropathy of the shoulder. *J Bone Joint Surg* 1983;65A:456–460.
64. Neer CS II, Watson KC, Stanton FJ: Recent experience in total shoulder replacement. *J Bone Joint Surg* 1982;64A:319–337.
65. Hawkins RJ, Angelo RL: Glenohumeral osteoarthrosis: A late complication of the Putti-Platt repair. *J Bone Joint Surg* 1990;72A:1193–1197.
66. Harryman DT II, Sidles JA, Clark JM, et al: Translation of the humeral head on the glenoid with passive glenohumeral motion. *J Bone Joint Surg* 1990;72A:1334–1343.
67. Janevic J, Craig EV, Hsu KC, et al: Biomechanics of repair of anterior glenohumeral instability. *Trans Orthop Res Soc* 1992;17:495.
68. Soslowsky LJ, Flatow EL, Bigliani LU, et al: Quantitation of in situ contact areas at the glenohumeral joint: A biomechanical study. *J Orthop Res* 1992;10:524–534.
69. Kelkar R, Newton PM, Armengol J, et al: Three-dimensional kinematics of the glenohumeral joint during abduction in the scapular plane. *Trans Orthop Res Soc* 1993;18:136.
70. Bigliani LU, Flatow EL, Kelkar R, et al: The effect of anterior capsular tightening on shoulder kinematics and contact. *J Shoulder Elbow Surg* 1994;3(suppl):S65.
71. Ebara S, Kelkar R, Bigliani LU, et al: Bovine glenoid cartilage is less stiff than humeral head cartilage in tension. *Trans Orthop Res Soc* 1994;19:146.

Chapter 12

The Biomechanics of Soft Tissue: Normal, Injured, and Healed States

Savio L-Y Woo, PhD
John W. Xerogeanes, MD

Introduction

Ligaments and tendons are complex, dynamic structures that are important for both joint stabilization and joint movement. Because of their importance in initiating and guiding joint motion, they are exposed to large repetitive forces and, thus, are frequently injured. These injuries often result in joint instability or dysfunction that, in turn, has serious pathologic sequelae. However, these structures are living, and many are capable of hypertrophy, atrophy, and healing responses. The ligaments and tendons around the shoulder and knee joints are the most commonly studied because these structures are injured frequently. The focus of research has been on their histologic, biochemical, and biomechanical properties. This chapter will focus on the biomechanical aspects of these tendons and ligaments in the normal, injured, and healing states.

Although the shoulder joint accounts for the greatest percentage of soft-tissue damage of any joint in the body,[1] both the clinical and basic science literature have focused primarily on the knee and its associated ligamentous and tendinous structures. Thus, throughout this chapter, we will refer to studies using knee ligaments and tendons to illustrate important concepts that can be correlated with similar structures in the shoulder. We will present the basic experimental methods used to study the mechanical behavior of these soft tissues and then discuss the known biomechanical properties of the normal, injured, and healed states.

Tensile Properties of Tendons and Ligaments

Tensile testing is the experimental method of choice to evaluate the mechanical behaviors of parallel-fiber connective tissues, such as ligaments and tendons. These tissues generally are tested in tension because their main physiologic function is to resist tensile loads and act as a force conduit during joint motion. Tensile testing involves securing the specimen, then applying a deforming force while measuring this force and the corresponding specimen elongation. Thus, a load-elongation curve is obtained to represent the structural properties of the specimen. Data on cross-sectional area and specimen length are used to generate a stress-strain curve of the ligament or tendon substance, which represents the mechanical properties of the tissue.

Tensile testing of ligaments involves rigidly clamping a bone-ligament-bone specimen. For tendons, specialized clamps are used to secure the tendon origin, free from muscle. Therefore, specimen slippage at the clamp site can occur during testing. The resulting load-elongation curve represents the structural properties of the entire composite, which includes the ligament or tendon substance and its insertions into bone. These components have different biomechanical properties, and each contributes a different amount to the elongation of the complex. From the load-elongation curve, parameters such as the linear stiffness (slope of the load-elongation curve), ultimate load, ultimate elongation, and energy absorbed to failure (area under the load-elongation curve) are used to represent the structural properties (Fig. 1).

When discussing the biomechanical characteristics of ligaments or tendons, it is important to consider all of the parameters obtained from the entire load-elongation curve, rather than considering only the ultimate load. Figure 2 compares the load-elongation curves for two hypothetical ligament-replacement grafts together with that for a human femur-anterior cruciate ligament (ACL)-tibial complex (FATC). The ultimate load of graft B is equal to that of the FATC, but one half that of graft A. However, the load-elongation curves indicate that graft A is much more stiff than the human FATC and that graft B is considerably less stiff. Therefore, during physiologic function, neither will perform in the same manner as the ACL. As a result, neither graft would serve well as an ACL replacement during physiologic loading, when it is required to undergo a large number of cyclic elongations. An implanted graft that is too stiff or too compliant would not guide the motion of the knee joint properly before the large muscle forces act on the joint.

Although the structural properties of the bone-ligament-bone complex or bone-tendon complex provide valuable information, they cannot describe specifically the material that composes the ligament or tendon. Therefore, the mechanical properties of the ligament or tendon substance must be determined. To do this, we obtain both a stress-strain curve and a load-elongation curve during the same test. Stress is defined as force per unit area and strain as the ratio of change in length versus the original length. The values of stress are calculated from the information on the load by using the cross-sectional area of the ligament, and the values of strain are calculated from a stress-strain curve. Parameters such as modulus, ultimate stress or tensile strength, and ultimate strain, as well as strain energy density are obtained (Fig. 3).

Before embarking on an in-depth discussion of biomechanical testing, some basic principles of soft-tissue mechanics are helpful. Ligaments and tendons ex-

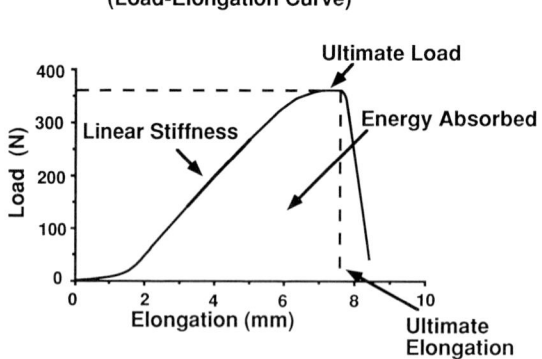

Fig. 1 Structural properties of femur-medial collateral ligament-tibial (FMT) complex (load-elongation curve). Typical results of tensile testing to failure. The structural properties are obtained from the load-elongation curve. (Adapted with permission from Woo SL-Y, Smith BA, Livesay GA, et al: Why do ligaments fail? *Curr Orthop* 1993;7:73–84.)

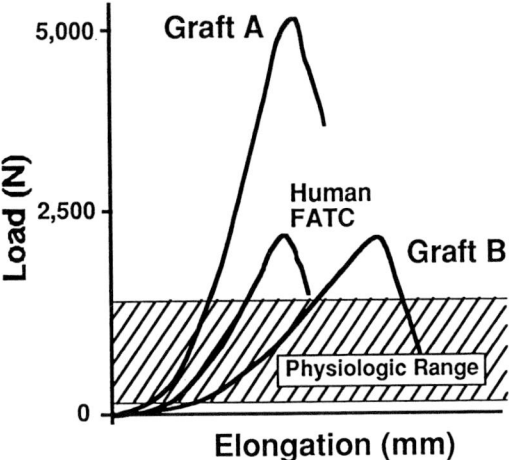

Fig. 2 Schematic diagram of the structural response of the human femur-anterior cruciate ligament-tibial complex (FATC) with two idealized grafts. Note that although graft A would allow the same elongation to failure, and graft B would allow the same load to failure, they are both ill-suited replacements due to their drastically different stiffnesses in the physiologic range. (Reproduced with permission from Woo SL-Y, Adams DJ: The tensile properties of human anterior cruciate ligaments (ACL) and ACL tissue grafts, in Daniel D (ed): *Knee Ligaments: Structure, Function, Injury and Repair.* New York, NY, Raven Press, 1990, pp 279–289.)

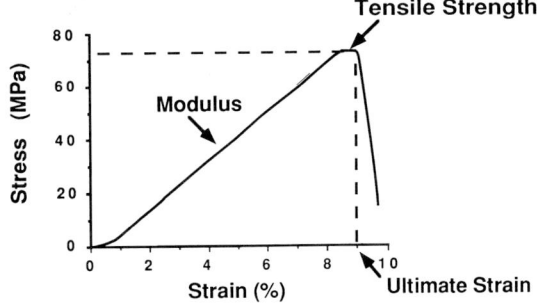

Fig. 3 Mechanical properties of ligament substance (stress-strain curve). Typical results of tensile testing to failure. The mechanical properties are obtained from the stress-strain curve. (Reproduced with permission from Woo SL-Y, Smith BA, Livesay GA, et al: Why do ligaments fail? *Curr Orthop* 1993;7:73–84.)

hibit nonlinear properties. In terms of tensile testing, this means that the tissue will deform in a nonlinear manner when subjected to differing loads. This is exemplified in Figure 4, in which identical increments in length are correlated with different load increments. This nonlinear deformation results from the microstructural property known as collagen crimping. As a load is place on a ligament, the ligament lengthens and the crimp is removed from the ligament. Under relatively small tensile loads, crimped fibrils begin to straighten out. Initially, there is little resistance to tension. This correlates with the initial section or "toe" region of the curve noted in Figure 4, where only a small load was needed to induce the length change. With increasing load, the soft tissue becomes progressively taut. This change is depicted in the latter, more linear part of the curve in which a larger load is needed to induce the same length change exhibited in the initial region of the curve. This phenomenon is very important in vivo. In low-energy states (passive movement), the ligaments act to guide the joint through the proper motion. However, in increased energy

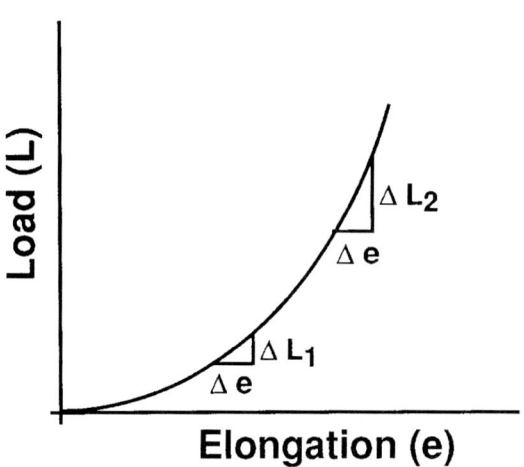

Fig. 4 Schematic representation of nonlinear structural response. Identical increments will result in differing load increments.

states, when muscle forces are acting across the joint, the nonlinear characteristics of the ligamentous tissue maintain correct joint motion.

Ligaments and tendons also exhibit time- and history-dependent viscoelastic characteristics. When a ligament or tendon is elongated to a specific length and remains at this position over time, the load supported by the tissue progressively declines. This property is termed stress relaxation (Fig. 5, *left*). Conversely, soft tissues such as ligaments and tendons also exhibit a time-dependent increase in elongation when subjected to a constant load. This is known as creep (Fig. 5, *right*). These behaviors are different from those of purely elastic materials in which there is no time-dependent load or elongation.

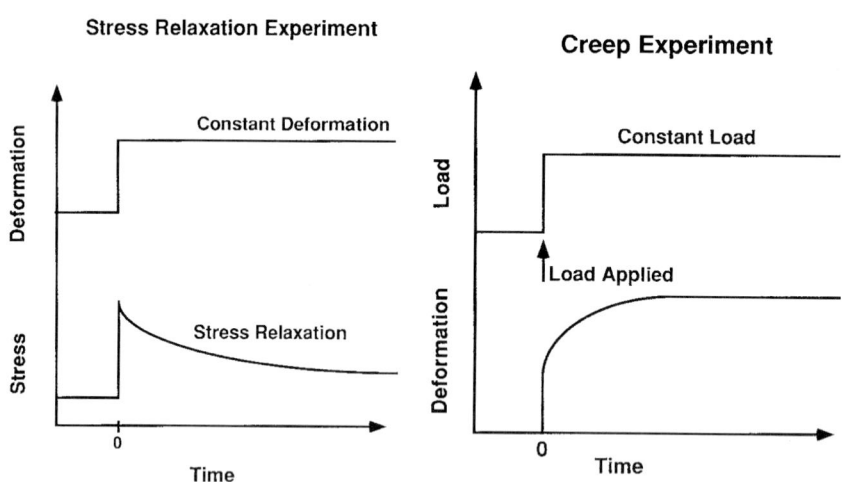

Fig. 5 Left, Schematic representation of stress relaxation (decreasing stress over time under a constant deformation). **Right**, Schematic representation of creep behavior (increasing deformation over time under a constant load). (Reproduced with permission from Woo SL-Y, Young EP: Structure and function of tendons and ligaments, in Mow VC, Hayes WC (eds): *Basic Orthopaedic Biomechanics*. New York, NY, Raven Press, 1991, pp 199–243.)

The viscoelastic response of soft tissue depends not only on time, but also on the strain history of the material. The amount of stress-relaxation can be minimized by exposing the tissue to multiple cycles of elongation, known as cyclic preconditioning. Thus, in biomechanical testing, preconditioning is a common part of the testing protocol to help ensure that the tissues have a relatively uniform strain history and, therefore, reach a similar initial condition prior to testing. This phenomenon also has clinical relevance. For example, in a capsular shift procedure, the amount of tension remaining in the graft during recovery is vital to the success of the procedure. Thus, for optimal results, the viscoelastic properties of the capsular tissue must be considered during the operation.

Factors Affecting Tensile Properties

Specimen Orientation

Because of the geometric complexity of some ligaments and tendons, the orientation of the specimen is very important during tensile testing. The direction of both the ligament or tendon fibers and of their insertion sites, in relation to the applied tensile force, can significantly affect the experimental results. This is best exemplified in the case of the ACL. The ACL contains fiber bundles of different lengths joined together and attached to the bone in a complex geometric arrangement, which makes uniform loading of the entire ligament in simple uniaxial tension difficult, if not impossible. When tensile testing is conducted, as much of the ACL as possible should be loaded simultaneously in order to minimize underestimation of its structural stiffness and strength. Effects of specimen orientation on the tensile properties have been well illustrated by testing the FATC of rabbits in two different orientations: anatomic and tibial.[2]

In the anatomic orientation, the tensile load is applied along the axis of the ACL, preserving the normal anatomic angles of the insertion with respect to the bone. In the tibial orientation, the tensile load is applied in line with the tibial and femoral insertion site, distorting the original anatomic angles of the ACL insertion.

In a follow-up study, our laboratory studied 27 pairs of human cadaver knees. The FATC pairs were tested at 30° flexion, one in anatomic orientation and the other in tibial orientation.[3] The linear stiffness, ultimate load, and energy absorbed at failure for the FATC were found to be significantly higher in specimens in which the tensile load was applied along the anatomic orientation than in those in which the tensile load was applied along the tibial orientation. Therefore, by maintaining the anatomic angles of the femoral and tibial insertions, a greater portion of the ACL fibers were loaded simultaneously.

For younger donors (22 to 35 years of age) tested in the anatomic orientation, the ultimate load was 2,160 ± 157 N, which was significantly greater than for those tested in the tibial orientation, 1,602 ± 167 N. The latter value was closer to values previously reported in the literature.[4] However, it is believed that for the structural properties of the FATC, the higher values obtained (over 30% higher) by testing in the anatomic orientation are most representative of the native ACL.

The specimen orientation also affected failure mode. The FATCs tested in the tibial orientation had a higher incidence of insertion failure by sequentially peeling off individual fiber bundles (48%) than did those tested in the anatomic orientation (4%). These findings suggest that special consideration should be given in tensile testing of the ligaments and tendons of the shoulder girdle because the fiber orientation and length of the structures are highly nonuniform.

Specimen Age

The biomechanical, biochemical, and morphologic properties of connective tissues change with age.[3-6] Strocchi and associates[7] showed that in human Achilles tendons, collagen fibrils decreased in average diameter, maximum diameter, and density with increasing age. Similar findings were found in electron microscopic evaluation of the human ACL.[8] Biomechanical characteristics also follow a similar trend.

Reeves[9] evaluated the tensile strength of the anterior capsular structures of the shoulder in cadavers of humans whose age at death ranged from 28 weeks to 92 years. Two structures were tested, the subscapularis with humeral insertion and the scapula-anteroinferior capsule-humerus complex. Results showed that 78% of the failures occurred at the anteroinferior labral insertion in cadavers of subjects between the ages of 10 and 40 years. In specimens from older subjects, the subscapularis tendon and capsule failed more frequently than the insertion sites.

Kaltsas[10] compared the structural properties of cadaveric shoulder and elbow joint capsules. Each shoulder was dissected down to the joint capsule and mounted in a tensile testing machine with a joint orientation of 90° of abduction. The strength of the joint capsule varied inversely with age. In all specimens, the anteroinferior capsule of the shoulder ruptured first at an ultimate load of approximately 2,000 N.

In our laboratory, we have also investigated the effect of age on the structural properties of the FATC.[3] When the FATC was tensile tested in its anatomic orientation, significant decreases in stiffness and strength were seen with increasing specimen age. For the younger specimens, linear stiffness (242 ± 28 N/mm) and ultimate load (2,160 ± 157 N) values were significantly higher than for the older specimens (180 ± 25 N/mm and 658 ± 129 N, respectively). These values are higher than those reported by Trent and associates[11] and Noyes and Grood,[4] but the age-dependent trend is similar.

There were also age-related differences in the failure modes of the FATC. The older specimens had a higher incidence of substance failures (67%) than the younger (28%) or middle-aged (44%) specimens. Of the younger specimens, 50% tested failed by tibial avulsion. These differences in failure modes show that ligament substance may deteriorate with age at a faster rate than bone.

Tendon Injuries

The biomechanics of tendon injuries is very important, although at present it is poorly understood. Tendons in the upper extremity are particularly at risk for injuries termed overuse injuries, which may result in inflammatory disorders (tendinitis) or degenerative disorders (tendinosis). These types of injuries represent approximately 30% to 50% of all sports-related injuries.[12] Yet, the clinical data on tendinitis and tendinosis are limited, and only a few experimental models are available.

Tkach and associates[13] used collagenase injection to initiate tendinosis. Collagenase was injected into one patellar tendon, and normal saline was injected into the contralateral patellar tendon. The animals were sacrificed at 4, 10, and

16 weeks postinjection. Each patellar tendon specimen then underwent tensile testing. The authors[13] reported a significant decrease in tensile strength at 4, 10, and 16 weeks and a significant decrease in stiffness at 4 weeks. Upon analysis of the experimental specimens, the histology of most was found to be consistent with that of chronic tendinosis. The authors believed that the variability in their data was related partially to the technical aspects of injecting the collagenase into the patellar tendon.

Work has begun in our laboratory to develop an animal model of tendinosis. As in the previously cited study, we are using a rabbit model in which a chemical substance is injected into the patellar tendon. Two tendinosis-producing substances are being investigated: collagenase and the interleukin-1 based cytokine model termed cytokine activating factor (CAF). Ultrasound imaging is used as a noninvasive means to ensure the injection of the solution into a specific intratendinous site. The study also uses both histologic evaluation and magnetic resonance imaging (MRI) to document the cause of tendinosis.

The biomechanical effect of the tendinosis was assessed at 4 and 16 weeks. The means and standard deviations of the structural and mechanical properties of the control, collagenase-injected, and CAF-injected tendons are shown in Tables 1 and 2. Although the trends in this study indicate that both collagenase and CAF injection produce a tendinosis-like condition as well as negatively affect the biomechanical properties of the patellar tendon, the only significant difference between treated and control specimens was found in the collagenase injected tendons at 4 weeks. In these tendons, the cross-sectional area significantly increased in size with a significant decrease in tensile strength. These results correlate with the MRI and ultrasound findings, which show that most of the observable tendon damage occurred at 1 to 2 weeks postinjection and then slowly began to resolve. These results correlate with the findings of earlier animal studies. The preliminary data exemplify the need to further develop the animal model and to focus our biomechanical evaluation on the initial phases of the tendinosis.

Table 1 Properties of 4-week control and injected tendons

Treatment*	Area (mm²)	Ultimate Load (N)	Stiffness (N/mm)	Elongation (%)	Stress (MPa)
CAF	14.8 ± 2.7	568.7 ± 89.2	173.1 ± 38.0	26.0 ± 10.5	40.0 ± 11.8
CON	16.6 ± 3.8	523.5 ± 102.6	169.7 ± 34.1	23.6 ± 12.8	32.4 ± 6.5
COL	27.8 ± 10.3*	424.5 ± 125.4	138.3 ± 58.4	23.9 ± 7.9	17.3 ± 10.6*
CON	14.5 ± 0.7	521.0 ± 91.0	180.6 ± 44.3	24.3 ± 16.2	36.1 ± 6.9

*CON, control; CAF, cytokine activating factor injected; COL, collagenase injected

Table 2 Properties of 16-week control and injected tendons

Treatment*	Area (mm²)	Ultimate Load (N)	Stiffness (N/mm)	Elongation (%)	Stress (MPa)
CAF	14.8 ± 5.0	412.8 ± 91.2	175.5 ± 36.3	21.2 ± 4.7	32.4 ± 11.3
CON	13.9 ± 2.1	518.8 ± 218.0	151.2 ± 49.1	27.8 ± 11.5	37.6 ± 18.9
COL	27.2 ± 13.1	498.0 ± 172.3	125.5 ± 35.7	28.5 ± 5.3	20.9 ± 12.2
CON	16.5 ± 3.6	513.3 ± 173.4	166.9 ± 45.1	30.5 ± 7.2	32.9 ± 9.4

*CON, control; CAF, cytokine activating factor injected; COL, collagenase injected

From the literature and our own laboratory, we can postulate a possible etiology of tendinosis. We hypothesize that tendon injury may be the result of cumulative failures following repetitive application of subfailure loads. Data from our laboratory revealed that application of a tensile load of 75% of the ultimate failure load to the rabbit medial collateral ligament (MCL) resulted in microscopic tears in its substance with no noticeable disruption of the gross ligament structure.[14] Fibril failure is conceivable for tendons that are subjected to higher physiologic loads. This type of microdamage, unlike the frank tears, will involve little or no disruption of the vasculature, and the reparative process may have to rely on a limited number of resident cells alone. Naturally, this type of reparative process is expected to be limited as well as ineffective. Recent data from our laboratory have shown that ligament fibroblasts alone have only a limited amount of factors/cytokine available to stimulate proliferation.[15] It is only with additional growth factors that a cascading effect can result and significantly increase fibroblast proliferation and repair of the collagen structure.

Theoretically, microdamage to the midtendon may not elicit a significant proliferative response, because significant bleeding and clot formation would not exist. A reparative response of this nature is not comparable to the higher concentration of growth factors or cytokines needed to initiate an inflammatory response for tissue repair. Therefore, repeated microfibril tears may eventually develop into tendinosis if sufficient time is not allotted between tears for the fibrils to heal. Further experimental studies will need to be done to test these hypotheses.

Healing of Ligaments and Tendons

The biochemical and histologic characteristics of healing tissue have been evaluated in many studies. Although less attention has been given to the biomechanical aspects, it is our contention that the biomechanical characterization of healing soft tissue is imperative in order to assess its quality as well as its quantity. This information can then be directly applicable to the clinician's functional assessment. As a result, improved surgical and rehabilitation protocols can be developed.

The MCL is one of the most commonly injured ligaments in the body. Because of its susceptibility to injury and its ability to heal, it is often used as a model for ligament healing studies. The canine and rabbit MCLs frequently have been used as experimental models. Woo and associates[16] used a canine model to investigate the healing properties of surgically transected MCLs. The subjects were treated conservatively with no immobilization. The MCLs were tested at 6, 12, and 48 weeks posttransection. The structural properties of the transected femur-MCL-tibial complex (FMTC) were significantly decreased at 6 weeks posttransection, but they were nearly recovered by 12 weeks. Figure 6 illustrates the increased healing and stiffness of the FMTC with time using load deformation curves. Similar findings are noted when evaluating the ultimate load data. At 6 weeks postinjury, the ultimate load was significantly less than that of the control FMTC. However, at 12 weeks the ultimate load values approach those of the controls (Fig. 7). Although the structural properties returned to normal with time, the same was not true for the mechanical properties. At 6 weeks the tensile strength of the transected FMTC was approximately 20% that of the control FMTC. The tensile strength of the transected MCLs increased steadily up to 48 weeks, when it reached approximately 62% that of the control FMTC.

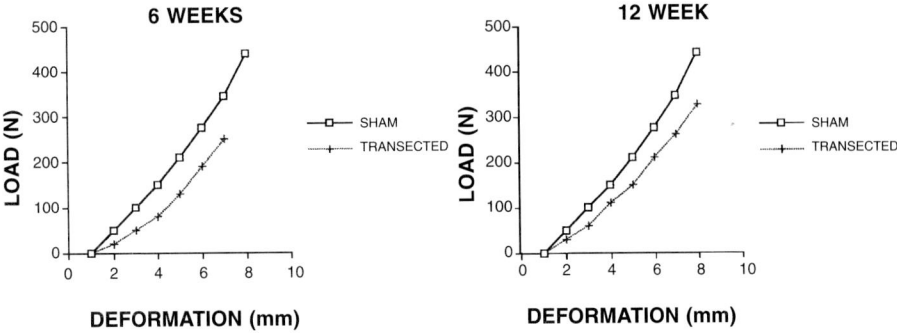

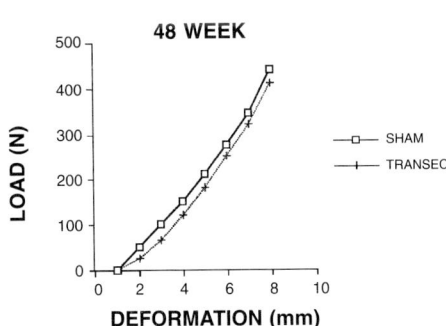

Fig. 6 Change to the structural properties of the femur-medial collateral ligament-tibial complex (FMTC) for sham-operated controls and experimental (surgically transected) knees at 6, 12, and 48 weeks postsurgery. (Adapted with permission from Woo SL, Inoue M, McGurk-Burleson E, et al: Treatment of the medial collateral ligament injury: II. Structure and function of canine knees in response to differing treatment regimens. Am J Sports Med 1987;15:22–29.)

The full recovery of the FMTC structural properties without like recovery of the mechanical properties gives insight into the healing mechanism of ligaments. It was noted that the cross-sectional area of the transected ligament was significantly larger than that of the control at 6 weeks after surgical transection; at 12 and 48 weeks, transected ligaments were still larger than their contralateral controls, but not significantly so. Thus, it appears that initially larger amounts of tissue, of inferior quality, serve to restore function and normal structural properties. Over time the tissues remodel, leaving smaller amounts of tissue of superior quality.

In the model discussed above, a scalpel cut was used to simulate a traumatic MCL disruption. However, with a traumatic midsubstance MCL disruption, a "mop-end" midsubstance injury is usually seen and is accompanied by concomitant insertion site injuries. Thus, a new model was developed in our laboratory to mimic the natural injury.[15] The MCL is ruptured by placing a rod beneath the ligament and pulling medially. The result is a consistent mop-end tear of the ligament substance with simultaneous injury to the insertion site.

Using the above technique, a mop-end tear (with concomitant injury to the insertion sites) of the rabbit MCL substance was created.[17] Two methods of treatment were evaluated: primary repair and nonsurgical treatment. There were no significant differences in the tensile properties of the FMTC between

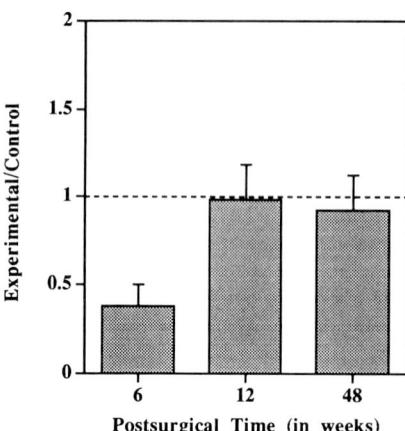

Fig. 7 Change to ultimate load of the medial collateral ligament midsubstance for surgically transected specimens at 6 weeks (**left**), 12 weeks (**center**), and 48 weeks (**right**) after surgery. The mean values of 35 sham-operated control MCLs are shown. (Reproduced with permission from Woo SL, Inoue M, McGurk-Burleson E, et al: Treatment of the medial collateral ligament injury: II. Structure and function of canine knees in response to differing treatment regimens. Am J Sports Med 1987;15:22–29.)

the primary repair group and the group treated nonsurgically. However, postoperative healing time improved the FMTC properties of both treatment groups. Differences in failure modes were noted at different times in the study. At 12 weeks, over half of the FMTCs failed by tibial avulsion but at 52 weeks, all of the specimens failed by midsubstance tears. Thus, the failure mode of these complexes indicates that, in this type of injury, the rates of recovery between the ligament substance and insertion sites are asynchronous. Further, the ultimate load of the healing FMTC increases with healing time but remains significantly lower than that of the control, and the mechanical properties of the healing ligament substance are different from those of the control up to 52 weeks.

Controversy exists as to whether immobilization or motion of torn ligaments is beneficial to their healing. Studies have shown that immobilization caused ligaments to exhibit loss of normal collagen fiber orientation, changes in mechanical properties of the midsubstance, and a decrease in the strength of the FMTC, particularly at the tibial insertion site secondary to osteoclastic activities.[18,19] However, positive effects of passive motion on healing have been shown in several studies. Fronek and associates[20] showed that passive motion of healing rabbit MCLs resulted in an ultimate load at 6 weeks that was four times greater than that of immobilized ligaments. Similar findings were demonstrated by Long and associates.[21]

Woo and associates[16] demonstrated that normal levels of activity have a positive effect on MCL healing when compared to immobilization. The study compared the healing of transected canine MCLs from two groups: one group underwent 6 weeks of immobilization and the other group underwent 6 weeks of normal activity. The immobilized group fared worse in all aspects of biomechanical testing. Even at 12 weeks postinjury, with 6 weeks of activity following the immobilization, the average load at failure was 54% that of their contralateral controls.

Less has been studied in the area of tendon healing. Most of the work has been done on hand flexor tendons. Bishop and associates[22] compared the effects of immobilization, tenorrhaphy, and repair on flexor tendon healing. They found that both immobilization and tenorrhaphy adversely affected the ultimate load and stiffness of the 60% transected canine flexor tendons. In our laboratory, unpublished data comparing the effect of surgical versus nonsurgical treatment of 30% and 70% flexor tendon lesions showed no difference in ultimate load or stiffness between the surgery groups. Although there are studies evaluating the healing process of Achilles and patellar tendons, very little has been written about the biomechanics of these healing tissues.

Summary

Understanding the biomechanical properties of normal, injured, and healing soft tissue is very important for improving the treatment of injuries to tendons and ligaments. The documentation of a tissue's structural and mechanical properties allows the formation of a database from which we can compare other tissues as well as prospective replacement grafts. Although more data are needed, much insight into the mechanical performance of ligaments and tendons in general has already been gained.

The biomechanical properties of normal soft tissue have been explored in the most depth. The fundamental properties of this tissue are similar to those of soft tissues in the injured and healing states. Ligaments and tendons are viscoelastic tissues that exhibit nonlinear biomechanical properties. These properties can be affected significantly by specimen orientation during testing as well as by specimen age. Thus, the knowledge gained about normal tissue can be applied to the study of the alternative tissue states.

The mechanical characterization of tendon injury is an area of great importance and interest, but our knowledge in this area is limited. To expand our understanding, new animal models for tendinosis are being explored. The use of intratendinous injections of collagenase or CAF in a rabbit model to induce a tendinosis reaction is very promising. However, more study is needed, especially of the initial phases of the tendinosis response.

The healing of ligaments has been intensely studied over the last decade. Ligaments like the MCL exhibit a good healing response when injured. In lacerated or ruptured MCLs, the structural properties of the ligament return to normal over time, and the mechanical properties of the tissue midsubstance recover much more slowly and incompletely. It is also evident that immobilization of the tissue after injury is detrimental to the healing of the tissue.

We have made great strides in understanding the mechanics of ligaments and tendons, but our current fund of knowledge is based primarily on studies of the tendons and ligaments of the knee. Although we can extrapolate (as we did in this chapter) many of the general biomechanical principles for soft tissues of the knee to the upper extremity, specific studies of the tendons and ligaments in the arm need to be undertaken. This is both an interesting and challenging goal for future investigations.

References

1. Kazar B, Relovszky E: Prognosis of primary dislocation of the shoulder. *Acta Orthop Scand* 1969;40:216–224.
2. Woo SL-Y, Hollis JM, Roux RD, et al: Effects of knee flexion on the structural properties of the rabbit femur-anterior cruciate ligament-tibia complex (FATC). *J Biomech* 1987;20:557–563.
3. Woo SL-Y, Hollis JM, Adams DJ, et al: Tensile properties of the human femur-anterior cruciate ligament-tibia complex: The effects of specimen age and orientation. *Am J Sports Med* 1991;19:217–225.

4. Noyes R, Grood ES: The strength of the anterior cruciate ligament in humans and rhesus monkeys. *J Bone Joint Surg* 1976;58A:1074–1082.
5. Woo SL-Y, Ohland KJ, Weiss JA: Aging and sex related changes in the biomechanical properties of the rabbit medial collateral ligament. *Mech Ageing Dev* 1990;56:129–142.
6. Viidik A (ed): Age-related changes in connective tissues, in *Lectures on Gerontology: On Biology of Ageing Part A*. London, UK, Academic Press, 1982, vol 1, pp 173–211.
7. Strocchi R, De Pasquale V, Guizzardi S, et al: Human Achilles tendon: Morphological and morphometric variations as a function of age. *Foot Ankle* 1991;12:100–104.
8. Parry DA, Barnes GR, Craig AS: A comparison of the size distribution of collagen fibrils in connective tissues as a function of age and a possible relation between fibril size distribution and mechanical properties. *Proc R Soc Lond [Biol]* 1978;203:305–321.
9. Reeves B: Experiments on the tensile strength of the anterior capsular structures of the shoulder in man. *J Bone Joint Surg* 1968;50B:858–865.
10. Kaltsas DS: Comparative study of the properties of the shoulder joint capsule with those of other joint capsules. *Clin Orthop* 1983;173:20–26.
11. Trent PS, Walker PS, Wolf B: Ligament length patterns, strength, and rotational axes of the knee joint. *Clin Orthop* 1976;117:263–270.
12. Herring SA, Nilson KL: Introduction to overuse injuries. *Clin Sports Med* 1987;6:225–239.
13. Tkach LV, Nguyen VDN, Coutts RD, et al: A model of experimentally induced tendonosis. *Trans Orthop Res Soc* 1993;18:366.
14. Peterson RH: *The Effect of Strain Rate on the Biomechanical Properties of the Medial Collateral Ligament*. San Diego, CA, University of California, 1986. Thesis.
15. Schmidt C, Georgescue HI, Kwoh CK, et al: The effect of growth factors on the proliferation of medial collateral and anterior cruciate ligament fibroblasts. *J Orthop Res*, in press.
16. Woo SL, Inoue M, McGurk-Burleson E, et al: Treatment of the medial collateral ligament injury: II. Structure and function of canine knees in response to differing treatment regimens. *Am J Sports Med* 1987;15:22–29.
17. Weiss JA, Woo SL, Ohland KJ, et al: Evaluation of a new injury model to study medial collateral ligament healing: Primary repair versus nonoperative treatment. *J Orthop Res* 1991;9:516–528.
18. Woo SL, Gomez MA, Sites TJ, et al: The biomechanical and morphological changes in the medial collateral ligament of the rabbit after immobilization and remobilization. *J Bone Joint Surg* 1987;69A:1200–1211.
19. Woo SL, Gomez MA, Woo YK, et al: Mechanical properties of tendons and ligaments: II. The relationships of immobilization and exercise on tissue remodeling. *Biorheology* 1982;19:397–408.
20. Fronek J, Frank C, Amiel D, et al: The effect of intermittent passive motion (IPM) on the healing of the medial collateral ligament. *Trans Orthop Res Soc* 1983;8:31.
21. Long ML, Frank C, Schachar NS, et al: The effects of motion on normal and healing ligaments. *Trans Orthop Res Soc* 1982;7:43.
22. Bishop AT, Cooney WP III, Wood MB: Treatment of partial flexor tendon lacerations: The effect of tenorrhaphy and early protected mobilization. *J Trauma* 1986;26:301–312.

Directions for Future Research

Develop, refine, and validate laboratory and field methods for measurement of "external" exposure.

Physical exposure parameters are important factors in tissue stress-strain patterns. They are needed as input variables for biomechanical models and for epidemiologic studies. Ultimately, they are needed for evaluation and design of jobs to prevent upper limb disorders.

Methods to be developed include observations, ratings, rankings, checklists, video-based motion analysis, electromechanical goniometers, electromyography, accelerometers, and instrumentation of work objects. The purpose of these methods is to provide time-based assessments of force, posture, velocity, acceleration, vibration, temperature, and work tasks. Accurate and precise methods should be developed and the joints, tasks, and settings (eg, laboratory, field, keyboard, and assembly line work; finger; wrist; elbow; and shoulder) for which each method is best suited should be determined.

Methods would be first evaluated under controlled conditions in laboratories where standardized work tasks are used. These tasks should be selected to represent "real world" work. Measurements then can be compared with known task parameters and with each other. In some cases, analytic models can be developed and used to compare theoretical calculations with measurements; eg, pinch strength required to transfer a known weight. Ultimately, measurement systems must be evaluated in different work settings (eg, office, meat plants, assembly lines), to determine their suitability for routine use under those conditions.

Develop, refine, and validate models for predicting structural changes in soft tissues based on external exposure.

Repetitive motion injuries are directly related to the repetitive activities that induce static and/or dynamic loading of the living tissues. Developing appropriate models to describe the loading effects on the living tissue can provide insight into the tissue behavior and the dominant parameters that lead to progressive tissue damage. Numerous mechanisms come into play in human activity. Development of appropriate models of these mechanisms and their interactions can provide information about the factors that lead to tissue damage and the eventual modeling of the damage process. Much can be learned at all levels of this functional modeling process.

The rigid body models (nondeformable models) assume that the bony segments, tendons, and ligaments do not deform under load. The resulting biomechanical models provide a good understanding of the force and motion interaction with the work task. The models provide forces and motion (position, velocity, and acceleration) acting on the tendons, ligaments, and joints. The models can be used to evaluate the tissue loading in order to assess the resulting biomechanical stresses caused by the activity, set limits on the activity, modify the task to reduce the loading, develop task training methods, and provide resultant forces to incorporate into deformable body models of calculating stress/strain at the tissue level.

Develop, refine, and validate methods for measuring biomechanical and biochemical changes in soft tissue.

It is necessary to better define the biomechanical and biochemical changes secondary to repetitive injuries to the dense connective tissues and to correlate these findings to the morphologic changes. Once this is achieved, the history and tissue responses of the mechanical environment that results in inflammatory responses can be defined and studied. To this end, the excessive levels and duration of stresses and strains in this tissue, whether tensile, compressive, shear stresses or strains, or combinations thereof, are the most likely cause(s) of these injuries. This needs to be evaluated from the cellular to tissue levels in order to understand the etiology.

Sample clinical problems related to this discussion include impingement at the shoulder, carpal tunnel syndrome, and tennis elbow. This study will require that currently available tissue culture loading devices be expanded to include other loading conditions; that tissue testing be carried out at more complex and combined loading modes; that new experimental design/apparatus for the epitendon and epiligament be developed; that better characterization of viscoelastic properties and the associated theories be developed to accommodate the time- and history-dependent behavior; and that biomechanical modeling of the cells and tissues be undertaken to understand the stress/strain fields and to apply the model for more complex or combination loading conditions not available from experiments.

Obstacles to this process are the difficulty of computing stress/strain field without detailed knowledge of tissue and cell properties, confirmation experiments that do not start from simple conditions, and tissue-to-tissue and cell-to-cell variations.

Develop, refine, and validate models for calculating stress/strain at the tissue level (deformable body mechanics).

The functional units of the upper extremity are often repetitively loaded and sometimes these loads may reach high magnitudes. The biomechanical response of these functional units depends not only on their anatomic form but also the stress/strain behavior of each constituent comprising the unit. These stress/stain behaviors in turn depend on the composition (eg, collagen, fibrin, water, electrolyte, etc) and on the microstructural arrangement of these elements within the tissues. From the experimentally determined stress and strain behaviors of the tissues, emphasizing their cyclical and fatigue behaviors, as well as failure characteristics, there is a need to develop mathematical models that can represent these mechanical behaviors with high fidelity. Reliable predictive models could be created using these mathematical laws.

Deformable body mechanics is needed for this specific objective. Constitutive laws should be developed to calculate the stresses, strains, flows, and pressures within tissues. Micromechanical models of tissues should be developed to represent organizational arrangement of tissues and to predict microdamage under repetitive or traumatic loading. A damage accumulation theory should be developed that emphasizes the balance between the rate of biologic repair and the rate of mechanical microdamage.

Compare biologic and healing response of tissues to acute loading versus chronic loading.

The similarities and differences between the healing responses of repetitive injuries of the dense connective tissues and those resulting from frank tears of these tissues must be defined. Much of the literature concentrates on frank tears and also on those tissues in the lower extremity. More knowledge on the upper extremity tendons/ligaments is needed in addition to the healing of lacerated flexor tendons. It is assumed that repetitive injuries are more localized and focal (ie, could occur either at the tissue substance or near the insertion site, or could occur at the center and not necessarily involve the entire cross-section). In comparison, frank ruptures are distributed throughout the bone-ligament-bone/muscle-tendon-bone complex. Furthermore, one injury is chronic and the other is acute. Therefore, the environment of the reparative process needs to be studied, ie, the differences in biomechanical environment (stress/strain field, loading in the healing process) as well as the biochemical environment (localized growth factors versus multiple factors brought in by blood and new cells and repair mechanisms). Furthermore, localized inflammation will have the disadvantage that diffusion of the reparative agent to the site would require much effort and time. The healthy tissue surrounding the injured site could further lessen the signals to the cells to repair. Hence, many hypotheses could be tested to gain a better understanding of the healing processes on repetitive injuries, and many rational and appropriate treatment approaches could be designed based on the results of these studies.

New biomechanical testing technique for nonhomogeneous tissue cross-section and localized variation of material properties will be required. Collaboration between biomechanicians and biochemists is required to evaluate cascading effects of growth factors and cellular responses under these chronic conditions. Animal models could be considered for the study.

Identify thresholds of physiologic injury to soft tissue under repeated loading conditions.

It seems that the mechanism of repetitive motion disorder (RMD) is a "fatigue failure" phenomenon that may exhaust the repair mechanism. RMD is more likely to occur with more repetitions and longer duration of applied loads. The occurrence of RMD also seems proportional to the sum of energy absorbed. The more force applied, the more likely RMD will occur. To have a fundamental understanding of the etiology and of the biomechanical effects that influence the risk, an appropriate animal model should be developed to determine the injury threshold.

Animal models are used to answer the following questions. Where does RMD occur (origin, insertion, or tissue substance)? How much load and how many repetitions based on muscle contraction are needed to develop injury? During repetitive loading, how is the strain change correlated with the degree and pattern of microdamage? How do aging and degeneration affect RMD?

In vivo and in vitro animal models should be developed in association with experimental techniques, such as an electric stimulator to simulate repetitive muscle contraction, an in vivo strain measurement technique, histologic and biochemical techniques to determine pathophysiologic changes, and a molecular biology technique to show tissue reaction for treatment. The in vivo model that is developed should address etiologic factors and also serve as a test for clinical protocols developed for prevention and treatment. Treatment modalities such as the resting interval, immobilization, moderate immobilization, mobilization with mild exercise, strenuous exercise, and growth factors should be considered.

Determine the repetitive or constant loading "safety threshold" of soft tissue.

The process leading to repetitive loading failure may involve the mechanical engineering concept called damage accumulation theory or may involve increasing weakness of tissue through a physiologic healing process. The "safety load threshold" is less than acute failure load levels. An understanding of safety threshold is needed in models to establish limits for external body loading. Without these limits, planning prevention and treatment solutions will be limited to guessing.

Mechanical testing of the soft tissues under repetitive loading is required to establish material fatigue and endurance characteristics. Tissue failure will be defined based on macrodamage as well as microdamage, such as localized tears of the fiber bundle.

Develop models of the relationship between work design and physical exposure attributes.

Models are needed that describe the relationship between work design parameters and physical exposure parameters. These models can be used to determine the upper limb posture- and force-time patterns for a given production standard (method and rate), workstation, and tool. Combined with physiologic, biomechanical, and epidemiologic models, the proposed models can be used to prescribe job designs that control the risk of upper limb disorders, assess the risk of further injuries when placing medically restricted workers, and assess exposure in further epidemiologic studies.

The proposed work entails surveying and cataloging common tasks from representative industries, eg, use of hand tools, hand transfer of work objects, and keyboard work. Physical exposure and work design parameters would be documented and compared using biomechanical and empirical models. Surveys would be supplemented with laboratory simulations of selected tasks to evaluate the full range of task design parameters and intersubject variability.

Field and laboratory studies should also be performed to evaluate possible design interventions for upper limb disorders. Both laboratory and field studies would examine such factors as exposure, repetition, force, posture, and short-term work response (eg, user acceptance, comfort and fatigue effects of the interventions). In addition, field studies would examine short- and long-term health effects.

Develop models for specific musculoskeletal disorders.

Some activity-related musculoskeletal disorders appear to occur more frequently than others, yet occur at very different locations and involve different soft tissues. Examples of these disorders are rotator cuff disease, acquired glenohumeral instability, carpal tunnel syndrome, carpometacarpal arthrosis, cubital tunnel syndrome, de Quervain's tenosynovitis, medial and lateral epicondylitis, ganglion cysts, extensor compartment tenosynovitis, and trigger finger.

Pathophysiologic models using these specific disorders are needed in order to evaluate common and different mechanisms of the disease process. Whether all of these disorders are truly repetitive strain injuries due to repeated musculoskeletal activity or whether they are triggered by other factors (eg, job related stress, deconditioning, obesity, aging, etc) needs to be determined. Understanding the pathophysiology based on specific disorders will assist in addressing issues of methods of prevention, causation and, therefore, influence the use of intervention dollars. The implications to the worker's compensation system and product liability tort system are obvious.

For the development of carpal tunnel syndrome, is "tethering" the median nerve an important factor? The restriction of median nerve movement could be evaluated in normal fresh cadaver hands, as could the gliding of the median nerve at varying angles of wrist and digital motions. Nerve strain and pressure changes could be measured in both dynamic and static wrist motion. Tendon strains and stress could be measured intraoperatively with the subjects performing finger motions. A nerve/tendon gliding exercise program and its place in conservative management of CTS could be evaluated. The transverse carpal ligament itself has inadequately been studied. Thickening of the ligament has been observed intraoperatively, similar to the changes of Dupuytren's contractures. The relative importance of traction versus tissue compression in symptom production could be determined.

To understand the development of digital stenosing tenosynovitis, it would be important to know the gliding fractions of tendons and the surrounding tissues at sites of disease in normal subjects and patients with disease. The model developed could also be used to examine effect of medication, such as "cortisone," on the gliding of tendons. A model should also be developed to relate the stress environment to biologic response responsible for tendon/sheath thickening.

Rotator cuff disease is associated as one of the major repetitive motion disorders. Tears of the rotator cuff are nearly always found to be initiated in the same region, at the supraspinatus insertion. Future studies should quantitate intrinsic tendon properties of the supraspinatus, as well as factors in the external local mechanical environment. Information about stress and strain fields in various regions of the tendon under tensile and compressive loading might help to determine why the undersurface of this tendon usually fails first. Studies of the extrinsic geometric factors, such as correlating acromial/tendon contact with acromial morphology and with sites of tendon damage may yield further information about the role of subacromial impingement in this tendon disorder.

For the lateral epicondylitis, it is necessary to know a number of factors: the incidence and prevalence in tennis and nontennis players; the occupational risk exposures leading to occupational epicondylitis; the differences of load transmission; and the anatomic structure of soft-tissue insertions to bones at the proximal and distal ends of the same muscle or tendon.

Capsiloligamentous constraint to joint stability could significantly be related to the RMD as well. In the shoulder, acquired glenohumeral instability appears to develop on the basis of stretching of the capsular ligaments from high-demand overhead activities. The inferior glenohumeral ligament has been cited as a stabilizer that is damaged or deficient in this disorder. A future study might determine whether there is plastic deformation of this tissue with repetitive high-demand use. Specifically, nondestructive or subfailure mechanical testing with corresponding histomorphologic studies could be performed to investigate this issue. A similar situation could be applied to the development of arthrosis of the carpometacarpal of the thumb.

Section 3

Pathophysiology: Connective Tissue

Section Editor:
Kathryn G. Vogel, PhD

Louis C. Almekinders, MD
David Amiel, PhD
Albert J. Banes, PhD
Michael Benjamin, PhD
Scott Boitano, PhD
Robert C. Bray, MD
Brian Brigman, MD
Thomas D. Brown, PhD
Constance R. Chu, MD
Tom Fischer, PhD
Cyril B. Frank, MD

David A. Hart, PhD
Peiqi Hu, MD
W. Thomas Lawrence, MD
Joe Lee, MD
James R. Ralphs, PhD
Michael J. Sanderson, PhD
H. Ralph Schumacher, Jr, MD
Mari Tsuzaki, DDS, PhD
Kathryn G. Vogel, PhD
Hong Xiao, MD

Overview

This section is dedicated to Michael Flint, FRCS, FRACS (1927–1992). His perceptive clinical observations of connective tissue changes were experimentally pursued with vigor and insight, providing a firm basis for concluding that collagenous connective tissues are formed and remodeled in response to changing environmental stresses. His energy was boundless. Flint was trained in general surgery, orthopaedics, and plastic surgery at University College, London. During this period he became interested in investigative research, particularly hypertrophic scarring and wound healing, and published his first paper in 1951. He went to New Zealand in 1965 as a senior plastic surgeon and began studying the changes in rabbit tendon after sciatic neurectomy, an interest that grew from an observation that surgical manipulation apparently induced the fibrous bands of Dupuytren's contracture to soften. The studies include pioneering observation of changes in tendon glycosaminoglycan content, cellular morphology, collagen staining with Masson's trichrome, and collagen fiber ultrastructure, as related to load. He also developed hypotheses relating charge distribution on the collagen fibers with regulation of cellular synthesis. Many of the subjects presented in the following chapters build directly on the work he carried out between the late 1960s and early 1980s.

Upon cursory observation, tendons and ligaments may appear to be uncomplicated mechanical structures. They are, after all, just a collection of collagen fiber bundles with some fibroblastic cells among the collagen. The significant message of Section 3 is that this is a deceptive view. Tendon is capable of modifying substantially both its composition and structure when subjected to varying load conditions. These modifications are apparently carried out by resident cell populations in response to environmental stress on the tissue. As such, the modifications, and the mechanisms by which they are stimulated and enacted, may be relevant to understanding the pathophysiology of repetitive motion syndromes.

Benjamin and Ralphs provide an overview of the gross, microanatomic, and developmental characteristics of tendons and ligaments. They point out that there are several aspects to tendon function in addition to transmission of force from muscle to bone, such as allowing muscle located some distance from the site of action to pull through a narrow space and enabling a change in the direction of muscle pull by wrapping around a bony pulley. Modifications of the general structure of tendons and ligaments occur at points where they attach to bone or where they are compressed against a neighboring structure. In both cases, a fibrocartilaginous tissue is found.

Evidence supporting the generation of fibrocartilage within tendon by metaplasia, induced by transverse mechanical load, is presented by Vogel. Studies conducted by Michael Flint and associates demonstrated a biochemical correlation between tendon composition and mechanical load in vivo. They showed that glycosaminoglycan accumulated at high levels in the rabbit flexor digitorum profundus tendon in a region of that wrapped around bone, and that the level was reduced when transverse loading on the tendon was eliminated by surgical translocation. Regions of proteoglycan-rich fibrocartilage at the point where tendons receive transverse compression have now been described in many tendons from several species, including humans. The belief that this transition is induced by mechanical load is strengthened by experiments showing that repeated in vitro transverse loading of segments of cultured fetal bovine tendon increased synthesis of aggrecan (the high molecular-weight proteoglycan known to provide compressive stiffness in cartilage).

Although tendons and ligaments share many structural features there are differences as well. The chapter by Amiel and associates points out distinctions in composition, fibril diameter, and cellular morphology between tendons and ligaments and also notes distinctions between one ligament and another. For example, the rabbit anterior cruciate ligament (ACL) has ovoid cells with many processes that project into a surrounding area of amorphous ground substance, whereas the medial collateral ligament (MCL) has spindle-shaped cells with little or no surrounding amorphous matrix. Immunostaining for various cell-associated integrins showed the presence of β1, α5, and αv integrin subunits in rabbit ACL and MCL. Interestingly, increased staining was noted in both ligaments after 12 weeks of immobilization. Passive movement has a positive effect on tendon and ligament repair processes. Overall, these studies suggest that mechanical forces affect metabolism and repair of injury at both cellular and tissue levels.

If tissues are responding to changes in mechanical load by altered synthesis of matrix components, then their cells must be capable of detecting and responding to this load. Banes and associates have investigated the response of cells isolated from epitenon and from the internal tendon compartment to mechanical stimuli. They report that indentation of the tendon cell membrane stimulates a wave of increased intracellular [Ca^{2+}] that is passed through gap junctions to nearby cells. Additional studies suggest that the mitogenic response of tendon cells to mechanical load may not occur unless growth factors are present. These important studies begin to explore both the capacity of individual tendon cells to detect mechanical load and the ability to regulate their response, by two types of stimuli acting synergistically. According to this model, stimulation of a connective tissue by mechanical load, but without the corresponding growth factor environment, could have detrimental effects.

Joints are lined by a vascular connective tissue called synovium that produces synovial fluid. A similar tissue lines bursae and tendon sheaths. It is clear that the synovium plays a role in nourishing articular cartilage and may also contribute to nourishing the less-vascular parts of tendons and ligaments within joints. By virtue of its location, blood supply, and content of potentially reactive cells, the synovium may be an important factor in the maintenance of tendons and ligaments and could play a role in tissue changes that accompany repetitive stress. The normal synovial microvasculature allows particulate materials injected into the bloodstream to escape. These can be subsequently localized histologically. Schumacher discusses experiments in which it is shown that passive movement of a joint greatly increased diffusion of fluid into (and out of) the joint space. This synovial "leakiness" could be a route for migration of inflammatory cells into the synovial fluid. In addition, the response of synovial tissue to mechanical irritation could result in cytokine production that affects cellular migrations and metabolic processes in nearby tissues.

An acute inflammatory response to overt tissue injury is well documented. It contributes to the removal of damaged tissue components and stimulates the migration and proliferation of fibroblasts that will generate and remodel scar tissue. The inflammatory phase ends long before tissue remodelling is complete. In contrast to these beneficial effects of inflammation, Hart and associates suggest that the repetitive motion, or overuse, syndromes may result from too much, or too little, inflammation. For example, tissue degeneration as a result of overuse could be due to chronic inflammation, perhaps because microinjuries occur faster than they can be repaired. On the other hand, the minor trauma of overuse syndromes may not stimulate a full array of inflammatory signals and produces unsatisfactory repair as a result. Units consisting of a neural cell in proximity to a mast cell are implicated in an "endogenous" inflammatory system in which mast cell degranulation is the effector mechanism. It is postulated that this neurogenic inflammation could be mechanically stimulated. Because the paratenon and epiligment have more nerve cells and mast cells than the tendons and ligaments they surround, it could be important to focus attention on these tissues when assessing a response to repetitive motion.

The overall message in this section is that tendons and ligaments have the capacity to change their structure and composition in response to mechanical stimulation. Because the tissues are often surrounded by paratenon or epiligament and often are located in a joint surrounded by synovial tissue, factors outside the tendon and ligament itself may be involved in regulating their response. In most cases, the experimental results demonstrate that mechanical loading within the tissue's normal range is beneficial for maintaining cell activity and tissue function. The changes that occur as a result of altered loading (such as fibrocartilage formation at the site of transverse loading in tendon) appear to be adaptive. Nonetheless, recognizing that tendons and ligaments show a cellular response to loading introduces the possibility that under some circumstances this response can generate nonadaptive changes. It is these nonadaptive changes that may underlie development of repetitive motion syndrome.

Chapter 13

Functional and Developmental Anatomy of Tendons and Ligaments

Michael Benjamin, PhD
James R. Ralphs, PhD

This chapter presents general principles of the structure, function, and development of tendons and ligaments. We have avoided undue overlap with *Injury and Repair of the Musculoskeletal Soft Tissues*[1–3] and have minimized the use of specialized anatomic terminology.

Functions of Tendons and Ligaments

As a general rule, tendons attach muscles to bones and transmit the movement generated by them. A typical tendon extends from a myotendinous junction to an enthesis (ie, the bone-tendon junction). Ligaments attach bone to bone and guide and limit joint movements. A typical ligament extends from one enthesis (ie, the bone-ligament junction) to another. Tendons and ligaments are dense connective tissues dominated by regularly arranged collagen fibers and both have high tensile strength.

Tendons

In transmitting the pull generated by a muscle, a tendon is part of a continuum of connective tissues that links contractile cells with their targets. Thus, the connective tissues of a muscle blend into a tendon, which attaches to a bone.

The force transmission role is well understood; however, several other important aspects of tendon function are not as well known. Tendons:

(1) allow the muscle belly to be some distance from its site of action and this permits the muscle to pull through a narrow space (eg, carpal tunnel);

(2) enable the pull of a muscle to be accurately focused onto single or multiple sites or for several muscles to act on one site;

(3) eliminate the need for an unnecessary length of muscle between origin and insertion, allowing the length of the muscle belly to be appropriate to the amount of movement required—thus, the longer the muscle belly, the greater the range of movement;

(4) change the direction of pull of a muscle by wrapping around a bony pulley;

(5) reinforce or replace part of a joint capsule;

(6) act as springs that store energy in locomotion;[4]

(7) hold other tendons in position (eg, the superficial flexor tendons of the digits hold the deep flexor tendons in position).

The position at which a tendon inserts is of key importance to its function. As a general rule, tendons in the upper limb are attached immediately distal to the joint on which they principally act. The consequent lack of mechanical advantage is compensated for by greater speed of action. Ultimately, this means that the hand can be moved with precision and speed in every direction.

Ligaments

All joints of the upper limb are synovial and their movements are guided and limited by ligaments that may be local thickenings of the capsule or separate accessory ligaments. The position, size, and shape of a ligament relate to the forces acting on the joint. The ligaments must limit allowable movements and prohibit unwanted ones.

As with tendons, there are other functions that are seldom appreciated.[5] Ligaments:

(1) provide attachment for muscles (eg, the interosseous membrane greatly increases the area available for the attachment of forearm muscles);

(2) send signals to the brain that are important in proprioception and allow ligaments to play an active role in the maintenance of joint stability;

(3) are modified to form articular disks that act as shock absorbers and provide articular surfaces in synovial joints;

(4) may act as guy ropes to tie down other soft tissues to bone, eg, tendons (the finger extensor tendons over the knuckles) or skin (the cutaneous ligaments holding the skin of the palm in position[6]).

Structure of Tendons and Ligaments

Tendons and ligaments can vary greatly in length and form (they can be rounded cords, straplike bands, or flattened ribbons). They commonly splay out near their entheses and interdigitate with the fibers of neighboring entheses (eg, the rotator cuff[7]). Cross connections link tendons together to coordinate their actions, eg, the extensor tendons on the back of the hand. Because most tendons are far thicker than is necessary to withstand the stresses their muscles can exert,[8] their tendency to stretch is reduced. If the tendons did stretch, the muscle would need longer fibers. However, very long tendons do stretch significantly in relation to the movement they produce.[9] Elastic fibers may return the tendon to its original length on relaxation10 and could account for the crimped appearance of a relaxed tendon (or ligament).[11,12]

Muscles with long tendons at one end usually have short tendons or aponeuroses (flattened tendons) at the other, but occasionally long tendons are present at both ends of a muscle (eg, biceps brachii). In pennate muscles, the tendon extends into the muscle belly, increasing muscle strength at the expense of range of motion.

General Principles and Terminology

Tendon and ligament cells are fibroblasts that lie in rows between longitudinally oriented bundles of collagen fibers. The cells appear elongated in longitudinal section, but stellate in cross section because of the numerous cell processes that are involved in laying down the oriented collagen matrix.

The terminology used for describing the hierarchical organization of the components of whole tendons or ligaments is inconsistent and conflicting and is based on studies of only a few sites. For the purposes of this review, we will define our use of terms.

Collagen *fibrils* visible with the electron microscope are grouped into fibers that are visible with a light microscope. Type I collagen predominates in the extracellular matrix (ECM), but other collagens are also present (eg, III, IV, and VI).[1,2,13] Considerable variations in the diameter of collagen fibrils have been reported in relation to site, age, and repair and have been discussed in detail by Frank and associates.[2] It has been assumed that collagen fibers can run the whole length of a tendon,[14] but serial section studies have shown that this is not true.[15,16] The fibers are collected together to form *fiber bundles* that may run helically. The fiber bundles are grouped together into *fascicles* and a large number of fascicles form the whole tendon or ligament.

This hierarchical structure is more obvious in tendons.[10,17] The fiber bundles and fascicles of tendons are enclosed in thin films of loose connective tissue called the *endotenon*,[18] or *endoligament*.[19] This connective tissue contains blood vessels, lymphatic vessels, nerves, and elastic fibers and allows the fascicles to slide relative to one another. The whole tendon or ligament is wrapped in a connective tissue called the *epitenon*,[18] or *epiligament*.[19] Chowdhury and associates[19] have drawn an analogy between fiber organization of the epiligament and the woven shielding around a coaxial cable; both can resist tension in various directions. In some tendons, a further sheath, the *paratenon*, surrounds the tendon. The paratenon is merely a specialization of the areolar connective tissue through which many tendons run (eg, those in the forearm[20]). The paratenon has numerous loose connections to the tendon but firm attachments to the neighboring deep fascia (sheets of fibrous connective tissue wrapping around groups of muscles) or bone. A similar connective tissue sheet (the *paraligament*) surrounds certain ligaments.[21] The general structure of tendons and ligaments is modified at two regions: the sites where they attach to bone (entheses) and the regions where they are compressed against neighboring structures (Fig. 1).

Attachment Regions (Entheses)

Typically, entheses near the ends of long bones contain fibrocartilage, and those on the shafts are fibrous.[3,7,22–24] In fibrocartilaginous entheses, the fibrocartilage contributes to a gradual change in mechanical properties between the tendon or ligament and the bone.[3,24] Most tendons and ligaments approach the bone obliquely, yet the fibers meet the bone more or less perpendicularly. The fibrocartilage controls the bending of the fibers, and it ensures that bending does not occur at the hard tissue interface but is displaced through the fibrocartilage and into the tendon or ligament itself.[24]

It is useful to compare the role of the fibrocartilage with that of a rubber grommet, where an electric cable joins a plug. The grommet ensures that the cable bending occurs away from the electric connections. There is a good correlation between the amount of fibrocartilage at an enthesis and the degree of bending that occurs. For example, there is more fibrocartilage at the insertion of biceps brachii than at the insertion of either brachialis or triceps.[25] This is because of the greater range of motion of biceps at its attachment. Biceps both supinates the forearm and flexes the elbow, whereas brachialis and triceps act in one plane only, flexing and extending the elbow. Similar correlations between mobility and quantity of fibrocartilage have been found in the lower limb.[26,27]

188   Pathophysiology: Connective Tissue

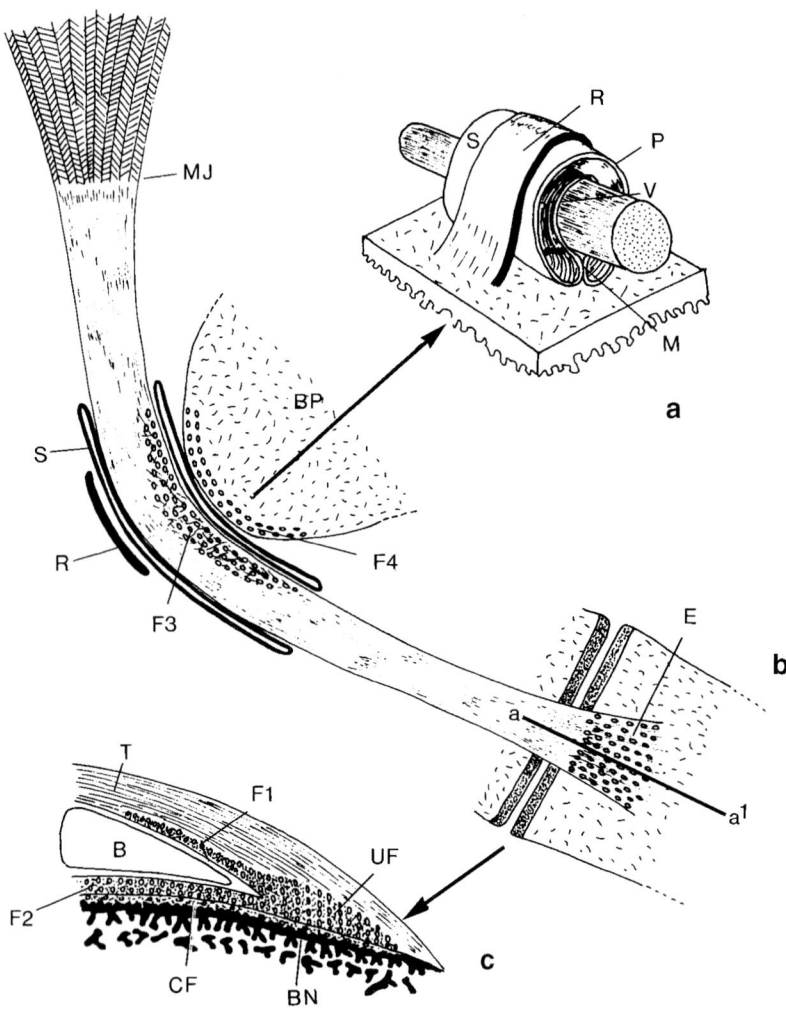

Fig. 1 Diagrammatic representations of a tendon to show its regional specializations (a) with close-up details of a tendon sheath (b) and the enthesis (c). **a**, The tendon is modified where it changes direction and wraps around a bony pulley (BP) and where it attaches to bone at its enthesis (E). At the pulley both the tendon and the periosteum are fibrocartilaginous (F1 and F2, respectively). The tendon is held in position by a fibrous retinaculum (R) and moves freely within a synovial sheath (S). Myotendinous junction (MJ). **b**, Detail of a tendon sheath in the region of a bony pulley. The tendon runs within a synovial sheath (S) and is held against the bone by a retinaculum (R). The sheath has an inner visceral layer (V) and outer parietal layer (P) joined by the mesotendon (M). (Reproduced with permission from Van de Graaff KM: *Human Anatomy*, ed 3. Dubuque, IA, WC Brown, 1992, p 199.) **c**, Enlarged view of a longitudinal section of the enthesis along the line of a to a^1 (in Fig. 1a). At the enthesis, there are a number of protective mechanisms to reduce wear and tear. These include a bursa (B) between the surface of the tendon and the bone, a layer of fibrocartilage on the deep surface of the tendon (F3) and on the bone itself (F4), and layers of calcified (CF) and uncalcified (UF) fibrocartilage between the tendon (T) fibers and the bone (B).

Fibrocartilage is part of a sequence of four tissues at the enthesis: dense regular connective tissue, uncalcified fibrocartilage, calcified fibrocartilage, and bone (Figs. 1 and 2, *top*).[3,24,28,29] The uncalcified fibrocartilage consists of rows of large rounded cells lying between parallel bundles of collagen fibers and is separated from the zone of calcified fibrocartilage by a calcification front, the tidemark. The calcified fibrocartilage has an irregular interface with the underlying bone that increases the surface area for attachment of the tendon and provides resistance to shear.[30] Both calcified and uncalcified fibrocartilage are rich in type II collagen, which is typical of hyaline cartilage, as well as types I, III, and VI collagen, which are typical of tendons or ligaments.[13,31–34] In the tendons so far examined, type II collagen is initially derived from the cartilage of the embryonic bone rudiment, representing cartilage that is left behind after endochondral ossification (Fig. 3).[32,35] However, at least some of the type II collagen may be the result of tendon cell metaplasia, because the type II collagen-containing region enlarges with age.[32,36] The fibrocartilage is also rich in chondroitin and keratan sulphate, as are other tendon fibrocartilages[31,32,37] (see chapter 18). Fibrocartilage at entheses is clinically important. In the fingers, it reappears in flexor tendons that have been reattached at surgery[38] and disappears from extensor tendons in severe rheumatoid arthritis.[33] The amount of fibrocartilage can increase in overuse injuries.[39,40]

Far less is known about fibrous entheses despite the fact that some of the most powerful muscles (eg, the deltoid) are attached in this manner. Fibrous insertions are said to attach to periosteum and eventually become incorporated into cortical bone.[41] However, little is known of their composition or of developmental and age-related changes. Woo and associates[3] have reviewed the findings in the literature on the histology, biomechanics, and biochemistry of insertion sites.

Despite the importance of enthesopathies in soft-tissue rheumatism, basic studies on the structure of entheses have been greatly neglected.[42] Tennis elbow, affecting the common origin of the forearm extensor muscles, is perhaps the best known enthesopathy, but many other entheses are implicated in repetitive motion syndromes.

Compressive Regions

Tendons that change direction around bony pulleys or fibrous retaining structures must withstand compression as well as transmit tension. Tendons are fibrocartilaginous where they press against the bone or fibrous tissue (Fig. 1).[31,43–46] Fibrocartilage is usually restricted to the side of the tendon facing the compressing structure, although it may extend throughout the tendon.[45] Compressive fibrocartilage is particularly prominent in the fingers. It is found where flexor tendons press against the fibrous pulleys[47,48] and where extensor tendons form the dorsal part of the finger joint capsules. In the latter instance, the extensor tendons press against the articular cartilage of the joint when the finger is flexed.[33,49] The presence of fibrocartilage in capsular tendons illustrates the important "articular" role that tendons can play in synovial joints.[50] At a few sites, for example, the annular ligament of the radius, ligaments may also pass around pulleys and become fibrocartilaginous. Fibrocartilaginous articular disks and menisci are also modified ligaments, notably the triangular fibrocartilage complex of the wrist.[51] The degree of fibrocartilaginous differentiation varies with site and probably relates to mechanical factors, such as the extent to which a tendon changes direction. Fibrocartilage changes in response to altered mechanical conditions. If tendons are rerouted under experi-

190　Pathophysiology: Connective Tissue

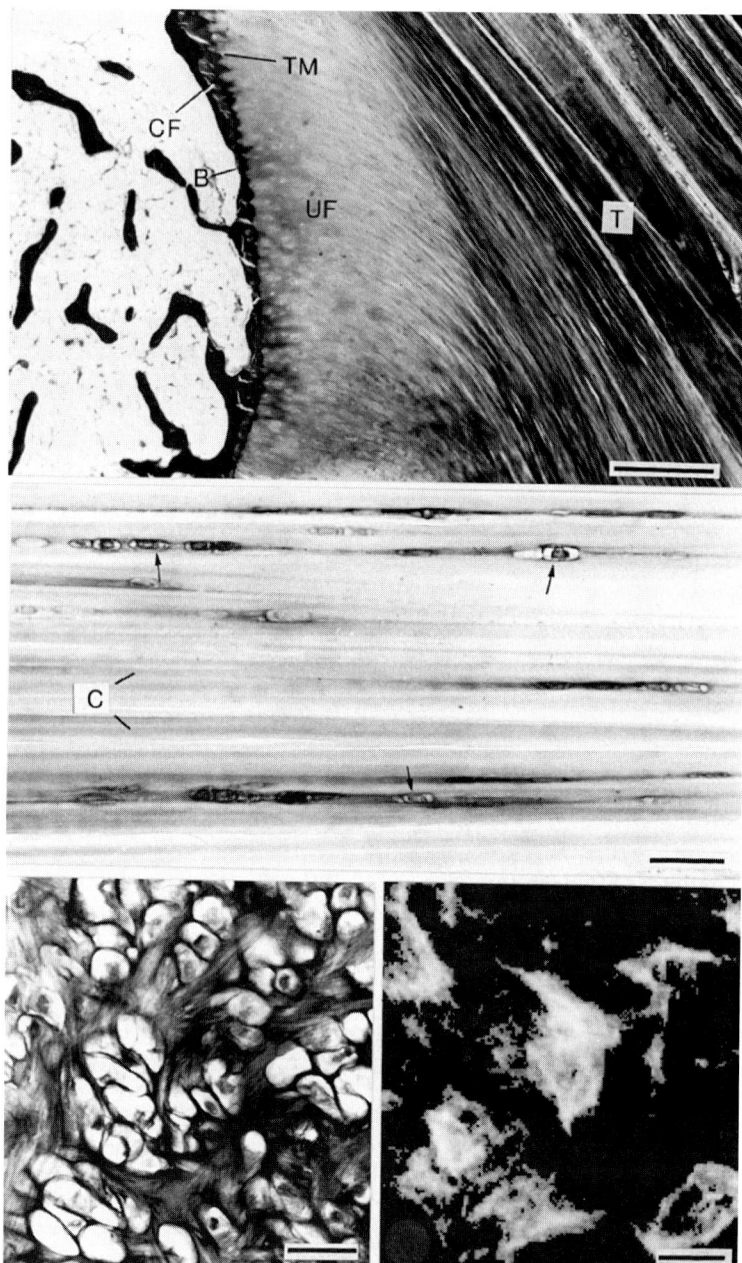

Fig. 2 Structural features of specialized regions of tendons. **Top**, A typical fibrocartilaginous enthesis showing the four zones of tissue: tendon (T), uncalcified fibrocartilage (UF), calcified fibrocartilage (CF), and bone (B). CF and UF are separated by a tidemark (TM). Note the change in the direction of the tendon fibers as they enter UF. Masson's trichrome: scale bar = 1mm. **Center**, Compressive fibrocartilage in which the cells (arrows) are arranged in rows between parallel collagen (C) fibers. Toluidine blue (metachromatic stain for glycosaminoglycans; note matrix staining); scale bar = 50 μm. **Bottom left**, Compressive fibrocartilage in which the cells are randomly distributed among interwoven collagen fibers. Toluidine blue; scale bar = 30 μm. **Bottom right**, Immunofluorescence labelling for vimentin in compressive fibrocartilage cells from a region similar to that in figure at bottom left. 3-D reconstruction of confocal laser scanning microscope section series. The dense fibrous mass of filaments extends throughout the cells. Scale bar = 5 μm.

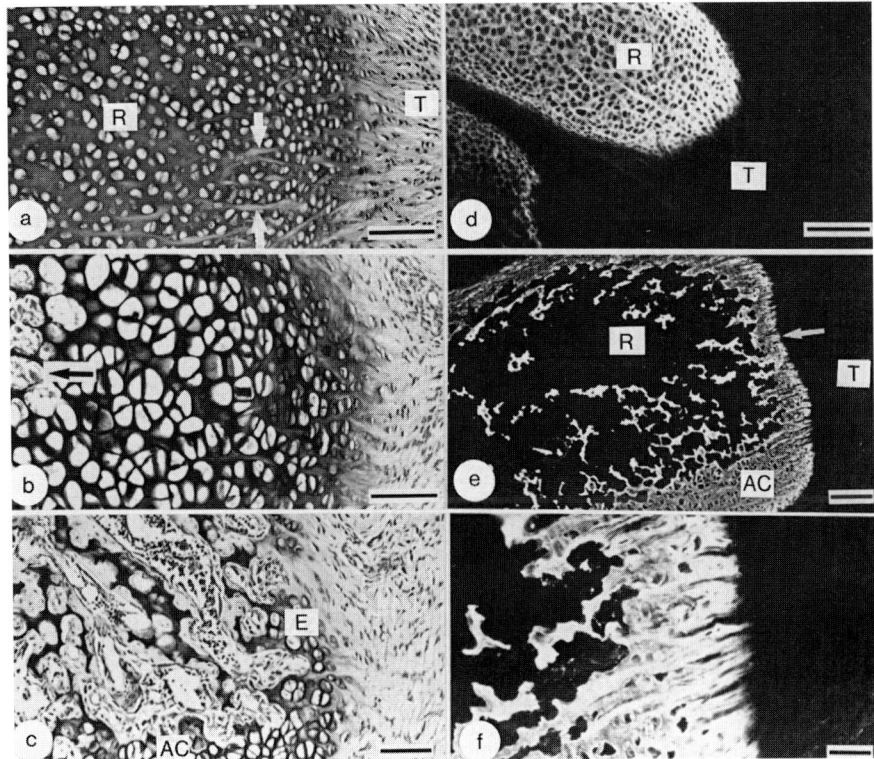

Fig. 3 The development of a typical fibrocartilaginous enthesis. **a-c**, Routine histology preparations stained with toluidine blue. **d-f**, immunohistochemical demonstrations of type II collagen. **a**, The tendon (T) initially attaches to the cartilaginous bone rudiment (R). Tendon fibers run into the cartilage matrix (arrows). Scale bar = 100 µm. **b**, The cartilage hypertrophies and is invaded by blood vessels (arrow). Scale bar = 100 µm. **c**, The hypertrophic cartilage calcifies and is replaced by bone, leaving behind the fibrocartilage of the enthesis (E) and articular cartilage (AC). Scale bar = 100 µm. **d**, At an early stage of development, type II collagen is visible in the cartilaginous bone rudiment (R) but not in the tendon (T). Scale bar = 100 µm. **e**, At a later stage (corresponding to **c**), most of the cartilage of the rudiment (R) has been replaced by bone, but a strip of extracellular matrix ECM containing type II collagen remains and forms the enthesis fibrocartilage (arrow). T, tendon; AC, articular cartilage. Scale bar = 200 µm. **f**, High power of **e**. Scale bar = 50 µm. (Reproduced with permission from Ralphs JR, Tyers RNS, Benjamin M: Development of functionally distinct fibrocartilages at two sites in the quadriceps tendon of the rat: The suprapatella and the attachment to the patella. *Anat Embryol* 1992;185:181–187.)

mental conditions, new fibrocartilage forms where the tendons press against new pulleys and existing fibrocartilage regresses where the tendon is no longer in contact with a pulley.[52,53] The same changes must occur following surgical rerouting of tendons—for example, in the treatment of nerve palsies.[54]

Compressive fibrocartilage contains rounded cells embedded in a collagenous matrix rich in glycosaminoglycans. There are two distinct types of fibrocartilage based on the arrangement of the cells and collagen fibers (Fig. 2b, c). In one type, the cells are arranged in rows between parallel collagen fibers. In the other, the cells are randomly distributed and the fibers are interwoven. The differences appear to be related to development. The first type of fibrocartilage is thought to arise by metaplasia of tendon cells,[32,55] whereas the second arises from a population of cells at the surface of the tendon (Fig. 4).[32]

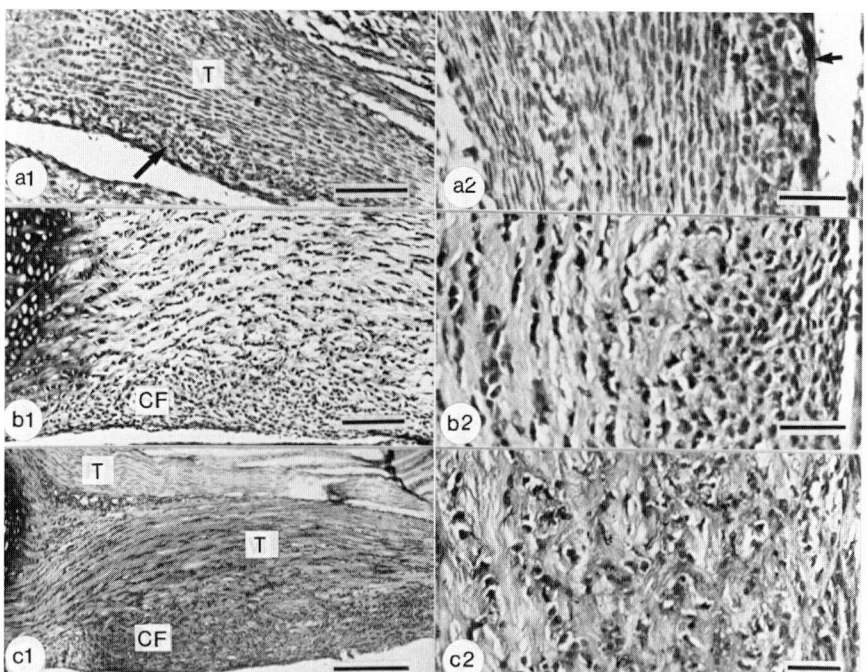

Fig. 4 The development of compressive tendon fibrocartilage (CF) from a population of cells (arrow) at the surface of the tendon (T). **a, b,** and **c,** Successive developmental stages. **a2-c2,** High powers of corresponding photographs **a1-c1** on the left. Scale bars **a1** and **b1** = 100 μm; **c1** = 0.5 mm; **a2, b2,** and **c2** = 50 μm. (Reproduced with permission from Ralphs JR, Tyers RNS, Benjamin M: Development of functionally distinct fibrocartilages at two sites in the quadriceps tendon of the rat: The suprapatella and the attachment to the patella. *Anat Embryol* 1992;185:181–187.)

However, it must be emphasized that few fibrocartilages have been studied developmentally. The composition of the ECM varies according to site, age, and loading. The dynamic response of tendons to compressive loading, particularly with reference to proteoglycans, has been discussed in chapter 18, whereas this chapter will focus on collagens. Types I, II, III, and VI collagens occur in compressive fibrocartilages. In some fibrocartilages, type II collagen is present from an early age; in others, it appears with advancing age; and in yet others, it is absent altogether.[33,36,44,56–60] The appearance of type II collagen (along with proteoglycans) makes the ECM more cartilage-like and presumably more tolerant of compressive loading. A striking feature of cells in certain compressive fibrocartilages is the presence of large quantities of intermediate filaments, notably vimentin (Fig. 2, *bottom right*).[31,43] These accumulate as the tissues differentiate, probably as a cellular response to increased loading.[35,61]

Neurovascular Supply

Both tendons and ligaments have a rich afferent nerve supply that mediates proprioception. They contain both nonencapsulated and encapsulated sensory nerve endings, the latter including Ruffini's corpuscles, Pacini's corpuscles, and Golgi tendon organs as mechanoreceptors.[62,63] The neurosensory function of ligaments is important in preventing overstretching of the ligament by controlling the reflex contractions of appropriate muscles.[2,50]

Vascular injection studies have shown that tendons have a significant blood supply.[46,64] The vessels run longitudinally in the endotenon and may be derived from several sources, including arterial branches from the muscle through the myotendinous junction and from nearby arteries supplying muscles and joints. The supply is supplemented by small vessels from the surrounding connective tissues or from the synovial sheath.[65] There is little or no communication between the blood supply of a bone and the associated tendon (or ligament) because the fibrocartilage of the entheses is virtually avascular.[24,28,66] In the upper limb, many of the tendons are so long that they are supplied by arteries from different sources at different points along their length.[64,67,68] Because long tendons often glide a considerable distance within tendon sheaths (notably in the hand and wrist[69,70]), their blood vessels must be long and coiled, so that they can stretch as the tendons move. However, some regions of tendons have a poor blood supply and may even be avascular, typically where the tendon is subject to friction, compression, or torsion. In the upper limb, this occurs in the fingers,[71] wrist,[67,72] and shoulder.[59,64,73] Hypovascular or avascular regions are more prone to tearing and calcification than vascular regions, but whether the difference relates directly to the absence of blood vessels or to other factors is unclear.[72-78] There is usually a poor repair response in such regions, and it seems reasonable to suggest that this is linked to the poor blood supply. A shortage of blood vessels could cause problems in mobilizing white blood cells, platelets, growth factors, and other agents of the repair response to the repair zone.[66]

Ligaments are normally supplied with blood vessels from periarticular arterial complexes,[62] some of which may be derived from a nearby synovium.[79] The importance of such a supply is indicated by deterioration in mechanical properties when the synovium is removed.[80]

Anatomic Variations The structure of tendons and ligaments can vary between individuals. For example, a tendon may insert in an unusual position or be linked anomalously to another, or it may run through unusual compartments beneath a retinaculum. Anatomic variations are often dismissed as tedious detail, but anomalies can be contributory factors in repetitive strain disorders and influence their subsequent treatment.[81,82] There are also variations in how adjacent tendon sheaths communicate with one another. The large synovial sheath surrounding the flexor tendons of the four fingers is sometimes linked to a smaller sheath for the thumb. This means that tenosynovitis can spread from the little finger to the thumb in some people but not in others.

Development of Tendons and Ligaments

Tendons have been studied more than ligaments, with tendons of the digits being the most commonly studied.

Early Development

The appearance of digital tendons is preceded by mesenchymal condensations that form at about the same time as those of the cartilaginous anlage of the phalanges.[11] The position of tendons in developing chick toes is marked by the accumulation of sheets of tenascin-rich ECM beneath the ectodermal basal lamina.[83,84] Mesenchymal cells condense on these sheets to form the tendons.

Experiments have shown that the initial development of a tendon is independent of its muscle belly. If tendons and muscles are prevented from interacting by grafting the presumptive "hand" regions of chick embryo limb buds onto the flank, the normal pattern of digital tendons appears, but then regresses.[85] When muscle precursor cells are ablated prior to migration into the limb, similar results are obtained.[86] If the tip of the limb bud is inverted rather than moved to a new site, the tendons develop normally but join to the wrong muscles: ventral tendons to dorsal muscles and vice versa.[85] This shows that attachment to a muscle is necessary for the further development and maintenance of a tendon, and that any muscle suffices, so long as its direction of pull matches that of the tendon. The conclusion that the development of tendons and tendon pattern is independent of muscle bellies is in line with Milaire's[87] observations that tendinous and muscle blastemae develop autonomously and join up later.

Postnatal Growth

Tendons must elongate after birth at a rate appropriate to the growth of the associated bones and muscles.[18] They grow most at myotendinous junctions and least at bone-tendon junctions.[88-90] Tendons also increase in thickness after birth, at a rate dependent on the duration and intensity of tension transmitted, ie, the muscle type (fast or slow) and size.[91,92] Ligaments grow more uniformly along their length, although their growth is enhanced where they cross a growth plate.[2] Tension is not necessary for ligament growth, but increasing tension can accelerate the growth rate.[93]

Because long bones only grow in length at their epiphyseal plates, a tendon or ligament attached to the shaft must migrate toward the nearest epiphysis to avoid being left behind as the bone grows.[2,94-96] The most commonly suggested mechanism of explaining the migration is that the tendon or ligament attaches to the periosteum, which moves relative to the underlying bone during growth.[95,96]

Matrix Deposition

Tendon cells condense in longitudinal rows that are pushed apart by the accumulating ECM. Procollagen synthesis begins within the rough endoplasmic reticulum of the fibroblasts and triple helix formation occurs in the Golgi apparatus, but procollagen is converted to tropocollagen in the ECM.[10]

Although the further assembly of collagen fibers occurs in the ECM, Birk and associates[15,16,97,98] have clearly shown that fibrillogenesis is completed under continuing cellular control. They describe three extracellular compartments, each of which is associated with a different level of matrix organization (Fig. 5). The first compartment is formed by small recesses in the cell surface that contain single or small groups of developing collagen fibers. The recesses are probably produced by multiple exocytoses that follow from the alignment of secretory vacuoles and are sites where procollagen processing occurs. The second compartment consists of folds of the cell surface that contain larger bundles of developing fibers. The folds are created when recesses fuse with each other. The third compartment is the general ECM space in which fiber bundles lie side-by-side and become grouped together as the folds retract. Thus, all of the extracellular compartments are formed by complex specializations of the cell surface that allow the influence of tendon cells to extend throughout the ECM.

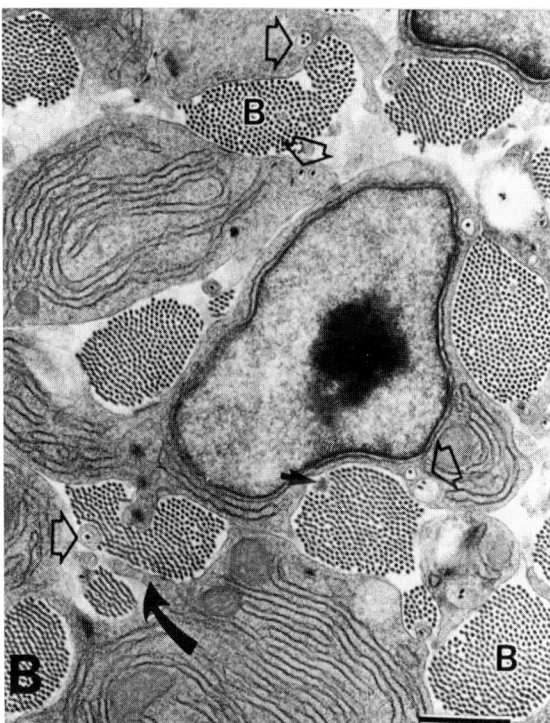

Fig. 5 The relationship of a fibroblast to the developing ECM. There are numerous collagen fibrils within membrane-delimited recesses (open arrowheads). The recesses usually contain a single fibril, but occasionally a few fibrils may be observed. Numerous fibril bundles (B) are also intimately associated with the cell and are generally separated from each other by cytoplasmic processes (curved arrow). The solid arrowhead highlights presumptive elastic elements at the surface of the fibril bundles. Scale bar = 1 μm. (Reproduced with permission from Birk DE, Trelstad RL: Extracellular compartments in tendon morphogenesis: Collagen fibril, bundle, and macroaggregate formation. *J Cell Biol* 1986;103:231–240.)

Control and Lubrication of Tendons

There are a number of structures associated with tendons that control and facilitate their movement. Where tendons wrap around bony pulleys or pass over joints they are held in place by retaining ligaments (retinaculae, fibrous pulleys, or fibrous sheaths). They glide easily beneath them because they are surrounded by lubricating synovial sheaths (Fig. 1). In some regions, tendons are prevented from rubbing against adjacent structures by bursae.

Retaining Ligaments

Flexor and extensor retinaculae in the wrist hold the tendons of the forearm muscles in position. They are implicated in such clinical conditions as carpal tunnel syndrome and De Quervain's tenosynovitis. Pulleys and fibrous sheaths in the fingers hold the flexor tendons in place and prevent them from moving out of line (bowstringing) in flexion. There is a whole succession of pulleys along the length of the finger, and the tendons are threaded through them like line through the eyelets of a fishing rod (Fig. 6).[99] The pulleys may be torn or avulsed by excessive load on the tendons, which is a common problem in competition rock climbers.[100] Pulleys may become too small for their tendons, leading to constriction and development of trigger finger.[81] Trigger fingers can also develop if a tendon has irregularities as a result of surgery or injury. It is intriguing that birds have a natural tendon "trigger" mechanism in their feet to aid in perching or grasping of prey, etc.[101]

In contrast to finger flexor tendons, extensor tendons do not have fibrous or synovial sheaths because they cannot bowstring. Nevertheless, they must stay

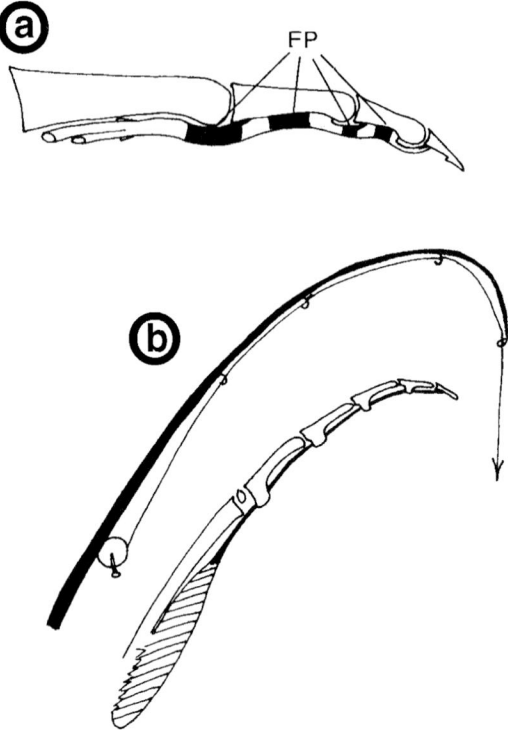

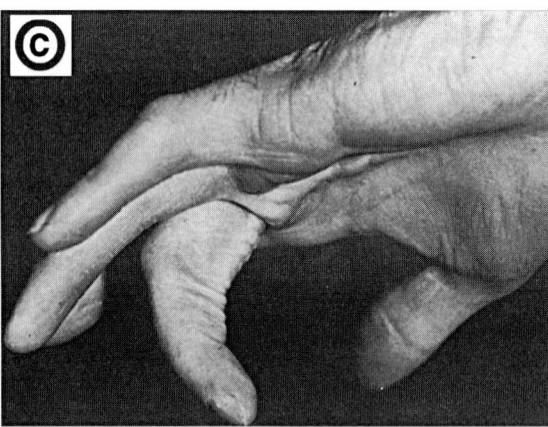

Fig. 6 a, The series of fibrous pulleys (FP) that holds the flexor tendons of the fingers in place. (Reproduced with permission from Semple C: The design of tendons and their sheaths, in Owen R, Goodfellow J, Bullough P (eds): *Scientific Foundations of Orthopaedics and Traumatology*. London, UK, Heinemann, 1980, pp 74–78.) The tendons are threaded through the pulleys like line through the eyelets of a fishing rod (**b**). (Reproduced with permission from Burton RI, Beasley RW, Littler JW: Anatomy of the hand, in McCollister EC (ed): *Surgery of the Musculoskeletal System*, ed 2. New York, NY, Churchill Livingstone, 1990, vol 1, pp 293–310.) If a pulley fails, the tendon bowstrings (**c**). (Reproduced with permission from Burke FD, Pulvertaft RG: Flexor tendons, in McFarlane RM (ed): *Hand and Upper Limb Volume 3: Unsatisfactory Results in Hand Surgery*. Edinburgh, Scotland, Churchill Livingstone, 1987, pp 232–249.)

central in the finger throughout the arc of flexion.[102] There are a number of mechanisms that ensure this, including the shape of the tendon as it passes over the knuckles and anchoring ligaments that act as guy ropes attaching the tendons to bone.

Retinaculae and fibrous pulleys may contain fibrocartilage of similar appearance to the compressive fibrocartilage of tendons and can contain type II collagen.[45,103,104] Indeed, they are sometimes more fibrocartilaginous than the tendon itself. Bony pulleys are commonly covered with fibrocartilage derived from the embryonic perichondrium/periosteum (Fig. 1).[32,45] As with tendons, the fibrocartilage is also dynamic, changing in response to altered mechanical conditions. For example, when the tendon of biceps is ruptured in the intertubercular sulcus, the fibrocartilage normally lining the sulcus is replaced by a loose connective tissue that resembles the tendon sheath.[105] Although the most conspicuous bony pulleys are associated with the midsubstance of a tendon, they also occur near certain entheses, depending on the shape of the bone near the attachment.[32,45]

Synovial Sheaths and Bursae

A tendon held by a retaining ligament must be able to glide freely beneath it when the muscle belly contracts. At such locations, tendons are surrounded by synovial sheaths (closed sacs that contain a thin film of lubricating synovial fluid [Fig. 1]). Sheaths often extend beyond the limits of their retaining ligaments so that the tendons can slide beneath them. Bursae are flattened synovial sacs that allow freedom of movement between a tendon or ligament and the structures against which they press (Fig. 1).[106] A synovial sheath may surround a single tendon or a group of tendons. The tendon(s) are surrounded by inner visceral and outer parietal layers of synovium linked by a fold called the mesotendon, which conveys blood vessels, lymphatics, and nerves. Tendons and ligaments may obtain nutrients not only from blood vessels but also by diffusion from synovial fluid.[107-109] There is considerable support for the idea that synovial diffusion is a more important source of nutrients than blood vessels for tendons with synovial sheaths.[110-112] The mechanism of lubrication of a tendon within its sheath differs from that of a synovial joint.[20] Only boundary lubrication can occur in tendons, whereas hydrodynamic lubrication occurs in synovial joints. In boundary lubrication, a film of synovial fluid coats the surfaces and fills in irregularities to minimize friction between them. In hydrodynamic lubrication, the joint surfaces ride on synovial fluid, which actually pushes the opposing joint surfaces apart. The friction created by the fast repetitive motion of tendons within their sheaths can result in tenosynovitis, but a similar problem does not seem to occur in the synovial joints that move at the same rate.[20] Synovial and fibrous sheaths are derived from the same population of mesenchymal cells as the tendon.[11,47,113] The sheaths develop from circumferential layers of cells wrapped around the tendon: tendon and sheath separate at the time the tendon first begins to move.[114,115] Local specializations of the fibrous sheath (ie, pulleys) appear at the same time as separation occurs. The timing of development ensures that the tendons are kept in position when they start to move.

Summary

Tendons are part of a continuum of connective tissue linking contractile cells to their bony targets. Ligaments generally connect bone to bone and may be thickenings of a synovial joint capsule or separate accessory ligaments around or within a joint. In both tendons and ligaments, collagen fibrils are grouped into fibers, the fibers into fiber bundles, and the fiber bundles into fascicles. The bundles and fascicles are enclosed in loose connective tissue (the endotenon or endoligament), and the whole structure is surrounded by an epitenon or epiligament. There are structural and compositional specializations where tendons and ligaments attach to bone (the enthesis) and where they are compressed against other structures. Some entheses are fibrocartilaginous (eg, at the ends of long bones), whereas others are fibrous, particularly on the shafts of long bones. The fibrocartilage is derived from cartilage of the bone rudiment and reduces bending of collagen fibers at the enthesis: the greater the bending, the greater the amount of fibrocartilage. Fibrous entheses blend with the periosteum and become incorporated into cortical bone during growth. Tendons also contain fibrocartilage where they press against other structures. This fibrocartilage develops either from a population of cells at the tendon surface or by metaplasia of tendon cells. Although tendons and ligaments generally have a good blood and nerve supply, regions of tendons subjected to friction, compression, or torsion are hypovascular or avascular.

Tendons develop as cellular condensations on a tenascin-rich template. Fibrillogenesis begins intracellularly but is completed in the extracellular matrix in distinct compartments formed by specializations of the cell surface. Early tendon development is independent of muscle, but development cannot proceed in its absence. The postnatal growth rate of tendons must match that of muscle and bones, and tendons must maintain the same relative position of attachment on the bone. Less is known about the development of ligaments. Capsular ligaments become apparent at the completion of joint cavitation, and intra-articular accessory ligaments develop from cell condensations that lie between the future articular surfaces before the joint is fully cavitated.

There are a number of structures associated with tendons that control and facilitate their movement. Where tendons pass over joints they are held in place by ligaments (retinaculae, pulleys, or fibrous sheaths) that prevent them from bowstringing. They glide easily beneath these retaining structures because they are surrounded by lubricating synovial sheaths. Sheaths are derived from the same population of mesenchymal cells as the tendons themselves and start to develop about the same time, probably in response to movement.

Acknowledgments

We would like to thank the following past and present members of our research group: Gary Dowthwaite, PhD, Lisa Durrant, Anthony Lewis, Ceinwen McNeilly, Aminu Rufai, MS, BS, Andrew Thornett, MB BCh, and Rachael Tyers, MB BCh. We also acknowledge the financial support of the Arthritis and Rheumatism Council, the Nuffield Foundation, and the Higher Education Funding Council for Wales.

References

1. Gelberman R, Goldberg V, An K-N, et al: Tendon, in Woo SL-Y, Buckwalter JA (eds): *Injury and Repair of the Musculoskeletal Soft Tissues*. Park Ridge, IL, American Academy of Orthopaedic Surgeons, 1988, pp 5–40.
2. Frank C, Woo SL-Y, Andriacchi T, et al: Normal ligament: Structure, function and composition, in Woo SL-Y, Buckwalter JA (eds): *Injury and Repair of the Musculoskeletal Soft Tissues*. Park Ridge, IL, American Academy of Orthopaedic Surgeons, 1988, pp 45–101.
3. Woo SL-Y, Maynard J, Butler D, et al: Ligament, tendon, and joint capsule insertions to bone, in Woo SL-Y, Buckwalter JA (eds): *Injury and Repair of the Musculoskeletal Soft Tissues*. Park Ridge, IL, American Academy of Orthopaedic Surgeons, 1988, pp 133–166.
4. Alexander R McN: Elastic energy stores in running vertebrates. *Am Zool* 1984;24:85–94.

5. Basmajian JV: The unsung virtues of ligaments. *Surg Clin North Am* 1974;54:1259–1267.
6. Schmidt H-M, Fritsch H: Cutaneous ligaments of the human hand. *Europ J Morph* 1990;28:3–13.
7. Clark JM, Harryman DT II: Tendons, ligaments, and capsule of the rotator cuff: Gross and microscopic anatomy. *J Bone Joint Surg* 1992;74A:713–725.
8. Ker RF, Alexander R McN, Bennett MB: Why are mammalian tendons so thick? *J Zool (Lond)* 1988;216:309–324.
9. Rack PM, Ross HF: The tendon of flexor pollicis longus: Its effects on the muscular control of force and position at the human thumb. *J Physiol (Lond)* 1984;351:99–110.
10. Butler DL, Grood ES, Noyes FR, et al: Biomechanics of ligaments and tendons. *Exerc Sports Sci Rev* 1978;6:125–181.
11. Greenlee TK Jr, R Ross: The development of the rat flexor digital tendon: A fine structure study. *J Ultrastruct Res* 1967;18:354–376.
12. Minns RJ, Soden PD, Jackson DS: The role of the fibrous components and ground substance in the mechanical properties of biological tissues: A preliminary investigation. *J Biomech* 1973;6:153–165.
13. Bray DF, Frank CB, Bray RC: Cytochemical evidence for a proteoglycan-associated filamentous network in ligament extracellular matrix. *J Orthop Res* 1990;8:1–12.
14. Viidik A: Biomechanics and functional adaptation of tendons and joint ligaments, in Evans FG (ed): *Studies on the Anatomy and Function of Bones and Joints*. New York, NY, Springer-Verlag, 1966, pp 17–39.
15. Birk DE, Southern JF, Zycband EI, et al: Collagen fibril bundles: A branching assembly unit in tendon morphogenesis. *Development* 1989;107:437–443.
16. Birk DE, Zycband E: Assembly of the tendon extracellular matrix during development. *J Anat* 1994;184:457–463.
17. Kuhlmann JN, Luboinski J, Laudet C, et al: Properties of the fibrous structures of the wrist. *J Hand Surg* 1990;15B:335–341.
18. Elliott DH: Structure and function of mammalian tendon. *Biol Rev* 1965;40:392–421.
19. Chowdhury P, Matyas JR, Frank CB: The "epiligament" of the rabbit medial collateral ligament: A quantitative morphological study. *Connect Tissue Res* 1991;27:33–50.
20. Brand PW, Thompson DE, Micks JE: The biomechanics of the interphalangeal joints, in Bowers WH (ed): *The Interphalangeal Joints*. Edinburgh, Scotland, Churchill Livingstone, 1987, pp 21–54.
21. Alm A, Stromberg B: Vascular anatomy of the patellar and cruciate ligaments: A microangiographic and histologic investigation in the dog. *Acta Chir Scand Supplementum* 1974;445:25–35.
22. Biermann H: Die Knochenbildung im bereich Periostaler-Diapysärer Sehnen-und Bandansätze. *Z Zellforsch* 1975;46:635–671.
23. Knese K-H, Biermann H: Die Knochenbildung an Sehnen-und Bandansätzen im Bereich ursprünglich chondraler Apophysen. *Z Zellforsch Mikrosk Anat* 1958;49:142–187.
24. Benjamin M, Evans EJ, Copp L: The histology of tendon attachments to bone in man. *J Anat* 1986;149:89–100.
25. Benjamin M, Newell RL, Evans EJ, et al: The structure of the insertions of the tendons of biceps brachii, triceps and brachialis in elderly dissecting room cadavers. *J Anat* 1992;180:327–332.
26. Evans EJ, Benjamin M, Pemberton DJ: Fibrocartilage in the attachment zones of the quadriceps tendon and patellar ligament of man. *J Anat* 1990;171;155–162.
27. Benjamin M, Evans EJ, Rao RD, et al: Quantitative differences in the histology of the attachment zones of the meniscal horns in the knee joint of man. *J Anat* 1991;177:127–134.
28. Cooper RR, Misol S: Tendon and ligament insertion: A light and electron microscopic study. *J Bone Joint Surg* 1970;52A:1–20.
29. Benjamin M, Evans EJ: Fibrocartilage. *J Anat* 1990;171:1–15.

30. Schneider H: Zur Struktur der Sehnenansatzzonen. *Ztschr Anat* 1956;119:431–456.
31. Ralphs JR, Benjamin M, Thornett A: Cell and matrix biology of the suprapatella in the rat: A structural and immunocytochemical study of fibrocartilage in a tendon subject to compression. *Anat Rec* 1991;231:167–177.
32. Rufai A, Benjamin M, Ralphs JR: Development and ageing of phenotypically distinct fibrocartilages associated with the rat Achilles tendon. *Anat Embryol (Berl)* 1992;186:611–618.
33. Benjamin M, Ralphs JR, Shibu M, et al: Capsular tissues of the proximal interphalangeal joint: Normal composition and effects of Dupuytren's disease and rheumatoid arthritis. *J Hand Surg* 1993;18B:371–376.
34. Tillmann B, Schünke M: Funktionelle Anpassungsvorgänge an Binde-und Stützgeweben, in Wirth CJ (ed): *Praktische Orthopädie*. Stuttgart, Georg-Thieme Verlag, 1993, pp 22–27.
35. Ralphs JR, Tyers RN, Benjamin M: Development of functionally distinct fibrocartilages at two sites in the quadriceps tendon of the rat: The suprapatella and the attachment to the patella. *Anat Embryol (Berl)* 1992;185:181–187.
36. Benjamin M, Tyers RN, Ralphs JR: Age-related changes in tendon fibrocartilage. *J Anat* 1991;179:127–136.
37. Vogel KG, Ordög A, Pogany G, et al: Proteoglycans in the compressed region of human tibialis posterior tendon and in ligaments. *J Orthop Res* 1993;11:68–77.
38. Jones JR, Smibert JG, McCullough CJ, et al: Tendon implantation into bone: An experimental study. *J Hand Surg* 1987;12B:306–312.
39. Ferretti A, Ippolito E, Mariani P, et al: Jumper's knee. *Am J Sports Med* 1983;11:58–62.
40. Ippolito E, Postacchini F: Rupture and disinsertion of the proximal attachment of the adductor longus tendon: Case report with histochemical and ultrastructural study. *Ital J Orthop Traumatol* 1981;7:79–85.
41. Matyas JR, Bodie D, Andersen M, et al: The developmental morphology of a "periosteal" ligament insertion: Growth and maturation of the tibial insertion of the rabbit medial collateral ligament. *J Orthop Res* 1990;8:412–424.
42. Littlejohn GO: Editorial: More emphasis on the enthesis. *J Rheumatol* 1989;16:1020–1022.
43. Merrilees MJ, Flint MH: Ultrastructural study of tension and pressure zones in a rabbit flexor tendon. *Am J Anat* 1980;157:87–106.
44. Vogel KG, Koob TJ: Structural specialization in tendons under compression. *Int Rev Cytol* 1989;115:267–293.
45. Benjamin M, Ralphs JR: The distribution of fibrocartilage associated with human tendons: A comprehensive survey of cadaveric material. *Trans Orthop Res Soc* 1994;19:640.
46. Tillmann B, Kolts I: Ruptur der Ursprungssehne des Caput longum musculi bicipitis brachii: Struktur und Blutversorgung der Bizepssehne. *Oper Orth Traum* 1993;5:107–111.
47. Greenlee TK Jr, Beckham C, Pike D: A fine structural study of the development of the chick flexor digital tendon: A model for synovial sheathed tendon healing. *Amer J Anat* 1975;143:303–313.
48. Abrahamsson SO: Matrix metabolism and healing in the flexor tendon: Experimental studies on rabbit tendon. *Scand J Plast Reconstr Surg Hand Surg* 1991;23:(suppl)1–51.
49. Slattery PG: The dorsal plate of the proximal interphalangeal joint. *J Hand Surg* 1990;15B:68–73.
50. Ralphs JR, Benjamin M: The joint capsule: Structure, composition, ageing and disease. *J Anat* 1994;184:503–509.
51. Benjamin M, Evans EJ, Pemberton DJ: Histological studies on the triangular fibrocartilage complex of the wrist. *J Anat* 1990;172:59–67.
52. Ploetz E: Funktioneller Bau und funktionelle Anpassung der Gleitsehnen. *Z Orthop Ihre Grenzgeb* 1938;67:212–234.

53. Gillard GC, Reilly HC, Bell-Booth PG, et al: The influence of mechanical forces on the glycosaminoglycan content of the rabbit flexor digitorum profundus tendon. *Connect Tissue Res* 1979;7:37–46.
54. Omer GE: Tendon transfers for combined traumatic nerve palsies of the forearm and hand. *J Hand Surg* 1992;17B:603–610.
55. Evanko SP, Vogel KG: Ultrastructure and proteoglycan composition in the developing fibrocartilaginous region of bovine tendon. *Matrix* 1990;10:420–436.
56. Okuda Y, Gorski JP, An K-N, et al: Biochemical, histological, and biomechanical analyses of canine tendon. *J Orthop Res* 1987;5:60–68.
57. Ralphs JR, Rufai A, Benjamin M: The development of the annulus fibrosus of the lumbar intervertebral disc. *Trans Orthop Res Soc* 1994;19:69.
58. Ralphs JR, Dowthwaite GP, Benjamin M: Developmental changes in extracellular matrix of fibrocartilage in the mouse quadriceps tendon. *Trans Orthop Res Soc* 1994;19:388.
59. Archer RS, Bayley JI, Archer CW, et al: Cell and matrix changes associated with pathological calcification of the human rotator cuff tendons. *J Anat* 1993;182:1–11.
60. Koch S, Tillmann B: Vergleichende Utersuchungen der Stuktur von Gleitsehnen im Hinblick auf die Inzidenz von Sehnenrupturen. *Annals Ann* 1994;76(suppl):44.
61. Benjamin M, Archer CW, Ralphs JR: Cytoskeleton of cartilage cells. *Microsc Res Tech* 1994;28:372–377.
62. Akeson WH, Woo SL-Y, Amiel D, et al: The biology of ligaments, in Funk FJ Jr, Hunter LY (eds): *Rehabilitation of the Injured Knee*. St Louis, MO, CV Mosby, 1984, pp 93–148.
63. O'Brien M: Functional anatomy and physiology of tendons. *Clin Sports Med* 1992;11:505–520.
64. Kolts I, Tillmann B, Lüllmann-Rauch R: The structure and vascularization of the biceps brachii long head tendon. *Anat Anz* 1994;176:75–80.
65. Edwards DAW: The blood supply and lymphatic drainage of tendons. *J Anat* 1946;80:147–152.
66. Wallace CD, Amiel D: Vascular assessment of the periarticular ligaments of the rabbit knee. *J Orthop Res* 1991;9:787–791.
67. Hergenroeder PT, Gelberman RH, Akeson WH: The vascularity of the flexor pollicis longus tendon. *Clin Orthop* 1982;162:298–303.
68. Zbrodowski A, Gajisin S, Grodecki J: Vascularization of the tendons of the extensor pollicis longus, extensor carpi radialis longus and extensor carpi radialis brevis. *J Anat* 1982;135:235–244.
69. Biddulph SL: Extensor tendons, in McFarlane RM (ed): *The Hand and Upper Limb: Unsatisfactory Results in Hand Surgery*. Edinburgh, Scotland, Churchill Livingstone, 1987, vol 3, pp 250–258.
70. Semple C: The design of tendons and their sheaths, in Owen R, Goodfellow J, Bullough P (eds): *Scientific Foundations of Orthopaedics and Traumatology*. London, UK, Heinemann, 1980, pp 74–78.
71. Lundborg G, Myrhage R, Rydevik B: The vascularization of human flexor tendons within the digital synovial sheath region: Structural and functional aspects. *J Hand Surg* 1977;2A:417–427.
72. Hirasawa Y, Katsumi Y, Akiyoshi T, et al: Clinical and microangiographic studies on rupture of the EPL tendon after distal radial fractures. *J Hand Surg* 1990;15B:51–57.
73. Rathbun JB, Macnab I: The microvascular pattern of the rotator cuff. *J Bone Joint Surg* 1970;52B:540–553.
74. Lohr JF, Uhthoff HK: The microvascular pattern of the supraspinatus tendon. *Clin Orthop* 1990;254:35–38.
75. Hermann B, Steiner D: Arterial supply of the human long biceps tendon. *Acta Anat (Basel)* 1990;137:129–131.
76. Chansky HA, Iannotti JP: The vascularity of the rotator cuff. *Clin Sports Med* 1991;10:807–822.

77. Brooks CH, Revell WJ, Heatley FW: A quantitative histological study of the vascularity of the rotator cuff tendon. *J Bone Joint Surg* 1992;74B:151–153.
78. Geppert MJ, Sobel M, Hannafin JA: Microvasculature of the tibialis anterior tendon. *Foot Ankle* 1993;14:261–264.
79. Hixson ML, Stewart C: Microvascular anatomy of the radioscapholunate ligament of the wrist. *J Hand Surg* 1990;15A:279–282.
80. Robinson D, Halperin N, Nevo Z: Devascularization of the anterior cruciate ligament by synovial stripping in rabbits: An experimental model. *Acta Orthop Scand* 1992;63:502–506.
81. Thorson E, Szabo RM: Common tendinitis problems in the hand and forearm. *Orthop Clin North Am* 1992;23:65–74.
82. Kiefhaber TR, Stern PJ: Upper extremity tendinitis and overuse syndromes in the athlete. *Clin Sports Med* 1992;11:39–55.
83. Hurlé JM, Hinchliffe JR, Ros MA, et al: The extracellular matrix architecture relating to myotendinous pattern formation in the distal part of the developing chick limb: An ultrastructural, histochemical and immunocytochemical analysis. *Cell Different Dev* 1989;27:103–120.
84. Ros MA, Hinchliffe JR, Macias D, et al: Extracellular material organization and long tendon formation in the chick leg autopodium: In vivo and in vitro study, in Hinchliffe JR, Hurle JM, Summerbell D (eds): *Developmental Patterning of the Vertebrate Limb*. New York, NY, Plenum Press, 1991, pp 211–213.
85. Shellswell GB, Wolpert L: The pattern of muscle and tendon development in the chick wing, in Ede DA, Hinchliffe JR, Balls M (eds): *Vertebrate Limb and Somite Morphogenesis*. Cambridge, MA, Cambridge University Press, 1977, pp 71–86.
86. Kieny M, Chevallier A: Autonomy of tendon development in the embryonic chick wing. *J Embryol Exp Morph* 1979;49:153–165.
87. Milaire J: Etude morphologique et cytochimique du développement des membres chez la souris et chez la taupe. *Arch Biol (Liege)* 1963;74:129–317.
88. Crawford GNC: An experimental study of tendon growth in the rabbit. *J Bone Joint Surg* 1950;32B:234–243.
89. Lowrance EW: Growth of the rabbit tendon calcaneus in relation to growth of the tibia and calcaneus. *Anat Rec* 1952;113:357.
90. Hughes H: An experimental study of the post-natal growth of tendon. *Anat Anz* 1956;103:192–197.
91. Elliott DH, Crawford GN: The thickness and collagen content of tendon relative to the cross-sectional area of muscle during growth. *Proc R Soc Lond Biol* 1965;162:198–202.
92. Elliott DH: Effects of tenotomy on the growth of muscle and its tendon. *Nature (London)* 1965;207:87–88.
93. Dahners LE, Sykes KE, Muller PR: A study of the mechanisms influencing ligament growth. *Orthopedics* 1989;12:1569–1572.
94. Grant PG, Buschang PH, Drolet DW: Positional relationships of structures attached to long bones during growth: Cross-sectional studies. *Acta Anat* 1978;102:378–384.
95. Dörfl J: Migration of tendinous insertions: I. Cause and mechanism. *J Anat* 1980;131:179–195.
96. Dörfl J: Migration of tendinous insertions: II. Experimental modifications. *J Anat* 1980;131:229–237.
97. Birk DE, Zycband EI, Winkelmann DA, et al: Collagen fibrillogenesis in situ: Fibril segments are intermediates in matrix assembly. *Proc Natl Acad Sci USA* 1989;86:4549–4553.
98. Birk DE, Trelstad RL: Extracellular compartments in tendon morphogenesis: Collagen fibril, bundle, and macroaggregate formation. *J Cell Biol* 1986;103:231–240.
99. Burton RI, Beasley RW, Littler JW: Anatomy of the hand, in Evarts CM (ed): *Surgery of the Musculoskeletal System*, ed 2. New York, NY, Churchill Livingstone, 1990, vol 1, pp 293–310.

100. Bollen SR, Gunson CK: Hand injuries in competition climbers. *Br J Sports Med* 1990;24:16–18.
101. Quinn TH, Baumel JJ: The digital tendon locking mechanism of the avian foot (Aves). *Zoomorphology* 1990;109:281–293.
102. Massengill JB: The boutonniere deformity. *Hand Clin* 1992;8:787–801.
103. Sampson SP, Badalamente MA, Hurst LC, et al: Pathobiology of the human A1 pulley in trigger finger. *J Hand Surg* 1991;16A:714–721.
104. Weiss A-PC, Kramer AA, Barrach H-J, et al: Variations in the quantity of type II collagen in carpal tunnel syndrome. *Trans Orthop Res Soc* 1994;19:389.
105. Benjamin M, Ralphs JR, Newell RL, et al: Loss of the fibrocartilaginous lining of the intertubercular sulcus associated with rupture of the tendon of the long head of biceps brachii. *J Anat* 1993;182:281–285.
106. Williams PL, Warwick R, Dyson M, et al (eds): *Gray's Anatomy*, ed 37. Edinburgh, Scotland, Churchill Livingstone, 1989.
107. Lundborg G, Myrhage R: The vascularization and structure of the human digital tendon sheath as related to flexor tendon function: An angiographic and histological study. *Scand J Plast Reconstr Surg* 1977;11:195–203.
108. Weidman KA, Simonet WT, Wood MB, et al: Quantification of regional blood flow to canine flexor tendons. *J Orthop Res* 1984;2:257–261.
109. Kleiner JB, Amiel D, Harwood FL, et al: Early histologic, metabolic, and vascular assessment of anterior cruciate ligament autografts. *J Orthop Res* 1989;7:235–242.
110. Manske PR, Lesker PA: Nutrient pathways of flexor tendons in primates. *J Hand Surg* 1982;7A:436–444.
111. Manske PR, Lesker PA: Nutrient pathways to extensor tendons within the extensor retinacular compartments: An experimental study in dogs. *Clin Orthop* 1983;181:234–237.
112. Manske PR, Ogata K, Lesker PA: Nutrient pathways to extensor tendons of primates. *J Hand Surg* 1985;10B:8–10.
113. Chaplin DM, Greenlee TK Jr: The development of human digital tendons. *J Anat* 1975;120:253–274.
114. Drachman DB, Sokoloff L: The role of movement in embryonic joint development. *Dev Biol* 1966;14:401–420.
115. Beckham C, Dimond R, Greenlee TK Jr: The role of movement in the development of a digital flexor tendon. *Am J Anat* 1977;150:443–459.

Chapter 14

Fibrocartilage in Tendon: A Response to Compressive Load

Kathryn G. Vogel, PhD

Tendon usually experiences purely longitudinal/tensional forces as it transmits muscle action to bone. However, in locations where the tendon changes direction as it wraps around bone, passes through a pulley, or is impinged upon by nearby structures, the tissue experiences transverse/compressive and frictional forces in addition to tension. A region of fibrocartilaginous tissue has been described at this location in many animal and human tendons.[1,2] This region is also discussed by Benjamin and associates and Amiel and associates in separate chapters in this volume. This chapter will briefly describe the biochemical changes that occur in tendon when it is subjected to compressive loads in vivo and in vitro. Evidence suggesting that these normal and appropriate responses to repetitive motion could lead to pathology will be discussed.

Histology and Biochemistry of Tendon Proteoglycan

A comparison of distinct regions of adult bovine deep flexor tendon illustrates the differences that can develop within one structure (Figs. 1 and 2). The proximal region of this tendon is subjected only to tensional forces. Collagen fibers in the proximal/tensional region are arranged in longitudinal bundles, and elongated cells are found among the fibers (Fig. 1A).[3,4] The fibrils in these fibers have a mean diameter of 158 ± 68 nm and the tissue does not stain with anionic dyes.[3] More-distal regions of this tendon pass under sesamoid bones of the metacarpophalangeal joint and are subjected to compressive and frictional forces in addition to tension. A fibrocartilaginous tissue extends through approximately one third of the tendon's thickness at this point. The collagen fibers in this region are arranged in a basket weave configuration with a great deal of interfibrillar space (Fig. 1B). Mean fibril diameter (109 ± 47 nm) is smaller than in the tensional region. Cells of the distal/compressed region are round and often appear to be enclosed in lacunae. This tissue stains intensely with dyes such as Alcian blue or Toluidine blue, indicating accumulation of negatively charged molecules (the glycosaminoglycans associated with proteoglycans).

Tensional regions of bovine deep flexor tendon contain very little extracellular proteoglycan. The predominant proteoglycan in adult bovine tendon is a "small" molecule called decorin.[5] Hardingham and Fosang[6] have published a good review of proteoglycan structure. When assessed by polyacrylamide gel electrophoresis, decorin migrates as a diffuse band with a molecular weight somewhat greater than 100 kDa (Fig. 2). The core protein of decorin has a

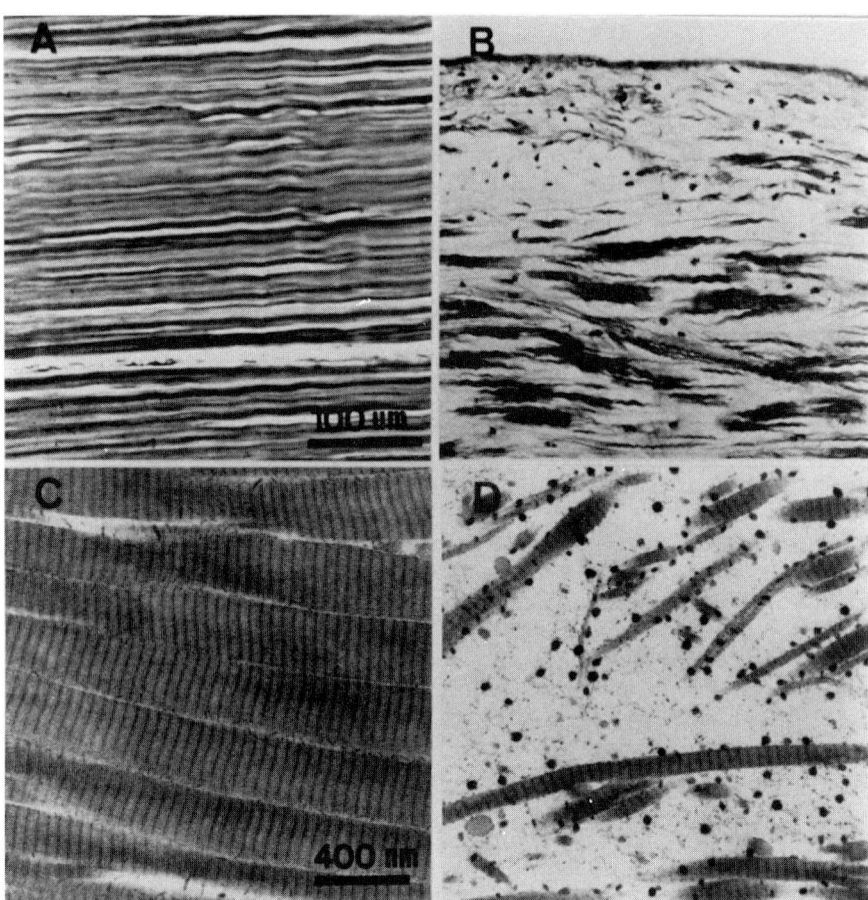

Fig. 1 Histology of tensional and compressed regions of adult bovine deep flexor tendon. Light microscopy of tensional (**A**) and compressed (**B**) regions stained with the Masson Trichrome procedure. Electron microscopy of tensional (**C**) and compressed (**D**) regions stained with cuprolinic blue and uranyl acetate. Short rod-like structures associated with collagen fibrils in **C** are believed to represent decorin. Large electron-dense deposits in the interfibrillar space of **D** are believed to represent aggrecan. (Courtesy of Dr. Stephen Evanko, University of Washington, Seattle.)

single dermatan sulfate chain, binds to type I collagen fibrils,[7,8] and has been located in virtually all tissues.[9,10] The compressed region of adult bovine tendon contains 5- to 10-fold more glycosaminoglycan than the tensional region, most of which is chondroitin sulfate associated with a large proteoglycan called aggrecan.[11,12] Aggrecan is best known as a major constituent of cartilage. It has a molecular weight greater than 10^6 Da, is substituted with both chondroitin sulfate and keratan sulfate glycosaminoglycan chains, and has a core protein that forms aggregates with hyaluronic acid. The very large complexes formed by aggrecan and hyaluronic acid constitute the fixed negative charges that are important in providing compressive stiffness to cartilage and to specific regions of tendon. This molecule remains in the stacking gel or at the interface of a 4% to 20% gradient SDS/polyacrylamide gel (Fig. 2). A third proteoglycan of intermediate size is found in the compressed regions of adult bovine tendon. The core protein of this proteoglycan, known as biglycan be-

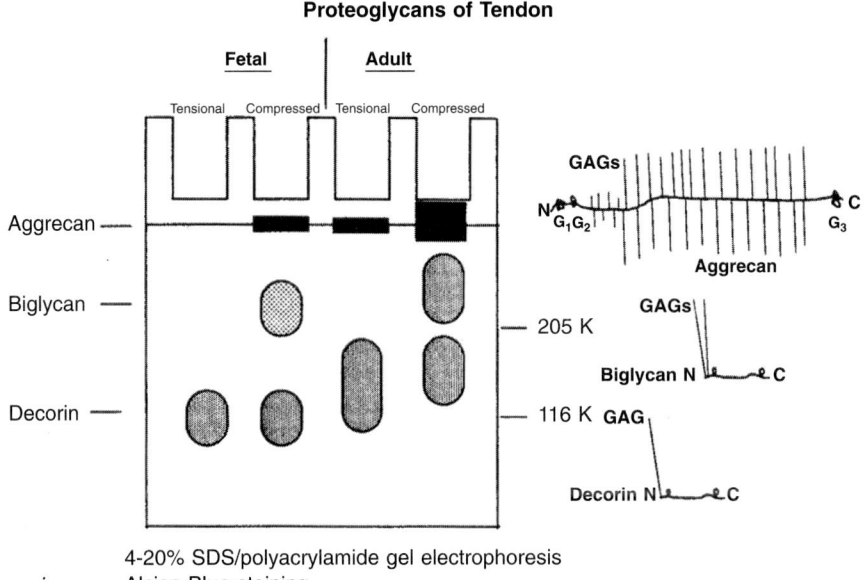

Fig. 2 The major proteoglycans of tendon. **Top,** This drawing shows an SDS/polyacrylamide gel after electrophoresis of proteoglycans from different regions of fetal and adult bovine tendon. A model of the molecular structure of each proteoglycan is shown at right. **Bottom,** Glycosaminoglycan (GAG).

cause it contains two dermatan sulfate chains, is structurally similar to decorin, but is a unique gene product.[13] The ultrastructural location and role of biglycan in tendon is not yet known. Type I collagen is the major constituent of both tensional and compressive regions of adult tendon. However, cells in the compressive region express messenger ribonucleic acid (mRNA) for type II collagen[14] and the presence of some type II collagen can be demonstrated in this region using immunohistochemistry.[1] Aggrecan and type II collagen synthesis is considered characteristic of chondrocytes, whereas synthesis of decorin and type I collagen defines a fibroblast. By these criteria, cells in the compressive region of tendon have changed from fibroblasts to chondrocytes.

The tensional region of fetal bovine tendon is much like the tensional region of adult bovine tendon in that total proteoglycan content is low and decorin is the most prevalent proteoglycan (Fig. 2). Interestingly, there is a small amount of aggrecan in the tensional region of adult tendon.[11] This aggrecan lacks the G1 domain of its core protein and does not show high aggregatability with hyaluronic acid. In the fetal tendon, decorin migrates somewhat farther on SDS/polyacrylamide gels than adult decorin because its glycosaminoglycan chain is shorter.[15] The compressive region of tendon undergoes notable changes during the late fetal period, including altered organization of the collagen fibers and accumulation of biglycan.[3] Cells from the region of fetal tendon that will become fibrocartilaginous express mRNA for aggrecan,[14] although the proteoglycan does not accumulate in substantial amounts until a few months after birth.[3]

Effects of Mechanical Loading on Tendon Composition

In Vivo Response to Mechanical Load

The ability of mechanical forces to affect tendon composition was demonstrated by Flint and associates in a series of seminal papers published between 1975 and 1980. A thickened "sesamoid-like pad" was described at the point where the rabbit flexor digitorum profundus tendon wraps under the calcaneum and talus. In this region, the tendon's collagen fibers stained green instead of red after the Masson trichrome staining sequence[16,17] and had a significantly shorter axial periodicity than collagen in the tensional region.[18] Glycosaminoglycan content (reported as micrograms uronic acid per milligram of tissue dry weight) was approximately 15-fold higher in the sesamoid region than in the tensional region and it was concluded, based on cellulose acetate electrophoresis and differential enzyme sensitivity, that most of this was chondroitin sulfate.[18] Cells in the pressure-bearing region were round and the cytoplasm was characterized by a dense array of intermediate microfilaments.[19]

The forces involved in maintaining these distinct regions of tendon were investigated by surgical translocation of the flexor digitorum profundus (FDP) tendon in 6- to 8-week-old New Zealand white rabbits, which were killed after times ranging from a few days to 9 months, and analysis of glycosaminoglycan amount and type.[20] When the tendon was translocated onto the extensor aspect of the leg, removing both tensional and compressive load, more than 60% of the glycosaminoglycan (mainly chondroitin sulfate) was lost from the pressure-bearing region in the first 8 days. The lower level of glycosaminoglycan content was held constant for the next 9 months. In contrast, translocation resulted in an increase in the total glycosaminoglycan (mainly dermatan sulfate) content of the tensional region that was maximal 14 days after surgery and was maintained for 3.5 months, followed by decline to presurgical levels as the tendon tension was regained. The glycosaminoglycan levels of the previously distinct regions became quite similar after translocation. These experiments established the capacity of tendon structure to modulate as a result of altered mechanical loading. Although these studies measured glycosaminoglycan type rather than proteoglycan type, they are consistent with subsequent analyses in bovine tendon indicating that the chondroitin sulfate prominent in compressive regions is associated with large proteoglycan (aggrecan), whereas dermatan sulfate in tensional regions is associated with small proteoglycan (decorin).[21]

Significant loss of glycosaminoglycan from the pressure-bearing region of tendon was measured under three conditions: 8 days after the Achilles tendon was severed and a 1-cm segment of the sciatic nerve was removed, after sciatic neurectomy alone, and 30 days after immobilization of one leg in a plaster cast.[20] Each of these procedures was expected to diminish compressive loading on the tendon. Thus, these findings further support the conclusion that biochemical change in the tendon was due to diminished compressive load. No significant change in the glycosaminoglycan content of either region of FDP tendon was found in control animals after making longitudinal incisions in the Achilles tendon or placing sutures in the Achilles tendon.[20]

Experiments designed to induce accumulation of tendon glycosaminoglycan in vivo, by imposing compressive loads on tissue that was not already under this load, indicated that the glycosaminoglycan-rich tissue could not be generated as readily as it was lost. Chondroitin sulfate content increased when tendon that had been translocated for 40 days (and had lost most of the glycosaminoglycan) was replaced to its original position.[20] Even after 6 months, however, the level of glycosaminoglycan was only about one third that of the original. Experimental attempts to induce a glycosaminoglycan-rich tissue by imposing compressive loading on tendon that would not normally experience this load were not successful. Glycosaminoglycan content did not increased in the posterior fibers of FDP tendon after the anterior two thirds of the tendon was split and translocated, although it would be predicted that the remaining tendon experienced direct contact with the calcaneum as a result. These negative results may indicate that there are special cells that respond to compressive loading, or that the response can only be developed in fetal or newborn tendon. However, because the surgery is damaging and subsequent load was not meaured, these experiments are not considered firm evidence against the possibility that a glycosaminoglycan-rich tissue can develop in adult tendon exposed to prolonged transverse loading.

In Vitro Response to Mechanical Load

Fresh pieces of fibrocartilage from adult bovine deep flexor tendon synthesize primarily large proteoglycans when placed in culture. After 2 weeks in culture, however, the synthetic pattern changes to synthesis of primarily small proteoglycans.[22] The capacity of mechanical loading to influence this synthesis was investigated by subjecting cultured pieces of newly isolated adult bovine tendon fibrocartilage in culture to a 2-week regimen of unconfined, cyclic, uniaxial compression (5 s/min, 20 min/day, force = 544 kPa, strain ~25%). Matched pieces of tendon were maintained in culture without loading. At the end of this period, nonloaded tendon synthesized predominantly small proteoglycans, whereas loaded tissue continued to produce predominantly large proteoglycan.[23] Autoradiography indicated that [^{35}S]-labeled large proteoglycans were synthesized by cells throughout the tissue, with a greater percentage of actively synthetic cells in the loaded tissue than in control, unloaded tissue. The results of these experiments indicate that synthesis of large proteoglycans in tendon fibrocartilage can be maintained by brief loading, but in the absence of loading, synthesis of large proteoglycans was lost. This result is consistent with the observation that tendon in vivo rapidly lost glycosaminoglycan content when transverse loading was removed.[20]

The capacity of fetal tendon to respond to mechanical loading also was investigated with in vitro experiments. Full-thickness segments from the region of fetal bovine deep flexor tendon that will develop fibrocartilage after birth were subjected to loading to 30% strain at a frequency of one cycle every 6 seconds for 3 days.[24] Matched tendon segments were cultured in the same vessel without loading as controls. This loading regimen consistently stimulated a 100% to 300% increase in incorporation of [^{35}S]sulfate into large proteoglycans compared to uncompressed controls (Fig. 3). A 50% to 100% increase in [^{35}S]sulfate incorporation into biglycan was also observed. Radiosulfate incorporation into decorin was not significantly affected. Northern blot analysis showed that the compression regimen stimulated a 5-fold increase in the level

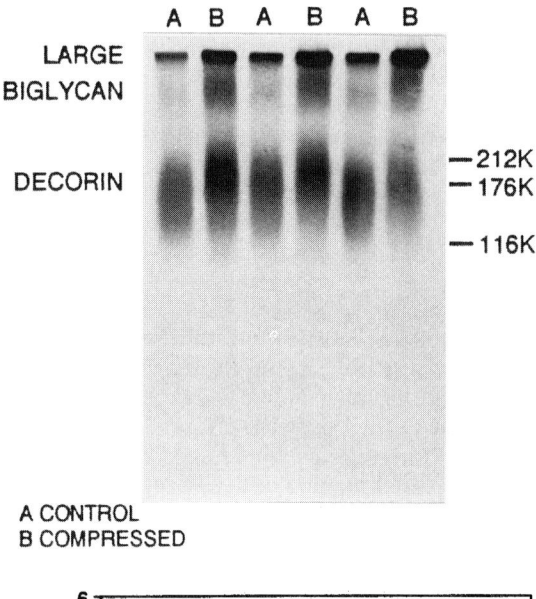

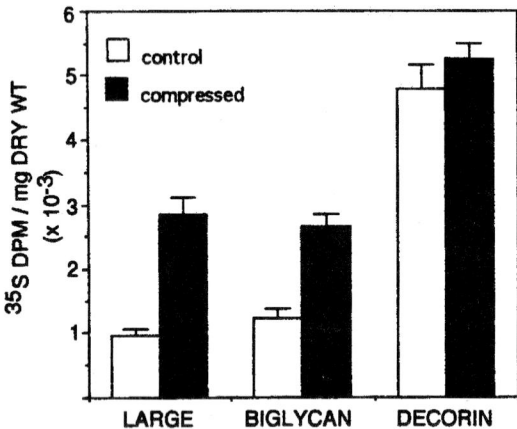

Fig. 3 Top, Sodium dodecyl sulfate/polyacrylamide gel electrophoresis (SDS/PAGE) and fluorography of proteoglycans synthesized by compressed fetal tendon segments. Segments of fetal tendon were subjected to 72 hours of cyclic compression and allowed to incorporate [^{35}S]sulfate for 12 hours. Radiolabeled proteoglycans were extracted from the tissue and separated by 5.5% to 20% SDS/PAGE. The migration positions of large proteoglycan, biglycan, and decorin are indicated. Molecular weight standards are myosin (212K), (α2-macroglobulin (176K), and (β-galactosidase (116K). A, control; B, compressed. **Bottom**, Quantitation of proteoglycan synthesis. Individual proteoglycans were separated by SDS/PAGE as shown at **top** and radioactivity quantitated by gel slicing and liquid scintillation counting. Error bars indicate SEM (n = 6). (Adapted with permission from Evanko SP, Vogel KG: Proteoglycan synthesis in fetal tendon is differentially regulated by cyclic compression in vitro. *Archiv Biochem Biophys* 1993;307:153–164.)

of mRNA recognized by an aggrecan probe.[24] Increased synthesis of aggrecan and biglycan as a response to compressive loading in vitro is consistent with the greater levels of aggrecan and biglycan found in compressive regions of the adult tendon in vivo. Because the in vitro experiments eliminate the influence of a systemic vascular or inflammatory response, this result constitutes strong evidence that the cells are responding to mechanical stress or deformation.

The effect of compression on segments from the tensional region of fetal tendon also was assessed. This region of tendon does not experience compressive forces in vivo. After 3 days of cyclic loading, the synthetic response of tensional tissue was similar to the response of tissue that will be compressed when the animal walks,[24] that is, loading selectively stimulated increased incorporation of [^{35}S]sulfate into large proteoglycans and biglycan while incorporation into decorin was not significantly affected. This suggests that cells in a region of tendon that would not normally experience transverse loads can nonetheless respond to this loading with development of a more cartilaginous matrix.

Fibrocartilage in Human Tendon

Regional differences in tendon morphology and composition, similar to what has been described above in bovine and rabbit tissue, has been also noted in a variety of dog, rat, and human tendons.[25-28] In each case, increased accumulation of proteoglycan was correlated with the presence of altered mechanical load on the tissue. For example, at the point where the human tibialis posterior tendon passes under the medial malleolus, the tendon develops a firm bump, which is characterized on histologic examination by rounded cells, a less regular arrangement of collagen fibrils, and staining with Alcian blue.[28] Glycosaminoglycan content in this region is 10-fold higher than in adjacent regions of the same tendon. The proteoglycans found in this region include large proteoglycans and biglycan as well as decorin, while adjacent regions contain only decorin (Fig. 4). A comparative histologic study of rotator cuff tendons and tendon biopsy specimens from cadavers with lateral epicondylitis suggests that fibrocartilage may occur in both shoulder and elbow tendons.[29] The most common histologic alteration was the presence of glycosaminoglycan (detected as Alcian blue staining) and fibrocartilaginous changes (characterized by rounded cells in rows between the collagen fibrils). Abnormal rotator cuff histology was present in more than 40% of specimens from patients older than 50 years of age.

A zone of hypovascularity was noted just distal to the medial malleolus in all of 28 cadaver specimens of posterior tibial tendon in which the relevant vasculature was injected with an India ink-gelatin mixture[30] (Fig. 5). This is the same place where fibrocartilage develops. The same site, just distal to the medial malleolus, has been reported as a common site of tears in the posterior tibial tendon.[31] Frey and associates[30] speculated that relative avascularity may predispose the tendon to rupture in this region, perhaps because of degenerative changes. It has been suggested that a similar relationship occurs in the rotator cuff of the shoulder where a zone of relative avascularity coincides with

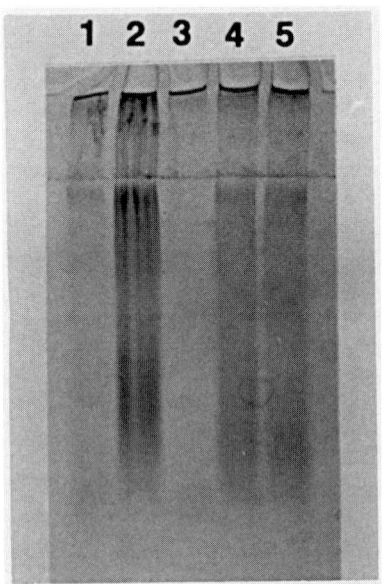

Fig. 4 Proteoglycan gel profiles of five connective tissues from a 28-year-old man. Tissue samples were extracted in SDS/glycerol and the extract assessed by 4% to 15% gradient SDS/PAGE stained only with Alcian blue. Each lane represents the content of 7.5 mg of tissue wet weight. Lane 1, tensional region of tibialis posterior tendon; lane 2, compressed region of tibialis posterior tendon; lane 3, patellar tendon; lane 4, lateral collateral ligament; and lane 5, anterior cruciate ligament. (Adapted with permission from Vogel KG, Ordog A, Pogany G, et al: Proteoglycans in the compressed region of human tibialis posterior tendon and in ligaments. *J Orthop Res* 1993:11:68–77.)

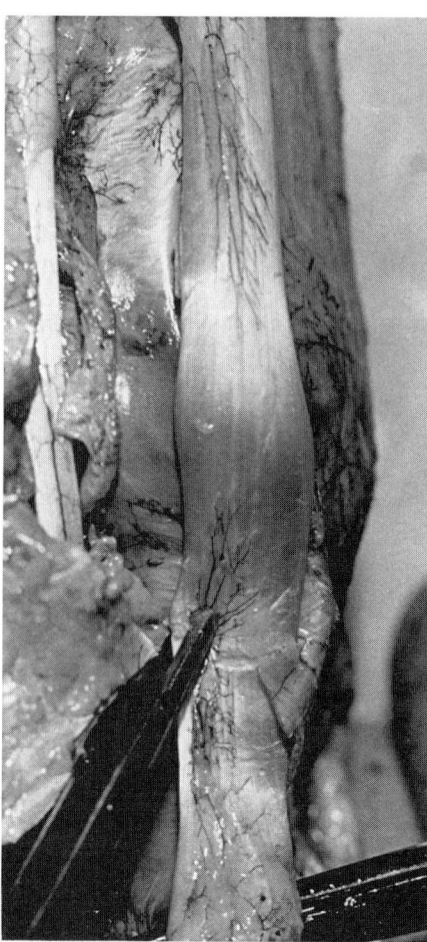

Fig. 5 A zone of hypovascularity in the mid-portion of the human posterior tibialis tendon. The zone was reported to start approximately 40 mm from the medial tubercle of the navicular bone and run proximally for an average of 14 mm.[29] A region of fibrocartilage was described on the opposite side of the tendon in the same location.[27] The vasculature was visualized by injection of the arteries with an India ink-gelatin suspension, as described by Frey and associates.[29] (Reproduced with permission from Frey C, Sheriff M, Greenidge N: Vascularity of the posterior tibial tendon. *J Bone Joint Surg* 1990;72A:884–888.)

the location of tears in the suspraspinatus tendon.[32] However, a quantitative histologic study showed that both supraspinatus and infraspinatus tendons were hypovascular in the distal 15 mm.[33] Because the most common site for rotator cuff tears is in the distal 10 mm of the supraspinatus, but not in the infraspinatus, the authors concluded that vascularity alone could not be the key factor generating pathology that leads to supraspinatus rupture.

Two significant questions are raised by the observation that zones of tendon fibrocartilage and hypovascularity are found in the same location. The first question is whether fibrocartilaginous changes in tendon subjected to transverse loading, changes which appear to be adaptive, could predispose a tendon to degenerative changes and/or rupture. There is some evidence supporting this suggestion. A lower modulus was measured in the fibrocartilaginous region of dog flexor digitorum profundus tendons compared to an adjacent tensional region.[34] The tendon might rupture more readily in this location. In a recent histologic study of Achilles tendon entheses in elderly humans, Rufai and associates[35] report frequent pathologic changes in a zone of compressive fibrocartilage that forms where the tendon presses on the calcaneus. Degenerative changes in this region, including fragmentation and delamination, were present in 73% of the tendons examined. This study suggests that fibrocartilage in tendon could predispose the tissue to degenerative changes. Because fibrocartilaginous changes in tendon may be induced by repetitive loading, this response could be a significant factor in the pathogenesis of repetitive motion syndrome.

The second question is whether there is a causal relationship between relative avascularity and the development of fibrocartilage, an avascular tissue, in tendon. There do not appear to have been any studies that directly address this developmental question. A chondrocyte-derived inhibitor of neovascularization has been described, however.[36] Even if a general correlation is established between the location of hypovascularity and fibrocartilage in tendon, this correlation does not necessarily imply a cause-and-effect relationship. Both changes could be independently induced by transverse loading of the tissue.

Summary

A region of fibrocartilage has been described in human and other mammalian tendons at the location where it changes direction around bone or passes through a restraining pulley. The tissue is characterized by rounded cells, a nonlinear organization of collagen fibrils, and the presence of increased amounts of large, aggregating proteoglycan. In vivo experiments using the rabbit flexor digitorum profundus tendon have demonstrated that maintenance of this fibrocartilage requires transverse/compressive loading of the tendon. When this loading was removed, the proteoglycans were lost rapidly. The direct connection between mechanical load and fibrocartilage development was further supported by experiments in which segments of fetal bovine deep flexor tendon were subjected to cyclic compression in vitro. This regimen resulted in increased synthesis of large proteoglycan (those proteoglycans capable of providing compressive stiffness to the tissue). There may be correlation between regions of relative hypovascularity and the presence of fibrocartilaginous tissue. Both characteristics are reported in the most common sites for pathology and rupture in the posterior tibial tendon and the supraspinatus tendon of the rotator cuff.

The development and disappearance of fibrocartilaginous tissue in tendon strongly suggests that it represents a response to transverse/compressional loading in a tissue that is also under tension. In this sense, it represents a response to repetitive motion. On the other hand, it must be acknowledged that the fibrocartilaginous regions of tendon are adaptive. Fibrocartilage in tendon should not be considered pathologic just because it is present. An important question is whether the presence of fibrocartilage alters the mechanical properties of tendon so that functional deficits or tissue degeneration are induced by overuse. If this proves to be the case, fibrocartilaginous changes could be a common precursor of tendon pathology induced by repetitive motion.

Acknowledgments

I would like to thank Dr. Stephen Evanko (University of Washington, Seattle) and Dr. James Robbins (University of New Mexico, Albuquerque) for their excellent work, and for many fruitful and pleasant discussions on this topic. Grant support was provided by the National Institutes of Health, through AR36110.

References

1. Vogel KG, Koob TJ: Structural specialization in tendons under compression. *Int Rev Cytol* 1989;115:267–293.
2. Benjamin M, Evans EJ: Fibrocartilage. *J Anat* 1990;171:1–15.
3. Evanko SP, Vogel KG: Ultrastructure and proteoglycan composition in the developing fibrocartilaginous region of bovine tendon. *Matrix* 1990;10:420–436.
4. Koob TJ, Vogel KG: Site-related variations in glycosaminoglycan content and swelling properties of bovine flexor tendon. *J Orthop Res* 1987;5:414–424.
5. Vogel KG, Heinegard D: Characterization of proteoglycans from adult bovine tendon. *J Biol Chem* 1985;260:9298–9306.
6. Hardingham TE, Fosang AJ: Proteoglycans: Many forms and many functions. *FASEB J* 1992;6:861–870.
7. Brown DC, Vogel KG: Characteristics of the in vitro interaction of a small proteoglycan (PGII) of bovine tendon with type I collagen. *Matrix* 1989;9:468–478.
8. Hedbom E, Heinegard D: Binding of fibromodulin and decorin to separate sites on fibrillar collagens. *J Biol Chem* 1993;268:27307–27312.
9. Bianco P, Fisher LW, Young MF, et al: Expression and localization of the two small proteoglycans biglycan and decorin in developing human skeletal and non-skeletal tissues. *J Histochem Cytochem* 1990;38:1549–1563.
10. Meyer DH, Krull N, Dreher KL, et al: Biglycan and decorin gene expression in normal and fibrotic rat liver: Cellular localization and regulatory factors. *Hepatology* 1992;16:204–216.
11. Vogel KG, Sandy JD, Pogany G, et al: Aggrecan in bovine tendon. *Matrix Biology* 1994;14:171–179.
12. Doege KJ, Sasaki M, Kimura T, et al: Complete coding sequence and deduced primary structure of the human cartilage large aggregating proteoglycan, aggrecan: Human-specific repeats, and additional alternatively spliced forms *J Biol Chem* 1991;266:894–902.
13. Fisher LW, Termine JD, Young MF: Deduced protein sequence of bone small proteoglycan I (biglycan) shows homology with proteoglycan II (decorin) and several nonconnective tissue proteins in a variety of species. *J Biol Chem* 1989;264:4571–4576.
14. Robbins JR, Vogel KG: Regional expression of mRNA for proteoglycans and collagen in tendon. *Eur J Cell Biol* 1994;64:264–270.
15. Vogel KG, Evanko SP: Proteoglycans of fetal bovine tendon. *J Biol Chem* 1987;262:13607–13613.
16. Flint MH, Lyons MF, Meaney MF, et al: The Masson staining of collagen: An explanation of an apparent paradox. *Histochem J* 1975;7:529–546.
17. Flint MH, Merrilees MJ: Relationship between the axial periodicity and staining of collagen by the Masson trichrome procedure. *Histochem J* 1977;9:1–13.
18. Gillard GC, Merrilees MJ, Bell-Booth PG, et al: The proteoglycan content and the axial periodicity of collagen in tendon. *Biochem J* 1977;163:145–151.
19. Merrilees MJ, Flint MH: Ultrastructural study of tension and pressure zones in a rabbit flexor tendon. *Amer J Anat* 1980;157:87–106.
20. Gillard GC, Reilly HC, Bell-Booth PG, et al: The influence of mechanical forces on the glycosaminoglycan content of the rabbit flexor digitorum profundus tendon. *Connect Tis Res* 1979;7:37–46.
21. Vogel KG, Heinegard D: Characterization of proteoglycans from adult bovine tendon. *J Biol Chem* 1985;260:9298–9306.
22. Koob TJ, Vogel KG: Proteoglycan synthesis in organ cultures from regions of bovine tendon subjected to different mechanical forces. *Biochem J* 1987;246:589–598.
23. Koob TJ, Clark PE, Hernandez DJ, et al: Compression loading in vitro regulates proteoglycan synthesis by tendon fibrocartilage. *Arch Biochem Biophys* 1992;298:303–312.
24. Evanko SP, Vogel KG: Proteoglycan synthesis in fetal tendon is differentially regulated by cyclic compression in vitro. *Arch Biochem Biophys* 1993;307:153–164.

25. Okuda Y, Gorski JP, An KN, et al: Biochemical, histological, and biomechanical analyses of canine tendon. *J Orthop Res* 1987;5:60–68.
26. Ralphs JR, Benjamin M, Thornett A: Cell and matrix biology of the suprapatella in the rat: A structural and immunocytochemical study of fibrocartilage in a tendon subject to compression. *Anat Rec* 1991;231:167–177.
27. Rufai A, Benjamin M, Ralphs JR: Development and ageing of phenotypically distinct fibrocartilages associated with the rat Achilles tendon. *Anat Embryol (Berl)* 1992;186:611–618.
28. Vogel KG, Ordog A, Pogany G, et al: Proteoglycans in the compressed region of human tibialis posterior tendon and in ligaments. *J Orthop Res* 1993;11:68–77.
29. Chard MD, Cawston TE, Riley GP, et al: Rotator cuff degeneration and lateral epicondylitis: A comparative histological study. *Ann Rheum Dis* 1994;53:30–34.
30. Frey C, Shereff M, Greenidge N: Vascularity of the posterior tibial tendon. *J Bone Joint Surg* 1990;72A:884–888.
31. Johnson KA: Tibialis posterior tendon rupture. *Clin Orthop* 1983;177:140–147.
32. Rathbun JB, Macnab I: The microvascular pattern of the rotator cuff. *J Bone Joint Surg* 1970;52B:540–553.
33. Brooks CH, Revell WJ, Heatley FW: A quantitative histological study of the vascularity of the rotator cuff tendon. *J Bone Joint Surg* 1992;74B:151–153.
34. Nessler JP, Amadio PC, Berglund LJ, et al: Healing of canine tendon in zones subjected to different mechanical forces: A biomechanical and histological analysis. *Trans Orthop Res Soc* 1990;15:10.
35. Rufai A, Ralphs JR, Benjamin M: The structure and histopathology of the insertional region of the human Achilles tendon. *J Orthop Res*, in press.
36. Moses MA, Sudhalter J, Langer R: Isolation and characterization of an inhibitor of neovascularization from scapular chondrocytes. *J Cell Biol* 1992;119:475–482.

Chapter 15
Effect of Loading on Metabolism and Repair of Tendons and Ligaments

David Amiel, PhD
Constance R. Chu, MD
Joe Lee, MD

Introduction

Epidemiology of Tendon and Ligament Overuse Injuries

Injuries ascribed to overuse and repetitive motion frequently result in pain and the inability to work or to participate in certain sports or activities. The cost to public health is great. Cumulative trauma disorders are the most frequently reported occupational injury, with upper extremity disorders making up the majority of those reported.[1,2] Among sports participants, 34% to 50% can expect to be injured, and 25% to 50% of these injuries will fall under the category of overuse injuries.[3]

Because the terms overuse syndrome, cumulative trauma disorder, repetitive strain injury, and permutations thereof have been used interchangeably, specific definitions are controversial. In general, these terms do not describe well-defined clinical entities. Instead, they include a wide variety of soft-tissue disorders characterized, most notably, by pain and generally associated with occupational conditions or repeated movements of the body. Although the terms imply etiology, the causal effect of cumulative trauma is not uniformly documented.[1]

Clinical entities most conclusively associated with repetitive trauma include tendinitis and carpal tunnel syndrome (CTS). Among sign language interpreters, tendinitis was the most frequently diagnosed occupational injury, with a prevalence of 48%, whereas CTS accounted for 12% of confirmed injuries.[4] Achilles tendinitis affects up to 18% of runners[5] and, being their most frequent lesion, it is diagnosed in approximately 31% of ballet dancers.[6] Analysis of the performance requirements of these populations at risk provide some etiologic clues.

Factors that increased the forces acting on the affected tendons tended to increase the incidence of tendinitis. In one group of dancers, the genesis of Achilles tendinitis was traced to dancing on cement surfaces 45% of the time and on more forgiving wooden surfaces only 4% of the time.[6]

Although tendinitis apparently is the most commonly reported result of cumulative trauma, it is important to understand that inflammatory changes to some ligaments in the upper and lower extremities, eg, the lateral collateral ligament (LCL) of the knee, have also frequently been diagnosed as tendinitis. A review of the normal properties of tendons and ligaments follows.

Normal Function and Physiology of Tendons and Ligaments

For many years tendons and ligaments have been classified together as dense, regularly arranged connective tissue.[7–9] It became common to think of these tissues as similar to the point that the terms tendon and ligament were sometimes used interchangeably in the literature.[10–12]

Although both are organized, regular connective tissues, they are entirely different functionally. Tendons are a conduit that connects muscle to bone. Because they have great tensile strength and some elasticity, they allow a joint complex to move through muscle contraction or relaxation. Ligaments are short bands of fibrous tissue which bind bone to bone and provide support for internal organs. Ligaments are relatively inelastic. In concert with the bony geometry and the dynamic effects of muscle and tendon,[13,14] ligaments limit and guide joint motion.

The functional differences between ligaments and tendons prompted a more thorough evaluation with regard to their histologic and biochemical properties. Substantial differences were noted in this assessment.[15]

Structure and Morphology Most histology texts include ligaments and tendons with the reticuloendothelial system and describe them as "dense, regular connective tissue."[16–19] This description is accurate but incomplete. Certain types of ligaments and tendons may be distinguished from each other based on their histologic appearance.[15] This distinction is analogous to the microscopic dissimilarity between cardiac and skeletal muscle tissues.

Some of the basic differences among a variety of tendons and ligaments are described here. The variables considered are collagen bundle width, cell morphology and size, and "crimp." Crimp, which is a feature of both tendons and ligaments, represents a regular sinusoidal pattern in the matrix. The periodicity and amplitude of crimp appear to be structure-specific, and they are best evaluated under polarized light. The simple functional explanation for this accordion-like pattern in the matrix is that it provides a buffer in which slight longitudinal elongation may occur without fibrous damage. Crimp also provides a mechanism for control of tension and acts as a shock absorber along the length of the tissue. When the physiologic mechanical limits of this crimp are exceeded, however, irreversible damage occurs and the physical properties of the tissue are changed.[20]

Although both ligaments and tendons have crimping within their fascicles, there appear to be differences in the crimp pattern between these two structures.[21]

Assessment of the anterior cruciate ligament (ACL) and the medial collateral ligament (MCL) by transmission electron microscopy (TEM) characterizes their ultrastructural differences and illustrates their heterogeneity.[22] The fibrils of the ACL exhibit a wide range of diameters. The fibroblasts are ovoid, lie in columns between layers of compact parallel bundles of collagen fibrils, and have abundant cellular organelles, which indicates a high level of cellular activity. The fibroblasts have multiple small cellular processes, or microvilli, which project into a surrounding area of amorphous ground substance with reticular fibers, but not into the compact parallel collagen fibrils.

The MCL has predominantly large diameter collagen fibrils. The MCL fibroblasts are spindle-shaped and lie in the midst of compact parallel collagen fibrils with little or no surrounding amorphous ground substance. These fibroblasts have an abundance of cellular organelles, indicating a high level of cellular activity. They also have long thin cellular processes (villi) extending from the main body of the cell out into the areas of densely packed collagen fibrils.

These substantial differences in morphology and ultrastructure may reflect both the functional and environmental differences between the ACL and the MCL. The cellular morphologic characteristics of the MCL are those of all fibroblasts, while the cellular characteristics of the ACL are similar to those of fibrocartilage cells. These observations lead to questions concerning the differences between these ligaments in terms of function, homeostasis, and repair.

Because tendons link muscle to bone, they have great tensile strength, a degree of pliability, and a component of elasticity. Although muscle can withstand mechanical forces up to 77 lbs/in^2 (531 KPa), the average tensile strength of human tendons ranges from 4,000 to 18,000 lbs/in^2 (27,600 to 124,000 KPa).[23]

In the patellar tendon, all the fascicles are found to undulate in the helical wave pattern. In contrast to the muscle and bone with which they associate, tendons have a relatively sparse supply of blood and lymphatic vessels. Their characteristic structural units are densely packed parallel bundles of fibrous collagen that extend between the myotendinous and osteotendinous junctions. A tendon fascicle consists of groups of collagen fiber bundles and associated tendon cells, surrounded by a fine layer of loose connective tissue referred to as the endotendon, or endotenon. Within each fascicle, rows of elongated and flattened fibroblasts extend the length of the collagen fiber bundles.

Groups of tendon fascicles are surrounded by a tendon sheath of epitenon. In certain specialized regions, the tendon sheaths form synovium. Synovial sheaths surround the tendons and lubricate and nourish them, especially where they pass over joints. Within the digital synovial sheath, the flexor tendon system has been described as a specialized joint allowing for finger movement.

Collagen fibrils of the tendon fascicles are bimodal in diameter; large fibrils are 150 to 200 nm in diameter and smaller fibrils are 40 to 80 nm in diameter. The relative proportions of the two sizes vary throughout a tendon. The collagen fibrils of tendon sheaths, however, have a narrower range of diameters and an average diameter of 60 nm. They do not align in parallel, but are loosely interwoven in multiple orientations.

Biochemistry of Normal Tendons and Ligaments Roughly 70% by dry weight of normal ligament is composed of collagen. The collagen is mainly type I (also found in tendon, skin, and bone) and it is the principal tensile-resistant substance present. The collagen in ligament is thought to remain relatively inert metabolically, with a half-life of 300 to 500 days (a turnover rate even slower than bone collagen).[24] Certain components of the collagen molecule, however, may turn over faster than others and may, therefore, be relatively more important in terms of adaptation to environmental, traumatic, or pathologic processes.[25]

Periarticular ligaments also have a small amount of type III collagen, which is about 9% to 12% of the total collagen.[26] Type III collagen is also observed in healing[27,28] and embryonic tissue.[29] Because the ratio of type I to type III collagen changes with age, and type III is predominant in fetal skin, it often is referred to as fetal or embryonic collagen.

The presence of a less mature form of collagen may reflect the tissue response to a broad range of stresses, with the percentage of type III collagen changing relatively rapidly as a function of applied forces. Alternatively, the type I/III ratio endows the tissue with specific structural properties, allowing it to cope with the wide varieties of force and force vectors to which ligaments are subjected.[26]

The ligamentous collagen obtains structural stability from its unique molecular coil configuration, the quarter-staggered packing of tropocollagen units,[30] and its ability to form covalent intramolecular and intermolecular cross-links.[31–36] The functional importance of glycosylation of hydroxylysine residues is uncertain, but various effects have been postulated, including aiding stability, regulating synthesis, controlling fiber diameter, and influencing collagen-proteoglycan interaction.

The cross-links are key to both tensile strength and resistance to chemical or enzymatic breakdown. Absence of such cross-links causes the collagen fibers to be extremely weak and friable.[26,37] Tendon has been shown to contain relatively large amounts of the intermolecular cross-links hydroxylysinonorleucine (HLNL) and histidinohydroxymerodesmosine (HHMD), whereas ligament contains mainly dihydroxylysinonorleucine (DHLNL) and lesser amounts of both HLNL and HHMD.[15]

The proteoglycan constituents of ligament make up only about 1% by dry weight of the total tissue. However, 60% to 80% of the total net weight is water and a significant part of that water is associated with the ground substance. The water and proteoglycans probably provide lubrication and spacing, which are crucial to gliding at intercept points where fibers cross in the tissue matrices. Gliding is an essential physical property of ligaments and other periarticular connective tissues. The water and proteoglycans also confer viscoelastic properties to ligaments. The movement of water in the system is inhibited by its entrapment between the large, highly charged proteoglycan molecules. Therefore, at high strain rates, the water cannot displace completely in the brief time of force application. At slow rates, water displacement is greater because force is applied more slowly, allowing greater ligament strain.

The concentration of glycosaminoglycans (GAGs) present in the rabbit ligamentous tissue studied differs significantly from that present in tendinous tissue of rabbits. The cruciate ligaments have the highest proportion of GAGs, two to four times the amount observed in the tendons studied. The MCL also has a higher GAG concentration than the tendons, about twice the amount found in tendons.

The importance of these differences is not known; however, the higher the GAG content, the more water is associated with the complex. This difference alters the viscoelastic properties of these tissues and may represent an additional shock absorbing feature in ligament, which is unnecessary in tendon.[11]

The integrins are a family of cell-surface adhesion receptors known to play critical roles in a number of cellular processes necessary for wound healing, including adhesion, migration, proliferation, differentiation, and elaboration of extracellular matrix (ECM).[38–42] They are heterodimeric molecules, each composed of noncovalently associated α and β-polypeptide subunits that span the plasma membrane and simultaneously bind to the ECM outside the cell and to cytoskeletal components within the cell.[43] Each member of the very late activation (VLA) subfamily of integrins consists of a common β-chain (β_1) associated with a specific α-chain (α_1–α_6), forming $\alpha_1\beta_1$ through $\alpha_6\beta_1$ heterodimers.[44] A number of ECM proteins present in ligaments, including collagen, laminin, and fibronectin, are ligands of the β_1 integrins.[45–47] These ligands are important in the physical attachment of the cell to the ECM, are instrumental in allowing the cell to sense and modify the extracellular environment,[48] and are important in the cell's wound healing response.[49]

Both ACL and MCL fibroblasts from normal human knees were found to bear the common β_1 chain, $\alpha_1\beta_1$, and $\alpha_5\beta_1$, but $\alpha_2\beta_1$, $\alpha_3\beta_1$, $\alpha_4\beta_1$, and the α_6 subunit were absent. Monoclonal antibodies (Mabs) specific for β_1 revealed strong staining of fibroblasts in both tissues, while Mabs specific for $\alpha_1\beta_1$ and $\alpha_5\beta_1$ stained less intensely (Table 1). The ACL and MCL did not appear to show any significant difference in the intensity of the staining with a particular Mab, indicating that $\alpha_1\beta_1$ and $\alpha_5\beta_1$ are present in roughly equivalent amounts on ACL and MCL fibroblasts. Similar studies of rabbit ACL and MCL using Mabs reactive with rabbit integrins revealed the presence of β_1 and $\alpha_5\beta_1$ and the absence of $\alpha_6\beta_1$ in both ligaments. Again, probes for β_1 stained more intensely than for $\alpha_5\beta_1$ and staining was comparable in ACL and MCL. The expression of $\alpha_1\beta_1$, $\alpha_2\beta_1$, $\alpha_3\beta_1$ and $\alpha_4\beta_1$ on rabbit ligaments is as yet undetermined because of the lack of appropriate rabbit cross-reactive Mabs. Moreover, both rabbit and human ACL and MCL fibroblasts stained intensely when probed with an α_v-chain Mab. This suggests that these ligament fibroblasts also bear a specific integrin receptor for fibronectin, such as $\alpha_v\beta_1$ or $\alpha_v\beta_6$, or for the protein vitronectin, such as $\alpha_v\beta_3$ or $\alpha_v\beta_5$. A summary of integrin expression in human skin and in human and rabbit ACL and MCL is shown in Table 2.

The Effect of Loading on Tendon and Ligament

It is now commonly known that Wolff's law can be extended to include the soft tissues of the musculoskeletal system.[10,50]

The effects of loading on the metabolism and structure of tendon and ligament have been studied at the gross, microscopic, and increasingly, the molecular level. Whole animal studies allow changes in connective tissue to be evaluated in response to immobilization, exercise, and the alteration of normal biomechanical loads. Kinematic and biomechanical studies analyze forces experienced by the intact tissue in situ. As tissue culture techniques evolved, researchers began to examine the effects of isolated experimental stresses on the excised tissue. Increasing interest in understanding cellular adaptation to stress at the molecular level has lead, in recent years, to the examination of strain fields

Table 1 Summary of monoclonal antibodies used, indicating their specificity, rabbit reactivity, and source

Monoclonal Antibody	Integrin Specificity	Rabbit Reactive	Antibody Source
A1A5	β_1 chain	No	M. Hemler
DH12	β_1 chain	Yes	J.J. Cassiman
TS2/7	$\alpha_1\beta_1$	No	M. Hemler
12F1	$\alpha_2\beta_1$	No	V. Woods
J143	$\alpha_3\beta_1$	No	C. Finstad
B-5G10	$\alpha_4\beta_1$	No	M. Hemler
BIIG2	$\alpha_5\beta_1$	Yes	C. Damsky
GOH3	α_6 chain	Yes	A. Sonnenberg
13C2	α_v chain	Yes	M. Horton

(Reproduced with permission from Gesink DS, Pacheco HO, Kuiper SD, et al: Immunohistochemical localization of β1-integrins in anterior cruciate and medial collateral ligaments of human and rabbit. *J Orthop Res* 1992;10:596–599.)

Table 2 Summary of staining patterns observed in human skin, ACL, and MCL, and rabbit ACL and MCL

Integrin Specificity	Human Skin		Human Ligament		Rabbit Ligaments	
	Epidermis	Fibroblasts	ACL	MCL	ACL	MCL
β_1	+	+	+	+	+	+
α_1	–	±	+	+	NT	NT
α_2	+	–	–	–	NT	NT
α_3	+	±	–	–	NT	NT
α_4	–	–	–	–	NT	NT
α_5	–	+	+	+	+	+
α_6	+	±	–	–	–	–
α_v	+	+	+	+	+	+

+, structures that demonstrated a clearly positive staining pattern
±, structures that demonstrated a minimal or scattered staining pattern
–, structures that demonstrated no significant staining pattern
NT, rabbit ligaments that were not tested because there was a lack of appropriate rabbit cross-reactive antibodies
ACL, anterior cruciate ligament
MCL, medial collateral ligament
(Reproduced with permission from Gesink DS, Pacheco HO, Kuiper SD, et al: Immunohistochemical localization of β1-integrins in anterior cruciate and medial collateral ligaments of human and rabbit. J Orthop Res 1992;10:596–599.)

on individual cultured cells. The effects of biomechanical stresses on the digital flexor tendon, a connective tissue with easily identifiable regions subjected to different biomechanical forces, will be discussed to illustrate many of the current concepts on the metabolic response to loading. We will focus in this chapter on in vivo physiologic loading.

In Vivo Physiologic Loading

The mechanical environment of a tendon or ligament is affected by numerous factors, including muscle strength and joint position, the individual physical properties of the connective tissue components of the joint, external forces, and other factors. Thus, muscle-tendon forces, joint-articulating forces, and capsuloligamentous forces during physiologic static or dynamic loading are difficult to measure. However, useful information can be obtained from isolated studies of tissue.[51]

A series of studies was conducted of the structural and metabolic differences between tension and compression regions of the rabbit flexor digitorum profundus tendon.[52-54] The authors described the compression region as the area of the rabbit hindlimb flexor that passes around the bony pulley below the ankle.[52] During physiologic loading, this region of the tendon is subject to both compression and friction forces. The region of maximal tension was determined to be the portion of tendon on the outside curve of the pulley.[55] These regions were analyzed separately and after surgical translocation to alter the pattern of loading exerted on each region.

Ultrastructural examination revealed marked differences in cell shape, collagen fibril structure, and matrix content between tension and pressure zones of this tendon.[54] The cells of the tension region were elongated and had cytoplasmic flanges that appeared to contact neighboring cells. The cell surface was scalloped and conformed to the adjacent positively charged and tightly packed collagen fibrils of long periodicity (63 nm) and varying diameters. In contrast, round fibrochondrocytic cells with dense arrays of microfilaments and numerous lipid droplets were seen in the pressure zone. These cells were surrounded by loosely packed, small diameter collagen fibrils of short periodicity (53 nm) and a GAG-rich matrix.

The GAG content and profile were also found to be significantly different between the tension and compression regions.[52] In tension regions, the GAG content was approximately 0.2% of dry weight with a predominance of dermatan sulfate. These values were comparable to that of the simultaneously studied rabbit Achilles tendon and to other tension transmitting tendons.[56] In the region of the tendon subject to compressive and frictional forces, the proteoglycan content was elevated to approximately 3.5% of tissue dry weight. There was a two- to threefold increase in chondroitin sulfate content compared to that of the tension region, along with a corresponding decrease in the proportion of dermatan sulfate. The GAG content approached that of articular cartilage, a tissue that has a proteoglycan content rich in chondroitin sulfate moieties and is subject to compressive forces (J Buckwalter, unpublished data, 1994).

The Effects of Exercise and Immobilization

The effect on ligaments of exercise and immobilization have been studied extensively. In 1975, Tipton and associates[57] demonstrated that a 10-week endurance training regimen resulted in a heavier, thicker, wider ligament but was not associated with any change in water content or with more collagen per weight/length unit. A schedule of sprint training of 2 minutes duration followed by 3 seconds of rest for 2 h/day also led to increases in weight and weight/length ratio of ligaments, but did not increase the junction strength. Rat ACL had increased resistance to failure after 8 weeks of endurance training.[58] Immobilization without exercise led to decreases in the width of fiber bundles of knee ligaments in dogs or hypophysectomized rats.[57]

Biochemical changes also occur in ligament and tendon following immobilization; greater changes are seen in ligaments, especially in the cruciate ligaments of the knee.[59] There is decreased collagen synthesis, increased degradation, and, in certain types of collagen, cross-linking as the period of immobilization is increased. The patellar tendon was less susceptible to immobilization, with only slight decreases in hydroxypyridinoline.[60] The concentrations of reducible collagen cross-links DHLNL, HHMD, and HLNL were also greater in the immobilized MCL and ACL.[60,61] These cross-links are associated with new collagen synthesis, and increases in them indicate greater amounts of immature collagen in the affected ligaments.[62,63] There are also losses in water content (up to 6%), hyaluronic acid (40%), dermatan sulfate (8%), and chondroitin -4- and -6-sulfates (20%).[64] These changes cause a decrease in the spacing between fibers and reduced lubrication of the ligament matrix, which seem to affect the mechanical properties of the ligament.[62]

Cellular changes in ligaments can also be observed with immobilization. Fibroblasts in 9-week stress-deprived mature ACL and MCL have a predominance of spindle-shaped cells.[65] More recently, increased expression of cell adhesion molecules, integrins, in immobilized ACL and MCL in acute flexion has been demonstrated using immunostaining and Western blot analysis with monoclonal antibodies. Increased staining was found for the β_1, α_5 and α_v integrin subunits, and Western blot study of sodium dodecyl sulfate-polyacrylamide gel (SDS-PAGE) extracted proteins showed an increase in β_1 subunit in 9- and 12-week stress-deprived ACL and MCL. The results support the hypothesis that integrins may play a role in the tissue remodeling that occurs in these stress-deprived knee ligaments.[66]

The Effects of Loading on Repair

Tendons

Early attempts to repair injured flexor tendons uniformly failed to return useful active motion to the involved finger. For decades, the prevailing concept was that the gliding surface could not be maintained after tendon injury and repair because adhesion formation was an undesirable but necessary part of the healing process. The triad of digital sheath injury, tendon suture, and immobilization were identified as factors that both contributed to adhesion formation and were essential components of the injury and repair process. With development of a grasping suture technique,[67] investigators began to consider the effects of loading on flexor tendon repair. In a series of studies, Gelberman and associates[68] demonstrated the positive effects of early controlled passive motion on the healing process of primarily repaired lacerated digital flexor tendons in a canine model. The results of these studies led to a revolution in clinical options and rehabilitation protocols for the treatment of flexor tendon injuries.[69]

In experimental and clinical evaluations of injured flexor tendons repaired primarily and treated postoperatively with early passive motion, significant improvements in the quality of tendon healing were reported.[69,70] Although the former gliding surfaces of immobilized tendons were obliterated by vascularized connective tissue adhesions, the gliding surfaces of tendons treated with early motion were restored (Fig. 1). Early mobilization appeared to stimulate an intrinsic healing response originating from surface epitenon cells. This early epitenon response was accompanied by accelerated collagen formation and remodeling at the repair site as compared to a delayed proliferative response originating from the endotenon in immobilized tendons.[70] Both the tensile strength and excursion properties of the mobilized repaired tendon were significantly higher than that of similarly repaired but immobilized flexor tendons.[51,70] A multicenter prospective randomized clinical study evaluating the effects of daily passive motion on finger function following primary repair of lacerated digital flexor tendons revealed significantly improved active motion in patients treated with greater duration and number of passive motion cycles.[69] More recently, mobilized intrasynovial tendon grafts were also found to incorporate through an intrinsic healing process that allowed for preservation of gliding function (Fig. 2).[71,72]

Ligaments

Several investigators have demonstrated the beneficial effects of loading on ligament healing.[73–75] Tipton and associates[73] examined the effects of exercise and immobilization on healing canine MCLs. The results indicated that immobilization of intact or incised MCLs weakened the ligaments and decreased the collagen content. Exercise, however, increased the strength and the collagen content of the MCL.[73]

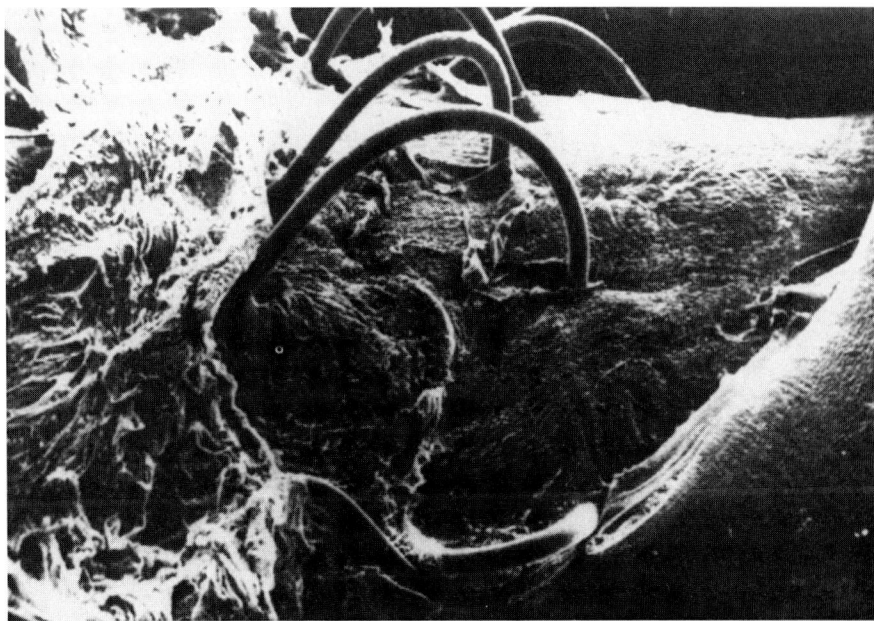

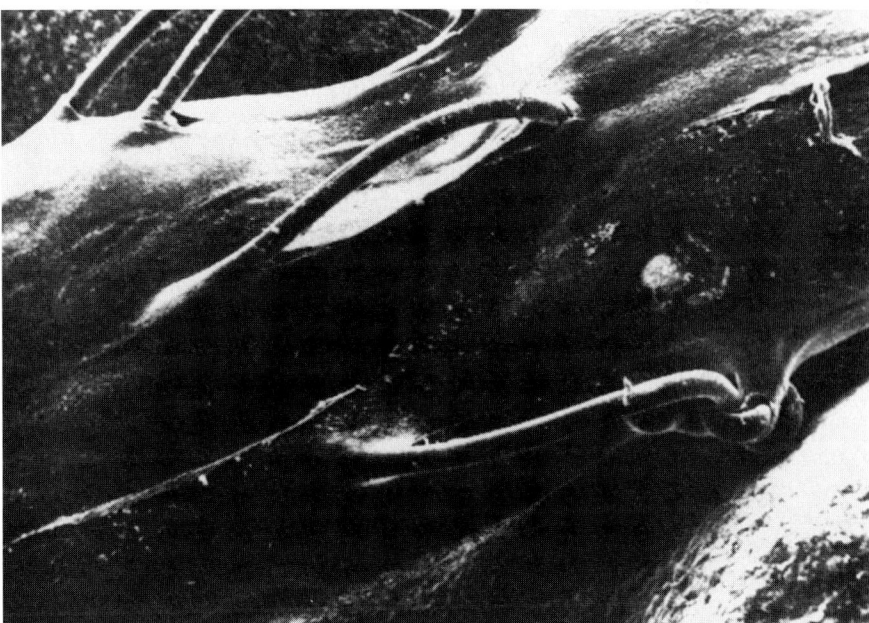

Fig. 1 Effects of loading on flexor tendon repair. Institution of postoperative controlled passive motion led to decreased adhesion formation following primary repair of lacerated digital flexor tendons. **Top,** Ten-day immobilized tendon revealing marked surface irregularity from adhesion formation, 60X; **Bottom,** Smooth, adhesion-free repair surface in a 42-day mobilized tendon, 60X. (Reproduced with permission from Gelberman RH, Vande Berg JS, Lundborg GN, et al: Flexor tendon healing and restoration of the gliding surface: An ultrastructural study in dogs. *J Bone Joint Surg* 1983;65A:70–80.)

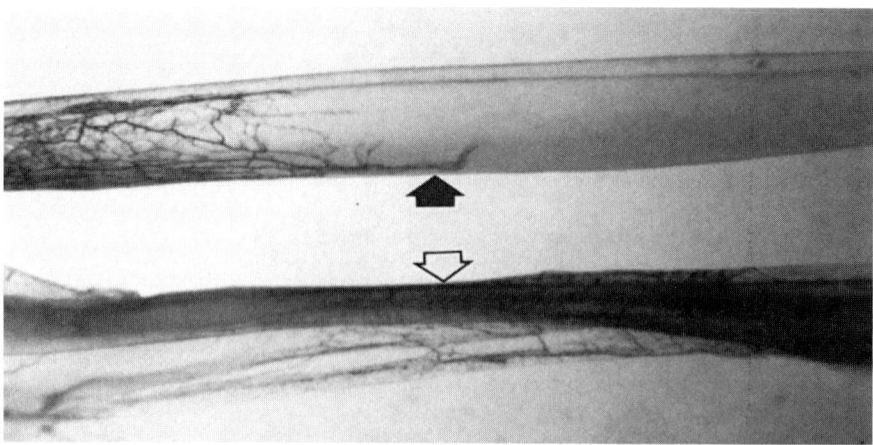

Fig. 2 Mobilized autogenous intrasynovial flexor tendon graft. Protected mobilization stimulated an intrinsic healing process within the intrasynovial tendon graft allowing for preservation of gliding function. The superficialis tendon (open arrow) is seen below the adhesion-free surface (closed arrow) of a 4-week intrasynovial tendon graft. (Reproduced with permission from Gelberman GH, Chu CR, Williams CS, et al: Angiogenesis in healing autogenous flexor-tendon grafts. *J Bone Joint Surg* 1992;74A:1207–1216.)

In 1981, Vailas and associates[74] used a rat model to further demonstrate Tipton and associates' findings. They compared incised MCLs that were subjected to repair, exercise, and various periods of immobilization. The tensile strength and total collagen were 2.06-fold and 2.35-fold, respectively, greater for the exercise group than for the immobilized group. The DNA and collagen synthesis of the exercise group were similar to that of the control group (ie, normal, intact tissue). They concluded that exercise returned the repaired MCL to normal cell division and collagen synthesis more rapidly than immobilization.

In 1991, Gomez and associates[75] demonstrated that increasing the mechanical stress on a healing ligament by the insertion of a pin underneath the healing MCL leads to improved biomechanical, biochemical, and morphologic properties. The valgus-varus laxity in the joints with increased stress was found to be similar to control after 12 weeks. The total collagen and the ratio of DHLNL/HLNL collagen cross-links were also the closest to normal of any transected group after 12 weeks. Histologic examination revealed decreased cellularity and more longitudinal arrangement of collagen fibers in the increased stress group.

Discussion

As load-bearing and load-transmitting connective tissues, tendons and ligaments have structural and metabolic mechanisms to serve as "buffers" to physiologic loads. Distinct collagen crimp patterns provide for the control of tension forces experienced by different connective tissues. Analyses of the biochemical composition of tension- and compression-bearing tissues demonstrate characteristic differences in extracellular matrix constituents. Although the functional importance of these differences is unknown, cellular responses to a change in mechanical loading include altered proteoglycan synthesis, as well as that of other proteins, ie, collagen and fibronectin. At high forces exceeding the mechanical limits of the collagen crimp pattern or at high load frequencies, which result in suboptimal viscoelastic strain patterns, tissue injury may occur.

Whereas injury often results from excessive loading, repair processes are enhanced by the application of physiologic forces either through passive motion protocols or through controlled exercise regimens. Conversely, immobilization both weakens the load-bearing capacity of normal tissues and contributes to inadequate wound healing.

These studies demonstrate that changes in mechanical forces applied to tendons and ligaments directly affect metabolism, repair, and injury at both tissue and cellular levels. High forces exceeding the mechanical limits of the tissue lead to irreversible damage, whereas physiologic forces allow for normal maintenance and enhanced wound healing. A middle zone in which normal but submaximal loading, as seen in repetitive motions performed for work or recreation, may overwhelm the adaptive responses of tendons and ligaments and result in chronic injuries.

Acknowledgment

We acknowledge the financial support of NIH grants AG07996, AR41151, AR34264, AR07464, AR33097, and the Malcolm and Dorothy Coutts Institute for Joint Reconstruction and Research.

References

1. Gerr F, Letz R, Landrigan PF: Upper-extremity musculoskeletal disorders of occupational origin. *Annu Rev Public Health* 1991;12:543–566.
2. Thorson E, Szabo RM: Common tendinitis problems in the hand and forearm. *Orthop Clin North Am* 1992;23:65–74.
3. Kiefhaber TR, Stern PJ: Upper extremity tendinitis and overuse syndromes in the athlete. *Clin Sports Med* 1992;11:39–55.
4. DeCaro JJ, Feuerstein M, Hurwitz TA: Cumulative trauma disorders among educational interpreters: Contributing factors and intervention. *Am Ann Deaf* 1992;137:288–292.
5. Clain MR, Baxter DE: Achilles tendinitis. *Foot Ankle* 1992;13:482–487.
6. Fernandez-Palazzi F, Rivas S, Mujica P: Achilles tendinitis in ballet dancers. *Clin Orthop* 1990;257:257–261.
7. Bloom W, Fawcett DW (eds): *A Textbook of Histology*, ed 8. Philadelphia, PA, WB Saunders, 1962, pp 85–111.
8. Copenhaver WM, Bunge RP, Bunge MB (eds): *Bailey's Textbook of Histology*, ed 16. Baltimore, MD, Williams & Wilkins, 1971, pp 109–135.
9. Ham AW (ed): *Histology*, ed 6. Philadelphia, PA, JB Lippincott, 1969, pp 374–387.
10. Akeson WH, Woo SL-Y, Amiel D, et al: The biology of ligaments, in Hunter LY, Funk FJ (eds): *Rehabilitation of the Injured Knee*. St. Louis, MO, CV Mosby, 1984, pp 93–148.
11. Amiel D, Abel MF, Kleiner JB, et al: Synovial fluid nutrient delivery in the diathrial joint: An analysis of rabbit knee ligaments. *J Orthop Res* 1986;4:90–95.
12. O'Donoghue DH, Rockwood CA Jr, Zaricznyj B, et al: Repair of knee ligaments in dogs: I. The lateral collateral ligament. *J Bone Joint Surg* 1961;43A:1167–1178.
13. Noyes FR, Grood ES, Butler DL, et al: Clinical biomechanics of the knee: Ligament restraints and functional stability, in *American Academy of Orthopaedic Surgeons Symposium on The Athlete's Knee: Surgical Repair and Reconstruction*. St Louis, MO, CV Mosby, 1980, pp 1–35.
14. Palmer I: On the injuries to the ligaments of the knee joint: A clinical study. *Acta Chir Scand* 1938;(suppl 53):8–282.

15. Amiel D, Frank C, Harwood F, et al: Tendons and ligaments: A morphological and biochemical comparison. *J Orthop Res* 1984;1:257–265.
16. Amenta PS: *Histology*, ed 3. New Hyde Park, NY, Medical Examination Publishing, 1983, pp 64–73.
17. Bailey FR: The connective tissues, in Kelly DE, Wood RL, Enders AC (eds): *Bailey's Textbook of Microscopic Anatomy*, ed 18. Baltimore, MD, Williams & Wilkins, 1984, pp 160–193.
18. Leeson CR, Leeson TS, Paparo AA (eds): *Textbook of Histology*, ed 5. Philadelphia, PA, WB Saunders, 1985, pp 97–124.
19. Snell RS (ed): *Clinical and Functional Histology for Medical Students*, ed 1. Boston, MA, Little Brown & Co, 1984, pp 107–153.
20. Viidik A: Simultaneous mechanical and light microscopic studies of collagen fibers. *Z Anat Entwicklungsgesch* 1972;136:204–212.
21. Yahia LH, Drouin G: Microscopical investigation of canine anterior cruciate ligament and patellar tendon: Collagen fascicle morphology and architecture. *J Orthop Res* 1989;7:243–251.
22. Lyon RM, Akeson WH, Amiel D, et al: Ultrastructural differences between the cells of the medial collateral and the anterior cruciate ligaments. *Clin Orthop* 1991;272:279–286.
23. Cronkite AE: The tensile strength of human tendons. *Anat Rec* 1936;64:173–186.
24. Neuberger A, Slack HGB: The metabolism of collagen from liver, bone, skin and tendon in the normal rat. *Biochem J* 1953;53:47–52.
25. Grant ME, Prockop DJ: The biosynthesis of collagen: 1. *N Engl J Med* 1972;286:194–199.
26. Amiel D, Billings E Jr, Akeson WH: Ligament structure, chemistry, and physiology, in Daniel DM, Akeson WH, O'Connor JJ (eds): *Knee Ligaments: Structure, Function, Injury, and Repair*. New York, NY, Raven Press, 1990, pp 77–91.
27. Clore JN, Cohen IK, Diegelmann RF: Quantitation of collagen types I and III during wound healing in rat skin. *Proc Soc Exp Biol Med* 1979;161:337–340.
28. Gay S, Vijanto J, Raekallio J, et al: Collagen types in early phases of wound healing in children. *Acta Chir Scand* 1978;144:205–211.
29. Epstein EH Jr, Munderloh NH: Isolation and characterization of CNBr peptides of human (a 1 (III))3 collagen and tissue distribution of (a 1 (I))2 a 2 and (a 1 (III))3 collagens. *J Biol Chem* 1975;250:9304–9312.
30. Petruska JA, Hodge AJ: A subunit model for the tropocollagen macromolecule. *Proc Natl Acad Sci USA* 1964;51:871–876.
31. Bailey AJ, Robins SP: Embryonic skin collagen: Replacement of the type of aldimine crosslinks during the early growth period. *FEBS Lett* 1972;21:330–334.
32. Bailey AJ, Robins SP, Balian G: Biological significance of the intermolecular crosslinks of collagen. *Nature* 1974;251:105–109.
33. Gallop PM, Blumenfeld OO, Henson E, et al: Isolation and identification of α-amino aldehydes in collagen. *Biochemistry* 1968;7:2409–2430.
34. Nimni ME: Collagen: Its structure and function in normal and pathological connective tissues. *Semin Arthritis Rheum* 1974;4:95–150.
35. Paz MA, Henson E, Rombauer R, et al: α-Amino alcohols as products of a reductive side reaction of denatured collagen with sodium borohydride. *Biochemistry* 1970;9:2123–2127.
36. Tanzer ML: Cross-linking of collagen. *Science* 1973;180:561–566.
37. Nimni ME, Harkness RD: Molecular structures and functions of collagen, in Nimni ME (ed): *Collagen: Biochemistry*. Boca Raton, FL, CRC Press, vol 1, pp 1–77.
38. Albelda SM, Buck CA: Integrins and other cell adhesion molecules. *FASEB J* 1990;4:2868–2880.
39. Buck CA, Horwitz AF: Cell surface receptors for extra-cellular matrix molecules. *Annu Rev Cell Biol* 1987;3:179–205.
40. Hynes RO: Integrins: A family of cell surface receptors. *Cell* 1987;48:549–554.
41. Ruoslahti E, Pierschbacher MD: New perspectives in cell adhesion: RGD and integrins. *Science* 1987;238:491–497.
42. Ruoslahti E: Integrins. *J Clin Invest* 1991;87:1–5.

43. Burridge K, Fath K, Kelly T, et al: Focal adhesions: Transmembrane junctions between the extracellular matrix and the cytoskeleton. *Annu Rev Cell Biol* 1988;4:487–525.
44. Hemler ME: VLA proteins in the integrin family: Structures, functions, and their role on leukocytes. *Annu Rev Immunol* 1990;8:365–400.
45. Santoro SA, Rajpara SM, Staatz WD, et al: Isolation and characterization of a platelet surface collagen binding complex related to VLA-2. *Biochem Biophys Res Commun* 1988;153:217–223.
46. Sonnenberg A, Modderman PW, Hogervorst F: Laminin receptor on platelets is the integrin VLA-6. *Nature* 1988:336:487–489.
47. Takada Y, Huang C, Hemler ME: Fibronectin receptor structures in the VLA family of heterodimers. *Nature* 1987;326:607–609.
48. Dejana E, Lampugnani MG, Giorgi M, et al: Fibrinogen induces endothelial cell adhesion and spreading via the release of endogenous matrix proteins and the recruitment of more than one integrin receptor. *Blood* 1990;75:1509–1517.
49. Clark RA: Fibronectin matrix deposition and fibronectin receptor expression in healing and normal skin. *J Invest Dermatol* 1990;94(suppl 6):128S-134S.
50. Amiel D, Kleiner JB, Roux RD, et al: The phenomenon of "ligamentization": Anterior cruciate ligament reconstruction with autogenous patellar tendon. *J Orthop Res* 1986;4:162–172.
51. Gelberman RH, Goldberg V, An K-N, et al: Tendon, in Woo SL-Y, Buckwalter JA (eds): *Injury and Repair of the Musculoskeletal Soft Tissues*. Park Ridge, IL, American Academy of Orthopaedic Surgeons, 1988, pp 5–40.
52. Gillard GC, Merrilees MJ, Bell-Booth PG, et al: The proteoglycan content and the axial periodicity of collagen in tendons. *Biochem J* 1977;163:145–151.
53. Gillard GC, Reilly HC, Bell-Booth PG, et al: The influence of mechanical forces on the glycosaminoglycan content of the rabbit flexor digitorum profundus tendon. *Connect Tissue Res* 1979;7:37–46.
54. Merrilees MJ, MH Flint: Ultrastructural study of tension and pressure zones in a rabbit flexor tendon. *Am J Anatomy* 1980;157:87–106.
55. Ploetz E: Funktioneller Bau und funktionelle Anpassung der Gleitsehnen (D25). *Z Orthop Ihre Grenzgeb* 1938;67:212–234.
56. Meyer K, Davidson E, Linker A, et al: The acid mucopoly-saccharides of connective tissue. *Biochim Biophys Acta* 1956;21:506–518.
57. Tipton CM, Matthes RD, Maynard JA, et al: The influence of physical activity on ligaments and tendons. *Med Sci Sports Exerc* 1975;7:165–175.
58. Cabaud HE, Chatty A, Gildengorin V, et al: Exercise effects on the strength of the rat anterior cruciate ligament. *Am J Sports Med* 1980;8:79–86.
59. Klein L, Player JS, Heiple KG, et al: Isotopic evidence for resorption of soft tissues and bone in immobilized dogs. *J Bone Joint Surg* 1982;64A:225–230.
60. Harwood FL, Amiel D: Differential metabolic responses of periarticular ligaments and tendon to joint immobilization. *J Appl Physiol* 1992;72:1687–1691.
61. Akeson WH, Amiel D, Mechanic GL, et al: Collagen cross-linking alterations in joint contractures: Changes in the reducible cross-links in periarticular connective tissue collagen after nine weeks of immobilization. *Connect Tissue Res* 1977;5:15–19.
62. Akeson WH, Amiel D, Abel MF, et al: Effects of immobilization on joints. *Clin Orthop* 1987;219:28–37.
63. Akeson WH, Amiel D, Woo SL: Immobility effects on synovial joints: The pathomechanics of joint contracture. *Biorheology* 1980;17:95–110.
64. Akeson WH, Woo SL, Amiel D, et al: The connective tissue response to immobility: Biochemical changes in periarticular connective tissue of the immobilized rabbit knee. *Clin Orthop* 1973;93:356–362.
65. Newton PO, Woo SL, Kitabayashi LR, et al: Ultrastructural changes in knee ligaments following immobilization. *Matrix* 1990;10:314–319.
66. Abiezzi SS, Gesink DS, Schreck PJ, et al: Integrin expression in the anterior cruciate (ACL) and medial collateral (MCL) ligaments after joint immobilization. *Trans Orthop Res Soc* 1994;19:299.

67. Kessler I, Nissim F: Primary repair without immobilization of flexor tendon division within the digital sheath: An experimental and clinical study. *Acta Orthop Scand* 1969;40:587–601.
68. Gelberman RH, Manske PR, Akeson WH, et al: Flexor Tendon Repair. *J Orthop Res* 1986;4:119–128.
69. Gelberman RH, Nunley JA II, Osterman AL, et al: Influences of the protected passive mobilization interval on flexor tendon healing: A prospective randomized clinical study. *Clin Orthop* 1991;264:189–196.
70. Gelberman RH, Vande Berg JS, Lundborg GN, et al: Flexor tendon healing and restoration of the gliding surface: An ultrastructural study in dogs. *J Bone Joint Surg* 1983;65A:70–80.
71. Gelberman RH, Chu CR, Williams CS, et al: Angiogenesis in healing autogenous flexor-tendon grafts. *J Bone Joint Surg* 1992;74A:1207–1216.
72. Seiler JG III, Gelberman RH, Williams CS, et al: Autogenous flexor-tendon grafts: A biomechanical and morphological study in dogs. *J Bone Joint Surg* 1993;75A:1004–1014.
73. Tipton CM, James SL, Mergner W, et al: Influence of exercise on strength of medial collateral knee ligaments of dogs. *Am J Physiol* 1970;218:894–902.
74. Vailas AC, Tipton CM, Matthes RD, et al: Physical activity and its influence on the repair process of medial collateral ligaments. *Connect Tissue Res* 1981;9:25–31.
75. Gomez MA, Woo SL, Amiel D, et al: The effects of increased tension on healing medial collateral ligaments. *Am J Sports Med* 1991;19:347–354.

Chapter 16

Tendon Cells of the Epitenon and Internal Tendon Compartment Communicate Mechanical Signals Through Gap Junctions and Respond Differentially to Mechanical Load and Growth Factors

Albert J. Banes, PhD
Peiqi Hu, MD
Hong Xiao, MD
Michael J. Sanderson, PhD
Scott Boitano, PhD
Brian Brigman, MD
Tom Fischer, PhD
Mari Tsuzaki, DDS, PhD
Thomas D. Brown, PhD
Louis C. Almekinders, MD
W. Thomas Lawrence, MD

Introduction

Tendons are fibrous connective tissue structures that transmit the force of muscle contraction to bone to achieve limb movement. The surface paratenon and epitenon are subjected to shear stress, tension, and compression, whereas the internal compartment is subjected to tension and some compression. Cells that reside in these two anatomic locations also are subjected to force; however, the load placed on cells in vivo is difficult to measure. Early papers have indicated that cells in tendon are subjected to load in vivo.[1-4] Merrilees and Flint[1] showed that the surfaces of internal tendon cells from flexor digitorum profundus tendons subjected to a tensile load and fixed while in tension were scalloped, with impressions of parallel collagen fibrils deforming their membranes. They hypothesized that the charge on collagen changed with tension and delivered information to cells about the load magnitude. They also conjectured that the intermediate filaments and lipid droplets might resist compression to protect the cells from excessive load.[1] Banes and associates[2] later demonstrated that flexor tendon cells subjected to cyclic compression of 0.13% at 0.05 Hz for 5 days (3,500 cycles) decreased tubulin expression. They hypothesized that to survive the load regimen, the tendon cells increased their plasticity by reducing expression of the more rigid tubulin in favor of actin. Gillard and associates[3] demonstrated that the rabbit flexor digitorum profundus tendon, which passes over the talus and calcaneous, is subjected to compression and that cartilage-like cells in the tendon down-regulated glycosaminoglycans (GAG, largely chondroitin sulfate) expression when the load was surgically relieved. Stopak and Harris[4] indicated that during development, tendons may be formed by tractional structuring in which cells attached at muscle and bone initiate intrinsic load on their matrices in addition to the passive load of muscle and bone growth and the simultaneous active load of muscle contraction.

These reports indicate that tendon cells detect applied load, interpret it, and respond biochemically and biologically to load signals. How cells detect, interpret, and respond to mechanical load are questions of intense interest. Possible mechanisms by which tendon cells may detect mechanical load involve integrins, which are connected to the cytoplasmic filament complex of the nucleus.[5,6] Deformation of the matrix would place an instantaneous strain on the mechanically linked complex. The level of prestress in the filament network or the number of integrin molecules in contact with it may regulate the degree of strain sensitivity. Intercellular communication through gap junctions is one of the most probable mechanisms for inositol triphosphate (IP_3)-mediated recruitment of contacting cells in response to a strain signal.[7-10] IP_3 signaling occurs through these conduits, and the IP_3 receptor blocker, heparin, abrogates propagation of a mechanical stimulus-induced release of IP_3 and intracellular calcium.[11,12] Other possible mechanisms for detecting strain signals include stretch-activated channels, other ion channels, and activation of kinase pathways and genetic response elements.[13-17] Understanding the relevant mechanisms through which load acts may lead to discovery of new therapeutic strategies to treat tendon injury and to improve healing during convalescence after surgery.

We have used two in vitro models of load application to determine which pathways are involved in the tendon cells' response to load. The first is a single-cell membrane deformation model, which tests the response of the target cell and the ability to recruit neighboring cells in the response via gap junctions. The second is a culture substrate deformation, which transmits the load signal to most of the cells in a culture plate well.

Results of Recent Studies

The Target Cell Membrane Deformation Model: Testing the Response of Individual Cells to a Mechanical Load

Figure 1, *top*, shows the membrane challenge model and the mechanism by which the mechanical deformation is transduced to communicating cells. A micropipet was advanced into the target cell plasma membrane. No membrane rupture occurred, as indicated by the lack of extracellular fura-2. The membrane deformation resulted in an increase in intracellular calcium ion ($[Ca^{2+}]_{ic}$), which may have been initiated by an influx of extracellular calcium ions shown as open triangles at the pipet tip and inside the cell. In Figure 1, *bottom*, panel 1 shows an epitenon synovial cell (TSC) target cell in which $[Ca^{2+}]_{ic}$ has increased within milliseconds after a single membrane indentation from a pipet. The basal calcium ion concentration was approximately 50 nM and increased to over 1,000 nM in the target cell. Adjacent cells were recruited in the response within seconds (panels 2 and 3). Calcium ion increase was detected as a decrease in fluorescence emission at 510 nm with excitation at 380 nm. A calcium wave was propagated to adjacent cells connected through gap junc-

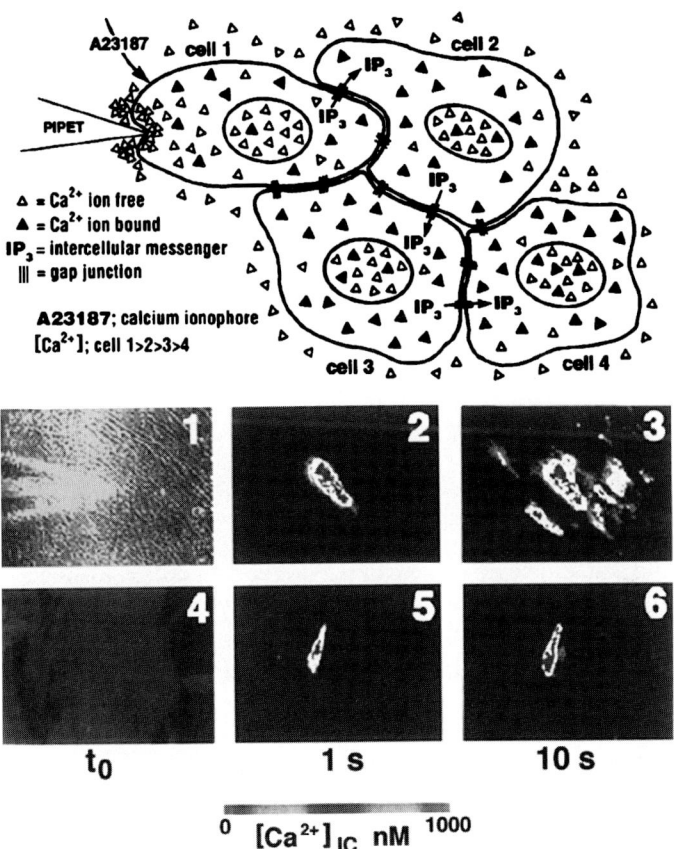

Fig. 1 Top, Single-cell membrane deformation paradigm. A micropipet indents the plasma membrane of the target cell, previously loaded with fura-2. Extracellular calcium may diffuse into the target cell increasing the intracellular calcium ion concentration ($[Ca^{2+}]_{ic}$). The target cell sustains an increase in intracellular calcium ion and IP_3, which diffuses through gap junctions to recruit adjacent cells in the calcium ion response. Treatment of the cells with the calcium ionophore, A23187, induces general diffusion of extracellular calcium into the cell, resulting in an increase in intracellular calcium. **Bottom,** Panel 1 shows a phase contrast photo of a micropipet advancing into a fura-2-loaded tendon epitenon synovial cell (TSC). Panel 2 shows the target cell responding to the membrane deformation by increasing $[Ca^{2+}]_{ic}$, which also increases in adjacent cells within seconds (Panel 3). Cells in Panel 4 have been electroporated with heparin, a substance known to bind and inhibit IP_3 receptors. Stimulating a heparin-loaded target cell with a micropipet results in an increase in $[Ca^{2+}]_{ic}$ but a failure to recruit adjacent cells in the response due to an inhibition of IP_3 binding (Panels 5 and 6). Tendon internal fibroblasts cells responded in a similar way.

tions. The calcium wave propagated for a 4- to 7-cell radius, after which the signal strength dropped below the threshold for continued propagation. Tendon internal fibroblasts (TIFs) responded in the same manner. Panel 4 shows that TSCs in which heparin was introduced before they were challenged with a membrane indentation, increased $[Ca^{2+}]_{ic}$ but failed to propagate the wave to adjacent cells (panels 5 and 6). Heparin is an IP_3 receptor antagonist and blocks IP_3 diffusion from a target cell to adjacent cells.[18] A similar result was obtained if the gap junction inhibitor, halothane, was applied to the cells.[19–21] The responses of TIFs to heparin and halothane were similar to those of TSCs. In initial experiments, TSCs or TIFs in whole tendon ex vivo, loaded with fura-2, did not respond to a membrane deformation stimulus by increasing $[Ca^{2+}]_{ic}$ stores. TSCs or TIFs cultured on flexible Biflex membranes, with 85% uniform radial strain, and subjected to increasing cycles of 0.05 strain (1, 10, 100, 1,000 cycles at 1 Hz) or increasing strain (0.01, 0.05, 0.1, 0.2 strain) at 1 Hz for 1 minute did not increase $[Ca^{2+}]_{ic}$.

Figure 2 indicates that both TSCs and TIFs express messenger molecule and protein for connexin 43 (CXN-43), a gap junction protein, from quiescence through days 1 to 5 in growth phase (Table 1). The level of messenger molecule is moderately high; it is detectable in cells 24 hours after plating and increases in abundance with time in culture. Peak messenger molecule expression for TSCs and TIFs occurred on days 2 and 3 for both cell types. CXN protein expression followed messenger molecule expression, with protein peaks occurring for both cell types on days 3 to 5. CXN exists in a nonphosphorylated, approximately 43-kd form (CXN-43), as well as two phosphorylated 45- and 47-kd forms (CXN-43P, and CXN-43PP, respectively).[22–26] TSCs at quiescence expressed principally the nonphosphorylated form and some of the phosphorylated 45-kd form. TIFs expressed about equal amounts of phosphorylated and nonphosphorylated CXN-43 at quiescence and throughout the 5 days of culture. TIFs also expressed three- to five-fold more total CXN-43 protein than did TSCs. TSCs expressed increased CXN-43 over the 5 days in culture and had a greater percentage of the phosphorylated form than did the TIFs.

Growth Factors Can Modulate Gap Junction Protein Phosphorylation in Tendon Cells

Figure 3 demonstrates the effect of 8 hours of growth factor treatment on CXN-43 protein expression in TSCs and TIFs. These experiments were designed to simulate early wound conditions in which tendon cells are in contact with active growth factors. TSCs contained predominantly the nonphosphor-

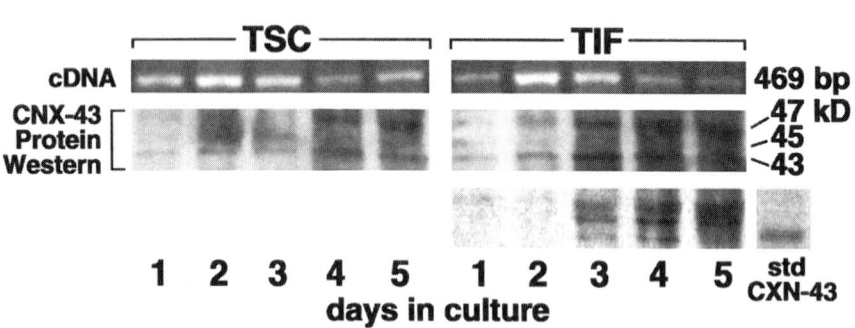

Fig. 2 Connexin 43 (CXN-43) expression increases in cultured tendon epitenon synovial cells (TSCs) and tendon internal fibroblasts (TIFs) throughout a 5-day culture period. Expression of CXN-43 mRNA measured by RT-PCR as a 469-base pair cDNA product was maximal on days 2 and 3 in both cell types (TSC and TIF) with protein expression, detected by Western analysis, increasing thereafter.

Table 1 Kinetics of intracellular calcium $[Ca^{2+}]_{ic}$ release in response to a poke and connexin 43 (CXN-43) expression in tendon epitenon synovial cells (TSCs) and tendon internal fibroblasts (TIFs) in culture

Stimulus*	Q	Day 1	Day 2	Day 3	Day 4	Day 5
TSCs†						
Ca^{2+} poke	+/+	+/−	+/−	+/−	+/+	+/++
Ca^{2+} 4 Br	+++	+++	+++	+++	+++	+++
CXN cDNA	−	1,661	2,491	2,324	1,269	1,518
CXN-47P	−	115	1,856	852	3,421	4,473
CXN-45P	−	160	3,436	1,622	1,840	1,521
CXN-43	−	357	1,021	489	1,811	2,207
Total P	−	275	5,292	2,474	5,261	5,994
Total CXN	−	632	6,313	2,963	7,072	6,201
% P	−	44	84	84	74	97
IF/SC P	−	−	−	−	−	−
IF/SCT Tot	−	−	−	−	−	−
TIFs†						
Ca^{2+} poke	+/+	+/−	+/−	+/−	+/+	+/++
Ca^{2+} 4 Br	+++	+++	+++	+++	+++	+++
CXN cDNA	−	1,263	3,340	2,865	1,121	690
CXN-47P	−	993	1,893	3,529	3,122	3,560
CXN-45P	−	820	602	1,718	1,738	1,478
CXN-43	−	1,003	1,152	3,296	3,707	3,025
Total P	−	1,813	2,495	5,247	4,860	5,038
Total CXN	−	2,816	3,647	8,543	8,567	8,063
% P	−	64	68	61	57	63
IF/SC P	−	6.6	0.47	2.1	0.92	0.84
IF/SCT Tot	−	4.5	0.58	2.9	1.2	1.3

*CXN cDNA is a 469-bp PCR amplified product from CXN mRNA; CXN-45P and CXN-47P are phosphorylated CXNs; poke is a membrane indentation; 4 Br is 4Br A23187; IF/SC P is the ratio of band intensities for phosphorlylated connexins in IF/SC; IF/SCT is the ratio of band intensities for total connexins

†TSC, epitenon synovial cell; TIF, tendon internal fibroblast; +/+ means target and adjacent cells released $[Ca^{2+}]_{ic}$; +/− means target cells released $[Ca^{2+}]_{ic}$ and adjacent cells did not; Q is quiescent; and all numbers are image-analyzed quantitations (relative band intensities)

ylated form of CXN-43 and less protein at quiescence than did TIFs. In the quiescent TIFs, 68% of the CXN was in the phosphorylated form; whereas in the TSCs, only 28% was CXN-43P. Treatment of TSC with 160 pM platelet-derived growth factor-BB (PDGF-BB), a mitogenic dose, stimulated CXN expression slightly, but treatment with 1 nM insulin-like gowth factor-I (IGF-I) stimulated expression to a greater degree with or without PDGF. TIFs had sixfold more phosphorylated CXN at quiescence than did the TSCs. Treatment of TIFs with PDGF-BB slightly diminished the amount of CXN-43P and CXN-43. IGF-I, with or without PDGF-BB, diminished expression of both forms of CXN-43. Treatment with serum-containing medium preserved both forms of CXN protein.

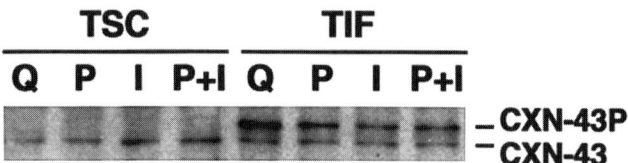

Fig. 3 Quiescent tendon internal fibroblasts (TIFs) have more of the phosphorylated form of connexin 43 (CXN-43) than do tendon epitenon synovial cells (TSCs). Both cell types have the nonphosphorylated proteins. Treatment of TSC with insulin-like growth factor-I (IGF-I) or with platelet-derived growth factor-BB (PDGF-BB) and IGF-I increased expression of CXN-43 protein after 24 hours, whereas treatment of TIF diminished the presence of the phosphorylated form. Because dephosphorylation results in greater abundance of the nonphosphorylated form, an increase should have been detected in the CXN-43 band. Slightly less CXN-43 was detected, indicating that both forms probably were degraded in response to the growth factors in TIF. The phosphorylation state of CXN-43 may be related to the ability to pass ions through a gap junction pore.

Cyclic Loading and Growth Factors Act Synergistically to Stimulate Tendon Cell DNA Synthesis

Figure 4, *left*, indicates that the mitogenic response to PDGF-BB of TSCs cultured on type I collagen on a flexible substrate without mechanical loading was only moderate. However, when TSCs were treated with both 100 pM PDGF-BB and 8 hours of 1 Hz, 5% average strain cyclic mechanical load, then rested for 16 hours and collected at 24 hours after treatment (to simulate a daily activity regimen for tendon), DNA synthesis was increased 15-fold ($p < 0.001$) more than the static control and 2.5-fold ($p < 0.05$) more than values for the PDGF-BB-treated group without load. Results for TIFs were similar with respect to PDGF-BB alone. TIF DNA synthesis was increased 10.5-fold by treatment with 100 pM PDGF-BB, as compared with the medium only control value ($p < 0.001$). TIFs responded mitogenically to PDGF-BB and load at approximately the same level as did TSCs.

Discussion

Tendon is principally a structural tissue that is overdesigned to contend with repetitive motion. The forces applied to most flexor tendons do not exceed 18% elongation, and more commonly do not exceed 4%.[27-29] Tendon also experiences a compressive force that is normal to the principal tensile force or is a more pronounced component if the tendon glides over a bone or through a pulley.[3] While gliding through sheaths, pulleys, or extratendinous tissues without sheaths, the tendon surface experiences shear stress. The tendon exterior comprises the paratenon and epitenon, a modest anatomic structure consisting in width of two to eight plump cells that are connected loosely to each other.[30-32] The epitenon matrix is 23% collagen (73% type I and 27% type III) and less than 1% fibronectin.[33] The major component in the tendon surface covering is lipid, which makes up 43%, with the remaining 34% composed of proteoglycan and elastin (2% to 4% elastin or more in the elastic wing tendon).[33,34] The TSCs contain and secrete Sudan black, lipid positive vesicles that may serve boundary lubrication as well as pulse dampening functions.[1,35,36] Application of cyclic strain to cultured TSCs stimulated release of ^{14}C-labeled lipids into the medium (a 27-fold increase compared to the non-

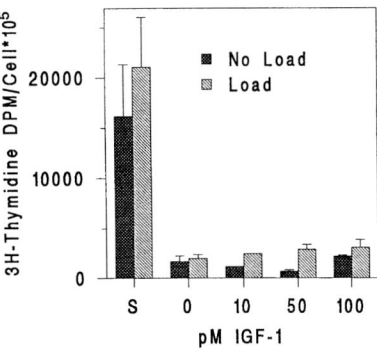

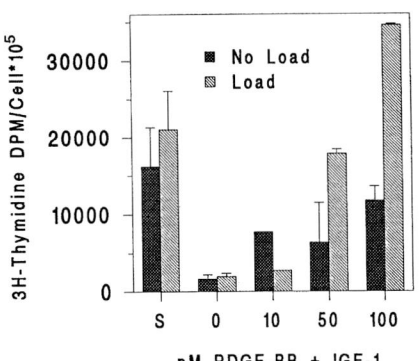

Fig. 4 Top Left, The effects on quiescent avian tendon epitenon synovial cells (TSC) of an increasing dose of platelet-derived growth factor BB homodimer (PDGF-BB) and/or mechanical load (5% average elongation at 1 Hz for 8 hours) with sample collection at 24 hours. Tritiated thymidine incorporation in mechanically loaded TSC was not different from that in the control, nonloaded counterpart unless PDGF-BB was given in concert with load at 50 or 100 pM. The data indicate that cyclic load acts synergistically with PDGF-BB to stimulate DNA synthesis in TSC. **Top right,** IGF-I and load were only slightly growth stimulating. **Bottom,** PDGF-BB, IGF-I, and load stimulated TSC maximally, however.

loaded counterpart), which suggests that repetitive mechanical loading triggers lipid release.[36] A similar but smaller response was found for TIFs, which suggests that TSCs are the primary cells that serve a lubricating function in tendon. Growth factors, principally IGF-I and transforming growth factor-beta (TGF-β, have also been identified in the epitenon (M Tsuzaki, DDS, PhD and associates, unpublished data, 1995).[37] The internal compartment of tendon is 80% collagen of which greater than 90% is type I with some type III and a trace amount of types V and VI.[33] Resident TIFs are aligned in linear arrays of ten to 20 cells that seem ideal for facilitated signaling. Each TIF array may be in contact with other arrays through tenuous pseudopods, as reported in electron microscopy studies.[1,32]

Tendon Cells Contain Functional Gap Junctions Comprised of Connexin 43

Gap junctions are 1.2-nm spaces between plasma membranes from two adjacent cells in which hemichannels, or connexons, comprising six CXN monomers appose each other to form a functional ion channel (Fig. 1, *top*).[38–42] The external face of a connexon of one cell links with a corresponding connexon of a second cell (Fig. 1 top). The Ca^{2+} and phosphorylation states of the CXN-43 monomers may regulate the channel conformation.[25] Gap junctions often appear in clusters in freeze-fracture specimens. Confluent TSC and TIF contain both phosphorylated and nonphosphorylated forms of the CXN monomer; however, at quiescence, TSCs have a preponderance of nonphosphorylated CXN-43, whereas TIFs contain about equal amounts of the phosphorylated and nonphosphorylated forms. In growth curve experiments, although CXN-43 protein is detectable on day 1, cells are unable to communicate a mechanical signal that elicits a $[Ca^{2+}]_{ic}$ increase in adjacent TSCs or TIFs until days 4 to 5. Under the latter growth conditions, cells are in physical contact with each other after day 1, but are not functionally communicating as evidenced by a lack of ability to propagate a calcium wave. CXN-43 expression intensifies in quiescent cells (mainly TIFs), thereby suggesting that maintenance of gap junctions is particularly important in nondividing cells. The phosphorylation state of CXN-43 most likely is related to the capacity to pass ions through the channel (open state) or to the stability of the protein.[43,44]

Concordance between the amounts of steady-state [mRNA] and detectable net protein suggests that the increase in CXN-43 protein in either TSCs or TIFs results from an increase in messenger molecules. An increase in CXN expression over a period of days in culture is in agreement with the observation that intercommunication through functional gap junctions also requires at least 4 to 5 days in culture. It is likely that the assembly of gap junctions from connexons that cluster at regions of intercellular communication requires substantial time.

Quiescent cells have readily detectable CXN-43, which is degraded within hours if the cells are plated at subconfluence. However, if the cells are plated at confluence, the cells maintain a greater level of CXN-43 protein and maintain the ability to propagate a calcium wave when mechanically challenged. The latter observation indicates that connexons from one cell may be stabilized by alignment with connexons of an adjacent cell. If connexons disengage, as occurs during cell disaggregation, connexon degradation may occur rapidly. Little has been reported to date on this subject. Wounding a tendon may disrupt intercellular communication breaking gap junction CXN hemichannels. Re-establishing gap junction channels may occur only after days and may be accelerated by motion therapy. Recently, Benjamin and associates have demonstrated the presence of connexin-43-containing gap junctions in chick and rat digital flexor tendons (M Benjamin, PhD, unpublished data, 1995).

Tendon Cells Detect, Interpret, and Respond to Mechanical Load Signals Under Defined Conditions

Both TSCs and TIFs can detect and transduce a mechanical signal delivered by a micropipet or by deformation of the culture substrate surface, and the cells respond by producing a variety of second messenger molecules that may elicit a mitogenic response, depending on the growth factor environment (AJ Banes, PhD, unpublished data, 1994). Membrane indentation stimulates both TSCs and TIFs to increase $[Ca^{2+}]_{ic}$ and propagate a calcium wave through four to seven cells in all directions from the target cell. This number of cells is similar to the maximum number of cells in an array of TIFs in whole tendon, but it probably is less than the number of TSCs that may communicate in vivo in paratenon or epitenon. In other systems, intercellular communication in response to mechanical stimulation is believed to increase after inositol phosphate lipids at the cytoplasmic side of the membrane have been hydrolyzed to release IP_3 and internal calcium stores.[45] In addition, influx of Ca^{2+} may be an important event that triggers $[Ca^{2+}]_{ic}$ release (calcium-induced calcium release, CICR) via the IP_3 receptor.[11] Consequently, in view of the similar responses of TIFs and TSCs to mechanical stimulation in the presence or absence of heparin, we suggest that these cells also transduce and communicate mechanical signals by the formation and diffusion of IP_3 through gap junctions. In addition, introduction of heparin into tendon cells inhibits the ability of a mechanical signal to be transduced. Heparin binds to the IP_3 receptors on the endoplasmic reticulum (ER) and inhibits binding of IP_3. In this way, IP_3 action is inhibited and an intercellular calcium wave is not produced.[11] Moreover, treatment of target cells with halothane, a gap-junction blocker, also inhibits calcium wave propagation.[10] Therefore, it is hypothesized that IP_3 is the messenger molecule that traverses the cell and activates adjacent cells by passing through gap junction channels and effecting liberation of intracellular calcium stores in the ER. Data from physical chemistry experiments involving the diffusion rates of Ca^{2+} and IP_3 in cytosol further support this view. Calcium ion has a long half-life but a short (0.2 µ) diffusion distance because it is readily bound, whereas IP_3 has a long diffusion distance but a short half-life. Likewise, the concentration of phosphoinositol in the membrane or enzymes that hydrolyze it may be rate limiting for IP_3 generation.

Tendon Cells Are Refractory to Mechanical Load in Vitro Unless Growth Factors Are Present

Cells in normal tendon are in a maintenance state with respect to cell division.[46] Most cells appear to be in the G_0 phase of the cell cycle (AJ Banes, PhD, unpublished data, 1994). When stimulated to exit G_0, tendon cells synthesize D cyclins.[47] Stimulation of whole tendon with serum stimulates cells to leave G_0, traverse G_1, and enter S phase. Cultured TSCs and TIFs stimulated with serum, PDGF-AA, PDGF-BB, TGF-β1, or a combination of PDGF, IGF-I, and TGF-β1 exhibit the same response. TGF-β1 alone is only a mild mitogen, but does not inhibit tendon cell DNA synthesis (AJ Banes, PhD, unpublished data, 1994). Moreover, tendon cells in ex vivo preparations or cultured TSCs and TIFs that do not receive growth factors in serum or in pure form do not exit the G_0 phase. Mechanical load applied to quiescent cells in ex vivo tendon or to cultured cells grown on flexible substrates does not stimulate cells to exit G_0 and divide. This lack of a mitogenic response to mechanical load is reasonable in that tendon cells must be matrix intensive rather than highly cellular to withstand the forces applied by muscle. If the opposite were true, tendons would be highly cellular, contain less matrix, and fail under peak load demands.

Tendon cells respond mitogenically to load only in the presence of 50 to 100 pM concentrations of PDGF-BB with or without 100 pM IGF-I (Fig. 5). Higher doses of PDGF but not IGF-I may stimulate cell division in tendon cells. Mitogenesis in the presence of growth factor and load is in the order of two- to three-fold greater than the growth factor effect alone. This type of growth promotion effect is reasonable because it is during wounding that platelets release PDGF and TGF-β.[48-53] Plasma can provide IGF-I but it may be a limiting factor because tendons are not well vascularized, and tendon injuries can occur without florid bleeding and clot formation. IGF-I is also synthesized by TIFs and accreted in the internal compartment, and it is synthesized to a lessor extent by TSCs and stored in the epitenon (M Tsuzaki, DDS, PhD, unpublished data, 1995). The epitenon contains a fine capillary network so that when injury occurs, blood clot may provide the necessary growth factors needed to heal a defect by stimulating cell migration and division.

Mechanical load may act passively by hydraulically distributing growth factors and plasminogen to activate endogenous IGF-I and TGF-β present in both

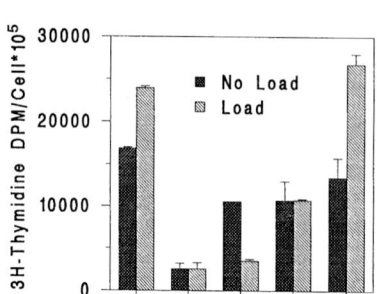 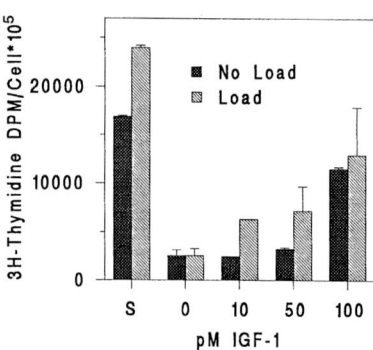

Fig. 5 Left, Avian tendon internal fibroblasts (ATIFs) respond to platelet-derived growth factor BB (PDGF-BB) and load in a similar manner to that of tendon epitenon synovial cells (TSCs). Treatment of ATIFs with 100 pM PDGF-BB and load stimulated DNA synthesis approximately twice as much as the nonloaded but growth factor-treated counterpart. **Right,** IGF-I and load were only slightly growth-stimulating. PDGF-BB, IGF-I, and load-treated cells responded maximally (data not shown).

the epitenon and the internal compartment (M Tsuzaki, DDS, PhD, unpublished data, 1995). Load may actively stimulate second messenger substances, such as Ca^{2+} and IP_3, that recruit other cells to respond. Excessive load application, which may occur in repetitive motion injury to tendon, may stimulate production of degradative enzymes that initially activate stored growth factors, but then degrade matrix and elicit production of inflammatory mediators such as prostaglandin E_2 (PGE_2).[54]

Variables in Mechanical Treatment Regimens for Tendon Cells: A Theory of Mechanical Load Discrimination

Our group[55] was the first to publish a mathematical expression that described how a cell's response, R, was related to a summation of a nonlinear function of A, the amplitude of the applied strain, t_1 the duration of the strain event, t_2 the time between strain events, t_3 a long rest period after many strain events, e^*_1, the strain rate to achieve maximum deformation, e^*_2, the strain rate declining to rest, t, the shear stress, and S, a substrate chemistry term. An inertial loading term, I, can now be added to this expression to account for the inertial force of medium overlying cells or cells in tissue deformed by inertia (T Brown, PhD, personal communication, 1994).[56]

$$R5f\{[A,(t_1,t_2,t_3),(e^*_1,e^*_2,T),I,S]_n$$

This expression can be used to model load regimens to ascertain which specific component of the load event produces a biologic or biochemical effect. Under these conditions, our group[57–60] used frequency modulation (10, 15, and 40 cycles/min or 0.17, 0.25, and 0.67 Hz, respectively) with tendon cells grown in complete medium and assayed for DNA synthesis. There was no difference between control and loaded cultures. A negative impact on DNA synthesis and cell division was found for porcine smooth muscle cells[57] and dental pulpal fibroblasts.[58] At the same time, we[59,60] found that osteoblasts and endothelial cells responded in a positive way to cyclic deformation. These results led us to conclude that some cells perceive strain but do not interpret the signal as mitogenic. The theory of mechanical load discrimination by cells indicates that cells can discriminate some part of the load regimen and elect to not respond by dividing. We feel that a refractoriness to load is a protective effect to prevent cell proliferation during unfavorable conditions.

Tendon Maintenance, Healing, and Overuse: Positive and Negative Modulation by Mechanical Load

The model in Figure 6 provides a hypothetical explanation of mechanisms for mechanical loads as positive and negative modulators of tendon cell responses. Under normal conditions, active loading of tendon by muscle and passive load-

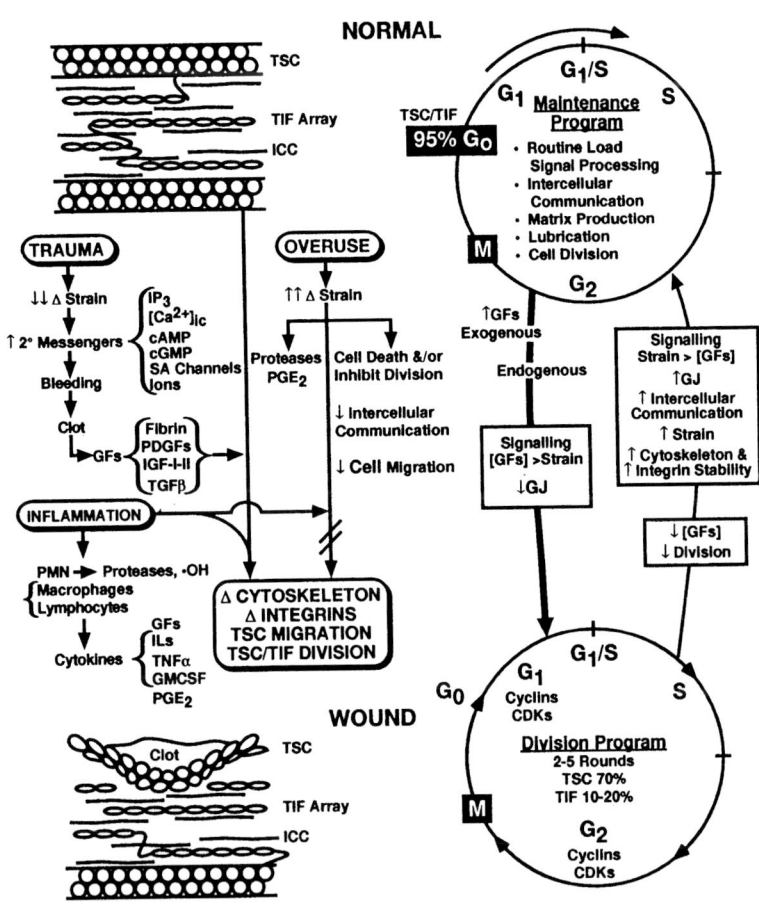

Fig. 6 A hypothetical model describing how mechanical load and growth factors may act on tendon cell division after trauma and bleeding or overuse injury. Although in this model tendon cells are normally mechanically active and communicate via gap junctions, they remain in a G_0 nondividing state until after a traumatic event, when they are stimulated to enter S phase by PDGF derived from platelets. The hierarchy of growth factor signal strength mandates that tendon cells migrate to the wound area and divide until the level of growth factor diminishes. Once the migratory and mitogenic responses to PDGF and other factors decrease, normal intercellular communication is restored and cells re-enter the maintenance program with cells in the G_0 state. Overuse of tendon may result in decreased intercellular communication and cell death, causing a focal necrotic area.

ing result in intercellular communication to achieve a homeostasis of matrix maintenance and cell replacement. Injury alters the normal balance, superceding maintenance conditions by introducing growth factors that drive cells to migrate and divide. Cell division occurs for two to five growth cycles over several weeks, then the hierarchy of signaling returns growth control from a growth factor-driven state to a load-regulated maintenance state. Overuse or continuous cyclic loading without growth factors may result in direct cell death or cell death by inhibition of cell division and production of enzymes that degrade matrix. This imbalance leads to a necrotic lesion in which cells die, matrix fails, and the environment does not favor repopulation.

Summary

Single tendon cells can detect and respond to mechanical deformation by communicating an intracellular calcium wave to a limited number of adjacent cells. Wave propagation appears to be mediated by the diffusion of IP_3 through gap junctions. A principal gap junction protein in tendon cells is CNX-43. The expression of this connexin correlates with the ability to propagate a calcium wave. Normally, tendon cells do not respond to mechanical load by dividing, but if cells are subjected to growth factors and mechanical load simultaneously, mitogenesis is initiated. Therefore, mechanical load and growth factors appear to act synergistically to stimulate cell division. However, continuous cyclic load at high strain levels in vitro may down-regulate DNA synthesis and cell division, resulting in repetitive motion injury.

Acknowledgments

Funding for this project was provided by NIH grants AR38121 (AJ Banes) and HLY9288 (MJ Sanderson), Plastic Surgery Research Fund (AJ Banes), and The Hunt Foundation (AJ Banes). S Boitano was supported by a fellowship from the Parker B. Francis Foundation.

References

1. Merrilees MJ, Flint MH: Ultrastructural study of tension and pressure zones in rabbit flexor tendon. *Am J Anat* 1980;157:87–106.
2. Banes AJ, Gilbert J, Taylor D, et al: A new vacuum-operated stress-providing instruments that applies static or variable duration cyclic tension or compression to cells in vitro. *J Cell Sci* 1985;75:35–42.
3. Gillard GC, Reilly HC, Bell-Booth PG, et al: The influence of mechanical forces on the glycosaminoglycan content of the rabbit flexor digitorum profundus tendon. *Conn Tiss Res* 1979;7:37–46.
4. Stopak D, Harris AK: Connective tissue morphogenesis by fibroblast traction: I. Tissue culture observations. *Devel Biol* 1982;90:383–398.
5. Ingber DE: Cellular tensegrity: Defining new rules of biological design that govern the cytoskeleton. *J Cell Sci* 1993;104:613–627.
6. Wang NJ, Butler P, Ingber DE: Mechanotransduction across the cell surface and through the cytoskeleton. *Science* 1993;260:1124–1127.
7. Sanderson MJ, Dirksen ER: Mechanosensitivity of cultured ciliated cells from the mammalian respiratory tract: Implications for the regulation of mucociliary transport. *Proc Natl Acad Sci USA* 1986;83:7302–7306.
8. Sanderson MJ, Chow I, Dirksen ER: Intercellular communication between ciliated cells in culture. *Am J Physiol* 1988;254:C63–C74.

9. Sanderson MJ, Charles AC, Dirksen ER: Inositol triphosphate mediates intercellular communication between ciliated epithelial cells. *J Cell Biol* 1989;109(suppl): 304A.
10. Sanderson MJ, Charles AC, Dirksen ER: Mechanical stimulation and intercellular communication increases intracellular Ca^{2+} in epithelial cells. *Cell Regul* 1990;1: 585–596.
11. Boitano S, Dirksen ER, Sanderson MJ: Intercellular propagation of calcium waves mediated by inositol trisphosphate. *Science* 1992;258:292–295.
12. Berridge MJ, Irvine RF: Inositol phosphates and cell signalling. *Nature* 1989;341: 197–205.
13. Sachs F: Baroreceptor mechanisms at the cellular level. *Fed Proc* 1987;46:12–16.
14. Sachs F: Mechanical transduction in biological systems. *Crit Rev Biomed Eng* 1988; 16:141–169.
15. Komuro I, Katoh Y, Kaida T, et al: Mechanical loading stimulates cell hypertrophy and specific gene expression in cultured rat cardiac myocytes: Possible role of protein kinase C activation. *J Biol Chem* 1991;266:1265–1268.
16. Komuro Y, Kaida T, Shibazaki Y, et al: Stretching cardiac myocytes stimulates protooncogene expression. *J Biol Chem* 1990;265:3595–3598.
17. Resnick N, Collins T, Atkinson W, et al: Platelet-derived growth factor B chain promoter contains a cis-acting fluid shear-stress-responsive element. *Proc Natl Acad Sci USA* 1993;90:7908.
18. Hirata M, Sasaguri T, Hamachi T, et al: Irreversible inhibition of Ca^{2+} release in saponin-treated macrophages by the photoaffinity derivative of inositol-1, 4, 5-trisphosphate. *Nature* 1985;317:723–725.
19. Peracchia C: Effects of the anesthetics heptanol, halothane and isoflurane on gap junction conductance in crayfish septate axons: A calcium- and hydrogen-independent phenomenon potentiated by caffeine and theophylline, and inhibited by 4-aminopyridine. *J Membr Biol* 1991;121:67–78.
20. Mody I, Tanelian DL, MacIver MB: Halothane enhances tonic neuronal inhibition by elevating intracellular calcium. *Brain Res* 1991;538:319–323.
21. Randriamampita C, Giaume C, Neyton J, et al: Acetylcholine-induced closure of gap junction channels in rat lacrimal glands is probably mediated by protein kinase. C *Pflugers Arch* 1988;412:462–468.
22. Musil LS, Cunningham BA, Edelman GM, et al: Differential phosphorylation of the gap junction protein connexin43 in junctional communication-competent and -deficient cell lines. *J Cell Biol* 1990;111:2077–2088.
23. Crow DS, Beyer EC, Paul DL, et al: Phosphorylation of connexin-43 gap junction protein in uninfected and Rous sarcoma virus-transformed mammalian fibroblasts. *Mol Cell Biol* 1990;10:1754–1763.
24. Laird DW, Puranam KL, Revel JP: Turnover and phosphorylation dynamics of connexin43 gap junction protein in cultured cardiac myocytes. *Biochem J* 1991;273:67–72.
25. Moreno AP, Campos de Carvalho AC, Christ G, et al: Gap junctions between human corpus cavernosum smooth muscle cells:gating properties and unitary conductance. *Am J Physiol* 1992;264:C80–C92.
26. Moreno AP, Fishman GI, Spray DC: Phosphorylation shifts unitary conductance and modifies voltage dependent kinetics of human connexin43 gap junction channels. *Biophys J* 1992;62:51–53.
27. Abrahams M: Mechanical behaviour of tendon in vitro: A preliminary report. *Med Biol Engin* 1967;5:433–443.
28. Walker LB, Harris EH, Benedict JV: Stress-strain relationship in human cadaveric plantaris tendon: A preliminary study. *Med Elect Bio Engin* 1964;2:31–38.
29. Walker P, Amstutz HC, Rubinfeld MJ: Canine tendon studies: II. Biomechanical evaluation of normal and regrown canine tendons. *Biomed Matls Res* 1976;10:61.
30. Greenlee TK Jr, Ross R: The development of the rat flexor digital tendon, a fine structure study. *J Ultrastr Res* 1967;18:354–376.

31. Greenlee TK Jr, Beckham C, Pike D: A fine structural study of the development of the chick flexor digital tendon: A model for synovial sheathed tendon healing. *Am J Anat* 1975;143:303–313.
32. Caplin DM, Greenlee TK: The development of human digital tendons. *J Anat* 1975;120:253–274.
33. Tsuzaki M, Yamauchi M, Banes AJ: Tendon collagens: Extracellular matrix composition in shear stress and tensile components of flexor tendons. *Conn Tiss Res* 1993;29:141–152.
34. Banes AJ, Link GW, Bevin AG, et al: Tendon synovial cells secrete fibronectin in vivo and in vitro. *J Orthop Res* 1988;6:73–82.
35. Banes AJ, Donlon K, Link GW, et al: Cell populations of tendon: A simplified method for isolation of synovial cells and internal fibroblasts: Conformation of origin and biologic properties. *J Orthop Res* 1988;6:83–94.
36. Brigman BE, Shapiro I, Lawrence WT, et al: Mechanical loading of tendon cells increases phospholipid secretion in vitro. *Trans Orth Res Soc* 1994;19:494.
37. Tsuzaki M, Brigman BE, Xiao H, et al: IGF-I and TGF-beta drive tendon cell DNA synthesis. *Trans Orth Res Soc* 1994;19:18.
38. Robertson JD: The occurrence of a subunit pattern in the unit membranes of club endings in Mauthner cell synapses in goldfish brains. *J Cell Biol* 1963;19:201–221.
39. Revel JP, Karnovsky MJ: Hexagonal array of subunits in intercellular junctions of the mouse heart and liver. *J Cell Biol* 1967;33:C7–C12.
40. Beyer EC, Paul DL, Goodenough DA: Connexin family of gap junction proteins. *J Membrane Biol* 1990;116:187–194.
41. Bennett MV, Barrio LC, Bargiello TA, et al: Gap junctions: New tools, new answers, new questions. *Neuron* 1991;6:305–320.
42. Beyer EC, Kistler J, Paul DL, et al: Antisera directed against connexin43 peptides react with a 43-kD protein localized to gap junctions in myocardium and other tissues. *J Cell Biol* 1989;108:595–605.
43. Trautmann A: Functions of gap junction channels in the open and closed states. *Biochem Soc Trans* 1988;16:534–536.
44. Unwin N: The structure of ion channels in membranes of excitable cells. *Neuron* 1989;3:665–676.
45. Sanderson MJ, Charles AC, Boitano S, et al: Mechanical and function of intracellular calcium signalling. *Molec Cell Endocrinology* 1994;98:173–187.
46. Banes AJ, Enterline, Bevin AG, et al: Effects of trauma and partial devascularization on protein synthesis in the avian flexor profundus tendon. *J Trauma* 1981;21:505–512.
47. Hu P, Xiao H, Brigman B, et al: G1 D cyclins are differentially regulated in tendon epitenon and internal fibroblasts. *Trans Orth Res Soc* 1994;19:639.
48. Ross R, Glomset J, Kariya B, et al: A platelet-dependent serum factor that stimulates the proliferation of arterial smooth muscle cells in vitro. *Proc Natl Acad Sci USA* 1974;71:1207–1210.
49. Ross R, Raines EW, Bowen-Pope DF: The biology of platelet-derived growth factor. *Cell* 1986;46:155–169.
50. Raines EW, Ross R: Platelet-derived growth factor: I. High yield purification and evidence for multiple forms. *J Biol Chem* 1982;257:5154–5160.
51. Raines EW, Dower SK, Ross R: Interleukin-1 mitogenic activity for fibroblasts and smooth muscle cells is due to PDGF-AA. *Science* 1989;243:393–396.
52. Pledger WJ, Stiles CD, Antoniades HN, et al: An ordered sequence of events is required before BALB/c-3T3 cells become committed to DNA synthesis. *Proc Natl Acad Sci USA* 1978;75:2839–2843.
53. Pledger WJ, Stiles CD, Antoniades HN, et al: Induction of DNA synthesis in BALB/c 3T3 cells by serum components: Reevaluation of the commitment process. *Proc Natl Acad Sci USA* 1977;74:4481–4485.
54. Almekinders LC, Banes AJ, Ballenger CA: Effects of repetitive motion on human fibroblasts. *Med Sci Sports Exerc* 1993;25:603–607.

55. Banes AJ, Link GW, Gilbert JW, et al: Culturing cells in a mechanically active environment: I. The flexercell strain unit can apply cyclic or static tension or compression to cells in culture. *Am Biotech Lab* 1990;8:12–22.
56. Pederson DR, Bottlang M, Brown TD, et al: Hyperelastic constitutive properties of polydimethylsiloxane cell culture membranes. *Trans Amer Soc Mech Eng* 1993;26:607–609.
57. Sumpio BE, Banes AJ: Response of porcine aortic smooth muscle cells to cyclic tensional deformation in culture. *J Surg Res* 1988;44:696–701.
58. Levin LG, Banes AJ, Link W: Abstract: Reactions of human pulpal fibroblasts to cyclic mechanical stretching in vitro. *J Dental Res* 1988;67:215.
59. Buckley MJ, Banes AJ, Levin LG, et al: Osteoblasts increase their rate of division and align in response to cyclic, mechanical tension in vitro. *Bone and Min* 1988;4:225–236.
60. Sumpio BE, Banes AJ, Levin LG, et al: Mechanical stress stimulates aortic endothelial cells to proliferate. *J Vasc Surg* 1987;6:252–256.

Chapter 17

Inflammatory Processes in Repetitive Motion and Overuse Syndromes: Potential Role of Neurogenic Mechanisms in Tendons and Ligaments

David A. Hart, PhD
Cyril B. Frank, MD
Robert C. Bray, MD

Introduction

Over the past several years, the incidence and awareness of repetitive motion and overuse syndromes has increased. Athletics, life-style changes, and occupational factors have been implicated. Repetitive motion syndromes associated with sports or occupational factors can have a serious impact not only on quality of life and productivity but also on the health-care system. Repetitive motion is one mechanism by which overuse syndromes can be initiated.

In most instances, the growth in our understanding of the factors leading to these syndromes has not kept pace with the apparent increased incidence. This dichotomy is due to a number of factors, such as the unavailability of tissue to analyze early on in the course of the disease, a paucity of animal models, and the unavailability, until recently, of technology to study the regulation of function in relatively hypocellular tissues, such as tendons and ligaments. However, considerably more is being learned about the biochemistry, cellular and molecular biology, and biomechanics of these tissues. Furthermore, a new understanding of structure-function relationships in these tissues, their responses to acute injury, and the role of inflammatory processes in wound healing has enabled researchers to address central issues in repetitive motion syndromes and to integrate this information into general knowledge about inflammatory and noninflammatory processes in other tissues.

This chapter is not intended to cover in detail aspects of repetitive motion or overuse syndromes that have been addressed in other chapters of this book or in recent reviews and monographs.[1-5] Rather, we will attempt to integrate recent findings regarding ligament and tendon biology into what is known about common mechanisms of inflammation, wound healing, and biologic regulation.

Role of Inflammatory Processes in Acute Wound Healing in Ligaments and Tendons

Acute, gross injury to ligaments or tendons, such as complete or partial rupture, usually leads to a rapid initiation of the healing response. The inflammatory response plays an important role in both the initiation of this response and the early development of the fibrotic phase of healing.[6–8] Bleeding into the wound site, caused by disruption of the microvasculature, activates the clotting cascades and platelets, with fibrin deposition, generation of biologically active peptide fragments, and release of growth factors (eg, plate-derived growth factors, PDGF), cytokines, and chemotactic factors. The early involvement of inflammatory cells, such as macrophages, neutrophils, and mast cells, contributes to the removal of damaged matrix and cells and the chemotaxis and proliferation of fibroblast populations that will repopulate the wound site and generate the scar matrix.

The early inflammatory phase probably also plays an active role in the angiogenesis required to maintain the healing response. Recent investigations by Eng and associates[9] have demonstrated that early ligament scar tissue is hypervascular and more recent experiments using fluorescent microspheres[10,11] have also led to quantitative assessment of this vascularity during the process of wound healing. Both cellularity and vascularity decrease as the inflammatory phase of healing makes way for the remodelling phase, which in tissues such as ligaments and tendons appears to be a protracted process that leads to mature scars but not tissue regeneration.

An important point is that the effectiveness of the inflammatory response described above is not static and can be influenced by a variety of factors, including age, gender, and the presence of diseases such as diabetes. In addition, tissue-specific factors and genetics can also contribute to the intensity and diversity of the inflammatory response to an injury or insult. Interestingly, a recent report by Beck and associates[12] has indicated that a single systemic injection of the growth factor transforming growth factor-β1 (TGF-β1), which is made by macrophages and other cell types, restores the wound healing potential of aged or glucocorticoid-treated rats to that found in young rats. Because TGF-β1 is effective in influencing early ligament scar cell phenotype but not late scar tissue,[13–15] the findings of Beck and associates[12] may partially explain the mechanism of age-dependent decline in the effectiveness of the inflammatory phase of wound healing.

Genetics may be a factor predisposing to connective tissue injuries as well as to the response to inflammatory stimuli or mediators released as a consequence of the inflammatory process.[16,17] Wahl and Renström[16] recently reviewed the regulation of fibrosis in soft-tissue injuries and discussed the incidence of individuals in whom an excess reaction to injury caused a large mass of scar tissue and adhesions that could interfere with joint function. This outcome was found in approximately 5% of the injured population seen by clinicians in this study. It is not yet clear what mechanisms are responsible, but they could involve dysregulated expression of growth factors and cytokines or an increased sensitivity to "normal" levels of mediators. Relevant to this point is the recent finding that TGF-β responsive elements in the collagen I gene of skin fibroblasts from patients with scleroderma, a disease of extensive fibrosis, are different from those of a control population.[17] It remains to be determined whether subsets of patients exhibiting hypertrophic scar responses also have similar or related changes in their genome.

Nirschl[18] uses the term "mesenchymal syndrome" to describe the subset of patients (estimated to be approximately 15% of patients) who may have multiple sites of tendon pain. Not all of these patients are subjected to repetitive motion or overuse conditions. This syndrome is more common in women than men and the typical patient is older than 30 years of age. Such patients appear to be likely to develop upper extremity tendon problems, which in certain cases may be influenced by estrogens.[18] Thus, gender-related variables may influence susceptibility and outcome. Whether these findings are also related to gender-dependent influences on inflammatory processes is unknown.

Although much of this discussion has focused on acute inflammatory responses to overt injury, some aspects are relevant to the subsequent analysis of inflammation associated with repetitive motion syndromes. A primary goal in acute injury is to mobilize inflammatory elements extrinsic to the tissue in order to facilitate a rapid return to at least partial function. The inflammatory response is beneficial, if not necessary. In only a minority of cases could an overexuberant response be considered detrimental to tissue function. This is in contrast to situations in which degeneration may be associated with a lack of inflammation-induced repair or in which chronic stimulation of an inflammatory reaction can lead to loss of function. Examples of the latter probably include chronic synovial inflammation and pannus formation in rheumatoid arthritis and possibly some of the repetitive motion or overuse syndromes discussed in the following sections.

Inflammatory Processes in Chronic Tendon and Ligament Injury

The inciting event(s) that lead to chronic ligament and tendon pathology are neither well defined nor understood. Because tendons and ligaments require mechanical stimulation for both maturation and maintenance of function,[19,20] it is likely that circumstances leading to functioning in the "upper limit" of biologic adaptation responses have an increased risk of incurring acute tissue failure or chronic tissue dysfunction (pathology). This can occur in what are commonly called "overuse" syndromes (Fig. 1). Repetitive motion syndromes fall into this category. However, because repetitive motion syndromes affect a subset of individuals, there may be a spectrum of individual factors that contribute to make their normal function lower than a significant percentage of the population (Fig. 2).

The potential mix of individual factors coupled with the percentage of individuals presenting with pathology has made it difficult to define the mechanisms responsible for repetitive motion syndromes. Even more difficult has been defining the role of inflammatory processes in the inciting events leading to the *development* of pathology because patients usually present well after the problem has become chronic, a point in the disease process that probably reflects a state quite distinct from the early phases.[21] Despite these limitations, a number of possibilities can be suggested: ischemia (or possibly ischemia-reperfusion injury) in these hypovascular tissues, thermal denaturation or damage resulting from limitations in heat transfer during repetitive motion, microinjuries incurred at a rate that exceeds repair potential, dysregulation of paratenon-tendon or epiligament-ligament function (see *Cellular and Structural Features of Ligaments and Tendons That Could Contribute to Inflammatory Processes*) and induction of inflammatory processes secondary to some of these other factors. Although this list is by no means exhaustive, it is a point from which to begin discussing some of the clinical and experimental findings assessed below.

Overuse Syndromes Involving Tendons

Overuse or repetitive motion syndromes have been reported to involve a variety of tendons in contrast to comparisons in ligaments. Involvement of the medial collateral ligament (MCL) of the knee has been described.[22] This dif-

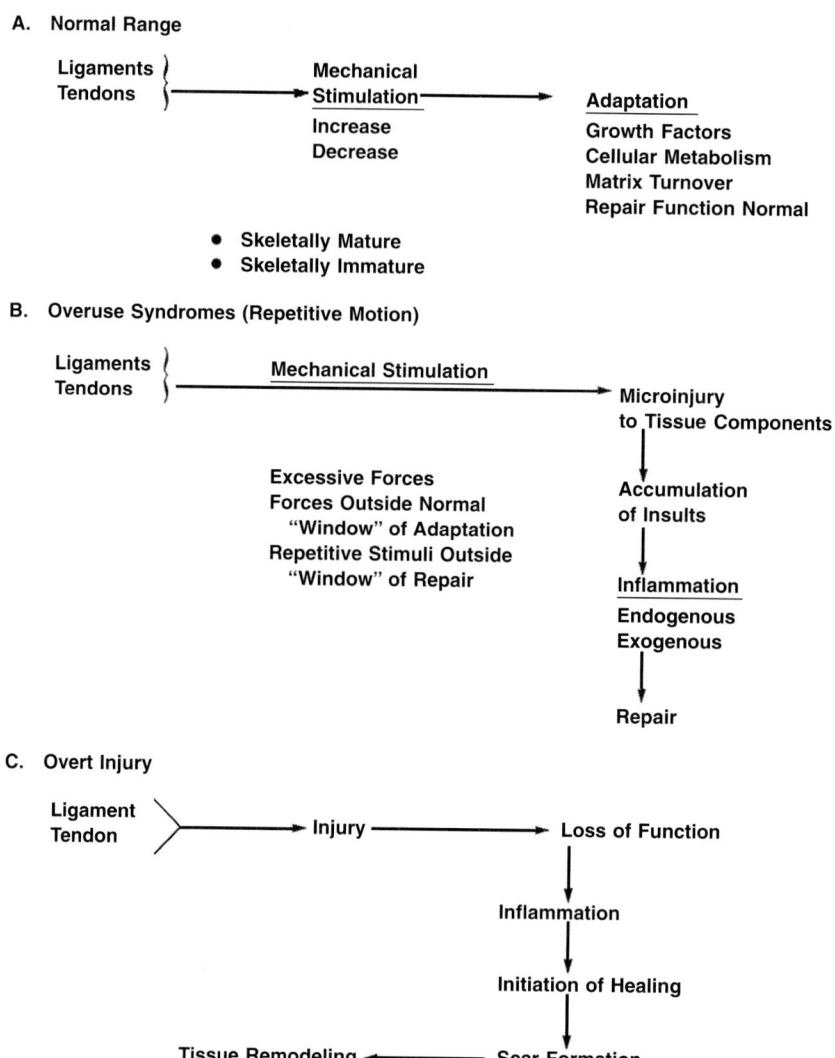

Fig. 1 Schematic of the regulation of ligament and tendon function in different mechanical and biological environments. The normal range for skeletally immature (growing) animals is probably different than that for skeletally mature animals.

ference between tendons and ligaments may be partly related to anatomic aspects or could be related to mechanical and biological environment in which they are required to function. This spectrum of variables has led to the application of a variety of terms to these overuse syndromes and the associated histologic and clinical assessments. For the purposes of this discussion, the definitions reviewed by Clancy[22] will apply. Paratenonitis (peritendonitis, tenosynovitis) is inflammation of the structure with edema, thickening, hyper-

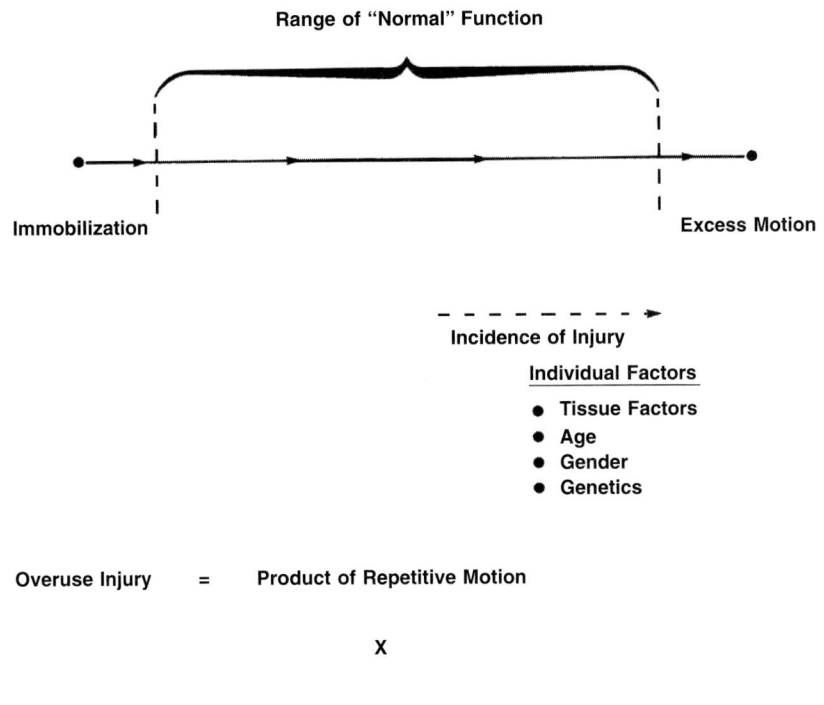

Fig. 2 Schematic of the relationship between motion and incidence of injury in ligaments and tendons.

vascularity, and inflammatory cell infiltrates. Tendinitis occurs when the primary site of injury is in the tendon; there is an inflammatory healing response and a secondary reactive paratenonitis. Tendinosis occurs when there are degenerative changes within a tendon without evidence of inflammation.

Because most conditions are treated conservatively and many cases respond to rest and/or anti-inflammatory medications, histologic changes have been documented in only a subset of patients whose cases proceed to surgery. Thus, many cases are defined as tendinitis based on presentation of pain and impaired function.

Achilles Tendinitis

The Achilles tendon is a common site for injury in a number of athletes and is considered an overuse/repetitive motion syndrome associated with pain and inflammation. Conservative treatment usually involves the use of anti-inflammatory drugs (steroids, nonsteroidal anti-inflammatory drugs [NSAIDs]) and surgical intervention very commonly shows "degeneration" of the tendon in relatively avascular areas of the tissue.[23] In contrast, paratenonitis is a commonly observed inflammation of the paratenon.[23–25] Repetitive motion or over-stimulation of the paratenon apparently leads to chronic inflammation and fibrosis of this structure.[1,23-25] In the Achilles tendon, the inflammatory involvement in tendinitis and paratenonitis may be due to different inciting mechanisms. Tendinitis may involve a response to tissue damage that cannot adequately heal because of repetitive mechanical stress, while paratendinitis may be due to other mechanisms because this area of the tendon is organized differently. The paratenon may perceive loads differently and probably responds to repetitive motion differently than the tendon itself.

Hansson and associates[26] found that short-term exercise of rats leads to increased expression of insulin-like growth factor-1 (IGF-1), an anabolic growth factor in the Achilles tendon. Highest levels of expression were at the myotendinous junction and the insertion into bone. The same authors also found that overuse of one leg (as a consequence of denervation of the other leg) using the same 5-day exercise protocol led to a rapid and more-intense IGF-1 staining in the paratenon of the Achilles tendon of the exercised leg. Thus, in this model there is a distinct difference between "exercise" and "overuse" and a difference between paratenon and tendon in the response to overuse. In the short-term experiments reported in this paper, an overt inflammatory response was not readily apparent in the tissue sections presented.[26]

In contrast to the rat exercise model, Backman and associates[27] have developed a rabbit model of overuse tendon injury with defined conditions. These authors have used male and female New Zealand white rabbits 6 to 9 months of age (ie, skeletally immature to barely skeletally mature). One leg was exercised for 5 to 6 weeks, with a rate of 150 flexions and extensions per minute for 2 hours, 3 times per week. The animals were killed and the exercised and nonexercised legs compared histologically. Evidence for degenerative changes in the exercised tendons was documented in hematoxylin and eosin sections of the tissues. Increased capillaries, edema, inflammatory cell infiltrates, and fibrotic changes in the paratenon of the exercised tendon were also noted. A later study with cerium-labelled microspheres demonstrated that blood flow was increased twofold in the exercised tendon compared to the nonexercised tendon.[28] This was primarily in the paratenon area. Unfortunately, because exercise protocols of less than 5 to 6 weeks were not performed, it is not apparent whether the observed changes in the paratenon preceded or paralleled the development of degenerative changes in the tendon proper. Such studies are critical if we are to form mechanistic conclusions regarding the two types of pathology. It is possible that the two phenomena are independent effects of overuse or there could be an interdependence where changes in the paratenon influence the ability of the tendon to initiate and maintain repair functions.

Interestingly, the pattern of changes in the paratenon (edema, increased vascularization, fibrosis, inflammatory cell infiltrates) is similar to changes induced by mast cell products[29-31] or occurring as a consequence of neurogenic inflammation.[32-35] It should also be noted that mast cells can be found in high numbers in some inflamed tissues, as in rheumatoid synovium,[36-39] and as such might further increase the fibrotic process. Detailed analysis of the inflammatory cells in the Achilles tendon was not performed in the studies by Backman and associates.[27]

Patellar Tendon

Inflammation of the patellar tendon has been shown histologically, primarily on surgical specimens obtained from the advanced chronic stage of disease.[5,40]

This type of overuse is commonly observed in athletes involved in jumping sports. At the present time there are no good models of patellar tendinitis and, therefore, the role of inflammatory processes in either the development or progression of the disease cannot be well documented. However, the symptoms are treated with anti-inflammatory agents with some success, so elements of inflammatory processes may be involved.

Tendons of the Hand and Wrist

Pyne and Adams[41] have recently provided an extensive review of overuse injuries to the tendons of the hand and wrist, with particular emphasis on sports-induced overuse syndromes. These may involve a number of different tendon complexes. A common feature of some of these is a stenosing tenosynovitis (paratenonitis). Whether this inflammatory condition develops secondarily to chronic microinjury to specific areas of the tendon is not clear. In cases that are resistant to conservative treatment (rest, anti-inflammatory agents, steroid injections) and proceed to surgery, evidence for acute and chronic inflammation can be detected. Details of the cellular infiltrates, however, have not been elucidated in most cases. In such chronic circumstances, the stenosis appears to result from edema, fibrosis, and thickening of the paratenon.

Tendinosis of the Elbow

This area has also been recently reviewed by Nirschl.[18] A number of different tendon complexes can be involved. A common feature, which has been called "angiofibroblastic tendinosis" or chronic tendinosis,[18] appears to be an attempt to initiate a form of repair or scarring after repetitive microinjury. The hypercellularity (fibroblasts) and hypervascularity is usually devoid of inflammatory cells, but the lesions do appear to be edematous. Some evidence for inflammatory cells in the periphery of these lesions has been reported, but detailed analysis of these has not been made. However, as these are usually very chronic cases, the possible involvement of more intense inflammatory-based events early in the "angiofibroblastic" response cannot be eliminated. Inflammatory response elements are effective at stimulating both fibroblast proliferation and angiogenesis, but could be less prominent in the later stages of the condition.

Repetitive Motion and Overuse of Ligaments

Most repetitive motion syndromes appear to affect tendons rather than ligaments;[22] however, ligaments can adapt to changes in mechanical stimulation. They respond to immobilization with altered cellular function and biomechanical properties.[20,42] They also respond to exercise with increased mass and alterations in mechanical properties.[43] Following injury to a ligament, such as the medial collateral ligament (MCL) of the rabbit knee, the corresponding ligament in the contralateral leg cannot be considered mechanically and histologically normal.[44] This may involve mechanisms related to increased usage of the noninjured leg. Likewise, in a rabbit model of immobilization,[20,42] the ligaments of the nonimmobilized leg appear to adapt to the potential overuse of the limb. It is not known whether this overuse involves inflammatory processes or falls within a normal window of adaptation.

Injury to one of the stabilizing ligaments, such as the anterior cruciate ligament (ACL) of the knee, can lead to adaptive responses in other ligaments of the knee in what could be interpreted as an attempt to maintain joint function. Histologic examination of the MCL of ACL deficient canine knees 10 weeks postinjury (transection) demonstrated extensive changes to the epiligament of this complex with no discernible changes in the ligament itself (Dr. J. Matyas, personal communication). The ligaments exhibited normal cellularity and appearance of the matrix. In contrast, the epiligament was extensively thickened with increased cellularity and vascularity. No evidence for overt involvement of inflammatory cells or processes was evident. Thus, these findings may represent an adaptive response to overuse that falls within a normal window of response. However, these dogs were not exercised and exercise could exacerbate the overuse to the point of tissue changes and involvement of inflammatory processes. The existing canine results do, however, provide circumstantial evidence for a unique role of the epiligament in response to a type of overuse related to joint instability.

Summary of Repetitive Motion/Overuse Syndrome Findings

Evidence to date indicates that tendon and ligament responses to overuse or repetitive motion can involve adaptation as well as development of pathology. The development of pathology appears to be more prevalent in tendons than ligaments. Inflammatory processes appear to be involved in the repair of injury (microinjury) to the tendon itself, as well as in the response of the paratenon to repetitive motion/overuse. In some cases, degeneration of tendon appears to result from accumulated microinjuries that cannot be repaired by endogenous mechanisms. This can occur in the absence of inflammatory processes. This type of degeneration in a relatively noninflammatory environment has been reported in horses following intratendon injection of collagenase.[45] Surgical intervention with debridement and exposure of the affected areas to inflammatory involvement can lead to scar formation and healing of the tissue.[5,45–47]

Because the paratenon (and the epiligament) is not directly affected by a high percentage of the mechanical load in overuse syndromes, the changes in the paratenon may result from a sliding mechanism (eg, tissue movement within a sheath) or from microdamage to elements unique to this structure. In the case of paratenon, overuse/repetitive motion apparently leads to edema, hypercellularity, angiogenesis and inflammatory infiltrates.[27] Less intense overuse leads to increased expression of anabolic growth factors (eg, IGF-1)[26] and a noninflammatory thickening of the paratenon. Based on these somewhat circumstantial findings, one could hypothesize that the paratenon/epiligament serves unique functions in the regulation of tissue homeostasis and responsiveness to changes in the biomechanical environment.

Cellular and Structural Features of Ligaments and Tendons That Could Contribute to Inflammatory Processes

Ligaments and tendons are relatively hypocellular tissues that consist of an extensive collagenous matrix plus cells such as fibroblasts, endothelial cells (microvascular system), axons (neural system), mast cells (inflammatory system), as well as other potential cell types that have not been well defined. Whether or not the "fibroblast" phenotype represents multiple subsets of cells is still being investigated; however, it is likely that cells at the insertions into bone or at myotendinous junctions differ from those in the midsubstance. Ligaments and tendons have an identifiable surface layer of cells and matrix termed the epiligament and paratenon, respectively.[48,49] There appears to be some differences in this surface structure between various ligaments and tendons. In the rabbit MCL, the fibroblast-like cells of the epiligament express a phenotype that is distinct from either ligament or synovial fibroblasts.[8,50] The matrix of the epiligament is also different from the ligament, and cells from the epiligament express an elevated ratio of type III/type I collagen compared to ligament cells.[8,15,51] The spatial arrangements of the cells and components, such as the innervation and microvascular elements, appear to be developmentally regulated, with the epiligament being more highly vascularized and innervated than the respective ligament tissues.[52-55] Thus, discrete areas of certain tendons and ligaments are relatively avascular and aneural, factors that, as discussed earlier, may contribute to development of tendonosis in repetitive motion syndromes. The apparent extent of total innervation and vascularization varies between ligaments[10,11,52-57] (and probably between tendons), a finding that may indicate that the potential for development of such neurovascular, inflammatory dysfunction also varies.

The finding that both the paratenon and epiligament are more highly innervated and vascularized than ligament and tendon, plus the observations indicating that epiligament fibroblasts (and likely paratenon cells) have a distinct phenotype, raises the possibility that epiligament and paratenon serve a unique role in both normal tissue regulation and responsiveness to stimuli (Fig. 3). The axons detected in ligaments contain the neurotransmitters substance P (SP) and calcitonin-gene related peptide (CGRP).[52,55] One of these, SP, is considered proinflammatory in certain concentrations and has been implicated in some aspects of the disease process in rheumatoid arthritis.[58-61] Recently, Murphy and Hart[62] demonstrated that SP can uniquely alter patterns of gene expression by fibroblasts cultured from epiligament and alter the biochemistry of epiligament explants. Furthermore, the patterns of innervation and the microvascular system are in close proximity in these tissues.[52-57] Because it is known that neurotransmitters can influence vascular cells,[63,64] it is generally believed that one

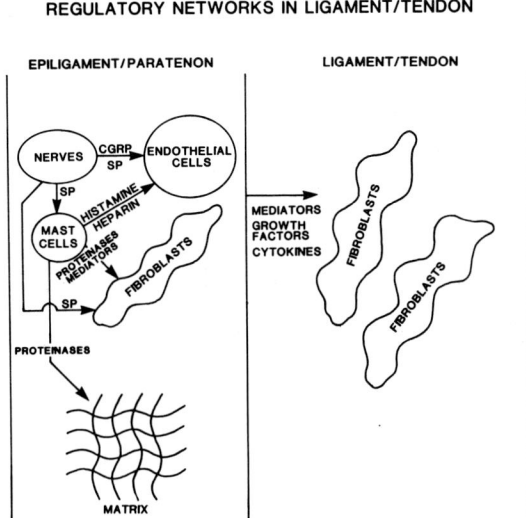

Fig. 3 Potential regulatory network in ligament and tendon based on the spatial arrangement of cells and components.

of the functions of the innervation is related to regulation of vascular control. Recent experiments have revealed that there is also close proximity between SP and CGRP-containing axons and tissue mast cells in epiligament (Fig. 4).

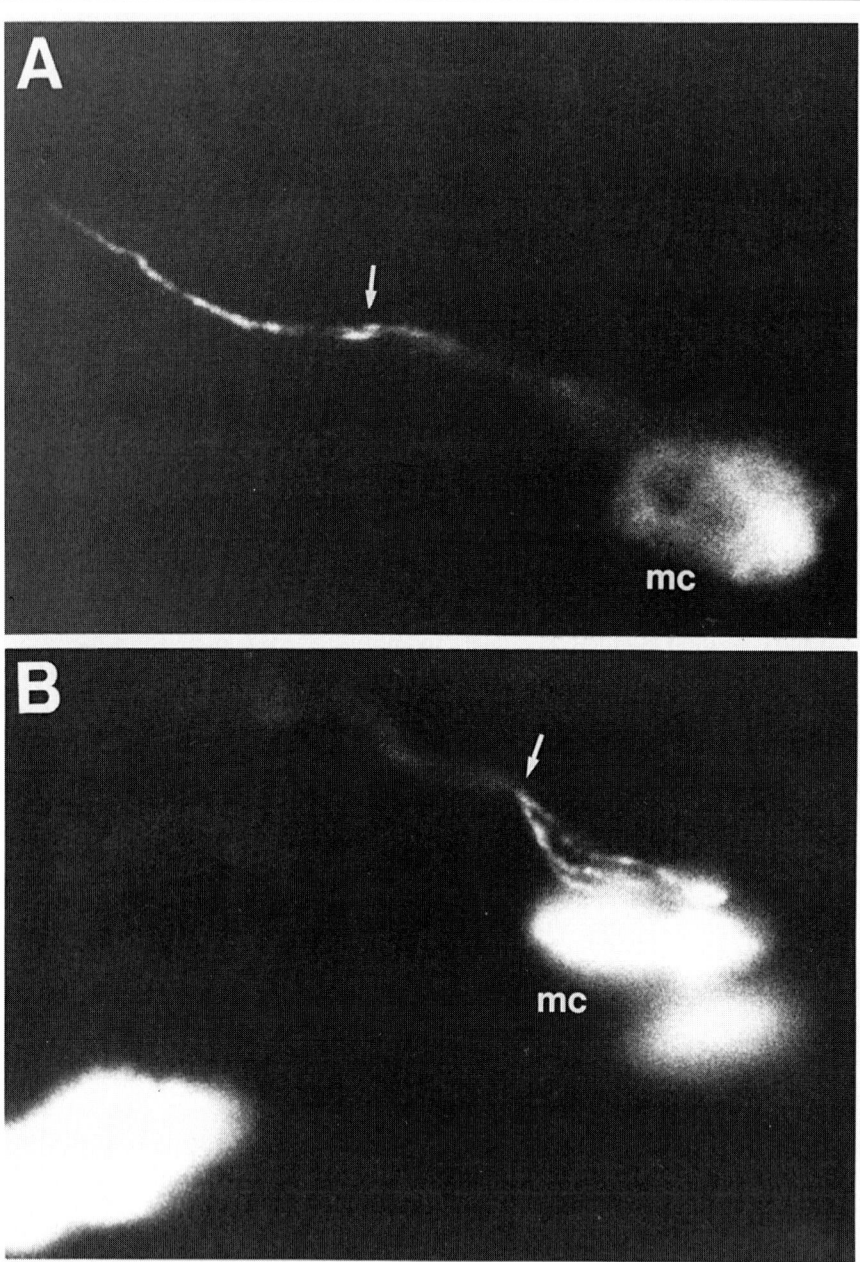

Fig. 4 A light micrograph showing association between axons (arrow) and mast cells (mc) in epiligament of the rabbit MCL. **A,** Axon demonstrating CGRP-like immunoreactivity neurite terminating in close proximity to a mast cell. **B,** An anti-SP stained axon (SP immunoreactivity) terminating in close proximity to mast cells.

NEUROGENIC INFLAMMATION

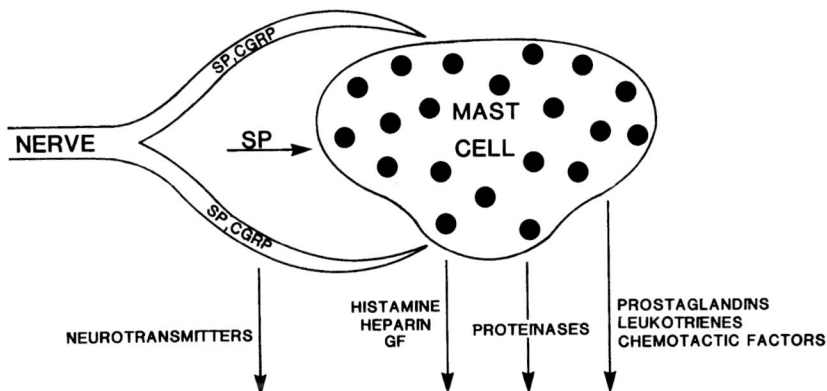

- Vascular Permeability (Edema)
- Angiogenesis
- Fibroblast Metabolism (Anabolic/Catabolic)
- Fibroblast Proliferation
- Chemotactic Factors (Eosinophils, etc.)
- Matrix Degradation (Biologically active fragments)
- Induction of Fibrosis (Wound healing?)

Fig. 5 Potential impact of mast cell-neurite "units" products on tissue responses as a consequence of neurogenic inflammation.

The close proximity between neural elements and tissue mast cells in ligament and tendon has also been detected in a number of other tissues, so the findings are not unique.[65–69] However, the finding in ligaments and tendons has a number of implications. First, because neurotransmitters such as SP can influence mast cell degranulation and secretory activity, neural activity could be amplified by inducing mast cells to release a panel of biologically active molecules that could impact on vascular elements, as well as fibroblasts (Fig. 5). As mast cells contain mediators (including growth factors and cytokines) that can influence edema, angiogenesis, fibroblast proliferation, as well as others which can function as chemotactic factors for specific inflammatory cells, their influence can be exaggerated in proportion to their numbers. Intra-articular injection of "arthritogenic" factors into rats leads to rapid mast cell degranulation and development of an inflammatory picture[70] not unlike what is seen in paratenonitis. Thus, these neural cell-mast cell "units" may contribute to normal ligament and tendon regulation and function when the tissues are operating within a defined set of normal biomechanical conditions (Fig. 6). The release of low amounts of some mediators such as granule components (histamine, heparin) and SP could be part of a normal regulatory system, while higher levels of mediators, due to more extensive degranulation and neurotransmitter release, may contribute to the adaptive response of these tissues.

Such "units" may also contribute to tissue dysfunction as such components have been implicated in what is termed neurogenic inflammation in a number

POTENTIAL ROLE OF NERVE-MAST CELL UNITS IN LIGAMENT/TENDON REGULATION

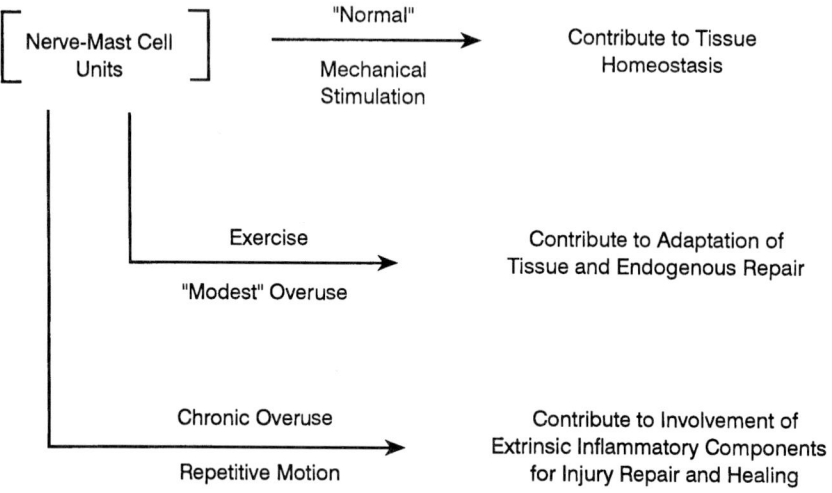

Fig. 6 Possible role of neurogenic mechanisms in ligament and tendon.

of tissues including synovium, skin, lung, intestine, and others.[32–35,65–69] In some respects, the neural-mast cell components could be considered an "endogenous" inflammatory system as compared to the "exogenous" inflammatory system composed primarily of blood borne cells (monocytes, neutrophils, eosinophils, lymphocytes) and cascades (complement, clotting, etc). Depending on the extent of the dysfunction to such an "endogenous" system, one may or may not observe evidence for involvement of the more classic "exogenous" system (Fig. 6). It could be speculated that dysregulation of mast cell degranulation in repetitive motion syndromes, occurring either indirectly through the neural component or directly through physical activation of mast cells, plays a critical role in these syndromes. Such possibilities are consistent with many of the features of paratenonitis described in earlier sections of this chapter; however, this interpretation may not explain the higher incidence of tendon involvement in repetitive motion syndromes compared to ligament. Ligaments, such as the MCL, have the neural-mast cell components in place and yet they appear to develop adaptation to overuse without evidence of exogenous inflammatory involvement. Thus, there may be as yet undiscovered unique features of the regulation of this system in tendons compared to ligaments. Confirmation of these hypotheses could lead to new treatment approaches for these conditions.

Acknowledgments

The authors thank Judy Crawford for excellent secretarial assistance in the preparation of the manuscript and Dr. John Matyas for helpful discussions. Investigations from the authors' laboratories were supported by the Medical Research Council of Canada and the Canadian Arthritis Society.

References

1. Kvist M: *Achilles Tendon Overuse Injuries.* Turku, Finland, Turku University, 1991. Dissertation.
2. Renström PAF, Leadbetter WB (eds): Tendinitis I: Basic concepts. *Clin Sport Med* 1992;11:493–677.
3. Renström PAF, Leadbetter WB (eds): Tendinitis II: Clinical considerations. *Clin Sport Med* 1992;11:679–904.
4. Pecina M, Bojanic I (eds): *Overuse Injuries of the Musculoskeletal System.* Boca Raton, FL, CRC Press, 1993.
5. Torstensen E, Bray RC, Wiley JP: Patellar tendonitis: A review of current concepts and treatment. *Clin J Sports Med* 1994;4:77–82.
6. Schurman DJ, Goodman SB, Smith RL: Inflammation and tissue repair, in Leadbetter WB, Buckwalter JA, Gordon SL (eds): *Sports-Induced Inflammation: Clinical and Basic Science Concepts.* Park Ridge, IL, American Academy of Orthopaedic Surgeons, 1990, pp 277–284.
7. Wilder RL, Lafyatis R, Remmers EF: Platelet-derived growth factor and transforming growth factor beta in wound healing and repair, in Leadbetter WB, Buckwalter JA, Gordon SL (eds): *Sports-Induced Inflammation: Clinical and Basic Science Concepts.* Park Ridge, IL, American Academy of Orthopaedic Surgeons, 1990, pp 301–313.
8. Murphy PG, Frank CB, Hart DA: The cell biology of ligaments and ligament healing, in Jackson DW, Arnoczky SP, Woo SLY, et al (eds): *The Anterior Cruciate Ligament: Current and Future Concepts.* New York, NY, Raven Press, 1993, pp 165–177.
9. Eng K, Rangayyan RM, Bray RC, et al: Quantitative analysis of the fine vascular anatomy of articular ligaments. *IEEE Trans Biomed Eng* 1992;39:296–306.
10. Butterwick D, Paul P, Bray R, et al: Abstract: Vascularity and blood flow in adult rabbit medial collateral and anterior cruciate ligaments. *Proc Can Orthop Res Soc* 1992;26:25.
11. Bray R, Butterwick D, Doschak M, et al: Quantitating blood flow to ligaments of the adult rabbit knee using coloured microspheres. *Trans Orthop Res Soc* 1994;19:790.
12. Beck LS, DeGuzman L, Lee WP, et al: One systemic administration of transforming growth factor-$\beta 1$ reverses age- or glucocorticoid-impaired wound healing. *J Clin Invest* 1993;92:2841–2849.
13. Murphy PG, Loitz BJ, Frank CB, et al: Influence of exogenous growth factors on the expression of plasminogen activators by explants of normal and healing rabbit ligaments. *Biochem Cell Biol* 1993;71:522–529.
14. Murphy PG, Hart DA: Influence of exogenous growth factors on the expression of plasminogen activators and plasminogen activator inhibitors by cells isolated from normal and healing rabbit ligaments. *J Orthop Res* 1994;12:564–575.
15. Murphy PG, Loitz BJ, Frank CB, et al: Influence of exogenous growth factors on the expression of plasminogen activators by explants of normal and healing rabbit ligaments. *Biochem Cell Biol* 1993;71:522–529.
16. Wahl S, Renström P: Fibrosis in soft-tissue injuries, in Leadbetter W, Buckwater JA, Gordon SL (eds): *Sports-Induced Inflammation: Clinical and Basic Science Concepts.* Park Ridge, IL, American Academy of Orthopaedic Surgeons, 1990, pp 637–647.
17. LeRoy EC: The control of fibrosis in systemic sclerosis: A strategy involving extracellular matrix, cytokines, and growth factors. *J Dermatol* 1994;21:1–4.
18. Nirschl RP: Elbow tendinosis: Tennis elbow. *Clin Sports Med* 1992;11:851–870.
19. Frank CB, Hart DA: Cellular Response to Loading, in Leadbetter WB, Buckwalter JA, Gordon SL (eds): *Sports-Induced Inflammation: Clinical and Basic Science Concepts.* Park Ridge, IL, American Academy of Orthopaedic Surgeons, 1990, pp 555–564.

20. Walsh S, Frank C, Shrive N, et al: Knee immobilization inhibits biomechanical maturation of the rabbit medial collateral ligament. *Clin Orthop* 1993;297:253–261.
21. Leadbetter WB: Cell-matrix response in tendon injury. *Clin Sports Med* 1992;11:533–578.
22. Clancy WG Jr: Tendon trauma and overuse injuries, in Leadbetter W, Buckwater JA, Gordon SL (eds): *Sports-Induced Inflammation: Clinical and Basic Science Concepts*. Park Ridge, IL, American Academy of Orthopaedic Surgeons, 1990, pp 609–618.
23. Galloway MT, Jokl P, Dayton OW: Achilles tendon overuse injuries. *Clin Sports Med* 1992;11:771–782.
24. Puddu G, Ippolito E, Postacchini F: A classification of Achilles tendon disease. *Am J Sports Med* 1976;4:145–150.
25. Kvist M, Jozsa L, Järvinen MJ, et al: Chronic Achilles paratenonitis in athletes: A histological and histochemical study. *Pathology* 1987;19:1–11.
26. Hansson H-A, Engstrom AM, Holm S, et al: Somatomedin C immunoreactivity in the Achilles tendon varies in a dynamic manner with the mechanical load. *Acta Physiol Scand* 1988;134:199–208.
27. Backman C, Boquist L, Friden J, et al: Chronic Achilles paratenonitis with tendinosis: An experimental model in the rabbit. *J Orthop Res* 1990;8:541–547.
28. Backman C, Friden J, Widmark A: Blood flow in chronic Achilles tendinosis: Radioactive microsphere study in rabbits. *Acta Orthop Scand* 1991;62:386–387.
29. Norrby K, Jakobsson A, Sörbo J: Mast-cell secretion and angiogenesis: A quantitative study in rats and mice. *Virchows Arch B Cell Pathol* 1989;57:251–256.
30. Gordon JR, Burd PR, Galli SJ: Mast cells as a source of multifunctional cytokines. *Immunol Today* 1990;11:458–464.
31. Ruoss SJ, Hartmann T, Caughey GH: Mast cell tryptase is a mitogen for cultured fibroblasts. *J Clin Invest* 1991;88:493–499.
32. Didier A, Kowalski ML, Jay J, et al: Neurogenic inflammation, vascular permeability, and mast cells: Capsaicin desensitization fails to influence IgE-anti-DNP induced vascular permeability in rat airways. *Am Rev Respir Dis* 1990;141:398–406.
33. Bienenstock J, MacQueen G, Sestini P, et al: Inflammatory cell mechanisms: Mast cell/nerve interactions in vitro and in vivo. *Am Rev Respir Dis* 1991;143:S55–S58.
34. Matucci-Cerinic M, Partsch G: Editorial: The contribution of the peripheral nervous system and the neuropeptide network to the development of synovial inflammation. *Clin Exp Rheumatol* 1992;10:211–215.
35. Kidd BL, Cruwys S, Mapp PI, et al: Role of the sympathetic nervous system in chronic joint pain and inflammation. *Ann Rheum Dis* 1992;51:1188–1191.
36. Wasserman SI: The mast cell and synovial inflammation: Or, what's a nice cell like you doing in a joint like this? *Arthritis Rheum* 1984;27:841–844.
37. Crisp AJ, Chapman CM, Kirkham SE, et al: Articular mastocytosis in rheumatoid arthritis. *Arthritis Rheum* 1984;27:845–851.
38. Bridges AJ, Malone DG, Jicinsky J, et al: Human synovial mast cell involvement in rheumatoid arthritis and osteoarthritis: Relationship to disease type, clinical activity, and antirheumatic therapy. *Arthritis Rheum* 1991;34:1116–1124.
39. Kopicky-Burd JA, Kagey-Sobotka A, Peters SP, et al: Characterization of human synovial mast cells. *J Rheumatol* 1988;15:1326–1333.
40. Blazina ME, Kerlan RK, Jobe FW, et al: Jumper's knee. *Orthop Clin North Am* 1973;4:665–678.
41. Pyne JI, Adams BD: Hand tendon injuries in athletics. *Clin Sports Med* 1992;11:833–850.
42. Walsh S, Frank C, Hart D: Immobilization alters cell metabolism in an immature ligament. *Clin Orthop* 1992;277:277–288.
43. Woo SL-Y, Maynard J, Butler D, et al: Ligament, tendon, and joint capsule insertions to bone, in Woo SL-Y, Buckwater JA (eds): *Injury and Repair of the Musculoskeletal System*. Park Ridge, IL, American Academy of Orthopaedic Surgeons, 1988, pp 133–166.

44. Frank CB, Loitz B, Bray R, et al: Abnormality of the contralateral ligament after injuries of the medial collateral ligament: An experimental study in rabbits. *J Bone Joint Surg* 1994;76A:403–412.
45. Henninger RW, Bramlage L, Bailey M, et al: Effects of tendon splitting on experimentally-induced acute equine tendinitis. *VCOT* 1992;5:1–9.
46. Anderson D, Taunton J, Davidson R: Surgical management of chronic Achilles tendonitis. *Clin J Sports Med* 1992;2:38–42.
47. Asheim A: Surgical treatment of tendon injuries in the horse. *J Am Vet Med Assoc* 1964;145:447–451.
48. Chowdhury P, Matyas JR, and Frank CB: The 'epiligament' of the rabbit medial collateral ligament: A quantitative morphological study. *Connect Tissue Res* 1991;27:33–50.
49. Smart GW, Taunton JE, Clement DB: Achilles tendon disorders in runners: A review. *Med Sci Sports Exerc* 1980;12:231–243.
50. Murphy PG, Frank CB, Hart DA: Characterization of the plasminogen activators and plasminogen activator-inhibitors expressed by cells isolated from rabbit ligament and synovial tissues: Evidence for unique cell populations. *Exp Cell Res* 1993;205:16–24.
51. Murphy PG: *Regulation of Plasminogen Activators and Their Inhibitors in Normal and Healing Connective Tissues*. Calgary, Alberta, Canada, University of Calgary, 1992. Thesis.
52. Bray RC: Blood supply of ligaments. *Int Orthop* 1995;3:39–48.
53. Bray R, Frank C, Miniaci T: Structure and function of diarthrodial joints, in McGinty JB, Caspari RB, Jackson RW, et al (eds): *Operative Arthroscopy*. New York, NY, Raven Press, 1991, pp 79–123.
54. Fisher AW, Bray R: The innervation of the collateral ligaments of the knee joint. *J Anat* 1989;164:245–246.
55. Sharkey K, Bray RC: Abstract: Innervation patterns of collateral knee ligaments as revealed by silver staining and immunohistochemistry. *Society for Neuroscience* 1991;16:882.
56. Schutte MJ, Dabezies EJ, Zimny ML, et al: Neural anatomy of the human anterior cruciate ligament. *J Bone Joint Surg* 1987;69A:243–247.
57. el-Bohy A, Cavanaugh JM, Getchell ML, et al: Localization of substance P and neurofilament immunoreactive fibers in the lumbar facet joint capsule and supraspinous ligament of the rabbit. *Brain Res* 1988;460:379–382.
58. Levine JD, Clark R, Devor M, et al: Intraneuronal substance P contributes to the severity of experimental arthritis. *Science* 1984;226:547–549.
59. Menkes CJ, Renoux M, Laoussadi S, et al: Substance P levels in the synovium and synovial fluid from patients with rheumatoid arthritis and osteoarthritis. *J Rheumatol* 1993;20:714–717.
60. Kimball ES: Substance P, cytokines, and arthritis. *Ann NY Acad Sci* 1990;594:293–308.
61. Lotz M, Carson DA, Vaughan JH: Substance P activation of rheumatoid synoviocytes: Neural pathway in pathogenesis of arthritis. *Science* 1987;235:893–895.
62. Murphy PG, Hart DA: Plasminogen activators and plasminogen activator inhibitors in connective tissues and connective tissue cells: Influence of the neuropeptide substance P on expression. *Biochim Biophys Acta* 1993;1182:205–214.
63. Kowalski ML, Kaliner MA: Neurogenic inflammation, vascular permeability, and mast cells. *J Immunol* 1988;140:3905–3911.
64. Khoshbaten A, Ferrell WR: Responses of blood vessels in the rabbit knee to acute joint inflammation. *Ann Rheum Dis* 1990;49:540–544.
65. Skofitsch G, Savitt JM, Jacobowitz DM: Suggestive evidence for a functional unit between mast cells and substance P fibers in the rat diaphragm and mesentery. *Histochem* 1985;82:5–8.
66. Levine JD, Coderre TJ, Covinsky K, et al: Neural influences on synovial mast cell density in rat. *J Neurosci Res* 1990;26:301–307.

67. Baraniuk JN, Kowalski ML, Kaliner MA: Relationships between permeable vessels, nerves, and mast cells in rat cutaneous neurogenic inflammation. *J Appl Physiol* 1990;68:2305–2311.
68. Barnes PJ, Belvisi MG, Rogers DF: Modulation of neurogenic inflammation: Novel approaches to inflammatory disease. *Trends Pharmacol Sci* 1990;11:185–189.
69. Hukkanen M, Grönblad M, Rees R, et al: Regional distribution of mast cells and peptide containing nerves in normal and adjuvant arthritis rat synovium. *J Rheumatol* 1991;18:177–183.
70. Caulfield JP, Hein A, Helfgott SM, et al: Intraarticular injection of arthritogenic factor causes mast cell degranulation, inflammation, fat necrosis, and synovial hyperplasia. *Lab Invest* 1988;59:82–95.

Chapter 18

Morphology and Physiology of Normal Synovium and the Effects of Mechanical Stimulation

H. Ralph Schumacher, Jr, MD

Normal Synovium

It has been tempting to ignore synovium when considering repetitive use syndromes. However, its location—lining tendons and joints—its vascularity and population of potentially reactive cells, and its continuity with fibrous capsules all speak for the importance of synovium.

Synovium, via the synovial fluid, plays an essential role in nourishment of the articular cartilage, and it also is likely to be involved in providing nutrition to less vascular parts of tendons and ligaments within joints and sheaths. Other well-defined functions of synovium include the phagocytic role of the macrophage-like cells in removing the debris from dead cells and in removing small cartilage fragments that are identifiable even in normal joint fluids. The type B lining cells are the main source for the joint fluid hyaluronate and a number of other molecules produced for export.[1,2]

Synovium is a vascular connective tissue with a discontinuous inner layer of mixed fibrocyte-like and monocyte-derived cells. This tissue lines the surface of synovial joints, and a very similar tissue lines bursae and tendon sheaths.[3] The deeper connective tissue structural components vary from site to site among joints and within the joint. Thus, some synovium is very fibrous and some has mostly fatty matrix (Fig. 1). In addition to water, prominent matrix molecules include collagen and proteoglycans. Vascular networks also vary and tend to be more extensive in looser areolar synovium.

Normal Synovial Microvasculature

The prominent microvascular bed in synovium is one of the obvious sites that is influenced by motion and mechanical effects.[1] Permeability of the synovial vessels to fluid and cells is important both in maintenance of a healthy joint and in either combating or spreading disease. Many superficial capillaries and small venules have thin fenestrated walls facing the joint space (Fig. 2); these walls seem ideal for fluid transit because similar vessels are seen in the kidney, intestine, and choroid plexus. The endothelium of deeper vessels is quite thick and can be acted upon by histamine to open gaps that allow emigration of leukocytes.

Intravenously injected carbon and ferritin have been used as tracers to examine the escape of particulate material from synovial vessels. In apparently healthy monkeys, which were obtained from the wild, leakage of carbon (mean

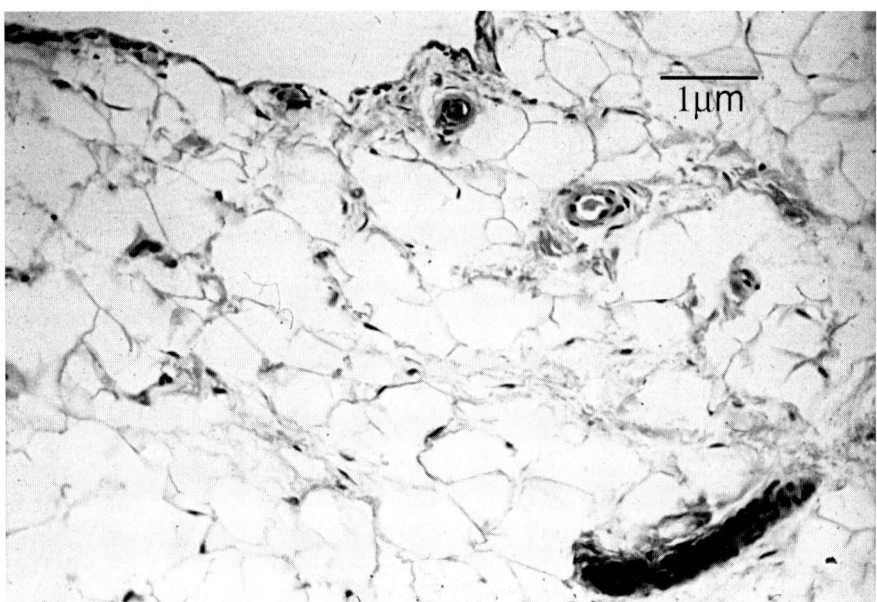

Fig. 1 Light microscopic view of areolar synovium with a single layer of synovial lining cells at the top. Small vessels can be seen among the matrix fat and loose connective tissue. × 400

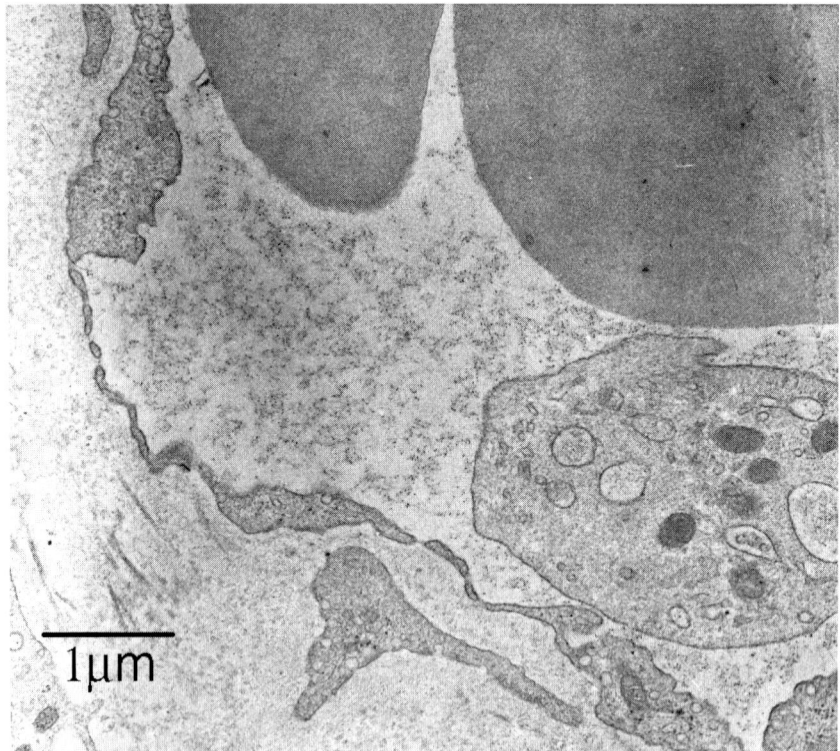

Fig. 2 Electron micrograph showing superficial synovial venule with red blood cells (RBCs) and platelets in lumen. The thin fenestrated endothelium is seen at the left. × 30,000 (Reproduced with permission from Schumacher HR: Normal anatomy of synovium, in Newton CD, Nunamaker DM (eds): *Textbook of Small Animal Orthopaedics*. Philadelphia, PA, JB Lippincott, 1985, pp 77–82.)

250 Å diameter) particles was identified at focal areas of a number of knee joints.[1] Using electron microscopy (EM), carbon was identified in vacuoles of the endothelial cells of deeper vessel, in gaps between endothelial cells, and lying in the vessel walls after escaping from the vessel. Leaky vessels were venules and not the most superficial fenestrated capillaries. This fact suggests some escape of small particles from normal joint vessels, although the monkey joints may have had some microtrauma (as do human joints). Data from earlier studies[4,5] had suggested that passage of circulating bacteria into joints was unusually prominent when compared to other sites.[4,5] Prompt staining of joints after intravenous injection of toluidine blue and rapid passage of intravenously injected proteins into joint fluid[6] also point to some potentially important permeability. In follow-up studies, carbon leakage was evaluated using light microscopy of glycerine cleared specimens from rabbits.[7,8] There was considerably more leakage from synovium at 1 and 2 hours than from any other site in the nonreticuloendothelial system. This is one of several observations which suggest that joints behave in some ways like reticuloendothelial tissue.

Microvascular physiology clearly varies among joints, as supported by the work of Simkin and associates,[9-11] who have extensively studied the permeability of small molecules. The microvascular beds also differ in the various types of synovium seen in different areas of the joint.[12,13] In an attempt to learn more about the role of synovial vessels, studies from different microvascular beds may become critical.

Free diffusion through the vessels and synovial matrix allows small solutes to equilibrate between plasma and the interstitial space.[10,11] Most therapeutic agents also seem to diffuse passively through the vessels. Normal plasma proteins also enter from the vessel into the joint fluid by passive diffusion, although levels tend to be lower in synovial fluid (SF) than in plasma. Smaller proteins pass more easily into the joint fluid, but it is not known whether they pass through intercellular junctions, vesicles, or fenestrae. Disease can alter not only vascular permeability but also clearance from the joint, and local production of some proteins can further complicate studies of permeability.

Effect of Exercise on Synovial Membrane and Its Microvascular Permeability

Passive manual flexion and extension 35 times per minute for 50 to 145 minutes produced a dramatic increase in the concentration carbon or ferritin leaking from this labeling in synovial vessels.[1] Again, all leaks were in the synovial venules (Fig. 3). No gross or light microscopic changes were detectable in most cases to parallel this increased permeability. In one tissue, EM showed actual vascular structural injury with a thrombus.

The effect of motion on acute urate crystal-induced arthritis in dog joints has also been studied.[14] Fairly subtle increases in joint motion, such as 5 minutes every 15 minutes over 4 hours, clearly increased leukocyte counts in synovial fluid. Carbon black labeling of synovial venules was increased. Xenon injected into the joint was cleared markedly more rapidly after joint motion, suggesting support for increased vascular or lymphatic clearance. Gross viewing indicated that vascular congestion was increased after exercise. In a single dog that had no urate crystals, exercise also produced increased evident synovial vascularity. In other dogs with effusions, rising intra-articular pressures of up to 60 mm Hg were demonstrated on knee flexion. Jayson and Dixon[15] had produced some similar findings on intra-artiular pressures in normal joints with and without effusions. Fam and associates[16] studied chronic joint motion

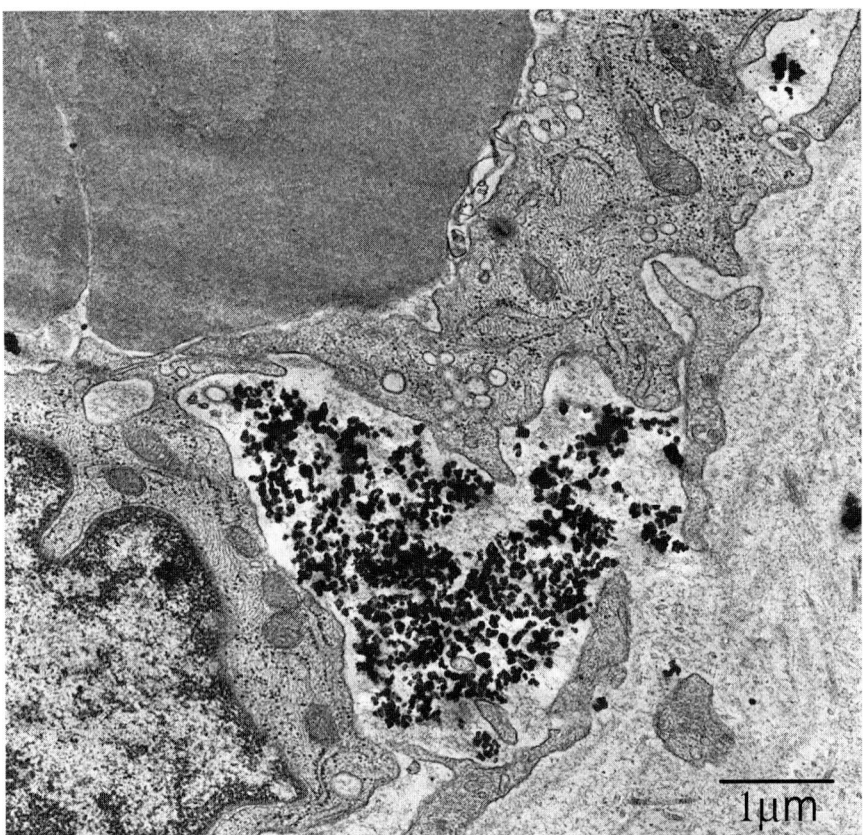

Fig. 3 Electron micrograph showing dark particles of intravenously injected carbon black that escaped from this deeper venule into the vessel wall after exercise. × 20,400 (Reproduced with permission from Schumacher HR: The microvasculature of the synovial membrane of the monkey: Ultrastructural studies. *Arthritis Rheum* 1969;12:387–404.)

in calcium pyrophosphate dihydrate (CPPD) crystal-induced inflammation in rabbits.[16] Although leukocyte counts rose with joint motion and decreased with immobilization, the cartilage was more adversely affected by the immobilization. Synovial edema and vasodilation increased with exercise.

Joint distention in rabbits, which was suggested to simulate changes seen with exercise and motion, moved lining cells apart, exposing more interstitium, and placed synovial vessels closer to the surface.[17] Thus, distention would appear to facilitate diffusion of various molecules into (and out of) the joint space. Geborek and associates[18] showed that raised intra-articular pressure decreased synovial flow. Different amounts and durations of joint distention may have different effects; antecedent synovial disease or effusion would also influence the effects of pressure. Recent studies on technetium diethylenetriamine pentaacetic acid clearance from knees with effusions showed that walking and cycling increased blood flow, straight leg raising had no effect, and flexion decreased flow.[19]

Exercise for 15 minutes has recently been shown by Farrel and associates[20] to raise plasma levels of von Willebrand factor in patients with rheumatoid arthritis (RA), whereas there was only an insignificant rise in normal controls.

The proposed mechanism for the change was that raised intra-articular pressure in the swollen RA joints exceeded capillary perfusion pressures, thereby causing hypoxia and then reperfusion injury to the capillaries with release of endothelial von Willebrand factor. The same group,[21] using nuclear magnetic resonance (NMR) spectroscopy, has also shown exercise-induced oxidative damage to hyaluronate and glucose in inflamed synovial fluid. Most such studies have been of knees, but NMR spectroscopic techniques can be applied noninvasively and may be ideal for studying the smaller joints in the upper extremities (G Keenan, MD, personal communication).

Adhesion molecule expression on the synovial microvasculature can certainly influence cell emigration and the associated permeability to a variety of other molecules. Studies are now being done to examine expression of various antigens on endothelium.[22-24] Normal synovial endothelium does express HLA DR, but not DQ. The HECA-452 antigen associated with high endothelial venules was not found in the few relatively normal specimens studied, although it was present in RA. Johnson and associates[23] showed expression of a number of selectins, integrins, and CD31 (platelet-endothelial cell adhesion molecule) on normal (from limb amputation) synovial endothelial cells. CD44 hyaluronate receptor was not expressed on endothelium, but was expressed in the vessel wall.

Fairburn and associates[12] have shown some E-selectin and intercellular adhesion molecule-1 (ICAM-1) expression on normal synovial venules, although there was less expression than in the skin. E-selectin was most prominently expressed on relatively superficial venules and ICAM on deeper vessels. These findings almost certainly have implications for the patterns of permeation by different cells. Whether joint, stress, motion, or various amounts of exercise have any effect on molecular expression on endothelium is not known, but it would be of great interest. Strenuous exercise in normal persons does appear to release several cytokines that can be measured in serum.[25] Tumor necrosis factor alpha (TNF-α) and interleukin-1 (IL-1) are known up-regulators of adhesion molecule expression.[26] Cytokines have also been considered as inducers of high endothelial morphology in vessels.[27] The mechanical effects of scraping synovial endothelial cells in vitro stimulated the release of fibroblast growth factors that, in turn, stimulated a proliferative response in synovial cells.[28]

Nerves and Other Features of Synovium

Synovium is also richly supplied with lymphatics, mast cells, and nerves.[29] Neuropeptides from these nerves can variously protect from or enhance the effects of diverse harmful stimuli. Neurologic deficits have been shown in several studies to spare joints from inflammatory disease.[30] Nerve fibers reactive for substance P and calcitonin gene-related peptide can be found throughout synovium; these fibers are often, but not invariably, related to vessels.[31,32] The peptides can be released into joint fluid. Large-diameter sensory afferent nerves that innervate identified receptor end organs (Pacinian, Ruffini) are not found in synovium, but they and thinly myelinated axons are present in the adjacent capsular tissue. The nonmyelinated C-type fibers in synovium are suggested to be both nociceptive and mechanoreceptive.[31,33] In reflex sympathetic dystrophy, which is presumed to produce swelling and vasomotor changes due to sympathetic nerve abnormalities, changes are also noted at joints distant from the initially traumatized or most symptomatic site. Either products from the primary joint or systemic predisposing factors seem to be important.

268 Pathophysiology: Connective Tissue

Lymphatics, which play a critical role in removing proteins and other materials from joints, have received very little study. Blockage of lymphatics can lead to chylous effusions. Mast cells are profuse in joints and provide the vasoactive substances that influence blood flow.[1,29]

Synovial Lining Cells

Different types of cells make up the synovial lining (Fig. 4). The type A phagocytic lining cell, which often appears to be most superficial, is now known to be monocyte-derived; the type B cell has fibrocyte-like features with profuse rough endoplasmic reticulum. A type C cell has been described as having intermediate features. Its significance is not yet clear.[29]

Some organelles common to synovial lining cells (SLC) and many other cells include the mitochondria, microtubules, 80- to 100-Å microfilaments, pinocytic vesicles, glycogen stores, centrioles, and occasional cilia, and lipid droplets. Mitotic figures are rare. Products known to be produced by SLC include

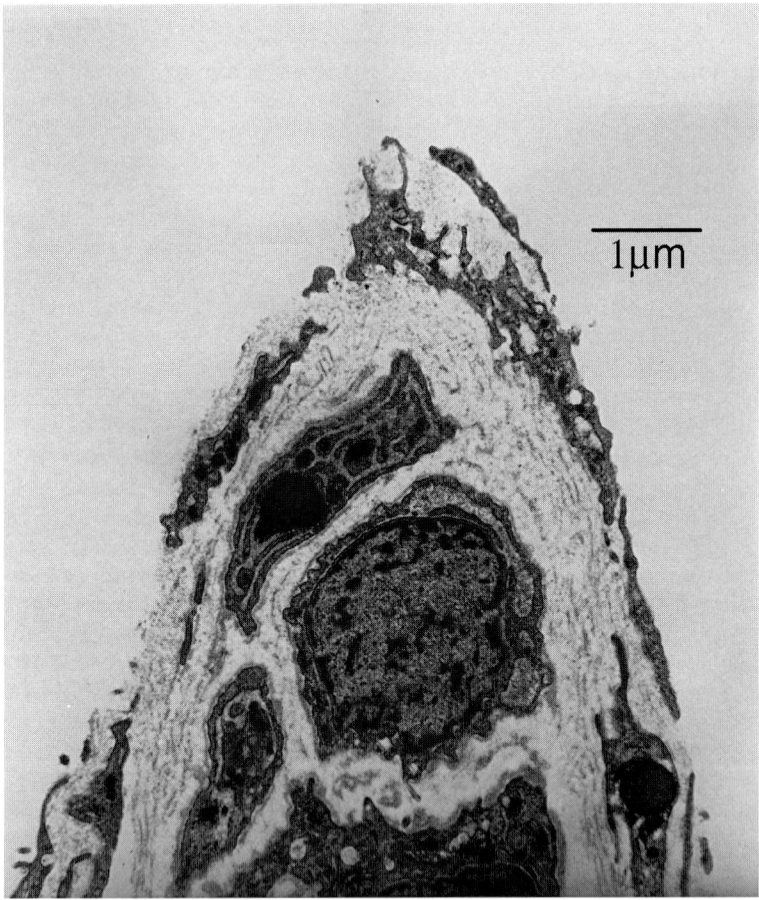

Fig. 4 Electron micrograph showing synovial villus with superficial type A phagocytic lining cells and deeper type B cells with prominent cisternae of endoplasmic reticulum. Note the intercellular matrix with wisps of basement membrane-like materials. × 30,000

a broad spectrum of molecules, such as hyaluronic acid, collagenase, other proteases, various proteoglycans, fibronectin, collagen, connective tissue activating peptide, diphosphopyridine nucleotide (DPN) diaphorase, lactate dehydrogenase (LDH), glucose-6-phosphate dehydrogenase, adhesion molecules, prostaglandins, and plasminogen activator. These very active cells and their products (as well as the deeper cells and their matrix) may well be affected in a variety of obvious and subtle ways by patterns of joint use. Synovium and the surface cells can heal and regenerate after wounding and synovectomy.[34–36] Synovial fibroblasts have been suggested as a source for cells aiding healing of injured tendons.[37]

Synovial Matrix

Small amounts of basement membrane (BM)-like material can occasionally be seen around SLC (Fig. 4) when using EM. This discovery is paralleled by recent identification of BM components, such as laminin, type IV collagen, heparan sulfate, entactin, and perlecan, in this area. Thus, although the synovium does not behave as a true BM-lined structure, many of the molecules that affect adhesion and emigration are present. Collagen in the synovium is predominantly types I and III. Areas of chondrometaplasia can occur and may produce typical cartilage collagens, such as type II. The collagen in areas of chondrometaplasia seems to be a preferential site for the calcification with calcium pyrophosphate crystals,[38] which occurs with aging and which may alter the joint's response to stresses tolerated earlier in life.

Joints Versus Bursae

The various normal synovium-bound spaces contain some fluid that, although often not in large enough amounts to be aspirated, has similarities and some differences between sites. Even different joints vary. Subatmospheric pressures in the joint space were found in dog shoulders and knees but not the wrists.[39] Hyaluronate, which is a major factor in joint fluid viscosity, is always present in joint fluid and in deep bursae but may not be present in all fluids in superficial bursae.[40,41] Part of the cavity of the retrocalcaneal bursa actually is molded over the posterior calcaneus and has more hyaluronate in its fluid than do prepatellar or olecranon bursae. In traumatic bursitis, fluid may be less viscous than in traumatic arthritis. In bursae, responses to various stimuli seem to produce lower leukocyte counts than do responses in joints. Bursal fluids often contain predominantly macrophages but also may have activated T lymphocytes, even after only local trauma.

Other Mechanical Effects on Synovium

There have been studies on a variety of mechanical insults to synovium, although few or none of these studies serve as satisfactory assessments of repetitive motion of upper extremities as it occurs in repetitive motion disorders. Some of these studies have been described under consideration of the microvasculature and exercise. It is hoped that information from the following studies can be extrapolated to repetitive use and to different sites.

It is not known whether certain amounts of nontraumatic repetitive joint motion can produce small joint effusions; although, as noted, effects of different types of exercise can be quite opposite in joints with or without effusions. Small effusions are seen by the bulge sign at the knees in some totally asymptomatic individuals in whom no other overt evidence of joint disease is seen on physical examination. Stiffness and tightness of a joint may be related to small effusions. The gaps opened between synovial vascular endothelial cells by passive motion in monkeys and dogs certainly could be a source of effusions and even escape of small numbers of red blood cells (RBCs) and white blood cells (WBCs). Even in idiopathic olecranon bursitis, which occurred without overt trauma or systemic disease, the small numbers of cells in the still noninflammatory fluid included both activated T lymphocytes and monocytes, with or without RBCs.[42] This finding suggests some role for cellular-immune reaction, even in local, presumably mechanical, problems. The effects of exercise on pain are complex. Some very physically active patients with rheumatoid arthritis, for example, seem to have less pain but still erode joints.

Study of small sutured and unsutured surgical defects in dog synovium[43] showed quick filling of even small wounds with polymorphonuclear leukocytes (PMNs), RBCs, platelets, and fibrin. Fibroblast-like cells were prominent in the wound base by 7 days (Fig. 5) and nearly healed all incisions by 10 days. Scattered lymphocytes, monocytes with phagocytized cell debris, and plasma cells appeared in the area. Some lining-cell proliferation occurred away from the incision. Adjacent vessels appeared to have more high endothelial cells early, and by 14 days, capillary sprouts with thin walled vessels were prominent. Thus, these experimental synovial wounds healed rapidly with some proliferative and mild inflammatory reaction. The cellular reaction to such wounds almost certainly would be accompanied by cytokine production; although this production was not studied in this older project. The production and expression of cytokine and growth factors would be interesting to examine in any presumably milder synovial injury that might occur with repetitive use. Tena-

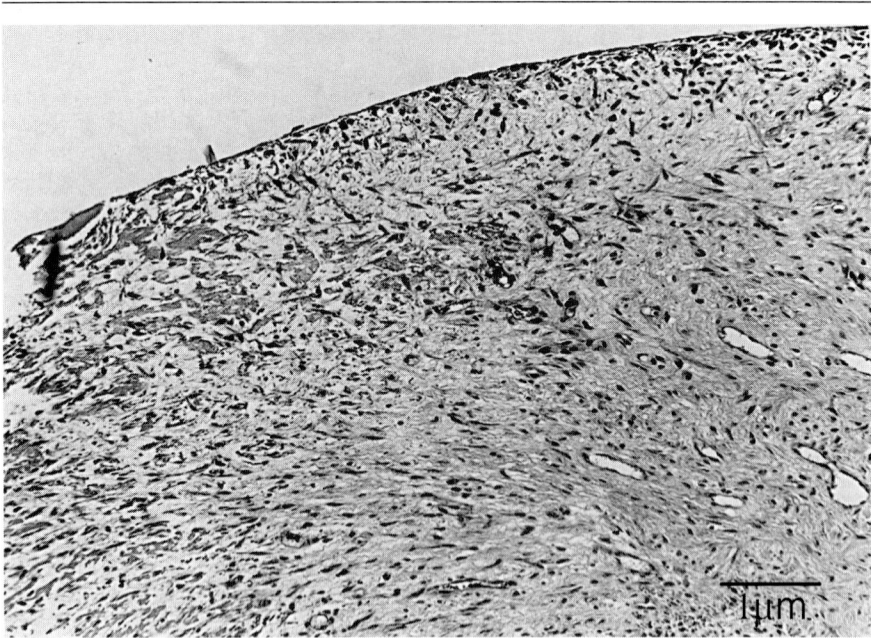

Fig. 5 Light microscopy showing fibroblasts growing into area of fibrin at approximately 1 week duration of a healing synovial wound. × 100

scin, an extracellular glycoprotein found in healing wounds in other tissues, is detectable in meniscectomy or overtly diseased synovium but not in normal synovium.[44]

Rest to the point of immobility also has effects, which can include suppressing the entry of inflammatory cell into the joint, but atrophy of cartilage and other adjacent structures. Some inflammatory response is part of normal healing and may be needed. Paralyzed joints develop bland effusions[45] without heat or redness or signs of significant inflammation or analysis. It is not known whether these effusions are related to loss of innervation with effects of this denervation on vessels or to the abuse of an unprotected joint. Complete immobilization of a normal joint actually may, in some cases, produce an inflammatory response. Any factors, including pain, posture, shoes, jobs, and so forth, that alter gait or use of a body part can change the adjacent (and opposite side) musculature, stresses on tendons and ligaments, and lines of weightbearing and, thus, can affect synovium. Heat and cold also affect synovium, with changes on blood flow most easily demonstrable. Heat over the joint may have an immediate opposite effect on intra-articular temperature of deep joints, but, at least with superficial joints, this effect is followed by intra-articular warming of synovial fluid (SF). Actual temperatures in synovium tissue have not been studied. Temperature is an obvious potential modulator of mechanical effects. Synovium and the physiologic responses to insults to synovium also change with age and with the minor or more severe diseases that accumulate with age.

Bland joint effusions attributed to a direct blow or forced inappropriate motion are often small and associated more with a tight sensation than with pain. Hyaluronate production may not keep up with transudation during the first days, thereby leading to decreased SF viscosity. Needle biopsies of synovium may show only vasodilation, edema, and mild focal increase in numbers of lining cells.[46] When dog joints were studied after blunt trauma, evidence was found of increased vascular permeability to intravenously injected carbon particles.[47] Potentially inflammatory lipid also was released,[48] although no inflammation was found.

The effects of some types of mechanical irritation on synovium do not appear to have been studied at all. These effects include vibration, such as that in jackhammer operators, which certainly does cause joint and periarticular disease, repetitions of normal motions, sustained forces, general conditioning, and relaxation techniques that might decrease intracapsular pressures. Synovial fibrosis, villous hyperplasia, vascular prominence, and multilaminated vascular basement membranes were found in three biopsy specimens from seven manual laborers with a metacarpophalangeal arthritis attributed to sustained tight gripping.[49] Because these joints also had cartilage change, it is not certain whether the synovial abnormalities were primary.

My coworkers and I are currently studying rotator cuff problems, which are generally attributed to repetitive motion, to examine the associated changes in synovial fluid and tissue. Joint fluids show little overt inflammation, but some fluids do contain apatite crystals. We hope to determine whether crystal presence influences progression. Necrotizing paratenonitis around Achilles tendons obtained from athletes at surgery[50] has shown mild inflammatory cell reaction and more dramatic proliferation, edema, and adhesion formation. Increased levels of lysosomal enzymes, increased anaerobic glycolysis, and decreased aerobic metabolism were reported. It would be of great interest to study tendon sheaths at an earlier stage.

In olecranon bursitis of presumed microtraumatic origin, cells in the bursal fluid have included RBCs, PMNs, and mononuclear cells, often with refractile droplets.[42] Erythrophagocytosis was noted as one likely stimulus to low-grade inflammation (mean 508 leukocytes/mm^3). In seven patients with painful shoulders (bursitis) attributed to calcific tendinitis, tight coracoacromial ligaments, or rotator cuff tear,[51] there was no cellular infiltration in the bursa, although proliferation of the lining cells, with increases in both types A and B cells, and thickened vascular endothelium were common. Some calcifications involved the bursal wall. Fibrin deposition was noted in one case, and lipid droplets were seen in cases with rotator cuff tear.

Erythrocyte products in the joint fluid can be released by very minor trauma and can induce synovial inflammation[52] (Fig. 6). The amounts needed to have some clinical impact have not been well defined. Mechanisms involved may include iron-induced oxidant tissue injury. Some of the experiments on effects of blood have been done using the rat subcutaneous air pouch[45,53] (derived from observations of Selye), which has a synovial-like lining around a space that is very similar to a bursa. The RBCs were found to contribute to the inflammation more than did the plasma.[52]

Medications and the Synovium

Many patients with musculoskeletal symptoms related to repetitive motion take medications on their own or on the advice of a physician. These medications may have complex effects on the healing and the response of synovium and

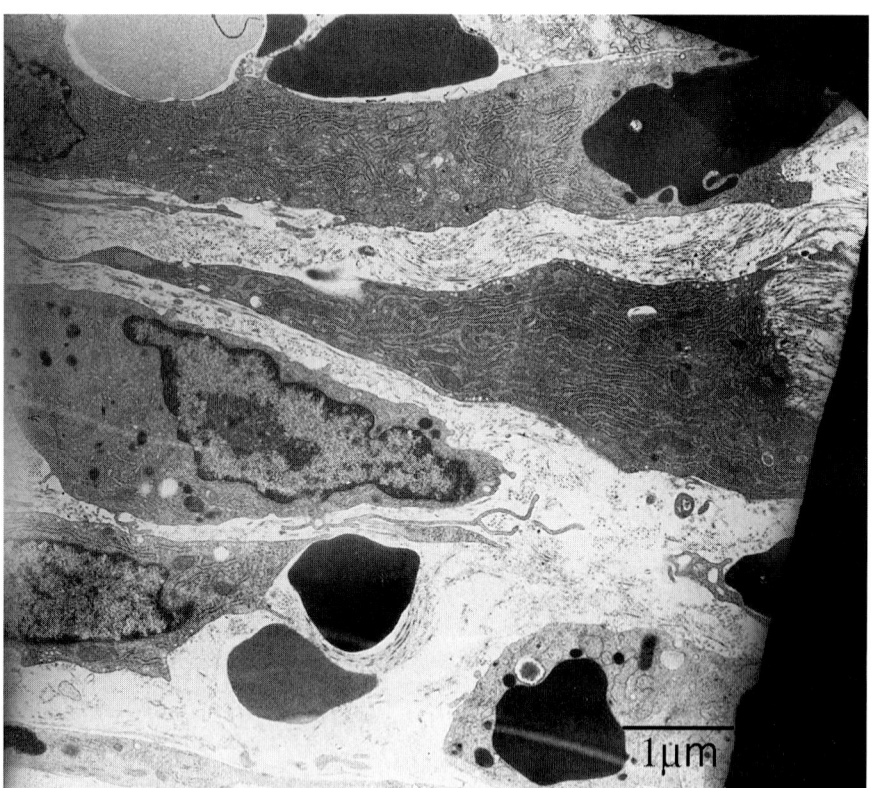

Fig. 6 Electron micrograph showing red cells being phagocytized by fibroblasts and other cells in a synovial wound. × 20,000

other tissues; these effects are just beginning to be explored. In inflamed synovial fluid, nonsteroidal anti-inflammatory drugs were found to actually increase the percentages of lymphocytes.[54] Piroxicam, when given to healthy individuals, had a variety of complex effects on cytokine production,[55] so that such agents almost certainly affect the low-grade inflammation and proliferative response that are expected with repetitive motion. Not all drug effects can be assumed to be beneficial.

Gender Differences

Gender differences are prominent in rheumatoid arthritis, systemic lupus, and other inflammatory rheumatic diseases. They have not been studied as far as tissue responses to most mechanical effects. The type A macrophage-like synovial lining cells appear to be the only or the predominant cells in synovium that express androgen receptors.[56,57] Any different responses of these cells in their production of cytokines in males versus females based on androgen or estrogen levels could modify response to inflammatory and injurious stimuli. In an inflammation induced by cartilage plugs, granulomatous tissue from female mice produced more IL-1 and degraded more cartilage than did tissue from male mice.[58]

Conclusions

Studies on synovium can be important both to ascertain the role of synovium in manifestations of repetitive motion syndromes and as an accessible connective tissue that probably reflects changes occurring at other sites.

Acknowledgments

The author thanks Gilda Clayburne, MLT, Susan Rothfuss, MLT, and Marie Sieck, MLT, for technical assistance throughout these studies.

References

1. Schumacher HR: The microvasculature of the synovial membrane of the monkey: Ultrastructural studies. *Arthritis Rheum* 1969;12:387–404.
2. Hamerman D, Rosenberg LC, Schubert M: Diarthrodial joints revisited. *J Bone Joint Surg* 1970;52A:725–774.
3. Rubens-Duval A: L'hygroma: Revision histologique. *Rev Rhum Mal Osteoartic* 1972;39:183–187.
4. Lewis GW, Cluff LE: Synovitis in rabbits during bacteremia and vaccination. *Bull Hopkins Hosp* 1965;116:175–190.
5. Shaffer MF, Bennett GA: The passage of type III rabbit virulent pneumococci from the vascular system into joints and certain other body cavities. *J Exp Med* 1939;70:293–302.
6. Bennett GA, Shaffer MF: The passage of proteins from the vascular system into joints and certain other body cavities. *J Exp Med* 1939;70:277–291.
7. Schumacher HR: Distribution of carbon after intravenous injection in the normal rabbit: Leakage into the synovium but not other non-reticuloendothelial tissues. *Experientia* 1972;28:1207.
8. Schumacher HR: Fate of particulate material arriving at the synovium via the circulation: An ultrastructural study. *Ann Rheum Dis* 1973;32:212–218.
9. Weinberger A, Simkin PA: Plasma proteins in synovial fluids of normal human joints. *Semin Arthritis Rheum* 1989;19:66–76.

10. Wallis WJ, Simkin PA, Nelp WB: Protein traffic in human synovial effusions. *Arthritis Rheum* 1987;30:57–63.
11. Simkin PA, Bassett JE: The microvascular physiology of IL-1 triggered synovitis differs between carpal and tarsal joints of adult goats. *Arthritis Rheum* 1991;34 (suppl):S142.
12. Fairburn K, Kunaver M, Wilkinson LS, et al: Intercellular adhesion molecules in normal synovium. *Br J Rheum* 1993;32:302–306.
13. Allard SA, Bayliss MT, Maini RN: The synovium-cartilage junction of the normal human knee: Implications for joint destruction and repair. *Arthritis Rheum* 1990;33:1170–1179.
14. Agudelo CA, Schumacher HR, Phelps P: Effect of exercise on urate crystal-induced inflammation in canine joints. *Arthritis Rheum* 1972;15:609–616.
15. Jayson MIV, Dixon AS: Intra-articular pressure in rheumatoid arthritis of the knee: 3. Pressure changes during joint use. *Ann Rheum Dis* 1970;29:401–408.
16. Fam AG, Schumacher HR Jr, Clayburne G, et al: Effect of joint motion on experimental calcium pyrophosphate dihydrate crystal induced arthritis. *J Rheumatol* 1990;17:644–655.
17. McDonald JN, Levick JR: Morphology of surface synoviocytes in situ at normal and raised joint pressure, studied by scanning electron microscopy. *Ann Rheum Dis* 1988;47:232–240.
18. Geborek P, Forslind K, Wollheim FA: Direct assessment of synovial blood flow and its relation to induced hydrostatic pressure changes. *Ann Rheum Dis* 1989;48:281–286.
19. James MJ, Cleland LG, Gaffney RD, et al: Effect of exercise on 99mTc-DTPA clearance from knees with effusions. *J Rheumatol* 1994;21:501–504.
20. Farrell AJ, Williams RB, Stevens CR, et al: Exercise induced release of vonWillebrand factor: Evidence for hypoxic reperfusion microvascular injury in rheumatoid arthritis. *Ann Rheum Dis* 1992;51:1117–1122.
21. Grootveld M, Henderson EB, Farrell A, et al: Oxidative damage to hyaluronate and glucose in synovial fluid during exercise in the inflamed rheumatoid joint: Detection of abnormal low-molecular-mass metabolites by proton n.m.r. spectroscopy. *Biochem J* 1991;273:459–467.
22. van-Dinther-Janssen AC, Pals ST, Scheper R, et al: Dendritic cells and high endothelial venules in the rheumatoid synovial membrane. *J Rheumatol* 1990;17:11–17.
23. Johnson BA, Haines GK, Harlow LA, et al: Adhesion molecule expression in human synovial tissue. *Arthritis Rheum* 1993;36:137–146.
24. Kaul A, Blake DR, Pearson JD: Vascular endothelium, cytokines, and the pathogenesis of inflammatory synovitis. *Ann Rheum Dis* 1991;50:828–832.
25. Northoff H, Berg A: Immunologic mediators as parameters of the reaction to strenuous exercise. *Int J Sports Med* 1991;12(suppl 1):S9–S15.
26. Cicuttini FM, Martin M, Boyd AW: Cytokine induction of adhesion molecules on synovial type B cells. *J Rheum* 1994;21:406–412.
27. Schrieber L, Manolios N, To SS, et al: Hypothesis: Lymphocyte trafficking in inflammatory rheumatic disease. A role for receptor mediated homing. *J Rheumatol* 1987;14:194–196.
28. Eguchi K, Migita K, Nakashima M, et al: Fibroblast growth factors released by wounded endothelial cells stimulate proliferation of synovial cells. *J Rheumatol* 1992;19:1925–1932.
29. Schumacher HR: Normal anatomy of synovium, in Newton CD, Nunamaker DM (eds): *Textbook of Small Animal Orthopaedics*. Philadelphia, PA, JB Lippincott, 1985, pp 77–82.
30. Courtright LJ, Kuzell WC: Sparing effect of neurological deficit and trauma on the course of adjuvant arthritis in the rat. *Ann Rheum Dis* 1965;24:360–368.
31. Hernanz A, De Miguel E, Romera N, et al: Calcitonin gene-related peptide II, substance P and vasoactive intestinal peptide in plasma and synovial fluid from patients with inflammatory joint disease. *Br J Rheumatol* 1993;32:31–35.

32. Marshall KW, Theriault E, Homonko DA: Distribution of substance P and calcitonin gene related peptide immunoreactivity in the normal feline knee. *J Rheumatol* 1994;21:883–889.
33. Goglia G, Skelenska A: Richerche ultra strutturali sopra i corpuscoli di Ruffini delle capsole articolari del coniglio. *Quaderni Anatomia Pratica* 1967;25:14–27.
34. Bentley G, Kreutner A, Ferguson AB: Synovial regeneration and articular cartilage changes after synovectomy in normal and steroid-treated rabbits. *J Bone Joint Surg* 1975;57B:454–462.
35. Patzakis MJ, Mills DM, Bartholomew BA, et al: A visual, histological, and enzymatic study of regenerating rheumatoid synovium in the synovectomized knee. *J Bone Joint Surg* 1973;55A:287–300.
36. Goldie I, Wellisch M: The presence of nerves in original and regenerated synovial tissue in patients synovectomised for rheumatoid arthritis. *Acta Orthop Scand* 1969;40:143–152.
37. Menon J, Frykman G, Swarm OJ: Role of synovial fluid cells in the healing of flexor tendons. *Clin Orthop* 1985;199:300–305.
38. Beutler A, Rothfuss S, Clayburne G, et al: Calcium pyrophosphate dihydrate crystal deposition in synovium: Relationship to collagen fibers and chondrometaplasia. *Arthritis Rheum* 1993;36:704–715.
39. Simkin PA, Benedict RS: Microvascular pressures in normal canine joints. *Arthritis Rheum* 1985;28(suppl):S90.
40. Canoso JJ, Stack MT, Brandt KD: On the content of subcutaneous and deep bursae. *Arthritis Rheum* 1982;25(suppl):S146.
41. Canoso JJ, Wohlgethan JR, Newberg AH, et al: Aspiration of the retrocalcaneal bursa. *Ann Rheum Dis* 1984;43:308–312.
42. Smith DL, Bakke AC, Campbell SM, et al: Immunocytologic characteristics of mononuclear cell populations found in nonseptic olecranon bursitis. *J Rheumatol* 1994;21:209–214.
43. Schumacher HR: Trauma and the healing process of synovium, in Newton CD, Nunamaker DM (eds): *Textbook of Small Animal Orthopaedics*. Philadelphia, PA, JB Lippincott, 1985, pp 82–90.
44. Salter DM: Tenascin is increased in cartilage and synovium from arthritic knees. *Br J Rheum* 1993;32:780–786.
45. Buschbacher R, Coplin B, Buschbacher L, et al: Noninflammatory knee joint effusions in spinal cord-injured and other paralyzed patients: Four case studies. *Am J Phys Med Rehabil* 1991;70:309–312.
46. Roy S, Ghadially FN, Crane WA: Synovial membrane in traumatic effusion: Ultrastructure and autoradiography with tritiated leucine. *Ann Rheum Dis* 1966;25:259–271.
47. Schumacher HR: Traumatic joint effusion and the synovium. *J Sports Med* 1975;3:108–114.
48. Weinberger A, Schumacher HR: Experimental joint trauma: Synovial response to blunt trauma and inflammatory reaction to intraarticular injection of fat. *J Rheumatol* 1981;8:380–389.
49. Williams WV, Cope R, Gaunt WD, et al: Metacarpophalangeal arthropathy associated with manual labor (Missouri Metacarpal Syndrome): Clinical, radiographic, and pathologic characteristics of an unusual degeneration process. *Arthritis Rheum* 1987;30:1362–1371.
50. Kvist M, Jozsa L, Jarvinen MJ, et al: Chronic Achilles paratenonitis in athletes: A histological and histochemical study. *Pathology* 1987;19:1–11.
51. Sarkar K, Uhthoff HK: Ultrastructure of the subacromial bursa in painful shoulder syndromes. *Virchows Arch A Pathol Anat Histopathol* 1983;400:107–117.
52. Tate G, Schumacher HR Jr, Reginato A, et al: Inflammation after blood injection into a synovial-like space is a result of the cellular component rather than the plasma. *J Rheumatol* 1988;15:1686–1692.
53. Edwards JC, Sedgwick AD, Willoughby DA: The formation of a structure with the features of synovial lining by subcutaneous injection of air: An in vivo tissue culture system. *J Pathol* 1981;134:147–156.

54. Bahremand M, Schumacher HR Jr: Effect of medication on synovial fluid leukocyte differentials in patients with rheumatoid arthritis. *Arthritis Rheum* 1991;34:1173–1176.
55. Rosenstein ED, Kunicka J, Kramer N, et al: Modification of cytokine production by piroxicam. *J Rheumatol* 1994;21:901–904.
56. Cutolo M, Accardo S, Villaggio B, et al: Evidence for the presence of androgen receptors in the synovial tissue of rheumatoid arthritis patients and healthy controls. *Arthritis Rheum* 1992;35:1007–1015.
57. Cutolo M, Accardo S, Villagio B, et al: Cultured synovial tissue macrophages from rheumatoid synovium contain androgen receptors and metabolize testosterone. *Eur J Histochem* 1993;37(suppl):76–77.
58. Da Silva JAP, Larbre J-P, Seed MP, et al: Sex differences in inflammation induced cartilage damage in rodents: The influence of sex steroids. *J Rheumatol* 1994;21:330–337.

Directions for Future Research

Study the structure-function relationships of human tendons and ligaments.

Determine the relationship between structural variations among tendons and ligaments and different functional demands.

It is clear that tendons and ligaments can be quite different from each other in terms of their collagen organization, cellular shape, and proteoglycan content. However, there is little comparative information on the basic anatomy of different tendons, and little understanding of how their distinct anatomic and compositional characteristics relate to the functional demands on the tissue. Even the basic parts of a tendon may vary greatly from one to another. A number of questions need to be answered. How are the cells of the surface/epitenon arranged, and how does this correlate with the environment of the tendon? What is the shape of tendon cells, and what is their relationship to other cells? Are the tendon cells in contact with cells of the epitenon or endotenon? Confocal microscopy is a new and promising tool for making these observations.

Determine the components of tendon that detect and resist load.

The structure and composition of tendon extracellular matrix (ECM) allow it to function under mechanical load, but there is little understanding of how components of this structure transmit load to the cells, how the load is detected, or how the cells resist being damaged by the load. What structures of the ECM are in a position to be affected by load (collagen cross linkages, specific cellular arrays)? What is the role of the cytoskeleton in resisting load? How do lipids aid in boundary lubrication in epitenon or entheses?

Investigate innervation of tendon.

Physiologic evidence indicates that innervation and nociception occur in tendons. There are insufficient morphologic studies on the nerves, however. Are there nerve endings in some or all tendons and, if so, what kinds of nerves are present and where are they located?

Elucidate the mechanisms by which cells perceive and respond to mechanical stimulation.

Studies in which tendon composition in vivo changes according to apparent mechanical environment, as well as studies that apply stress to tissue and to isolated cells in vitro, lead strongly to the conclusion that cells can perceive a mechanical load and will respond to this load. However, the mechanisms through which a cellular response to mechanical load is generated remain largely unknown. In no case are all cellular pathways defined by which mechanical stimulus is eventually transformed into a complex response (such as proliferation or synthesis of a new component). This question is a major current challenge in cell biology and connective tissue research, and understanding the mechanisms of cellular response will be highly relevant to understanding responses to repetitive motion. The following paragraphs do not suggest specific experiments but rather outline the scope of the problem.

Develop studies using tissue in vivo, explant culture, and cell culture.

Conducting research to elucidate cellular response to mechanical load is full of experimental difficulties. Ultimately, in vivo studies are the most relevant, but the types of cellular questions that can be asked are greatly limited, as is the feasibility of defining mechanical parameters experienced by the cells. Application of load to cells that remain associated with their ECM but are maintained in sterile culture (explant culture) has the advantage that the system is more accessible to mechanical manipulation and analysis. Even though cells remain in the structural environment of their tissue, however, systemic and soluble factors of the in vivo environment have been altered and key elements may be missing.

Studies on isolated cells in culture have the advantage of experimental accessibility and reproducibility with the greatest possible control. However, cells isolated from their ECM and maintained on plastic or coated substrata are not accurate models of cells surrounded by a natural tissue environment. Although it should be possible to define response mechanisms in cultured cells, the mechanisms defined may differ from those that actually occur in vivo because of missing cell-matrix interactions, lack of factors from other cell types, or inaccurate mechanical input. Carefully designed experimentation at all levels, taking advantage of the positive aspects of each experimental system, is required. It will be important to correlate the response with the type, magnitude, and duration of applied load, to the extent that this is feasible for each system.

Understand the time course of a cellular response.

A cellular response to mechanical load will involve intermediate steps that eventually lead to the major changes in cell number, cell behavior, or tissue composition that are noted in vivo. Understanding the individual responses within each time frame is a first step to constructing the complete pathway of a particular response. For example, the immediate response is detection of the mechanical signal and this may occur within seconds. Detection could involve receptors at the cell surface (such as integrins) or changes in ion channels at the cell membrane. The signal must be interpreted inside the cell by mechanisms that are activated within minutes, such as production of new second messenger molecules or phosphorylations that change the activity of key enzymes. These changes may then lead to transcriptional regulation, which generates changes that are measured over a period of hours or days, such as synthesis or degradation of matrix proteins, changes in the cytoskeleton, or mitosis. A measurable change in the tissue itself may take weeks or years.

Define the structure, composition, and pathology of the fibrocartilaginous regions of tendon.

A region of tendon that appears cartilaginous upon histologic examination and contains proteoglycans typical of cartilage has been described in many animal and human tendons. Most often this fibrocartilaginous tissue is found at the point of attachment of tendon to bone (attachment zone fibrocartilage) or at a region of tendon midsubstance where the tissue changes direction as it wraps around a bony pulley (compression zone fibrocartilage).

Determine where fibrocartilage is found and how it develops.

The histologic appearance, frequency of occurrence, composition, and development of fibrocartilage in human tendon are only minimally described at this point. A number of questions need to be addressed. How does fibrocartilage vary at different sites and is the appearance of this tissue correlated with repetitive motion? Do fibrocartilaginous regions calcify? Are fibrocartilages reestablished when tendon is surgically moved? How does the hypovascularity of fibrocartilge develop; ie, does lack of vascularity precede and/or induce fibrocartilage? Tendon entheses are particularly poorly described in terms of variation in relation to load and changes that may occur with overuse.

Determine whether the development of tendon fibrocartilage is associated with tendon pathology.

It seems unlikely, based on current studies of fibrocartilage distribution in tendons, that the appearance of fibrocartilage is a sign of pathology. It is more likely this tissue provides altered material properties, such as compressive stiffness, that are useful in that particular location. Fibrocartilage in tendon, however, may simultaneously be the site of degeneration and specific functional losses, causing, for example, localized diminished tensile strength, which could result in an increased probability of rupture. In addition, hypovascularity associated with fibrocartilage may diminish the capacity of the tissue to heal at that site. The key questions are whether tendon pathology is more prevalent at sites of fibrocartilage and whether development of fibrocartilage is a precursor to pathology. If either of these proves to be the case, it may then be reasonable to modify the patient's use of the affected joint or to surgically alter joint anatomy in order to diminish the accumulation of tendon fibrocartilage.

Study the effects of repetitive motion on synovium.

One way in which repetitive motion may produce injury and symptoms in certain individuals is via effects on the synovium of joints, tendon sheaths, and bursae. Studies to date on these tissues have been limited and have focused for the most part on short-term effects. Repetitive experimental passive motion in several animal species for times up to 3 hours increases venular permeability to small molecules. The mechanism for this change in permeability is not known. Each joint has different structural and functional properties and may respond differently to repetitive motion. Some effects of joint motion may be local, whereas others may be derived from circulating factors.

Future studies should examine the effects of a graded series of number and duration of joint excursions in different joints of several experimental animals. Potentially important parameters to be measured include microvascular permeability, radioisotope clearance from the joint, intra-articular pressure, inflammatory and resident cell populations identified by light and electron microscopy, and cell subsets identified in joint fluid and tissue by immunohistochemistry. Additional measurements that could prove significant include determining levels and gene expression for cytokines, growth factors, adhesion molecules, and proteases. Persistance of change at various times after repetitive motion also should be assessed. Although joint synovium is most easily studied, studies of the bursae and tenosynovium may have even greater implications for repetitive motion syndrome.

Develop an animal model for investigating the effects of repetitive use and overuse of tendons, ligaments, and synovium.

An appropriate animal model has not yet been developed for studying the etiology of repetitive motion syndrome. This may be because animals are so "overdesigned" that any motions that they will undertake regularly do not produce overuse injury, or perhaps we have simply not yet learned to recognize the symptoms without a verbal report by the subject. The model may be most successful if a way could be found to produce eccentric muscle loading, because this is a common condition under which overuse injuries occur.

When a model is available, there are several questions to be pursued concerning the development of tissue changes as correlated with time, force, and duration of the load. The model would be particularly useful in evaluating the physiologic changes that occur early but have disappeared by the time symptoms appear. These changes may be causally related to eventual development of symptoms. Much of the work in the orthopaedic literature has focused on determining the mechanical limits of various tissues. Relatively little attention has been paid to the characteristics of normal but submaximal loading on dense, regular connective tissues. This mechanical realm represents the likely source of chronic repetitive motion injuries.

A number of questions must be answered. How does repetitive use affect microvascular permeability of the synovium, bursae, and tenosynovium? What inflammatory and resident cell populations are present at various times? Which cytokines have been stimulated and how much? What protease levels are present? Can microstructural changes in tendons or ligaments be detected? A rodent model would be particularly valuable because transgenic mice that lack certain growth factors or have mutations in ECM components could be used to work out the molecular pathology.

Investigate host factors that influence development of repetitive motion syndromes.

The response of an individual to repetitive motion is variable and does not always lead to disease symptoms. This variability may be related to the differences between a response that is adaptive and a response that produces damage to the host tissues. A number of host factors can affect this balance. A great deal could be learned by epidemiologic investigation of correlations between development of repetitive motion syndrome and age, nutrition, gender, or the presence of previous injury. Furthermore, genetic factors affecting the inflammatory and immune responses of an individual may influence their response to repetitive motion.

Age. Aging is known to influence the repair process in connective tissues at the levels of fibroblasts and inflammatory processes. It is not known how this may influence the initiation or maintenance of microtrauma repair when there is a chronic state of injury.

Genetics. There are many examples of genetic influences on the quality of matrix molecules, the regulation of their synthesis in response to injury, the tendency for calcification, and the inflammatory system. In addition, more subtle changes in some components may put a subset of individuals at risk of developing repetitive motion syndrome. Identification of such prognostic indicators could be important in understanding repetitive motion syndrome as well as for knowing which individuals should avoid specific tasks.

Gender. There is an imbalance in frequency of certain repetitive motion syndromes in men and women. An influence of estrogens on connective tissue function and inflammatory processes has been described. Better definition of these factors may be critical to understand specific types of repetitive motion syndromes.

Develop criteria to distinguish between painful musculoskeletal syndromes having no physical findings and those with a structural mechanism.

Not all painful musculoskeletal syndromes are associated with demonstrable objective signs of tissue injury. Some symptoms are completely unexplained or have unclassifiable causes. The epidemiologic associations with occupational stresses may be weakened by failure to identify the contribution from nonoccupational factors, such as other activities, diseases, and host factors. Ideally, epidemiologic studies will include systematic studies both to establish specific repetitive use syndromes and to exclude symptoms with only biochemical or reversible microvascular causes. Investigations to do this should include physical assessments to supplement questionnaires. Precise physical examination can distinguish individuals with reported pain and tenderness from those with objective swelling and functional change. Techniques such as MRI and infrared spectroscopy might be considered. From such studies it may be possible to identify patterns of questions that could distinguish nonstructural causes of pain and thus avoid costly physical examinations. Careful identification of nonstructural causes of pain should also allow development of more cost-effective therapy.

Section 4

Pathophysiology: Muscle

Section Editor:
Richard L. Lieber, PhD

Robert B. Armstrong, PhD
Bruce M. Carlson, MD, PhD
Roger A. Fielding, PhD
Jan Fridén, MD, PhD

Richard L. Lieber, PhD
Dawn A. Lowe, PhD
Gordon L. Warren III, PhD

Overview

The precise etiology of repetitive strain injuries (RSI), such as carpal tunnel syndrome and lateral epicondylitis (tennis elbow), is not known. Because epidemiologic data suggest that these disorders result from cumulative effort at relatively low levels (see chapters 8 and 9) it is often presumed that muscles play some role in the etiology of RSI. Although there is not a clear scientific basis for this assumption, skeletal muscle does possess a remarkable ability to generate mechanical work and to recover from injury. Thus, in this section of the book we will synthesize the available information regarding skeletal muscle injury and recovery in response to perterbations that are, in many cases, analogous to those experienced by muscles in RSI.

Muscle Fiber Properties

Skeletal muscles convert chemical injury into mechanical work. Each individual muscle fiber possesses a unique ability to generate work over a certain period of time (endurance) and to generate work at a certain speed. Skeletal muscles are thus composed of fibers with a wide spectrum of contractile and metabolic properties.

Lieber and Fridén describe the metabolic properties of skeletal muscle fibers. It is demonstrated that the muscle fibers' metabolic properties are coordinated with the level of activation of the entire muscle. This coordination is a result of the fundamental structure of the peripheral nerve and the axons contained within that nerve. At low levels of exertion, muscle fibers that are slow contracting and have high endurance are activated. As the exertion level increases, faster, more fatigable units are activated and only during the all-out efforts are the fastest, strongest, and most fatigable fibers activated. Because repetitive motions in muscles are only possible at relatively low levels of exertion, the recruitment pattern in skeletal muscle suggests that the etiology involves slower and less fatigable muscle fibers.

Injury Models for Skeletal Muscle

There are a number of treatments that cause muscle injury. Mechanically, the so-called eccentric contraction is an excellent model for causing skeletal muscle injury. Fridén and Lieber present the available evidence that outlines the mechanical conditions under which the eccentric contraction causes injury. Because many normal movements involve the eccentric contraction, it is possible that one component of RSI involves cyclic eccentric contraction. Fridén and Lieber demonstrate that the fibers that appear most vulnerable to this type of injury are the fastest fibers with the lowest oxidative capacity. They describe the specific cellular changes that occur throughout the muscle itself. Specifically, it appears that the cytoskeletal structures (which include intermediate filaments and the sarcomere Z disk) are the mechanical structures most vulnerable to such injury. In a vibration-induced muscle injury model, they further characterize the injury process.

Armstrong and associates present a model that describes the very early events occurring in muscle injury after eccentric contraction. They demonstrate that a materials fatigue model fits the experimental data quite well in explaining muscle injury over time. Thus, if they are applied for a sufficient duration, whether continuously or cyclically, even low forces can produce injury in muscles. This information, integrated with the recruitment information contained in the chapter by Lieber and Fridén, point out that although muscle forces may be low, muscle fiber stress may be high because recruitment may involve only a few fibers. Armstrong and associates proceed with a series of elegant studies designed to elucidate the cellular basis of muscle fiber injury. They demonstrate that muscle force is the primary determinant of injury in the rat soleus muscle. They further demonstrate that, while force is obviously lost through disruption of the contractile apparatus, the inability to even activate the muscle is also a factor. In other words, excitation-contraction coupling is also affected in such situations. Finally, preliminary evidence is presented which suggests that loss of a muscle fiber's ability to maintain appropriate calcium homeostasis results in focal fiber injury. Because calcium influx into cells is known to result in activation of intracellular proteolytic enzymes, it is likely that mechanical events resulting in the loss of calcium homeostasis are involved in injury at the cellular level.

Carlson reviews the involvement of the satellite cell in repairing injured skeletal muscle. Satellite cells are muscle fiber precursor cells that remain quiescent in adult muscle fibers. After fiber injury, these cells proliferate to repair injured tissue. Interestingly, the number of satellite cells within a fiber decreases with age and this may explain why repetitive strain injuries as well as other musculoskeletal injuries become more severe with age and why recovery requires more time. Carlson also presents interesting data suggesting that the inability for aged skeletal muscle to regenerate does not result from any intrinsic properties to the skeletal muscle because, when aged muscle is transplanted into a young donor site, it regenerates as well as young muscle placed in the young donor site. Thus, some factors exist in the environment of the young versus the old tissue, which limits its ability to regenerate. Obviously, this has significant consequences with regard to RSI because it is primarily an adult disease. Further elucidations of factors that limit a muscle's ability to regenerate may provide insights into therapeutic methods for prevention or even recovery from RSI.

Inflammation in Muscle Injury

Fielding reviews available information describing the role of inflammation in muscle injury after cyclic eccentric contraction. He demonstrates in humans that inflammation itself can cause injury to muscle above and beyond that resulting from the original exercise protocol. He further demonstrates that the magnitude of the inflammation is related to the magnitude of the muscle injury in a direct way. Because anti-inflammatory medications are widely prescribed for RSI and do appear to alleviate symptoms, it is not clear the extent to which such anti-inflammatory medications prevent the adaptive process of skeletal muscle.

We have assembled a great deal of the available data on skeletal muscle and its ability to adapt to repetitive trauma. We hope that the reader will be able to apply what is known about muscle physiology research to the treatment and prevention of RSI in humans.

Chapter 19
Skeletal Muscle Metabolism, Fatigue, and Injury

Richard L. Lieber, PhD
Jan Fridén, MD, PhD

Introduction

Skeletal muscles are composed of fibers with a wide range of contractile speeds and with varying metabolic properties. Muscle fibers are integrated into the nervous system as motor units that have a wide range of functional and structural properties. The metabolic and contractile properties of muscle fibers and motor units and how these units are used during normal movement will be reviewed here.[1] Before discussing motor unit physiologic properties, a brief review of metabolism, along with the relevant features of carbohydrate and lipid metabolism, which form the basis of later discussions of fatigue, will be presented.

Skeletal Muscle Metabolism

Muscle cells, like any other body cell, require energy to function normally. In contrast to other cells that only have to generate enough energy to maintain normal cellular processes, muscle cells have the additional burden of providing energy for force generation. Glucose provides the major energy source for muscle cells. There are two main processes by which glucose can be oxidized to yield energy that is useable by the cell (Fig. 1). Of these, glycolysis does not require oxygen, while oxidative phosphorylation does. Glycolysis occurs within the soluble cytoplasm of the cell, while oxidative phosphorylation occurs within the mitochondria.

Glucose Metabolism

Glycolysis is the cellular process by which the glucose molecule is enzymatically broken down into pyruvate. The chemical reaction can be represented as: Glucose + 2ADP + 2 P_i → 2Pyruvate + 2ATP, where P_i represents the inorganic phosphate molecule; ADP, adenosine monophosphate; and ATP, adenosine triphosphate. Glucose breakdown occurs as a series of chemical reactions that permit cellular control of the rate and amount of glucose metabolized. For every molecule of glucose metabolized, two ATP molecules are created. If the glycolytic process is to occur continuously without oxygen, several intermediate molecules must be regenerated by further oxidizing the pyruvate molecule to lactate: Pyruvate + NADH → Lactate + NAD^+, where NADH and NAD^+ are the reduced and oxidized versions of nicotinamide adenine dinucleotide, re-

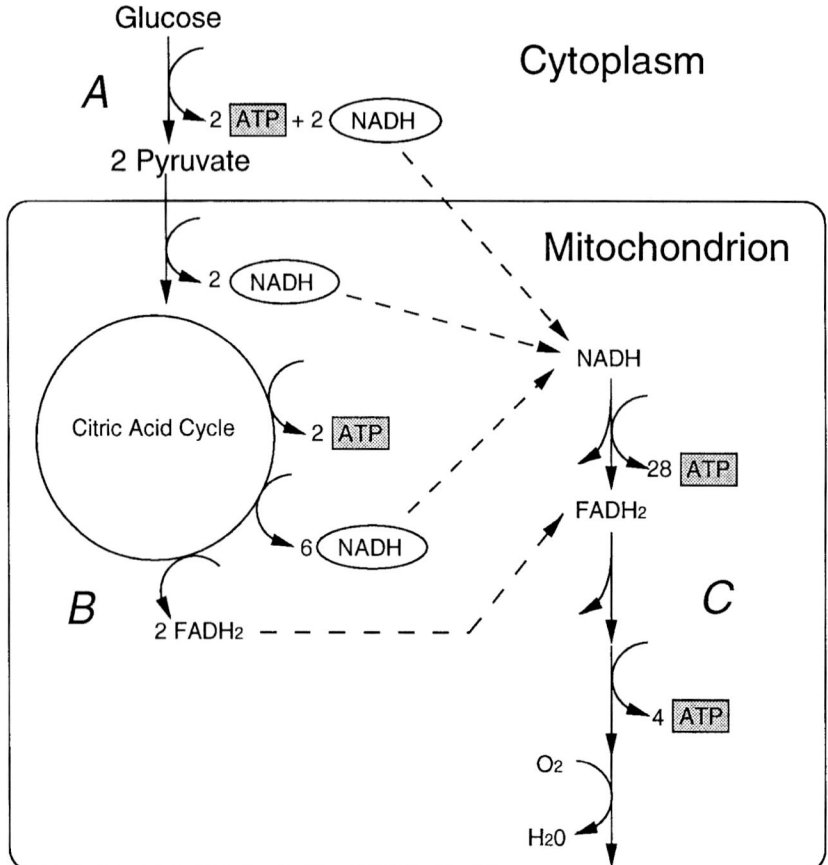

Fig. 1 Summary of glucose metabolism. **A**, Glycolysis represents the metabolism of glucose to two molecules of pyruvate. This process yields 2 ATP molecules and 2 NADH molecules (shown in shaded squares and ellipses), and occurs without oxygen. **B**, The citric acid cycle represents the conversion of pyruvate into acetyl Coenzyme A, which then passes through various intermediates (not shown), and yields one molecule of ATP, four molecules of NADH, and one molecule of $FADH_2$. The NADH and $FADH_2$ are available for further oxidation by the electron transport system, which yields much ATP. This process requires oxygen. **C**, Oxidative phosphorylation used to generate ATP from either NADH (three molecules of ATP per NADH) or $FADH_2$ (two molecules of ATP per $FADH_2$). If the NADH is derived from the cytoplasm via glycolysis, only 2 ATP are produced net, because 1 ATP is required to transport NADH into the mitochondrion. (Reproduced with permission from Lieber RL: Skeletal muscle physiology, in *Skeletal Muscle Structure and Function: Implications for Rehabilitation and Sports Medicine*. Baltimore, MD, Williams & Wilkins, 1992.)

spectively, a common reaction coenzyme. While glycolysis can supply the energy needs of the cell, it is not extremely efficient.

Lactate accumulates in skeletal muscle cells after prolonged anaerobic activity and can be measured in the blood. However, contrary to popular belief, lactate accumulation in muscle is not the cause of muscle soreness and injury after exercise. Lactate buildup after anaerobic glycolysis within the cell has two main drawbacks. First, because lactate is an acidic molecule, accumulation can alter the intracellular pH, thus altering subsequent contractile and metabolic activity of the cell. Second, lactate clearance from the cell requires further ATP to transport it via the blood and further metabolizing elsewhere in the body. When oxygen is present, the preferable metabolic pathway for glucose metabolism is to oxidize glucose completely to pyruvate and then, within the mitochondria, to further oxidize pyruvate into CO_2 and H_2O. These molecules are easily cleared from the cell via diffusion into the blood and CO_2 is exhaled via the lungs.

Oxidative phosphorylation can thus be further represented as: Pyruvate + $15ADP + 15P_i + 4OH_2 \rightarrow 3CO_2 + H_2O + 15ATP$. Thus, whereas anaerobic metabolism (glycolysis) of glucose yields 2 ATP per glucose molecule, oxidative metabolism yields 32 ATP per glucose molecule (15 ATP for each pyruvate and 2 ATP for glucose-to-pyruvate oxidation). Thus, when available, oxygen is a much more energy-efficient mechanism of generating cellular energy.

Fatty Acid Oxidation

Glucose is available from at least three sources: blood glucose, intracellular glucose, and muscle glycogen. Glycogen is a large polymer of chemically linked glucose molecules, which are stored in muscle cells to provide energy under anaerobic conditions. However, another source of energy, fats, is also available to meet cellular needs. Fats, or more properly, fatty acids, are metabolized by β-oxidation. β-Oxidation and oxidative phosphorylation occur in the mitochondria. From a simple 16-carbon chain of fatty acid (palmitate), two unit carbons are sequentially cleaved off to yield ATP:

$$\text{Palmitate 1 Acetyl CoA } 17OH_2 \rightarrow 7CO_2 1\ 4H_2O\ 1\ 129ATP$$

Clearly, oxidative metabolism yields great quantities of ATP from glucose and fatty acids, while metabolism under anaerobic conditions has a much lower energy yield.

Skeletal Muscle Fiber Types

Different skeletal muscle fibers have a range of metabolic properties. This enables the different fiber types to perform different types of tasks. Indeed, there is evidence that muscle fiber metabolic properties are strongly influenced by the tasks performed. Differences between fiber types in oxidative and glycolytic capacity are represented as large differences in the concentration of the metabolic enzymes. For example, in fast-contracting muscle fibers, the cytoplasm has a much higher concentration of all of the glycolytic intermediates compared with slow-contracting muscle fibers.

Motor Unit Physiologic Properties

A motor unit is defined as the α-motoneuron plus the muscle fibers it innervates. Motor units act as the muscle-nervous system interface. Motoneurons have their cell bodies in the ventral root of the spinal cord. The cell body is responsible for synthesis of the various nutrients needed for maintenance of neuronal integrity. An axon is a long projection that extends from the cell body. Each cell body projects one axon through the ventral root. The axon extends along with many other axons projecting from other cell bodies; together these axons, along with associated connective tissue and vasculature, form the peripheral nerve. As the axon (or neuron) approaches the muscle, it branches many times and normally each small terminal branch innervates a single muscle fiber. One muscle contains numerous motor units, each of which contains a single motoneuron and its composite muscle fibers.

Many classic motor unit physiology experiments were performed in the late 1960s and early 1970s. Burke and associates[2,3] isolated single cat hindlimb motor units (using intracellular motoneuron stimulation) and measured electrophysiologic properties of the motoneuron and mechanical properties of the motor units within the whole muscle. Interestingly (and fortunately), they found that motor units could be classified into three categories based on three physiologic properties of the contracting fibers (Fig. 2). In other words, motor units were most easily classified based on the physiologic properties of their muscle fibers. These physiologic properties were (1) the motor unit twitch tension; (2) the fatigability of the unit in response to a specific stimulation protocol; and (3) the behavior of the tetanic tension record at an intermediate stimulation frequency.

Motor Unit Twitch Tension

Early motor unit studies revealed that in response to a single electrical impulse, some units developed very high twitch tensions while others developed relatively low twitch tensions and still others generated intermediate tensions. The exact basis for this difference was not clear. However, the units with low twitch tensions also tended to have slow contraction times while those with higher tensions tended to have fast contractions. This provided some of the first evidence that the different properties of motor units might have profound physiologic significance. A second functional property used to distinguish between the various motor units was their "fatigue index," or how much the muscle tension declined upon repetitive stimulation. The fatigue index test required stimulation of the motor unit at approximately 40 Hz (generating about half-maximum tension) for one third of a second, allowing the muscle to relax for two thirds of a second, and then repeating the sequence. The stimulation protocol was continued for 2 minutes and the muscle tension measured. If the motor unit was highly fatigable, the tension dropped significantly compared with the initial tension. If the unit was not fatigable, the tension dropped only slightly or not at all. Using this approach, it was observed that units could be classified as highly fatigable (defined as units that generated less than 25% of the initial tension after 2 minutes), fatigue resistant (units that generated over 75% of the initial tension after 2 minutes), and fatigue intermediate (units that generated between 25% and 75% of the initial tension after 2 minutes).

Motor Unit "Sag" Property

A final and less well understood criterion for motor unit classification is based on the nature of the tension record in response to an unfused tetanic contraction. In some units, tension increases smoothly, while in other units, the tension record first increases and then decreases or "sags" slightly. The presence or absence of "sag," while not clearly understood in origin, is the final classification criterion.

Only three types of motor units are commonly observed: Those that have a fast contraction time, a low fatigue index, and sag are known as fast fatigable

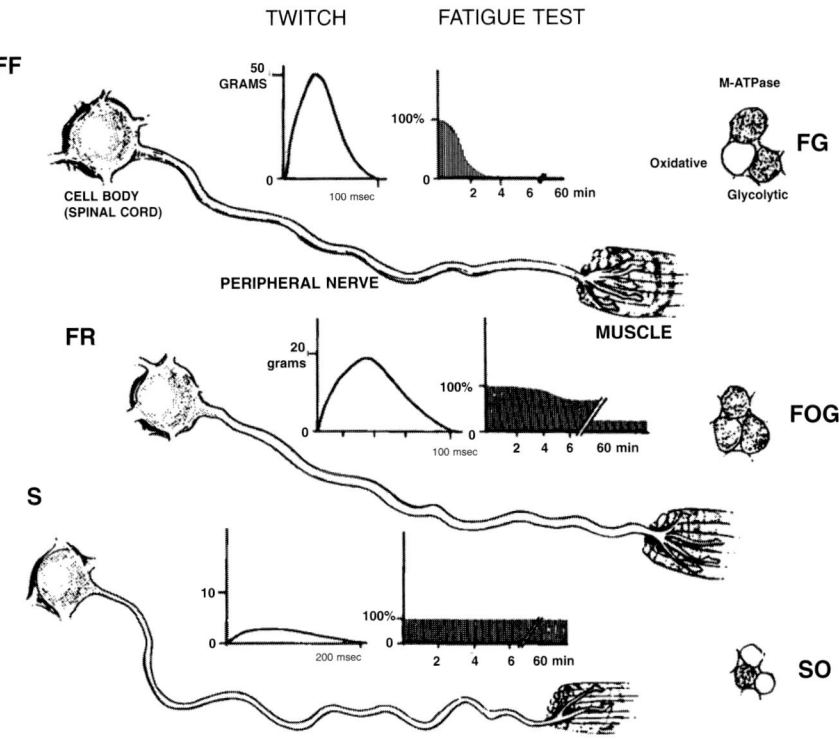

Fig. 2 Schematic representation of the anatomic, physiologic, and histochemical properties of the three motor unit types. FF units (**top**) have large axons that innervate many large muscle fibers. The units generate large tensions but fatigue rapidly (tension record insets). FR units (**middle**) have moderately sized axons that innervate many muscle fibers. The units generate moderate tensions and do not fatigue a great deal. S units (**bottom**) are composed of small axons that innervate a few small fibers. The units generate low forces but maintain force for a long time. Schematic diagram of histochemical staining pattern is shown on right of figure. (Reproduced with permission from Lieber RL: Skeletal muscle physiology, in *Skeletal Muscle Structure and Function: Implications for Rehabilitation and Sports Medicine*. Baltimore, MD, Williams & Wilkins, 1992.)

(FF) units. Those with a fast contraction time, a high fatigue index, and demonstrated sag are known as fast fatigue resistant (FR) units. Finally, those with slow contraction times, a high fatigue index, and no sag are known as slow (S) units.

Motor Unit Recruitment

One mechanism used to vary muscle force during normal movement is to change the number of motor units that are active at a given time. For relatively low-force contractions, few motor units are activated, while for higher force contractions, more units are activated. The process by which motor units are added as muscle force increases is known as recruitment. A classic study was performed by Henneman and associates[4] whereby motoneuron electrical activity was measured as a muscle was slowly stretched, therefore causing tension to slowly increase. The increase in passive tension applied to a muscle caused more motor units to be recruited (Fig. 3).[4,5] Henneman and associates

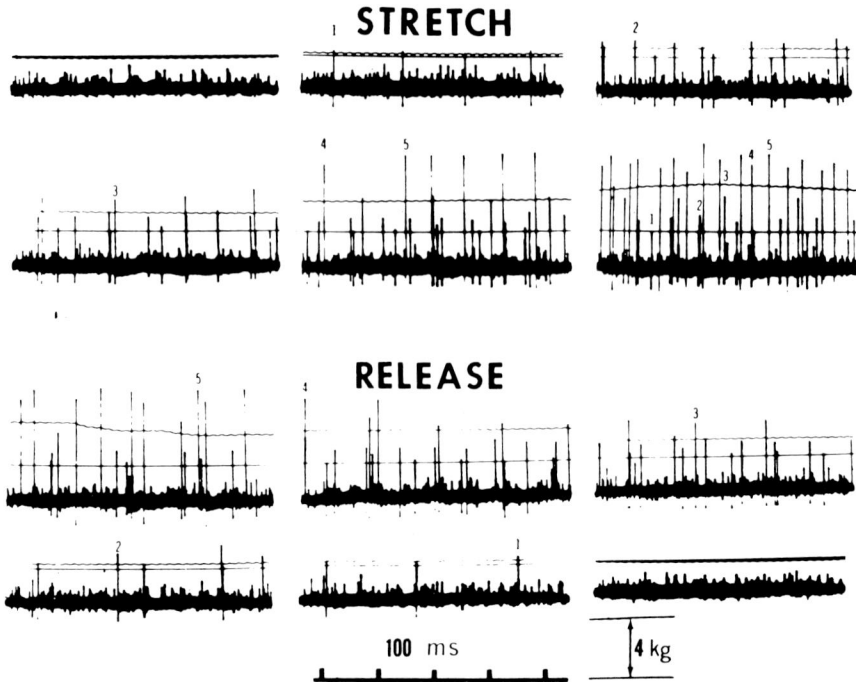

Fig. 3 Demonstration of orderly recruitment according to the size principle. As the muscle is passively stretched (**top panel**), axons of various sizes (labeled 1 to 5) are recruited. Continuous line across each trace represents muscle passive tension. As tension decreases (**bottom panel**) units drop out in the reverse order of recruitment. (Reproduced with permission from Henneman E, Somjen G, Carpenter DO: Functional significance of cell size in spinal motoneurons. *J Neurophysiol* 1965;28:560–580.)

found that at very low forces, electric spikes which were very low amplitude, were observed on the nerve. (It was already known at the time that the amplitude of the spike is related to the size of the axon.) As muscle force increased, the size of the spikes also increased in a very orderly fashion. In other words, as force continued to increase, the recruited units always had larger and larger spikes. The entire process was reversed as force decreased. This result was interpreted to mean that at low muscle force levels motor units with small axons were first recruited, and, as force increased, larger and larger axons were recruited. This became known as the "size principle" and provided an anatomic basis for the orderly recruitment of motor units to produce a smooth contraction. Based on other studies, it was generally determined that small motor axons innervated slow motor units and larger motor axons innervated fast motor units. In fact, the FF units had the largest axons of all.

Human Voluntary Motor Unit Recruitment

One method that has validated many of the results from animal studies has been developed to study human motor unit properties. Milner-Brown and associates[6] developed an ingenious method for measuring the contractile properties of human motor units. The experimental apparatus consisted of small needle electrodes placed in the muscle of interest, a force transducer placed on the joint of interest, and surface electrodes to measure muscle electrical activity (Fig. 4). After placement of the small electrodes in the muscle of interest, the subject was asked to attempt to activate a single motor unit voluntarily! With a little practice and feedback, this task can be performed. During these low-level voluntary activations, motor unit spike trains were recorded from the intramuscular electrodes. As voluntary activation levels increased, the size of

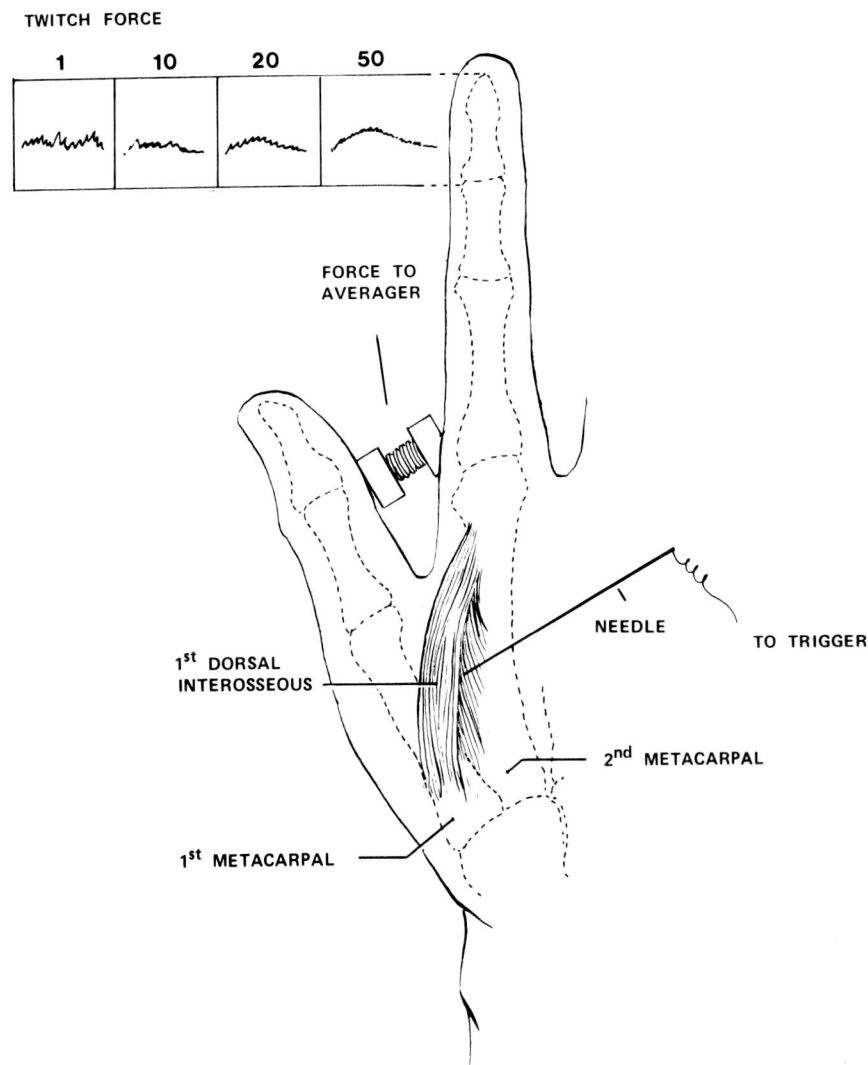

Fig. 4 Experimental method for demonstration of human motor unit properties according to the spike-triggered averaging method. A needle is placed into the first dorsal interosseous muscle to record motor unit spikes and connect to a trigger. After each spike, finger abduction force is recorded. Many records are recorded (**upper panels**), which decrease background noise and reveal motor unit twitch tension. (Reproduced with permission from Lieber RL: Skeletal muscle physiology, in *Skeletal Muscle Structure and Function: Implications for Rehabilitation and Sports Medicine*. Baltimore, MD, Williams & Wilkins, 1992.)

the motor unit spikes also increased. At very low contraction levels, the force recorded was a very noisy force record—nothing like the smooth twitches recorded from animal motor units. Thus the force recording was synchronized with the intramuscular electrical spikes recorded. Each time a spike of a particular size was recorded, the force recording equipment was triggered to measure tension. As more and more spikes triggered the recording equipment, the force records were averaged to yield records that looked like muscle twitches (Fig. 4)! This technique was named spike-triggered averaging for obvious reasons. Using this technique, it has also been shown that at low levels of voluntary effort, slow contracting motor units with low tensions are recruited. As effort increases, faster motor units with higher tensions are recruited. Numerous subsequent experiments on a variety of muscles have verified these initial studies. Thus, it appears that the size principle is applicable to human as well as animal subjects. Using all of this information, the following scheme was proposed for the manner in which motor units are recruited voluntarily (Fig. 5): At very low exertion levels, the smallest axons (which have the lowest threshold to activation) are first activated. Most of these small axons innervate slow oxidative (SO) muscle fibers within S units. As voluntary effort increases, most of the next-larger axons are recruited, which activates the fast oxidative glycolytic (FOG) fibers belonging to FR units. Finally, during maximal efforts, the largest axons are activated, most of which innervate fast glycolytic (FG) fibers and make up FF units. An appealing aspect of this concept is that the units most often activated (S units) are those with the greatest endurance. The FF units, which are rarely activated, have the lowest endurance. In addition, the S units develop the lowest tension, and thus as contractions begin, low tensions are generated. This provides a mechanism for smoothly increasing tension as first S, then FR, and then FF units are recruited.

Skeletal Muscle Fatigue

Nearly everyone is familiar with the *feeling* of muscle fatigue following prolonged exercise. However, a strict definition of fatigue has been more difficult to establish. This is partly the result of the complex nature of voluntary contractions themselves. At least three major components are involved in the production of voluntary contractions: the central nervous system (CNS), the pe-

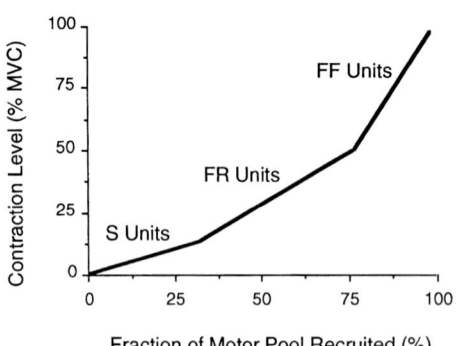

Fig. 5 Schematic demonstration of predicted orderly recruitment of motor units during voluntary activity as a function of contractile force. At lower forces S units are recruited, while as force increases FR and FF units are recruited. (Adapted with permission from Edgerton VR, Roy RR, Bodine SC, et al: The matching of neuronal and muscular physiology, in Borer KT, Edington DW, White TP (eds): *Frontiers of Exercise Biology.* Champaign, IL, Human Kinetics Publishers).

ripheral nerve and neuromuscular junction, and the skeletal muscles. Any one of these systems might be involved in the fatigue process. Several of the classic fatigue studies that add to current understanding of muscle fatigue will be examined.

Fatigue Caused by Substrate Depletion

Intuitively, it is obvious that low forces can be maintained longer than high forces. In fact, this relationship was quantified for a number of human muscles.[7] Subjects were asked to maintain a target force ranging from 5% to 100% of their maximum voluntary contraction (MVC) level. For contraction levels less than 15% MVC, subjects could maintain the target level indefinitely (>45 minutes). However, as the target force increased, endurance time rapidly decreased (Fig. 6). How can these changes in endurance time be explained? Why does muscle force decrease? Which of the different systems changes in response to prolonged contraction? ATP is the immediate energy source for force generation in muscle. However, under normal conditions, skeletal muscle only contains enough ATP to fuel two or three maximal contractions! What happens as ATP levels suddenly drop following contraction? An ATP regenerating system present in muscle is composed of the high-energy molecule creatine phosphate and the enzyme creatine phosphokinase (CK). Immediately after ATP depletion begins, it is replenished. The greater the workload, the greater the decrease in creatine phosphate. As cellular ATP levels continue to drop, cellular glycogen and fat are mobilized to replenish energy stores. The relative degree of glycogen and fat mobilized depends largely on the intensity of the exercise and the capability of the muscle fiber. In an experimental investigation of glycogen metabolism, the glycogen content was measured in muscle biopsy specimens obtained from the vastus lateralis muscles of cross-country skiers.[8] As exercise proceeded, muscle glycogen levels dropped dramatically. In fact, the amount of time these skiers could pedal a bicycle ergometer at an intense level was directly related to the amount of glycogen in their muscles (Fig. 7). In addition, following glycogen depletion, if the subjects were fed a high-carbohydrate diet, the amount of glycogen restored in the muscle actually exceeded the original amount. This overshoot was not seen if subjects were fed a diet high in fat and protein following glycogen depletion. The overshoot was

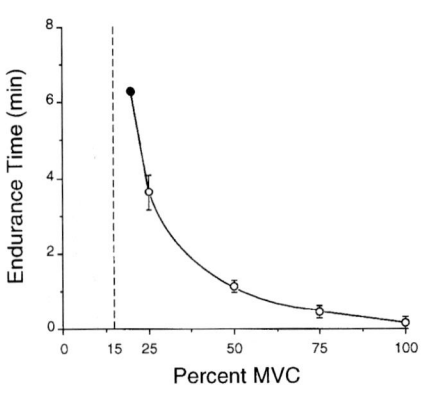

Fig. 6 Relationship between endurance time and contraction intensity (% MVC). Note that forces lower than approximately 15% MVC can be maintained indefinitely (defined here as >45 min). As force increases, endurance time rapidly decreases.[7] (Reproduced with permission from Lieber RL: Skeletal muscle physiology, in *Skeletal Muscle Structure and Function: Implications for Rehabilitation and Sports Medicine*. Baltimore, MD, Williams & Wilkins, 1992.)

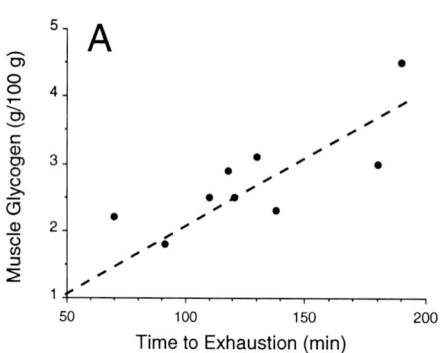
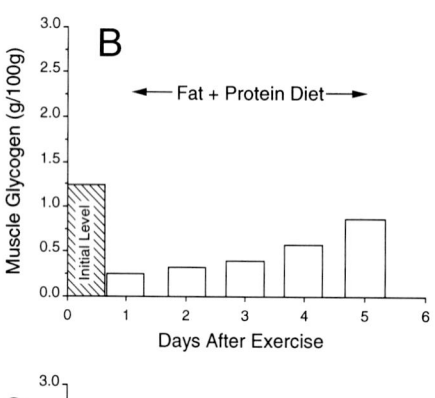
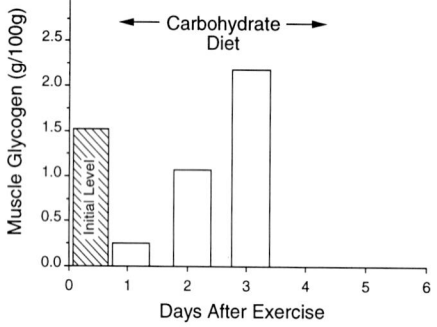

Fig. 7 A, Relationship between muscle glycogen content and endurance time for intense bicycle ergometry. Increased muscle glycogen enables greater exercise time before exhaustion occurs. **B,** Muscle glycogen content before exercise (**hatched bar**) and after exercise (**open bars**). Data are shown after a fat and protein diet (**upper panel**), and after a carbohydrate diet (**lower panel**). Note that after exercise and a high carbohydrate diet, muscles store more glycogen than prior to exercise while a fat + protein diet results in glycogen levels below the original level even for 6 days. (Adapted with permission from Hultman E: Physiological role of muscle glycogen in man, with special reference to exercise. *Circ Res* 1967;21(suppl 1):99–112).

also not seen in the contralateral leg, which indicated that the "control" of glycogen storage was at the muscle level rather than the systemic level. In intense anaerobic exercise, substrate availability can thus limit performance.

Neural Fatigue Mechanisms

When muscle force declines, can it be ascertained that the central drive from the CNS has not decreased? In a now classic study, Merton[9] measured muscle force decline during fatiguing contractions to determine whether muscle force declined because of a decrease in drive or intensity from the CNS (CNS fatigue). Periodically during the person's voluntary effort, a massive electrical stimulation was superimposed onto the voluntary contraction. It was then hypothesized that if muscle force decreased because of CNS fatigue, then electrical stimulation superimposed on the voluntary contraction would increase muscle force. In fact, no force increase was observed, and Merton concluded that CNS fatigue was not the cause for the muscle fatigue. This type of experiment has been confirmed by others, and it is generally agreed that muscle fatigue in highly motivated, trained subjects is not caused by CNS fatigue. Similar experiments have been performed to determine whether fatigue of the neuromuscular junction or sarcolemma occurs during muscle fatigue. In these experiments, during fatiguing MVCs, electrical stimuli were again superimposed and the muscle mass action potential (the M-wave) measured. Bigland-Ritchie and associates[10] demonstrated that almost no change in the M-wave occurred in spite of the force decrease. These data suggested that the weak link in fatigue was also not the neuromuscular junction or muscle sarcolemma.

Neuromotor Control and Muscle Fatigue

Recently, Bigland-Ritchie and associates[11,12] succeeded in measuring single muscle fiber action potentials in human adductor pollicis longus muscles during MVCs. They found that as muscle force declined during the MVC, the average motor unit firing rate decreased from approximately 30 Hz to approximately 15 Hz (Fig. 8). However, based on the well-established relationship between stimulation frequency and muscle force, should not this decreased firing frequency result in decreased muscle force? Interestingly, these investigators hypothesized a reasonable neuromotor control strategy to explain the rationale for the frequency decrease. By measuring the time course of the muscle twitch during fatigue, they found that the muscle actually contracted and relaxed more slowly. Because slower muscles generate higher forces at lower frequencies, a decreased firing rate combined with muscle slowing would have the

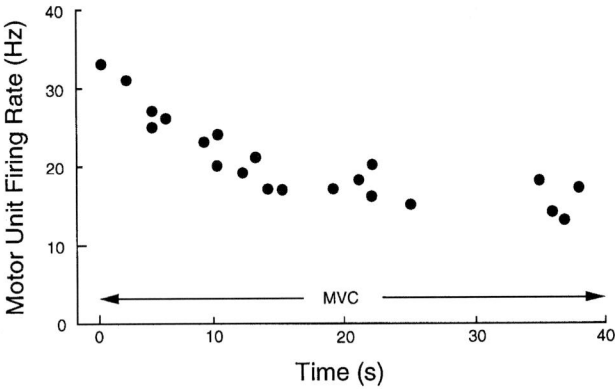

Fig. 8 Motor unit firing frequency during maximal voluntary activation of the adductor pollicis longus muscle. As fatigue occurs, firing rate decreases. (Adapted with permission from Bigland-Ritchie B, Johansson R, Lippold OC, et al: Changes in motoneuron firing rates during sustained maximal voluntary contractions. *J Physiol (Lond)* 1983;340:335–346).

net effect of maintaining approximately the same degree of force in the contractile record. It is as if the nervous system has a feedback system that senses muscle speed and drives it with the appropriate stimulation frequency. Support for this idea was obtained by comparing the average firing rate of fast muscles (biceps brachii) with that of slow muscles (soleus). They found that while the biceps firing rate was approximately 31 Hz, the soleus firing rate was only about 10 Hz. These firing rates varied in proportion to the relative speeds of the two muscles, providing support for the idea that firing rates are tailored to muscle contractile properties.

Relationship Between Muscle Fatigue and Injury

There is no evidence that repetitive muscle activation alone produces fiber injury.[13] If muscle is activated isometrically, force declines primarily because of a loss of internal energy stores and, in some cases, the ineffectiveness of the excitation-coupling mechanism. However, if muscles are activated while being forced to lengthen, ie, perform eccentric contractions, then force declines as a result of both fatigue and tissue injury.[14] We developed an animal model for eccentric contraction-induced muscle injury and one of our first observations was that not all muscle fiber types were equally injured. In fact, the fastest fibers with the lowest oxidative capacity (type FG or 2B fibers) were most often injured (Fig. 9) and demonstrated morphologic abnormalities.[15] In another model of tissue injury we measured muscle properties in the rabbit hindlimb after 30 minutes of ischemia and found contractile evidence that again supported the idea that type FG fibers were selectively damaged.[1] A similar con-

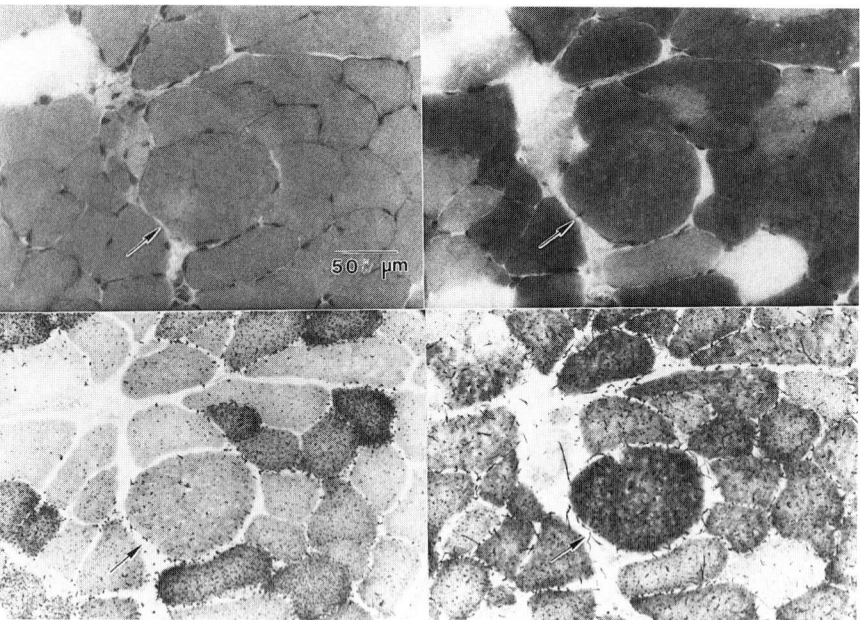

Fig. 9 Damage of FG fiber types after eccentric exercise. (Reproduced with permission from Lieber RL, Fridén J: Selective damage of fast glycolytic muscle fibres with eccentric contraction of the rabbit tibialis anterior. *Acta Physiol Scand* 1988;133:587–588.)

clusion has been reached by others.[16] Thus, some property of these fibers renders them vulnerable to injury. It can be speculated that these fibers are not able to metabolically deliver the required energy for cellular function and thus, because of ATP depletion, are vulnerable to injury by membrane oxidation, autodigestion, and increased fiber stiffness. However, because FG fibers have other unique properties (large size, narrow Z-disk, highly-developed sarcoplasmic reticulum), experiments must be performed to sort out these various factors.

Relevance to Repetitive Strain Injury

The data regarding muscle fatigue and injury described here do not have a direct relation to repetitive strain injury (RSI) as described in the rest of this book. However, a number of extrapolations can be made from the basic science information presented here. First, although there is evidence for selective damage of type FG muscle fibers in eccentric injury and ischemia, normal recruitment patterns activate these fibers only at high exertion levels. Muscle fiber damage may thus be different at physiologic (ie, submaximal) activation levels. This possibility needs to be clarified in future studies.

A second point relevant to RSI is that it is often stated that because muscle force is low during most repetitive tasks, tissue stresses must necessarily be low and probably would not result in injury. However, even though muscle force is very low during most repetitive tasks, muscle fiber stress may be relatively high because the low force is distributed across few muscle fibers. Therefore, even small muscle forces could result in high muscle fiber stresses that could be injurious to the tissue. Finally, it is obvious in the normal physiologic activation pattern, that the least fatigable muscle fibers are activated the most often and the most fatigable fibers are rarely activated. Therefore, the possibility exists for injury if recruitment patterns are reversed or altered because muscle fibers may be activated in an inappropriate amount or at an inappropriate time. Again, further studies are required to define normal recruitment patterns and whether they are altered secondarily to repetitive motions.

Acknowledgments

Some of the work described in this chapter was supported by the Veterans Administration, and NIH Grants AR35192 and AR40050.

References

1. Lieber RL: *Skeletal Muscle Structure and Function: Implications for Rehabilitation and Sports Medicine*. Baltimore, MD, Williams & Wilkins, 1992.
2. Burke RE: Motor unit types of cat triceps surae muscle. *J Physiol* 1967;193:141–160.
3. Burke RE, Levine DN, Zajac FE III, et al: Mammalian motor units: Physiological-histochemical correlation in three types in cat gastrocnemius. *Science* 1971;174:709–712.
4. Henneman E, Somjen G, Carpenter DO: Functional significance of cell size in spinal motoneurons. *J Neurophysiol* 1965;28:560–580.
5. Binder MD, Mendell LM (eds): *The Segmental Motor System*. New York, NY, Oxford University Press, 1990.
6. Milner-Brown HS, Stein RB, Yemm R: The contractile properties of human motor units during voluntary isometric contractions. *J Physiol (Lond)* 1973;228:285–306.

7. Rohmert W: Ermittlung von Erholungspausen für statische Arbeit des Menschen. *Int Z Angew Physiol* 1960;18:123–164.
8. Hultman E: Physiological role of muscle glycogen in man, with special reference to exercise. *Circ Res* 1967;20(suppl 1):I99–I114.
9. Merton PA: Voluntary strength and fatigue. *J Physiol* 1954;123:553–564.
10. Bigland-Ritchie B, Kukulka CG, Lippold OC, et al: The absence of neuromuscular transmission failure in sustained maximal voluntary contractions. *J Physiol (Lond)* 1982;330:265–278.
11. Bigland-Ritchie B, Johansson R, Lippold OC, et al: Changes in motoneurone firing rates during sustained maximal voluntary contractions. *J Physiol (Lond)* 1983;340:335–346.
12. Bigland-Ritchie B, Johansson R, Lippold OC, et al: Contractile speed and EMG changes during fatigue of sustained maximal voluntary contractions. *J Neurophysiol* 1983;50:313–324.
13. Lieber RL, Woodburn TM, Fridén J: Muscle damage induced by eccentric contractions of 25% strain. *J Appl Physiol* 1991;70:2498–2507.
14. McCully KK, Faulkner JA: Injury to skeletal muscle fibers of mice following lengthening contractions. *J Appl Physiol* 1985;59:119–126.
15. Lieber RL, Fridén J: Selective damage of fast glycolytic muscle fibres with eccentric contraction of the rabbit tibialis anterior. *Acta Physiol Scand* 1988;133:587–588.
16. Caiozzo VJ, Long SC, Gardner VO, et al: Fast muscle fibers are more susceptible to ischemia. *Trans Orthop Res Soc* 1990;15:145.

Chapter 20

Biomechanical Injury to Skeletal Muscle From Repetitive Loading: Eccentric Contractions and Vibrations

Jan Fridén, MD, PhD
Richard L. Lieber, PhD

Eccentric Contraction-Induced Muscle Injury

It is well known that skeletal muscle soreness and injury are associated with intense exercise. The soreness and accompanying muscle damage are even more pronounced if the exercise performed is new to the individual. Thus, even those individuals in excellent athletic condition may experience muscle soreness and damage when performing exercise to which they are unaccustomed. Recent experiments provide insights into muscle injury mechanisms that may lead to improved treatments and prevention of skeletal muscle injury of the upper extremity in environmental and occupational health.

Skeletal muscle injury is associated with intense exercise, especially if the exercise involves lengthening of an activated muscle. Recent[1-3] studies documented the mechanics of muscle injury as well as cellular events that follow the initial injury.

Mechanics of Muscle Injury

Because injury is especially associated with lengthening of activated muscles (eccentric contraction) and because active muscle lengthening produces extremely high forces, it has been hypothesized that muscle injury is the result of the high forces occurring during eccentric exercise. In two recent studies, skeletal muscles were subjected to eccentric contractions at different lengths and rates to determine whether it is the high muscle force associated with the eccentric contraction that produces damage, or whether the length change occurring during the eccentric contraction produces this damage.[1,3] In both cases, skeletal muscles were directly connected to motors that could induce length changes during muscle activation. In one case, muscle force was altered by varying the rate of the stretch; in the other, muscle force was altered by varying the timing of the stretch. Both studies measured the magnitude of the muscle force loss after eccentric exercise and used a stepwise regression model to explain the cause of the force deficit. In both cases it was shown that the greatest single predictor of magnitude of muscle injury was the length change imposed upon the muscle during the eccentric exercise. These data suggest that although high forces are associated with eccentric contractions, high force does not actually cause the muscle injury itself.

Although the length change during eccentric contraction explained muscle injury in the previous two examples, another recent study concluded that the high *force* change during eccentric exercise is responsible for injury.[3] The starting length of muscle contraction, velocity of muscle contraction, and length change occurring during muscle contraction were systematically varied to investigate the cause of muscle injury. The maximum tension occurring during the first eccentric contraction was most responsible for the damage observed. It is interesting to note that the two experiments in which strain was the major determinant of muscle injury were performed on skeletal muscles composed mainly of fast-contracting muscle fibers, while the study that demonstrated that high muscle force caused muscle injury was performed in a muscle composed primarily of slow fibers.

Fiber Type Specificity of Injury

In the study by Fridén and associates,[4] evidence was presented indicating that the fast-contracting fibers were selectively damaged during eccentric training. In that study the type 2/type 1 ratio of micrographs containing Z-band disturbances was 2.8:1 and 3.0:1 immediately and 3 days after exercise, respectively. The type 2B/2A ratio of injuries at these two occasions was 2.5:1. This fast-twitch fiber vulnerability was in contrast to the results of Armstrong and associates[5] in their study of downhill running rats. They showed that the deeply located predominantly slow-twitch fibers were affected, although no detailed ultrastructural fiber typing was performed in that study. This discrepancy may have had several causes. (1) In the human subjects, the exercise could be discontinued at any time. This was sometimes done when the subjective discomfort became too great. That is probably why the eccentric work in the humans never gave rise to true fiber necrosis. On the other hand, in the animals studied, an extended period of eccentric exercise surely put significant metabolic demands on the slow-twitch fibers. (2) Muscles with completely different functions were analyzed in these studies and the resistance and adaptation to eccentric exercise may be dependent on different, yet unknown, inherent structural properties. (3) It may also be that, although located predominantly in the deep type 1-dominated portion of the muscles, it actually was still the ultrastructurally defined type 2 fibers that showed lesions. (4) In the human muscles studied, type 2 fibers were the largest, whereas in the rat soleus type 1 fibers are the largest.[6]

Thus, perhaps the largest fibers are most vulnerable to injury. If muscle fiber oxidative capacity were a determining factor in fiber damage, we could hypothesize a damage scheme that occurs as follows: early in the exercise period (say within the first 10 minutes), fast glycolytic (FG) fibers fatigue. Then, based on their inability to regenerate adenosine triphosphate, they enter a rigor or high-stiffness state. Subsequent stretch of stiff fibers would mechanically disrupt the fibers, resulting in the observed cytoskeletal and myofibrillar damage (Fig. 1). This hypothesis is appealing because it explains the well-known "protective" effect of endurance training on eccentric contraction-induced damage. Endurance training is known to result in an increased muscle oxidative capacity, and therefore, FG to fast oxidative glycolytic (FOG) fiber subtype conversion. Because FOG fibers do not fatigue and enter rigor as readily as the FG fibers, eccentric contraction-induced damage would be expected to be lower following endurance training. This concept may be important in training regimes. Also, this hypothesis makes a testable prediction. We predict that the eccentric contraction-induced damage would occur early in the treatment

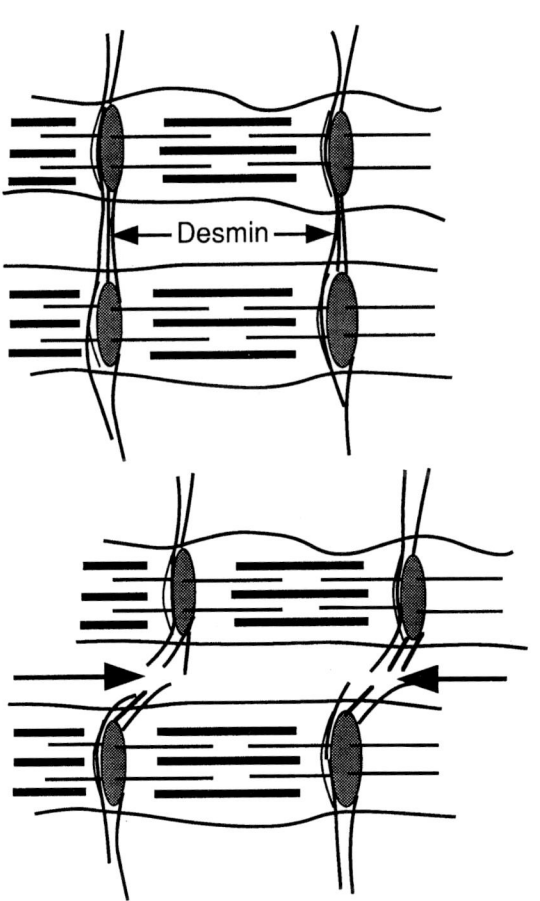

Fig. 1 Schematic drawing of a possible mechanical cause of disruptions of the intermediate filament desmin during forced lengthening. Slight differences in length and velocity pose no threat during muscle shortening because the force-velocity relationship near zero velocity for muscle shortening is not very "steep." However, for adjacent sarcomeres during lengthening, because of the steepness of the lengthening portion of the force-velocity relationship, the force in adjacent sarcomeres (or even in adjacent overlap regions within a sarcomere) may vary by more than 50% of maximal force. As such, it would not be surprising for an actin filament to experience dramatically different forces on each of its ends, which would place undue directional stress on the Z-disk. It is possible that this stress imbalance could lead to Z-disk streaming. **Top,** Normal sarcomeres. **Right,** Displaced sarcomeres after eccentric contraction.

period—within the first few minutes.[7] A second damage mechanism that could depend on fiber oxidative capacity relates to the other cellular processes, which rely on oxidative metabolism. For example, a large decrease in the adenylate charge of the muscle cell could reduce mitochondrial ability to buffer calcium, resulting in activation of the calcium-activated neutral proteases. Interestingly, these enzymes were recently implicated in the muscle fiber degeneration-regeneration process.[8]

Cellular Events of Injury

Following repetitive eccentric contractions, large and small fibers were found interspersed in histologic sections. This finding was thought to represent segmental hypercontraction of the fiber as demonstrated in longitudinal sections (Fig. 2). The phenomenon occurs adjacent to muscle fiber plasma membrane lesions and necrosis and manifests as very short sarcomere lengths. We conclude that differences of large fibers between sections are purely random, because the individual fiber structural integrity is frequently broken and, therefore, the cross-sectional fiber size is variable along the length of the fiber. In serial sections, the staining characteristics, sizes, and shapes of the same fiber may vary

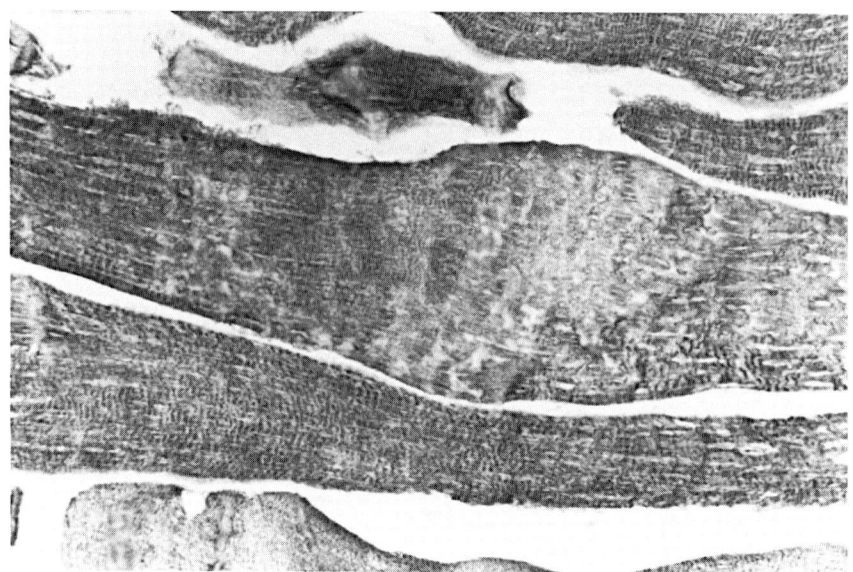

Fig. 2 Titin-stained longitudinal cryosection of a muscle biopsy obtained 2 days after repetitive eccentric activity. The striated band pattern is lost in many myofibrils as indicated by areas with loss of stain and highly variable fiber diameter and sarcomere lengths.

dramatically. Lieber and associates[9] found indications of variable fiber sizes on routine histologic sections after eccentric exercise in the 1-hour postexercise biopsies. The study by Fridén and associates[4] shows that such a morphologic feature is even more pronounced the subsequent days following eccentric exercise, as has been demonstrated by Stauber and associates[10] (Fig. 3).

Cytoskeletal Changes After Injury At the light microscopic level, the most prominent morphologic changes in the injured muscle fibers were the loss of

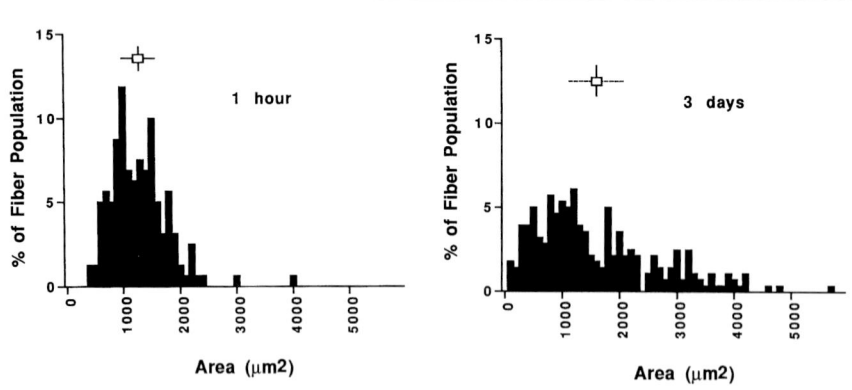

Fig. 3 Fiber area distribution of six rabbit extensor digitorum longus muscles (approximately 1,300 fibers) at 1 hour and 3 days after 30 minutes of repetitive eccentric contractions. Note the wide range of fiber sizes observed 1 hour (**left**) compared to 3 days (**right**) after exercise. Vertical and horizontal lines denote mean and standard deviation for each time period.

antibody staining for the desmin cytoskeletal protein and deposition of intracellular fibronectin indicating loss of cellular integrity (Figs. 4 and 5). Such changes were observable for several days, even when the muscle fibers retained their normal complement of contractile and metabolic proteins.

The fact that the muscle fiber cytoskeleton reveals complete disruption within 1 day of eccentric exercise further emphasizes its dynamic nature and ability to respond to severe mechanical events. We observed loss of desmin staining in cells where other contractile and metabolic enzymes appeared completely normal and in cells where the extracellular matrix was protein, fibronectin was still excluded. Thus, cellular disruption is not required for cytoskeletal derangement and may even represent a deliberate proteolytic event that permits rapid intracellular remodeling. In a subsequent study, loss of desmin staining was observed after exercise durations of only 5 and 15 minutes.[11] The morphologic evidence of damage seen at day 1 is believed to reflect an enhanced turnover of myofibrillar and cytoskeletal proteins,[12] while at 5 and 15 minutes of eccentric exercise it is most likely that the desmin disappearance is caused by mechanical disruption and extremely intensive protease activity between and during eccentric exercise (Fig. 1). The most dramatic cytoskeletal degeneration occurs between 5 and 15 minutes, whereafter the degradation proceeds at a slower rate. Much of the cytoskeletal degradation has been completed within 15 minutes. After this time, no further potentially damaging load would be expected to be imposed on the muscles even if the exercise proceeded for an additional 15 minutes. Thus, the dynamic nature of the cytoskeleton, which has proved important in regulating other cellular synthetic and degratory processes, may also be involved in sending messages to muscle cells to respond to an exercise stimulus. Embryonic myosin expression demonstrated the differential time course between the tibialis anterior (TA) and the extensor digi-

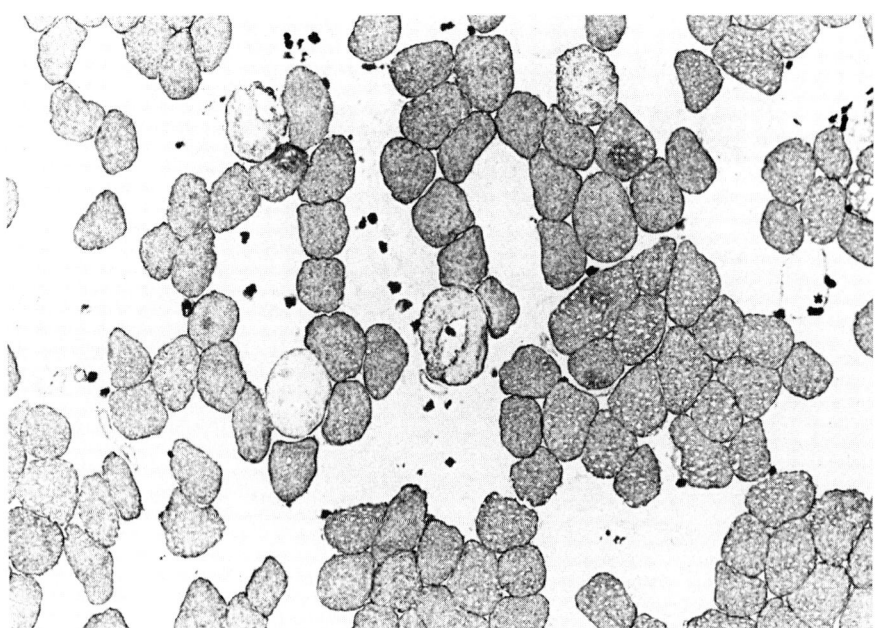

Fig. 4 Antidesmin stained cryosection of injured extensor digitorum longus muscle 3 days following eccentric exercise. Note the complete loss of desmin in some fibers.

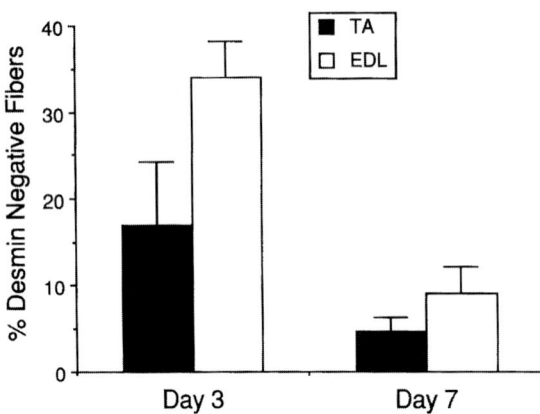

Fig. 5 Bar graph showing the percentage of negatively desmin-stained fibers 3 and 7 days after repetitive eccentric contractions. TA, tibialis anterior; EDL, extensor digitorum longus.

torum longus (EDL). This may simply indicate that the TA response, which appeared to be less severe in magnitude, is nearing resolution by 7 days while the more severe EDL response is still in the process of fully developing. The increased means and standard deviations of fiber cross-sectional area during the postexercise period also indicates that this process takes more than 1 week (Fig. 6). This finding was also reinforced with microscopic studies, where a great population of fibers was identified as either large or small.

Our present findings also elucidate the nonlethal fiber injuries in fibers of lower anti-desmin density but negative antifibronectin stainings. These fibers presumably correspond to the previously reported immediate ultrastructural consequence of eccentric load with distortion of the alignment of the A- and I-bands, irregular Z-disks and slippage of the thick filaments out of the thin filament lattice.[9,13] The structural integrity of the Z-disk and the transverse alignment of sarcomeric striations have been attributed to the existence of filamentous bridges between Z-disks and between M-lines across the fiber axis[14] (Fig. 1). Tokuyasu and associates[15] provided the first evidence that the inter-Z-band connections were composed of desmin. The region affected may very well be focal and with sarcolemma left intact as shown in the study by Fridén and associates.[12] This means that the fiber as an entity is essentially in good

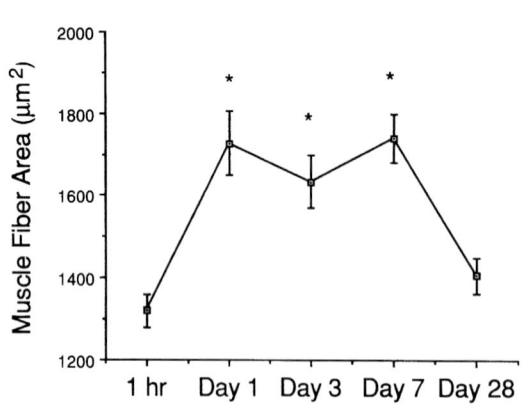

Fig. 6 Line chart demonstrating mean (± standard error) fiber areas at various intervals following 30 minutes of cyclic eccentric contractions. The fiber areas are increased by 25% during the first week after exercise. Asterisk indicates less than $p < 0.05$.

structural condition unless the focal injuries appear multiple times in the same fiber. This is, however, not likely because once a fiber is disrupted the remaining intact fibers supposedly take up the tension put on the muscle. That would mean that eventually fewer fibers will be subjected to forced lengthening, as has been proposed earlier.[4,16,17] Whether the longitudinally oriented intermediate filaments originating from the periphery of Z-disks in series as demonstrated by Wang and Ramirez-Mitchell[18] or the endosarcomeric mechanical integrator titin[19] play a role in transmitting tension in injured muscle is unknown. A commonly seen feature in the abnormal fibers as observed at the ultrastructural level was slippage of the A-band to one pole of the sarcomere (Fig. 7). This phenomenon is identical to the ultrastructure in dystrophic muscles as reported by Cullen and associates.[20] In this study, the slippage of the A-band was attributed to the breakdown of the titin molecules in the I-band. In our model, the high tensions could cause breakage of the elastic titin filaments and that instability would cause an asymmetrical movement of the A-filaments (Fig. 8). The result is a nonoverlap situation in half of the sarcomere, which consequently leads to inability to generate tension in the affected sarcomeres.

Using immunofluorescence localization of desmin in eccentrically exercised human vastus lateralis muscles, longitudinal extensions of fluorescent material were observed between successive Z-disks in biopsy specimens obtained 3 days postexercise.[12] These longitudinal extensions were randomly distributed throughout the depth of the sections. Such cytoskeletal changes were thought to be caused directly by the high strain, thus representing injury.

Myofibrillar Changes After Injury Myofibrillar alterations following repetitive eccentric contractions have been observed.[4,5,16,21,22] Fridén and associates[21]

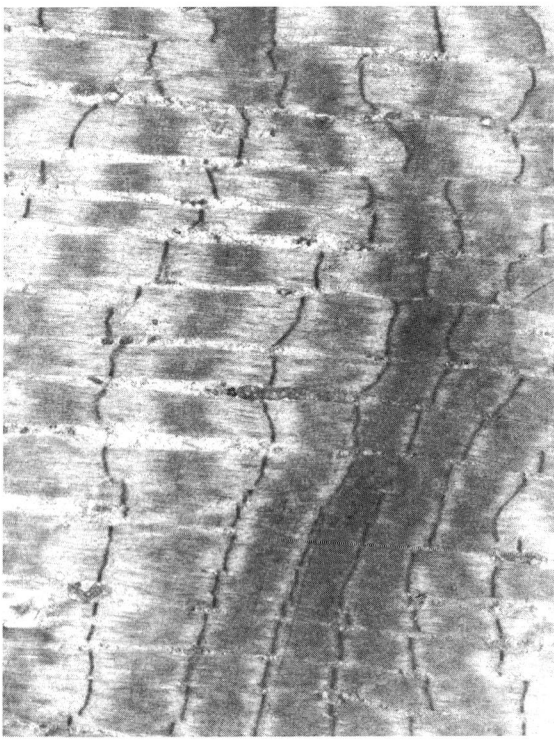

Fig. 7 Electron microscopic micrograph demonstrating several regions with slippage of the A-band all the way to the Z-disk.

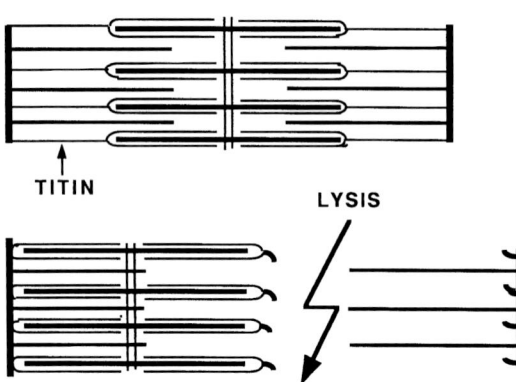

Fig. 8 Schematic drawing showing breakage of one set of titin filaments at one end of the sarcomere, resulting in sliding of the A-band to the contralateral side. (Reproduced with permission from Cullen MJ, Fulthorpe JJ, Harris JB: The distribution of desmin and titin in normal and dystrophic human muscle. *Acta Neuropathol* 1992;83:158–169.)

identified disorganization of the myofibrillar Z-band in human soleus muscles 3 days after downhill running. A characteristic pattern of changes in the contractile apparatus was established, including broadening, smearing, or even total myofibrillar disruption at the level of the Z-bands as has been shown elsewhere.[4,16] The Z-bands of adjacent myofibrils appeared out of register and followed a zigzag course that was referred to as "Z-band streaming." Additionally, some A-bands were out of register within affected sarcomeres and, in some cases, thick filaments were completely absent. Armstrong and associates[5] found that, immediately after downhill running in rats, fibers in the slow-twitch extensor muscles showed disruptions of the striation pattern. Ogilvie and associates[23] reported three types of lesions: (1) focal disruptions of the A-band; (2) Z-line dissolution; and (3) clotted fibers. They reported that 90% of the changes consisted of A-band disruptions. Newham and associates[16] showed that, in biopsy material obtained from eccentrically contracting human quadriceps muscles, extensive sarcomeric disruptions occurred. Taken together, this is clear evidence of dramatic structural deviations following eccentric exercise. Z-disk streaming appears to be a primary myofibrillar response to altered physical and metabolic situations. The composition of disorganized Z-disk material is not fully known but the Z-disk-associated proteins desmin and spectrin have been shown to be constituents of the electron dense filamentous material in areas of Z-disk streaming.[12,24] This fact has reinforced the need for a thorough investigation of the role of the cytoskeletal proteins in muscle injury.

Repetitive Motion Injury of the Wrist Extensor Muscles

Most of the morphologic studies of muscular overload and injury have been undertaken on leg muscles. There are, however, several reasons to believe that nonloadbearing muscles respond differently to repetitive motion-induced injury. From a work environment point of view, the shoulder, neck, and upper extremity muscles are particularly affected. In a morphologic study of extensor carpi radialis brevis muscle samples from patients with occupational lateral epicondylitis, we noted frequent fibers with multiple foci lacking mitochondrial enzyme activity (moth-eaten fibers) as well as occasional abnormally shaped fibers with clustering of mitochondria underneath the sarcolemma (ragged-red fibers) (Fridén and Lieber, unpublished data). These findings are similar to those observed in chronic trapezius myalgia[25] and are supposed to be related to overload of low-threshold motor units.[25] Both moth-eaten and ragged-red fibers have previously been observed in ischemic rat muscle[26] and have, consequently, been supposed to reflect temporary hypoxia and reduced oxygenation.[27] The morphometric analyses of these muscles revealed that all types of fibers were significantly smaller than controls (Fig. 9). We recently provided evidence that the passive shortening of the muscle following tendon lengthening results in approximately a 25% decrease in muscle passive tension.[28] This could lead to reduced insertional tension and decreased pain, and may cause a better circulatory condition during intermittent isometric contractions, known to be a causative component in the development of lateral epicondylitis.[29]

Morphologic Characteristics of Muscle Injury After Vibration

Reports regarding effects of vibration caused by habitual usage of hand-held tools have in most cases been focused on neurologic and vascular disorders, such as clinical signs of numbness, reduced tactile sensitivity, and intermittent finger blanching.[30] There are, however, also studies indicating that vibration may cause reduced hand-grip forces and endurance, which may be a sign of possible muscular damage.[31] The underlying pathophysiologic mechanisms are poorly understood. Therefore, an experimental model was recently developed to apply vibrations to the hindpaw of rats at any frequency, acceleration, and duration.[32] Initially, a frequency of 80 Hz was chosen because this frequency is common among tools used in the industry. Many of these tools, for example, grinding machines, work within the range of 4,000 to 6,000 rpm (ie, 80 to 100 Hz).[33] The acceleration was set to a comparatively high level (10 to 30 dB) and the vibration was applied for 5 hours per day and 5 consecutive days. The morphologic examination of the lower leg muscles demonstrated that injury, including necrosis, occurred (Fig. 10). The muscle damage was confined to muscles directly exposed to vibration (plantar muscles) while muscles far from the vibration-exciter (soleus and extensor digitorum longus) retained their normal structure. A similar distribution of vibration-induced injury was

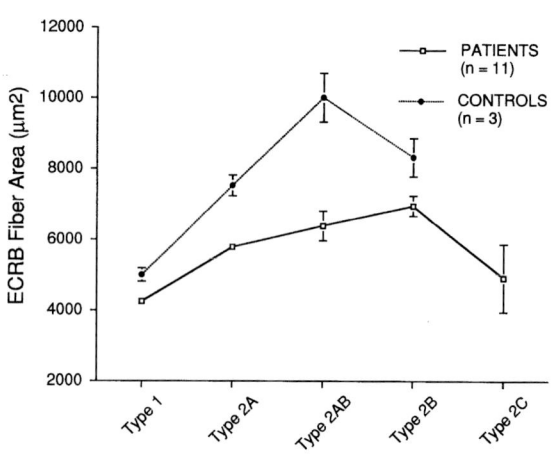

Fig. 9 Mean extensor carpi radialis brevis (ECRB) fiber areas in patients with radial epicondylitis. All types of fibers were significantly smaller than controls. Note also that no type 2C fibers were identified in control muscles.

also observed in peripheral nerves; ie, the peripheral part of nonmyelinated nerve fibers were affected by vibration.[34] Necking and associates,[35] applying the same protocol for only 2 days, found neither fiber necrosis nor regenerative activity. The mean area of vibration-exposed muscle fibers was, however, significantly increased compared with that of controls. Both type 1 and 2C fibers were significantly larger after vibration, while type 2A and 2B fibers were not significantly enlarged. The percentage of centrally located nuclei was significantly increased after vibration. Necking and associates[35] asserted that short-term vibration can induce changes of muscle fiber sizes and that this event is the first indication of a vibration-induced muscle injury that may develop into a chronic muscle function impairment if the exposure continues for an extended period. The reason the oxidative forms of type 2 fibers were relatively spared is still unclear. The regenerative activity in the damaged fibers after 5 days of vibration exposure implies that the muscle lesions have taken place some days prior to biopsy. This finding probably indicates that even the initial days of stress upon directly vibrated muscle exceed the critical limit for maintenance of structural integrity. An increased potential for regeneration of nerves has been shown to occur after vibration for as short a duration as 2 days (5 hours daily) and with the same frequency and acceleration as has been used in the present study.[36] Whether the present findings are the result of direct mechanical tearing of muscle fibers or secondary to a chronic vascular insufficiency has yet to be proved.

Motor impairment resulting from sustained vibration exposure is not only of neurologic but also of muscular origin, which may explain the decreased grip strength and hand control in patients exposed to vibration.[31]

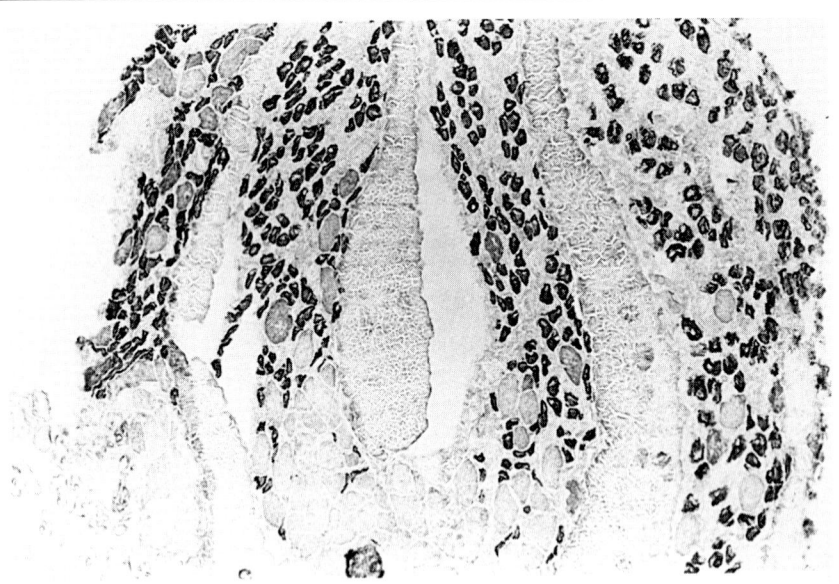

Fig. 10 Light micrograph of vibrated rat plantar muscle. The section is stained for visualization of neonatal myosin (NN_s). A significant number of fibers stain positively after 5 consecutive days of vibration. (Reproduced with permission from Necking LE, Dahlin LB, Fridén J, et al: Vibration-induced muscle injury: An experimental model and preliminary findings. *J Hand Surg* 1992;17B:270–74.)

Summary

Muscular activity involving lengthening of an activated muscle and vibration exposure are two examples of repetitive motion that may cause muscle injury in the upper extremity. Recent reports documented the mechanics of exercise-induced muscle injury as well as physiologic and cellular events and vibration-induced morphologic manifestations of injury. These studies indicate that the earliest events in muscle injury are probably mechanical in nature, while later events indicate that it may be more appropriate to conclude that intense exercise initiates a muscle remodeling process. Prolonged vibration appears to cause the same type of changes, although they are initially less dramatic. Vibration-induced muscle injury thus is believed to be the result of the cumulative trauma with only subtle indications of injury/remodeling during the very early phases.

References

1. Lieber RL, Fridén J: Muscle damage is not a function of muscle force but active muscle strain. *J Appl Physiol* 1993;74:520–526.
2. Zerba E, Faulkner JA: Abstract: Muscle injury after single lengthening contractions with variations in the magnitude and rate of displacement. *FASEB J* 1992;6:A297.
3. Warren GL, Hayes DA, Lowe DA, et al: Mechanical factors in the initiation of eccentric contraction-induced injury in rat soleus muscle. *J Physiol Lond* 1993;464: 457–475.
4. Fridén J, Sjöström M, Ekblom B: Myofibrillar damage following intense eccentric exercise in man. *Int J Sports Med* 1983;4:170–176.
5. Armstrong RB, Ogilvie RW, Schwane JA: Eccentric exercise-induced injury to rat skeletal muscle. *J Appl Physiol* 1983;54:80–93.
6. Lieber RL, Fridén JO, Hargens AR, et al: Long-term effects of spinal cord transection on fast and slow rat skeletal muscle: II. Morphometric properties. *Exp Neurol* 1986;91:435–448.
7. Fridén J, Lieber RL: Structural and mechanical basis of exercise-induced muscle injury. *Med Sci Sports Exerc* 1992;24:521–530.
8. Badalamente MA, Hurst LC, Stracher A: Neuromuscular recovery using calcium protease inhibition after median nerve repair in primates. *Proc Natl Acad Sci USA* 1989;86:5983–5987.
9. Lieber RL, Woodburn TM, Fridén J: Muscle damage induced by eccentric contractions of 25% strain. *J Appl Physiol* 1991;70:2498–2507.
10. Stauber WT, Fritz VK, Vogelbach DW, et al: Characterization of muscles injured by forced lengthening: I. Cellular infiltrates. *Med Sci Sports Exerc* 1988;20:345–353.
11. Lieber RL, Thornell L-E, Fridén J: Muscle cytoskeletal disruption occurs within the first 15 minutes of cyclic eccentric contractions. *J Appl Physiol*, in press.
12. Fridén J, Kjörell U, Thornell LE: Delayed muscle soreness and cytoskeletal alterations: An immunocytological study in man. *Int J Sports Med* 1984;5:15–18.
13. Dix DJ, Eisenberg BR: Redistribution of myosin heavy chain mRNA in the midregion of stretched muscle fibers. *Cell Tissue Res* 1991;263:61–69.
14. Price M, Sanger JW: Intermediate filaments connect Z-discs in adult chicken muscle. *J Exp Zool* 1979;208:263–269.
15. Tokuyasu KT, Dutton AH, Singer SJ: Immunoelectron microscopic studies of desmin (skeletin) localization and intermediate filament organization in chicken skeletal muscle. *J Cell Biol* 1983;96:1727–1735.
16. Newham DJ, McPhail G, Mills KR, et al: Ultrastructural changes after concentric and eccentric contractions of human muscle. *J Neurol Sci* 1983;61:109–122.
17. Armstrong RB: Initial events in exercise-induced muscular injury. *Med Sci Sports Exerc* 1990;22:429–435.

18. Wang K, Ramirez-Mitchell R: A network of transverse and longitudinal intermediate filaments is associated with sarcomeres of adult vertebrate skeletal muscle. *J Cell Biol* 1983;96:562–570.
19. Horowits R, Kempner ES, Bisher ME, et al: A physiological role for titin and nebulin in skeletal muscle. *Nature* 1986;323:160–164.
20. Cullen MJ, Fulthorpe JJ, Harris JB: The distribution of desmin and titin in normal and dystrophic human muscle. *Acta Neuropathol* 1992;83:158–169.
21. Fridén J, Sjöström M, Ekblom B: A morphological study of delayed muscle soreness. *Experientia* 1981;37:506–507.
22. Kuipers H, Drukker J, Frederik PM, et al: Muscle degeneration after exercise in rats. *Int J Sports Med* 1988;4:45–51.
23. Ogilvie RW, Armstrong RB, Baird KE, et al: Lesions in the rat soleus muscle following eccentrically-biased exercise. *Am J Anat* 1988;182:335–346.
24. Thornell LE, Eriksson A, Johansson B, et al: Intermediate filament and associated proteins in heart Purkinje fibers: A membrane-myofibril anchored cytoskeletal system. *Ann NY Acad Sci* 1985;455:213–240.
25. Lindman R, Hagberg M, Ängqvist K-A, et al: Changes in muscle morphology in chronic trapezius myalgia. *Scand J Work Environ Health* 1991;17:347–355.
26. Heffner RR, Barron SA: The early effects of ischemia upon skeletal muscle mitochondria. *J Neurol Sci* 1978;38:295–315.
27. Bengtsson A, Henriksson K-G, Larsson J: Muscle biopsy in primary fibromyalgia: Light-microscopical and histochemical findings. *Scand J Rheumatol* 1986;15:1–6.
28. Fridén J, Lieber RL: Physiologic consequences of surgical lengthening of extensor carpi radialis brevis muscle-tendon junction for tennis elbow. *J Hand Surg* 1994;19A:269–274.
29. Carroll RE, Jorgensen EC: Evaluation of the Garden procedure for lateral epicondylitis. *Clin Orthop Rel Res* 1968;60:201–204.
30. Pelmear PL, Taylor W: Clinical picture (vascular, neurological, and musculoskeletal), in Pelmear PL, Taylor W, Wasserman DE (eds): *Hand-Arm Vibration: A Comprehensive Guide for Occupational Health Professionals.* New York, NY, Van Nostrand Reinhold, 1992, pp 26–40.
31. Färkkilä M: Grip force in vibration disease. *Scand J Work Environ Health* 1978;4:159–166.
32. Necking LE, Dahlin LB, Fridén J, et al: Vibration-induced muscle injury: An experimental model and preliminary findings. *J Hand Surg* 1992;17B:270–274.
33. Lundström R, Burström L: Vibration in hand held tools. *The Swedish National Board of Occupational Safety and Health Investigation Report* 1984;84:1–111.
34. Lundborg G, Dahlin LB, Hansson H-A, et al: Vibration exposure and peripheral nerve fiber damage. *J Hand Surg* 1990;15A:346–351.
35. Necking LE, Lundborg G, Lundström R, et al: Vibration-induced muscle changes. *Scand J Plast Reconstr Surg Hand Surg*, in press.
36. Dahlin LB, Necking LE, Lundström R, et al: Vibration exposure and conditioning lesion effect in nerves: An experimental study in rats. *J Hand Surg* 1992;17A:858–861.

Chapter 21

The Satellite Cell and Skeletal Muscle Regeneration: The Degeneration and Regeneration Cycle

Bruce M. Carlson, MD, PhD

Introduction

There is ample evidence that, like bone, skeletal muscle is a dynamic tissue that regularly adapts to changing functional environments by undergoing reactions such as hypertrophy and atrophy.[1] Sometimes the functional environment is a stressful one that results in physical or ischemic damage to muscle fibers. In contrast to formerly held viewpoints, current research has shown that damaged skeletal muscle possesses a considerable capacity for regeneration. In fact, a contemporary view of muscle biology holds that throughout one's life muscles are subjected to circumstances that result in muscle fiber damage which is typically repaired by regeneration. Repetitive motion is one stimulus that can lead to muscle fiber damage and breakdown. This chapter will focus on cellular aspects of skeletal muscle regeneration.

The Muscle Fiber Complex

When viewed in the context of growth and repair, the skeletal muscle fiber is one part of a three-component complex consisting of (1) the multinucleated skeletal muscle fiber; (2) a surrounding basal lamina; and (3) a population of mononuclear stem cells, called satellite cells, which are interposed between the muscle fiber and its basal lamina (Fig. 1). The multinucleate muscle fiber itself is a postmitotic cell in which the nuclei have lost the capacity to divide. Therefore, if it is injured or destroyed, new nuclei must be derived from another source. Satellite cells retain the capacity to divide mitotically, and are a source of new myonuclei during growth, adaptation, and regeneration.

As part of its normal function and during regeneration, the muscle fiber complex constantly interacts with other tissue components, such as the axonal terminations of the motor nerve at the neuromuscular junction, connective tissue cells and fibers at the myotendinous junctions at both ends of the muscle fibers, and capillaries that run parallel to the muscle fiber. A tissue component that will not be discussed in this chapter is the mechanosensory apparatus, which includes the muscle spindle and the Golgi tendon organs.[2]

The Satellite Cell

The satellite cell is an undistinguished-looking mononuclear cell that is located between the muscle fiber and its surrounding basal lamina[3] (Fig. 2). Dis-

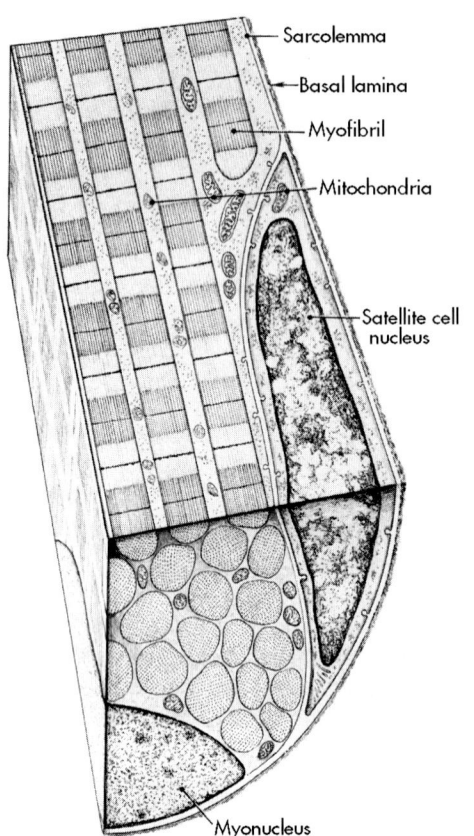

Fig. 1 Drawing of the muscle fiber complex, consisting of the muscle fiber, its basal lamina, and a satellite cell. (Reproduced with permission from Carlson BM, Faulkner JA: The regeneration of skeletal muscle fibers following injury: A review. *Med Sci Sports Exerc* 1983; 15:187–198.)

covered in 1961 by Mauro,[4] it cannot be recognized in an ordinary light microscopic preparation of muscle. Morphologically, the satellite cell is characterized more by what it lacks than by any specific identifying features. Although in recent years several antibodies have been reported to bind to satellite cells,[5,6] the binding is not confined to this cell type. Definitive electron microscopic demonstrations of exclusive binding of immunohistochemical markers to satellite cells in vivo have not been reported.

Embryonic Development

Evidence suggests that satellite cells arise from the somites, but as a separate lineage during embryonic development.[7,8] How they avoid fusing with the other embryonic myoblasts that form the primary and secondary muscle fibers in the embryo is not understood. Nevertheless, by the time of birth, the immature muscle fibers contain a large population of satellite cells.

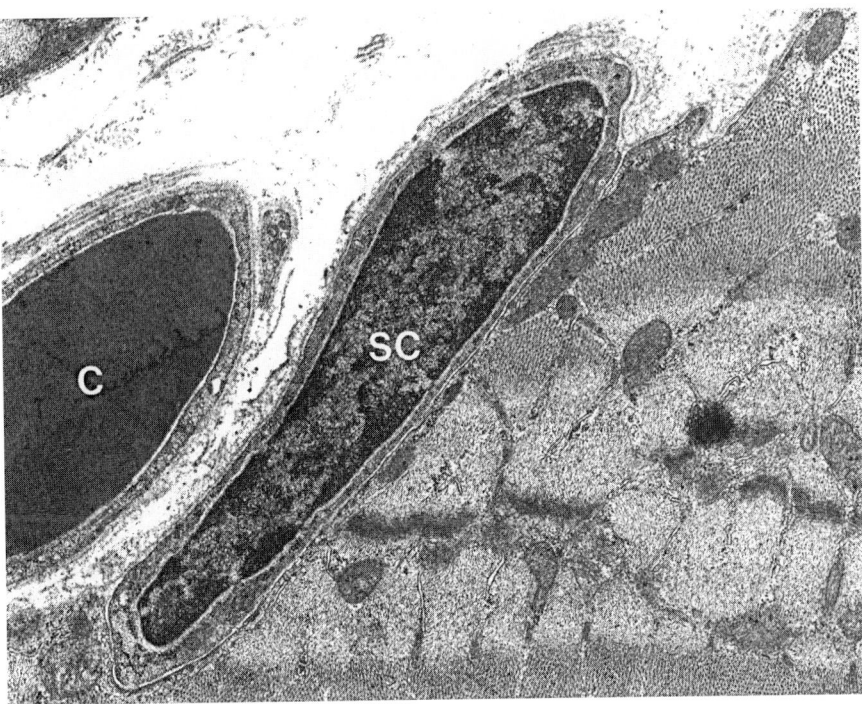

Fig. 2 Electron micrograph of a satellite cell from normal rat muscle. C, Cell; SC, Satellite cell.

Normal Postnatal Growth and Development

At the time of birth in rodents, satellite cells constitute nearly one third of the total nuclei within the muscle fiber complex.[9] The percentage of satellite cells rapidly declines during the early postnatal period, and steadily declines throughout the rodent's life span (Table 1). The number of satellite cells is related to the muscle type. In rats, the percentage of satellite cells in the slow soleus muscle is more than twice that of the fast extensor digitorum longus (EDL) muscle.[10]

Table 1 Numbers of satellite cells in rat muscles

Muscle	Age (Months)	Satellite Cells Percent*	Number ($\times 10^5$)
Soleus	1	9.6	5.2
	12	6.6	7.3
	24	4.7	5.4
Extensor digitorum longus	1	7.0	3.1
	12	2.9	1.5
	24	1.9	1.3

* Percent satellite cells refers to the percentage of the total nuclei within the myofiber complex identified as satellite cells

During postnatal growth of muscle fibers, myonuclear cells increase as the result of satellite cell proliferation and the incorporation of satellite cell progeny into the associated muscle fibers. During the early postnatal period in rats, the proliferative potential of satellite cells decreases, as measured by the number of progeny that are produced by clonal cultures of satellite cells.[11] During the rest of adult life the proliferative potential remains relatively stable, with a slight decrease into old age.[12] Throughout the life span, some satellite cells are capable of producing large numbers of progeny, whereas others divide only a few times in vitro.[11]

Muscle Adaptation

Satellite cells are highly responsive to changes in the functional environment of muscles. Under conditions leading to muscle fiber hypertrophy, satellite cells undergo increased proliferation and contribute nuclei to the enlarging muscle fibers.[13] Reduced activity (eg, hindlimb suspension) results in a rapid and profound decrease in the mitotic activity of satellite cells.[14] Denervation results in an increase in the percentage and absolute number of satellite cells up to 2 months postdenervation, but thereafter satellite cells decrease steadily up to 12 months after denervation.[15,16]

Muscle Damage

Satellite cells are also highly responsive to conditions leading to muscle damage. Within 1 day after an acute bout of eccentric treadmill running, satellite cell proliferation increased to 300% of control values in the rat soleus.[17] A lower peak of proliferation (250% of control values) occurred after 2 days in the EDL muscle.

At the time of its original discovery, Mauro[4] suggested that the satellite cell was a candidate for the myogenic precursor cell during muscle regeneration. After a number of years of intense controversy,[18] the satellite cell, rather than myonuclei, was shown to be the precursor cell for regenerating muscle fibers.[19] However, the possibility that certain mononuclear cells outside the basal lamina of the muscle fiber might have myogenic potential has not been definitely ruled out.

Muscle Fiber Regeneration

The regeneration of damaged muscle fibers has been demonstrated in virtually all species examined, including humans.[20-23] Although the mechanisms of initial damage differ and there is some topographical variation in the response depending on whether the muscle is totally versus focally damaged, the overall sequence of degeneration and regeneration of a muscle fiber is similar.

Muscle Fiber Damage and Degeneration

Muscle fibers can be damaged in many ways, and without a mechanism for repair there would be an increase in the level of muscular deficit caused by the loss of muscle fibers during the aging process. Among the demonstrated factors that produce muscle fiber degeneration are mechanical trauma, endurance events,[24,25] eccentric exercise,[26,27] ischemia,[28] a variety of snake toxins,[29,30] and local anesthetics.[31-33]

Most of these insults lead to a characteristic sequence of degenerative events. The first is a series of biochemical events that result in demonstrable intrinsic degeneration of the muscle fiber.[34] Although these events are not yet well understood, they typically begin with a net influx of extracellular Ca^{2+} and an increase in intracellular Ca^{2+}. This stimulates Ca^{2+}-activated proteases to selectively break down proteins, particularly in the region of the Z band. Morphologically, the loss of Z bands is a characteristic sign of the intrinsic phase of muscle degeneration.

The intrinsic changes previously described are often self-limiting. During ischemia, for instance, the intrinsic phase of muscle fiber degeneration appears to stabilize, and if not near a blood supply, the degenerated muscle fibers can remain in a stable state of ischemic necrosis for many weeks. During this period, viable myogenic cells are not demonstrable within the ischemic muscle, even though later in the regenerative process new muscle fibers are formed within the basal laminae of the formerly ischemic muscle fibers.[35,36] Free radicals have been implicated as agents of muscle fiber damage, especially under conditions of exhaustive or repetitive exercise.[37,38]

A second phase of cell-mediated degeneration occurs when macrophages from nearby or ingrowing blood vessels migrate into the degenerating muscle fiber. The macrophages penetrate the basal lamina that surrounds the muscle fiber and proceed to phagocytize the remainder of the original muscle fiber. The macrophages not only remove the remainder of the degenerating muscle fibers, but they are suspected of stimulating the activation of satellite cells through the action of the many growth factors that they secrete. Neutrophils, major elements of the first wave of a classic inflammatory response, are usually only minor components of the cellular reaction that attends muscle fiber damage. The presence of large numbers of neutrophils in an area of muscle fiber damage often inhibits to muscle regeneration, possibly because of free radical-induced damage inflicted upon satellite cells.

Satellite Cell Activation and the Initiation of Muscle Fiber Regeneration

Morphologically, there is a close spatiotemporal relationship between the macrophage-mediated removal of degenerating muscle fiber material and the activation of satellite cells beneath the basal lamina of the degenerating muscle fiber. On the other hand, Bischoff[39] was able to obtain the proliferation of satellite cells associated with muscle fibers cultured in vitro in the absence of macrophages. He demonstrated a satellite cell mitogen from crushed muscle fibers.[40]

It is likely that a variety of factors from different sources are involved in the activation of satellite cells in vivo. Grounds[22] has extensively reviewed the factors that could be involved in the activation of satellite cells (Outline 1), defining activation as the transition from the G_0 to the G_1 phase of the cell cycle. In vitro studies have shown that fibroblast growth factor (FGF) and insulin-like growth factor (IGF) strongly promote the proliferation of satellite cells derived from adult muscle.[41]

Acute injury to muscle also activates the expression of the muscle transcription factors, myogenin and MyoD. In normal adult rodent muscle the levels of expression of these factors is very low, but Grounds and associates[42] found transcription of these factors as early as 6 hours after muscle injury. Activity peaked at 24 to 48 hours and then subsided to normal levels after approximately 8 days. Fuchtbauer and Westphal[43] were not able to demonstrate increased levels of the MyoD and myogenin proteins by immunocytochemistry

Outline 1 Factors that may maintain the quiescent state of satellite cells in uninjured muscle or result in their activation after trauma to the myofiber*

Quiescent satellite cell (G_0)
  Intact plasmalemma (electric activity)
  Extracellular matrix: General composition
    Presence of negative growth factors (TGF-β?)
    Absence of available mitogens
  Receptors on satellite cells
    Absence of receptors for growth factors (eg, FGF?)

Trauma
  Membrane damage, Ca^{2+} influx
  Vascular coagulation, nerve injury
  Production of chemotactic agents that attract macrophages
    Complement activation products
    PDGF (mainly from platelets)
    TGF-β (from platelets and other cells)
  Production of angiogenic factors
    FGF
    Bischoff growth factor

Activation of satellite cells (G_0 to G_1)
  Proteases (mitogenic for satellite cells?)
  Extracellular matrix
    Decrease in many components may affect the shape and DNA synthesis of satellite cells
    Degradation of heparan sulfate
    Release of FGF by proteoglycans
    Fibronectin disappears first
    Slower disappearance of laminin from basal lamina

Growth factors and hormones
  Increase in nonspecific growth factors such as FGF (released from extracellular matrix and secreted by macrophages, endothelial and other local cells) and PDGF (secreted by platelets and other local cells)
  Increase in relatively specific satellite cell mitogens, such as Bischoff growth factor, and adrenocorticotrophic hormone glucocorticoids

Receptors on satellite cells
  Receptors become available for FGF and other mitogens

---

* TGF-β, transforming growth factor-β; FGF, fibroblast growth factor; PDGF, platelet-derived growth factor

until shortly before fusion of myoblasts, but these proteins persisted in the nuclei of regenerated muscle fibers for at least 2 weeks.

After initial activation, satellite cells undergo a phase of proliferation, followed by their fusion into myotube and ultimate differentiation into muscle fibers. In vitro studies have shown that fusion of satellite cells and their differentiation involves a different set of growth factors (transforming growth factor-β) from those that promote proliferation.[44] It is not unrealistic to assume that similar shifts in the humoral environment accompany the transition from proliferation to differentiation in vivo.

In most cases, the activation, proliferation, fusion, and early differentiation of satellite cells occur within the basal lamina of the original muscle fiber. However, if the basal lamina is torn, muscle fibers can form in the interstitial tissue. Among other possible functions, the basal lamina appears to serve as a selective cellular filter, keeping satellite cells in the basal lamina and keeping fibroblasts out. Macrophages have the ability to penetrate the basal lamina. A number of aspects of interactions between cells and the basal lamina remain obscure. In normal regeneration, the original basal lamina is occupied only by satellite cells and macrophages. If rat muscle is irradiated at the time of damage and muscle regeneration does not occur, the basal laminae persist but remain empty for up to 10 days. After that time, collagen fibers appear within the muscle basal laminae.[45] This process does not occur in normal muscle regeneration. The mechanism by which collagen fibers are prevented from forming within the original basal laminae during normal regeneration is not known.

Differentiation of the Regenerating Skeletal Muscle Fiber

Once myotubes have formed from fused myogenic precursor cells, the regenerating muscle fiber goes through a process of cellular differentiation that is remarkably similar to that which takes place during normal ontogenesis with respect to morphology, molecular events, and physiologic maturation.[46,47]

Reinnervation is a critical event in the differentiation of the regenerating muscle fiber. In the absence of reinnervation, the regenerating muscle fiber in many species undergoes a period of slow atrophy; it does not form the terminal set of isoforms of some of the important contractile proteins, and its contractile properties remain immature. Other species, such as the frog and mouse, are much more sensitive to the lack of innervation, and within 3 weeks, almost all noninnervated muscle fibers have disappeared.

If reinnervated and in an adequate functional environment, a regenerating muscle fiber returns to virtually normal morphology and function. The persistence of occasional central nuclei is a diagnostic sign of regenerating muscle fibers.

Age and Skeletal Muscle Regeneration

Muscle fiber injury occurs throughout an individual's life span, and its incidence may increase with age. Muscle fiber regeneration also occurs in older individuals, but most studies have reported that the success of posttraumatic muscle fiber regeneration decreases with age.[48,49] A fundamental question is whether the observed decrease in the success of muscle regeneration during aging is caused by an intrinsic decrease in the ability of the muscle fiber to regenerate or if it is caused by the environment in which the muscle fiber regenerates.

Carlson and Faulkner[50] tested this set of options in a cross-transplantation experiment. Extensor digitorum longus muscles from 24-month-old rats were grafted in place of EDL muscles in 4-month-old hosts; conversely, EDL muscles from the young rats were grafted in place of the EDL muscles of the old hosts. After the muscle grafts reached stability at 60 days, contractile properties of the cross-age grafts were compared with old-into-old and young-into-young grafts in the same hosts. The old-into-young grafts regenerated as well as young-into-young EDL grafts, whereas the young-into-old EDL grafts regenerated no better than old-into-old grafts. These results indicate that, in vivo at least, even an old muscle has the intrinsic capacity to regenerate well if it is placed in a favorable environment. The results of young-into-old grafting show that the graft environment of an old rat is not supportive of good regeneration of even a young muscle.

Why the limb of an old rat is not a good environment for muscle regeneration is not presently known, but a number of defective mechanisms, ranging from humoral environment to poor revascularization, or reinnervation are all possibilities to consider. Although deficiencies in reinnervation appear to be likely, other deficiencies cannot be ruled out. Little controlled research on the regeneration of aged human muscle has been done, but one study on the regeneration of extraocular muscles after damage by injections of local anesthetics has shown a couple of instances of nonregenerating lesions in subjects over 80 years of age.[51] In vitro studies of the proliferation potential of satellite cells have shown that satellite cells from young rats can produce more progeny than those from old rats,[12] but this does not seem to be a limiting factor in in vivo cross-age grafting experiments. It is possible that even an old muscle contains enough satellite cells with a total proliferative capacity that this is not a limiting factor to the success of regeneration of an old muscle.

Repetitive Motion and Skeletal Muscle Regeneration

Repetitive motion injuries often present initially as pathology of the connective tissues and joints, but in more severe cases or with certain stimulation (such as pronounced vibration) damage to muscle fibers can also result. Eccentric exercise (lengthening contractions) can also cause direct muscle damage. Regardless of the mechanism of injury, once the muscle fibers are damaged they initiate a similar sequence of repair and regeneration. If the regenerating muscle fibers are innervated, regeneration will typically be complete.

The response of muscle to repeated traumatic events is not well understood. Repetitive eccentric exercise (lengthening contractions) cause significant muscle fiber damage in untrained individuals, but after a period of training, such damage does not occur. Little is known about the protective mechanism effected by training. Serial damage to skeletal muscle results in repeated bouts of regeneration, but on occasion such repeated regeneration leads to excessive scarring.

Critical in the study of repetitive motion injuries is an increased knowledge of how multiple events that may result in subthreshold disturbances to muscle fibers produce a degree of cumulative damage that initiates the full sequence of muscle fiber degeneration and regeneration. The influence of advanced age on the success of the regenerative process needs further definition.

Summary

There is increasing evidence of damage to skeletal muscle fibers after repetitive exercise (such as long distance running) or situations involving eccentric (lengthening) muscle contractions. Once muscle fibers are damaged, regardless of the mechanism, they typically undergo a common degenerative reaction involving intrinsic cytoplasmic degeneration followed by macrophage-mediated phagocytosis of the degenerating muscle fibers. As the phagocytosis of the original muscle fiber is underway, the satellite cells located alongside the muscle fiber undergo activation and begin to proliferate. The progeny of these cells fuse to form a regenerating myotube within the basal lamina of the original muscle fiber. The myotube then differentiates in a manner recapitulating the ontogenetic differentiation of a muscle fiber. If innervated and in a good functional environment, a regenerated muscle fiber attains normal size and functional properties. Muscle fibers regenerate more poorly in older individuals, but this appears to be related to deficiencies in the environment.

References

1. Evered D, Whelan J (eds): *Plasticity of the Neuromuscular System*. Chichester, UK, John Wiley & Sons, 1988.
2. Hník P, Soukup T, Vejsada R, Zelená J: *Mechanoreceptors-Development, Structure and Function*. New York, NY, Plenum Press, 1988, pp 442.
3. Campion DR: The muscle satellite cell: A review. *Int Rev Cytol* 1984;87:225–251.
4. Mauro A: Satellite cell of skeletal muscle fibers. *J Biophys Biochem Cytol* 1961;9: 493–495.
5. Alameddine H, Sharp N, Dehaupas S, et al: Lymphocyte Leu-19 antigens expression in regenerating canine muscles. *J Neurol Sci* 1990;98(suppl):296.
6. Schubert W, Zimmermann K, Cramer M, et al: Lymphocyte antigen Leu-19 as a molecular marker of regeneration in human skeletal muscle. *Proc Natl Acad Sci USA* 1989;86:307–311.
7. Chevallier A, Pautou MP, Harris AJ, et al: On the non-equivalence of skeletal muscle satellite cells and embryonic myoblasts. *Arch d'Anat Microscop* 1986;75:161–166.
8. Miller JB: Myoblasts, myosins, myoDs, and the diversification of muscle fibers. *Neuromusc Disord* 1991;1:7–17.
9. Allbrook DB, Han MF, Hellmuth AE: Population of muscle satellite cells in relation to age and mitotic activity. *Pathology* 1971;3:223–243.
10. Gibson MC, Schultz E: Age-related differences in absolute numbers of skeletal muscle satellite cells. *Muscle Nerve* 1983;6:574–580.
11. Schultz E, McCormick KM: Cell biology of the satellite cell, in Partridge T (ed): *Molecular and Cell Biology of Muscular Dystrophy*. London, UK, Chapman and Hall, 1993, pp 190–209.
12. Schultz E, Lipton BH: Skeletal muscle satellite cells: Changes in proliferation potential as a function of age. *Mech Ageing Devel* 1982;20:377–383.
13. Snow MH: Satellite cell response in rat soleus muscle undergoing hypertrophy due to surgical ablation of synergists. *Anat Rec* 1990;227:437–446.
14. Schultz E: Satellite cell behavior during skeletal muscle growth and regeneration. *Med Sci Sports Exerc* 1989;21(suppl 5):S181–S186.
15. Lu D-X, Carlson BM: Abstract: A quantitative study of satellite cells in long-term denervated rat extensor digitorum longus (EDL) muscles. *Anat Rec* 1993;236 (suppl 1):78.
16. Viguie CA, Carlson BM: Abstract: Nuclear numbers in long-term denervated rat EDL muscle fibers. *FASEB J* 1994;8:60.
17. Darr KC, Schultz E: Exercise-induced satellite cell activation in growing and mature skeletal muscle. *J Appl Physiol* 1987;63:1816–1821.
18. Mauro A, Shafiq SA, Milhorat AT (eds): *Regeneration of Striated Muscle, and Myogenesis*. Amsterdam, Excerpta Medica, 1970.
19. Snow MH: Myogenic cell formation in regenerating rat skeletal muscle injured by mincing: II. An autoradiographic study. *Anat Rec* 1977;188:201–217.
20. Carlson BM: The regeneration of skeletal muscle: A review. *Am J Anat* 1973;137: 119–149.
21. Mauro A, Bischoff R, Carlson BM, et al: *Muscle Regeneration*. New York, NY, Raven Press, 1979.
22. Grounds MD: Towards understanding skeletal muscle regeneration. *Path Res Pract* 1991;187:1–22.
23. Grounds MD, Yablonka-Reuveni Z: Molecular and cell biology of skeletal muscle regeneration, in Partridge T (ed): *Molecular and Cell Biology of Muscular Dystrophy*. London, UK, Chapman and Hall, 1993, pp 210–256.
24. Armstrong RB: Muscle damage and endurance events. *Sports Med* 1986;3:370–381.
25. Hikida RS, Staron RS, Hagerman FC, et al: Muscle fiber necrosis associated with human marathon runners. *J Neurol Sci* 1983;59:185–203.
26. Armstrong RB: Initial events in exercise-induced muscular injury. *Med Sci Sports Exerc* 1990;22:429–435.

27. Friden J, Lieber RL: Structural and mechanical basis of exercise-induced muscle injury. *Med Sci Sports Exerc* 1992;24:521–530.
28. Carlson BM: A review of muscle transplantation in mammals. *Physiol Bohemoslov* 1978;27:387–400.
29. Couteaux R, Mira J-C, d'Albis A: Regeneration of muscles after cardiotoxin injury: I. Cytological aspects. *Biol Cell* 1988;62:171–182.
30. Pena J, Jimena I, Luqie E, et al: Muscle regeneration induced by snake venom: A histological and histochemical study. *Histol Histopathol* 1989;4:467–472.
31. Benoit PW, Belt WD: Destruction and regeneration of skeletal muscle after treatment with a local anaesthetic, bupivacaine (Marcaine). *J Anat* 1970;107:547–556.
32. Foster AH, Carlson BM: Myotoxicity of local anesthetics and regeneration of the damaged muscle fibers. *Anesth Analg* 1980;59:727–736.
33. Carlson BM, Shepard B, Komorowski TE: A histological study of local anesthetic-induced muscle degeneration and regeneration in the monkey. *J Orthop Res* 1990;8:485–494.
34. Jackson MJ: Molecular mechanisms of muscle damage, in Partridge T (ed): *Molecular and Cell Biology of Muscular Dystrophy*. London, UK, Chapman and Hall, 1993, pp 257–282.
35. Phillips GD, Lu DY, Mitashov VI, et al: Survival of myogenic cells in freely grafted rat rectus femoris and extensor digitorum longus muscles. *Am J Anat* 1987;180:365–372.
36. Schultz E, Albright DJ, Jaryszak DL, et al: Survival of satellite cells in whole muscle transplants. *Anat Rec* 1988;222:12–17.
37. Davies KJ, Quintanilha AT, Brooks GA, et al: Free radicals and tissue damage produced by exercise. *Biochem Biophys Res Comm* 1982;107:1198–1205.
38. Zerba E, Komorowski TE, Faulkner JA: Free radical injury to skeletal muscles of young, adult, and old mice. *Am J Physiol* 1990;258:C429–C435.
39. Bischoff R: Proliferation of muscle satellite cells on intact myofibers in culture. *Devel Biol* 1986;115:129–139.
40. Bischoff R: A satellite cell mitogen from crushed adult muscle. *Devel Biol* 1986;115:140–147.
41. Allen RE, Dodson MV, Luiten LS, et al: A serum-free medium that supports the growth of cultured skeletal muscle satellite cells. *In Vitro Cell Devel Biol* 1985;21:636–640.
42. Grounds MD, Garrett KL, Lai MC, et al: Identification of skeletal muscle precursor cells in vivo by use of MyoD1 and myogenin probes. *Cell Tissue Res* 1992;267:99–104.
43. Fuchtbauer E-M, Westphal H: MyoD and myogenin are coexpressed in regenerating skeletal muscle of the mouse. *Devel Dyn* 1992;193:34–39.
44. Allen RE, Boxhorn LK: Regulation of skeletal muscle satellite cell proliferation and differentiation by transforming growth factor-beta, insulin-like growth factor 1, and fibroblast growth factor. *J Cell Physiol* 1989;138:311–315.
45. Carlson EC, Carlson BM: A method for preparing skeletal muscle fiber basal laminae. *Anat Rec* 1991;230:325–331.
46. Carlson BM, Faulkner JA: The regeneration of skeletal muscle fibers following injury: A review. *Med Sci Sports Exerc* 1983;15:187–198.
47. Esser K, Gunning P, Hardeman E: Nerve-dependent and -independent patterns of mRNA expression in regenerating skeletal muscle. *Devel Biol* 1993;159:173–183.
48. Sadeh M: Effects of aging on skeletal muscle regeneration. *J Neurol Sci* 1988;87:67–74.
49. Brooks SV, Faulkner JA: Contractile properties of skeletal muscles from young, adult and aged mice. *J Physiol (Lond)* 1988;404:71–82.
50. Carlson BM, Faulkner JA: Muscle transplantation between young and old rats: Age of host determines recovery. *Am J Physiol* 1989;256:C1262–C1266.
51. Carlson BM, Emerick S, Komorowski TE, et al: Extraocular muscle regeneration in primates: Local anesthetic-induced lesions. *Ophthalmology* 1992;99:582–589.

Chapter 22

The Role of Inflammatory Processes in Exercise-Induced Muscle Injury: Implications for Changes in Skeletal Muscle Protein Turnover

Roger A. Fielding, PhD

Introduction

Physical activity has been shown to have differential effects on skeletal muscle protein turnover. For example, prolonged submaximal exercise increases the oxidation of several indispensable amino acids, and chronic endurance training has been shown to increase the daily requirement for dietary protein.[1,2] Conversely, high-intensity strength training has been shown to increase skeletal muscle mass despite resulting in increased myofibrillar proteolysis, suggesting a disproportionate increase in myofibrillar protein synthesis.[3] Eccentric exercise or active lengthening of muscle (a large component of high-intensity strength training) has been shown to initiate ultrastructural muscle damage, which results in a prolonged increase in the rate of protein degradation.[4,5] Exercise, particularly eccentric exercise, is also associated with a stereotypical acute phase response similar in many aspects to the acute phase response to infection, which is characterized by fever, complement activation, mobilization of neutrophils, redistribution of trace metals, and increased proteolysis.[6] Because skeletal muscle represents the largest organ mass in the body and is an important reserve of body protein, the mobilization and provision of amino acids from skeletal muscle for hepatic protein synthesis and whole body oxidation is an integral part of the acute phase response during starvation, burn injury, malignancy, and septicemia.[7] Along with the other similarities to the acute phase response to infection and trauma, the activators of protein turnover may be similar to those involved in the response to muscle damaging activity and subsequent repair processes.

The role of the inflammatory response to exercise as it relates to the activation of protein turnover following exercise-induced muscle damage will be discussed. Specific attention will be paid to the factors responsible for the "acute phase response to exercise" and their involvement in the activation of skeletal muscle protein turnover and subsequent remodeling. Because repetitive strain injury (RSI) may initially involve muscle trauma or injury, the models of exercise-induced muscle inflammation discussed in this chapter may shed light on the early course of these syndromes and their potential effects on skeletal muscle function.

Eccentric Exercise and Unaccustomed Activity

Before a discussion of the inflammatory mechanisms involved in muscle injury can begin, a brief summary of the type, magnitude, and time course of the ultrastructural alterations observed following eccentric exercise is necessary. A model of primarily eccentric muscle actions or muscle lengthening has been used to study exercise-induced muscle injury.[5,8–10] In general, the muscular effort of concentric exercise produces external work, while the muscular effort of eccentric exercise resists external force and "absorbs" the mechanical energy imposed by external forces. Most human movement has both an eccentric and a concentric component. An example of eccentric exercise is the action of the quadriceps muscle during descent on a flight of stairs. Nearly 50% of the force generated during a session of dynamic resistance training is performed by eccentric muscle actions. The eccentric component of exercise has been associated with delayed-onset muscle soreness, which appears 24 to 48 hours after strenuous exercise.[5,8,9,11] Because the injury process and delayed soreness are associated with this type of activity, eccentric exercise has been used to investigate the cause and associated metabolic events of delayed muscle soreness and damage.

Immediately following high-intensity eccentric exercise, disturbances of the cross-striated band pattern with disruptions of the Z-disk have been observed in human skeletal muscle.[8,12] Several key features need to be mentioned concerning the time course of these changes. In their early studies, Fridén and associates[8] observed more extensive lesions in muscle biopsy specimens obtained 3 days after eccentric exercise. Ten days after one bout of eccentric exercise, O'Reilly and associates[12] observed necrotic fibers with loss of myofibrillar organization, mitochondrial alterations, and inflammatory cell infiltration. These two studies indicate that there is a continued active degradation of skeletal muscle contractile units for a prolonged period of time following a single bout of eccentric exercise or activity with a large eccentric component. These reports suggest that there is an immediate exercise-induced lesion within muscle that appears to be a result of the mechanical strain of eccentric contractions followed on successive days by further increases in the extent of ultrastructural abnormalities. In attempting to examine the delayed effects of eccentric exercise on skeletal muscle injury, the change in the percentage of damaged Z-bands was measured using a grid system following a single bout of downhill treadmill walking or running in both young and older men and women.[13,14] In both studies, there was a significant increase in the percentage of damaged Z-bands following exercise that remained elevated in one study 5 days after exercise, and in a second study up to 12 days after the exercise bout (Fig. 1). These data reveal the prolonged residual effects of this type of activity and illustrate that the damaging effect of eccentric exercise is not fully restored by 2 weeks.

Exercise and Whole Body Protein Metabolism

The rate of oxidation of the indispensable amino acid leucine has been shown to increase several times during prolonged submaximal exercise,[15,16] while oxidation of the indispensable amino acid lysine increases by about 40%.[1] The exaggerated increase in the oxidation of leucine and potentially the other branched-chain amino acids may be caused by selective activation of the branched-chain ketoacid dehydrogenase enzyme during exercise,[17] which has also been shown to be induced by the cytokines interleukin-1 (IL-1) and tumor

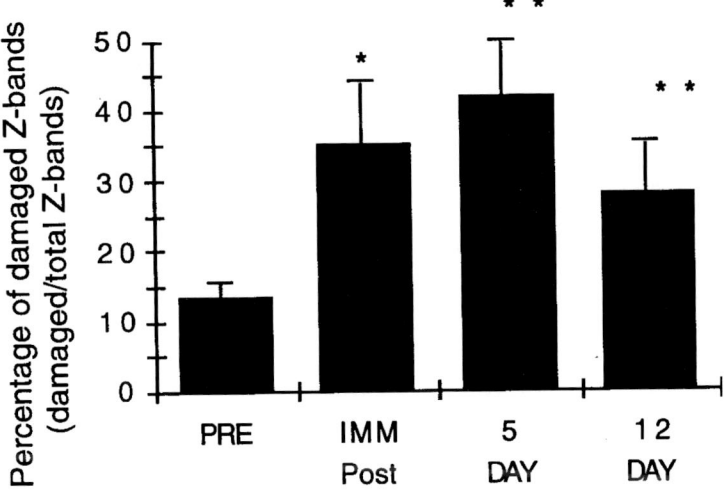

Fig. 1 Plot of the change in the percentage of damaged Z-bands following eccentric cycling or downhill running for 45 minutes at 78% of maximum heart rate in men and women (n=9; age 25 to 75 years). Asterisk indicates significantly different from preexercise ($p < 0.01$); double asterisk indicates significantly different from preexercise ($p < 0.05$).

necrosis factor (TNF).[18] Despite these increases in leucine and lysine oxidation, concomitant changes in urea flux have not been observed during low-intensity submaximal exercise, suggesting a redistribution of whole body protein synthesis and degradation.[1]

Several studies have examined protein turnover immediately following exercise. Devlin and associates[19] have reported a net uptake of branched-chain amino acids (BCAA) across the forearm following submaximal leg exercise to exhaustion, suggesting an increased oxidation of BCAAs or increased protein synthesis in inactive muscle in the postexercise recovery period. Carraro and associates[20] have observed a significant increase in the fractional rate of skeletal muscle protein synthesis following 4 hours of low-intensity exercise.[20] They have proposed that following exercise there is a redistribution of whole body protein synthesis from liver to skeletal muscle, which is in agreement with previous studies showing that exercise resulted in no change in whole body protein synthesis or an increased urea flux.[1,16]

Recent animal studies have confirmed the increase in muscle fractional protein synthetic rate following both prolonged concentric and eccentric muscle contractions.[21,22] These studies also demonstrated that relatively minor increases in selected contractile protein mRNAs occur immediately following electrically stimulated muscle contractions. This suggests that following contractile activity, translational and posttranslational events may regulate changes in muscle protein synthesis. These same studies also reported that eccentric muscle contractions induced a more prolonged increase in muscle protein synthesis than concentric muscle contractions and that with chronic bouts of electrical stimulation only the eccentrically contracting muscle groups demonstrated hypertrophy. In addition, using the same protocol, a 40% increase in immunoreactivity to insulin-like growth factor I has been observed in transverse sections of rat muscle 4 days after 192 electrically stimulated eccentric contractions.[23] In their study of the response of healthy older men to 12 weeks of progressive resistance training, Frontera and associates[3] reported a 12% increase in midthigh muscle cross-sectional area along with a 40% increase in urinary 3-methylhistidine excretion, illustrating the increased muscle protein degradation that occurs in conjunction with the resultant muscle hypertrophy.

Recent human studies have also confirmed that eccentric muscle actions during strength training contribute disproportionately to the resultant muscle hypertrophy and strength gains. Compared to concentric training, a combination of eccentric and concentric training results in a greater increase in peak torque, muscle strength, and type I muscle fiber hypertrophy in young male subjects.[24–26] The precise mechanism for the need for the performance of eccentric muscle actions in resistance training programs to maximize strength gains and hypertrophy is not clear, but the injury process itself may initiate or prime the subsequent remodeling.

The Acute Phase Response to Exercise: Effect of Cytokines and Neutrophils on Muscle Protein Turnover

Several studies have reported increased plasma levels of IL-1 3 to 6 hours after exercise.[5,27,28] Cannon and Kluger[27] reported that human subjects release endogenous pyrogen following 1 hour of submaximal cycling exercise. This pyrogenic factor was heat inactivated and had an apparent molecular weight of 14 kD. They concluded that endogenous pyrogen released following exercise may mediate a series of physiologic responses similar to the acute phase response to infection. Evans and associates[5] showed significant increases in IL-1 activity as measured by thymocyte proliferation (a biologic activity of IL-1) 3 hours following 45 minutes of eccentric cycling exercise. They also noted a prolonged increase in 24-hour urinary excretion of 3-methylhistidine, a marker of skeletal muscle protein breakdown, which peaked 10 days after exercise. They concluded that the systemic release of IL-1 following exercise may induce a delayed rise in myofibrillar protein breakdown that persists for many days. In addition, they observed that the increased plasma IL-1 activity was blunted in exercise-trained individuals. Cannon and associates[28] demonstrated that IL-1 activity appeared in plasma several hours after cycle ergometer exercise and was neutralized by a specific antiserum to IL-1. In addition, IL-1 secretion by monocytes was increased up to 48% by addition of physiologic concentrations of epinephrine in vitro. Low concentrations of hydrocortisone (1ng/ml) also augmented IL-1 secretion by 58%. These results indicate that IL-1 activity could be altered in vivo by the physiologic stress of exercise and in vitro by hormones associated with stress.

Cytokines and Muscle Protein Turnover

Early studies implicated leukocytic pyrogen or IL-1 as being the factor in serum responsible for the accelerated proteolysis and muscle wasting that occurred as a result of infection.[29,30] IL-1 was proposed to stimulate prostaglandin E_2 production that, in turn, degraded muscle protein. Animal studies also reported that administration of partially purified rabbit peritoneal exudate containing leukocytic endogenous mediator (LEM), increased tyrosine oxidation and urinary 3-methylhistidine excretion by 30%.[31] Since the completion of these studies, the biologic activity has been ascribed to IL-1 but LEM may also be composed of other important proteolytic stimulators, including TNF.

Using recombinant cytokine preparations and several different muscle preparations, the effects of IL-1 and TNF on muscle proteolysis have been inconsistent. Goldberg and associates[32] have reported that recombinant IL-1, TNF, interferon, and other cytokines failed to activate proteolysis or prostaglandin E_2 synthesis using isolated rat soleus and extensor digitorum longus muscle. However, peptides derived from activated human macrophages (*Staphylococcus albus* stimulation) were able to increase proteolysis to the same extent as reported in prior studies. Moldawer and associates[33] have also shown by using similar cytokine preparations that recombinant IL-1 and TNF did not increase muscle proteolysis despite stimulating prostaglandin E_2 production in vitro. In rats infused with recombinant IL-1 together with recombinant TNF, the rate of leucine release from protein was increased, suggesting an increase in muscle protein breakdown.[34] These effects were also reported for TNF alone but not IL-1. Goodman[35] has demonstrated an increase in myofibrillar and nonmyofibrillar protein degradation in rat muscle 8 hours after TNF injection. Interestingly, he noted a twofold increase in myofibrillar protein degradation compared to nonmyofibrillar proteins. In addition, another study has also shown that intraperitoneal administration of recombinant IL-1, coupled with the administration of a glucocorticoid receptor antagonist, induces a 49% increase in nonmyofibrillar and a 134% increase in myofibrillar protein breakdown, suggesting a disproportionate increase in myofibrillar proteolysis independent of cytokine effects on glucocorticoids.[36]

Some question also exists regarding the effects of the cytokines on muscle protein synthesis. In one study by Flores and associates,[34] there was no reported effect on muscle protein synthesis, although muscle protein breakdown was increased following combined infusion of IL-1 and TNF. In contrast, Fong and associates[37] have reported a decreased level of messenger RNA in rat gastrocnemius muscle following chronic administration of TNF or IL-1. More recently, Ballmer and associates[38] noted a significant decrease in the fractional rate of muscle protein synthesis following administration of recombinant human IL-1β in rat soleus and gastrocnemius muscles. Concomitant with decreased muscle protein synthetic rates, they observed increased fractional rates of liver protein synthesis illustrating the interorgan shift in the site of increased protein turnover following an experimentally-induced acute phase response.

Neutrophil Function and Muscle Protein Turnover

In addition to the systemic changes discussed previously, a correlation between exercise-induced muscle enzyme leakage (creatine kinase) and the activation and mobilization of circulating neutrophils has been observed after 45 minutes of downhill running.[39] Circulating neutrophils, which tend to increase 3 to 6 hours after downhill running exercise, may have a role in the response to exercise-induced muscle injury because of their ability to invade host tissues, generate superoxide radicals,[40,41] and release proteases such as elastase.[42] In an attempt to elucidate the role of neutrophil aggregation on exercise-induced muscle injury and subsequent activation of protein turnover, biopsy specimens obtained from the vastus lateralis muscles of young men were examined immediately following and 5 days after 45 minutes of downhill running exercise. Using a qualitative rating of neutrophil aggregation, there was a significant increase in intramuscular neutrophils immediately after exercise. The neutrophils also were present in the 5-day postexercise samples. Interestingly, neutrophil accumulation was positively correlated to intracellular Z-band damage ($\rho = 0.66$; $p < 0.001$). The disrupted muscle fibers may release fragments and other intracellular material that may form a chemotactic gradient that attracts neutrophils, and by their phagocytic and proteolytic capabilities may contribute to the clearance of damaged ultrastructural components. This hypothesis has been supported by Zerba and associates,[43] who showed that the reduction in maximal isometric force following lengthening contractions was attenuated in animals injected with superoxide dismutase (a free radical scavenger), suggesting a causal role for reactive oxygen molecules in the etiology of eccentric exercise-induced muscle injury. In the same subjects in which muscle neutrophils were measured, quantification of intramuscular accumulation of IL-1β was found to increase immediately after exercise but was increased even more by 5 days postexercise (Fig. 2). Staining for IL-1β was positively correlated to neutrophil accumulation, indicating that the increased IL-1β may be involved in chemoattraction of neutrophils to areas of injury. It has been postulated that IL-1β directs neutrophil chemoattraction and degranulation by inducing the neutrophil activating factor, interleukin-8.[44]

Eccentric Exercise and Muscle Protein Turnover

Because few studies have addressed the complex interactions between protein synthesis and degradation following acute exercise in human subjects and how these are altered in older individuals, a series of experiments were designed and performed to address the effects of a single bout of eccentric exercise on whole body and skeletal muscle protein turnover. Of particular interest are the factors that mediate exercise-induced changes in whole body protein turnover. The eccentric exercise model was used to examine these changes because it has been shown previously to result in the greatest amount of muscle damage following a single exercise session[8] and would provide an appropriate stimulus to examine these metabolic changes.

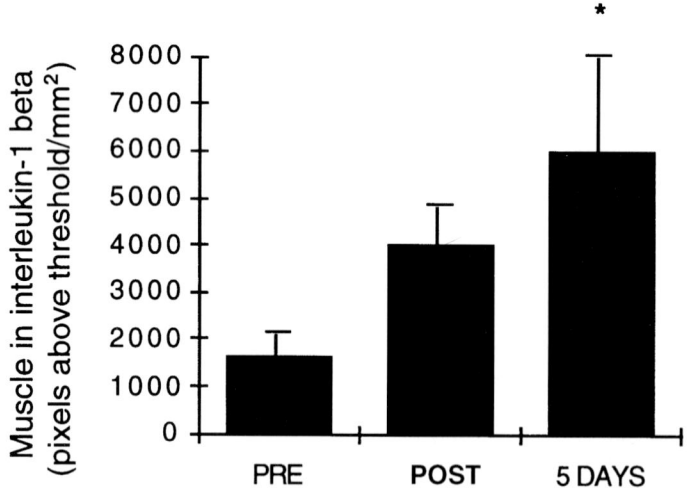

Fig. 2 Plot of muscle IL-1β expressed as the number of pixels above nonimmune staining background using nonimmune rabbit serum/mm². Asterisk indicates significantly increased above pre-exercise ($p < 0.03$; n=9). (Reproduced with permission from Fielding RA, Manfredi TJ, Ding W, et al: Acute phase response in exercise: III. Neutrophil and IL-1 beta accumulation in skeletal muscle. *Am J Physiol* 1993;265:R166–R172.)

Using a primed constant infusion of 1-^{13}C-leucine, there was a 9% increase in leucine flux following 45 minutes of eccentric cycling in young and older healthy men that persisted for 10 days after the exercise.[10] Along with these changes in flux, leucine oxidation rates were also increased approximately 16% up to 10 days after this single exercise bout (Fig. 3). Concurrent with these changes in whole body protein turnover, changes in urinary excretion of the posttranslationally modified amino acid 3-methylhistidine (3-MEH), which is exclusively found in contractile proteins and is used as an indirect measure of muscle protein degradation,[45] were examined. In the young men, urinary excretion of 3-MEH did not increase until 10 days postexercise, but in the older men, it increased 5 days after exercise and remained elevated through 10 days postexercise (Fig. 4). These data suggested that a single bout of eccentric exercise induces an increase in whole body protein turnover that persists for several days, and that there is a disproportionate increase in skeletal muscle protein breakdown in older men exposed to the same exercise stimulus. This increased response in the older men is also supported by examination of the degree of exercise-induced muscle injury in the older men, which revealed a significantly greater number of injured fibers compared to young subjects.[46] The increased muscle protein breakdown and injury in the older men may have been related to the smaller muscle mass activated during this exercise, along with lower aerobic fitness levels. Previous studies have demonstrated that exercise-trained individuals have an attenuated injury response to eccentric exercise.[5] The concept that individuals with a smaller muscle mass must absorb and withstand more eccentric force per cross section of muscle may have application to muscle injury in muscles of the upper extremity, which may also be forced to absorb relatively greater eccentric loads per cross-sectional area.

The reported changes in muscle protein turnover following eccentric exercise may be regulated by cytokine localization and function. Skeletal muscle IL-1β immunochemical reactivity has been shown to increase for up to 5 days after eccentric exercise in young untrained men and may be related to the prolonged increased muscle protein breakdown observed in other studies.[47] Cannon and associates[48] have also observed a significant relationship between IL-1β secretion 12 days after 45 minutes of downhill running (ρ = 0.479; p <0.05) (Fig. 5), suggesting a relationship between the ability of mononuclear cells to produce and release IL-1β and the magnitude of exercise-induced increases in muscle protein breakdown.

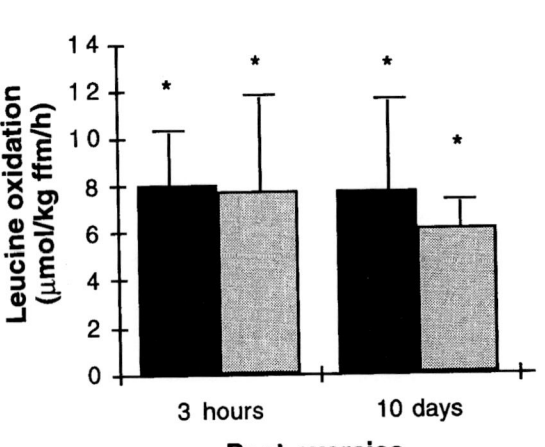

Fig. 3 Change in leucine oxidation in young and older men (n = 10) immediately and 10 days after 45 minutes of eccentric cycling exercise. Asterisk indicates significantly different from preexercise (p <0.04).

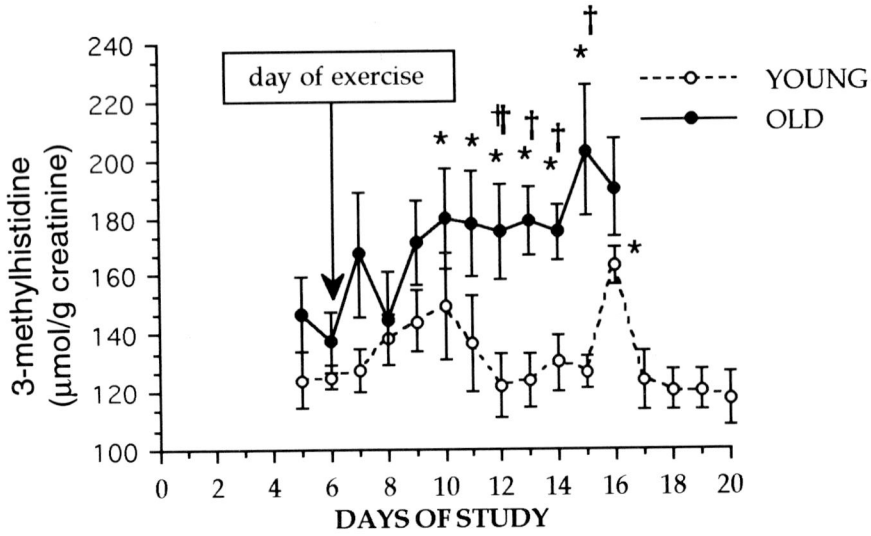

Fig. 4 Changes in excretion of urinary 3-methylhistidine during a study of eccentric exercise in young and older healthy men. Asterisk indicates increase over preexercise value (p <0.05). Difference between young and older men (p <0.05). (Reproduced with permission from Fielding RA, Meredith CN, O'Reilly KP, et al: Enhanced protein breakdown after eccentric exercise in young and older men. *J Appl Physiol* 1991;71:675–679.)

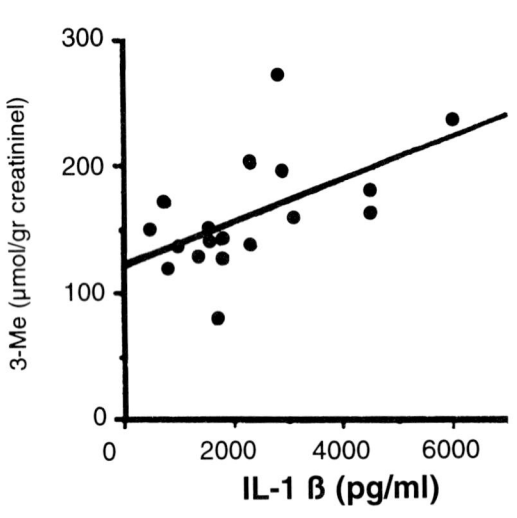

Fig. 5 Correlation between urinary 3-methylhistidine excretion and in vitro secretion of IL-1β from mononuclear cells 12 days after downhill running ($\rho = 0.479$; $p < 0.05$). (Reproduced with permission from Cannon JG, Meydani SN, Fielding RA, et al: Acute phase response in exercise: II. Associations between vitamin E, cytokines, and muscle proteolysis. *Am J Physiol* 1991; 260: R1235–R1240.)

Control of Muscle Protein Turnover Following Exercise

It is apparent from the previous discussion that following eccentric exercise in humans, there is an activation of muscle protein degradation and whole body protein turnover that may persist for several days. Evidence also indicates that activation of the acute phase response to exercise, which includes production and systemic release of IL-1β and mobilization and activation of neutrophils, may mediate these changes in protein turnover. However, few studies have examined the link between the release of these humoral factors and the pathways involved in skeletal muscle protein degradation. The following section will discuss the major proteolytic systems in skeletal muscle and their observed or potential roles in exercise-induced proteolysis.

The turnover of muscle proteins is regulated by a host of factors, including neurotrophic influences, steroid and peptide hormones, cellular nutrients, cytokines, and contractile activity. Many of these systems interact and it is clear that each may be more or less influential under a given set of metabolic circumstances. Proteolytic effector systems include the calcium-activated neutral proteases, lysosomal proteases, and ubiquitin-conjugated protein degradation. That eccentric exercise causes disruption of cellular proteins suggests that myofibrillar protein degradation may be activated to remove these damaged proteins and clear away cellular debris.

Lysosomal Proteases

Numerous studies have reported cellular infiltration and activation of lysosomal proteases following eccentric exercise. The initial edema that occurs during postexercise recovery from an acute bout of eccentric exercise[49] is followed by cellular infiltration of neutrophils and other leukocytes.[50] Costill and associates[51] have shown increases in leukocytes in transverse muscle sections obtained 24 hours after one-legged eccentric exercise.[51] Recently, Widrick and associates[52] also reported increases in mononuclear cells between 6 and 72 hours after one-legged eccentric exercise. The infiltration of these cells into areas of tissue damage may result in release of proteases such as elastase, cathepsin D, and β-glucoronidase.[53] Vihko and Salminen[53,54] have reported increases in the acid hydrolases and other lysosomal proteases after exhaustive exercise in untrained and in younger rats. No increases were seen in trained and older rats. They suggested that the increased proteolytic activity following exercise was a primary step in the cellular remodeling process and that older animals may have a reduced capacity for cellular repair. Recently, Kasperek and associates,[55] using the perfused rat hindquarter model, have noted an increased tyrosine release 30 minutes after electrically stimulated muscle contraction. They also reported a significant increase in cathepsin D levels following muscle contraction. They noted that the increased tyrosine release was suppressed by the lysosomal antagonist chloroquine. Results of this study indicate that the early rise in muscle protein degradation following electrical stimulation was caused by increased lysosomal enzyme activity.

Influence of Calcium Ion and Calcium-Activated Neutral Proteases on Proteolysis

Several studies have shown that Ca^{2+} or Ca^{2+} ionophores can induce muscle protein degradation in vitro.[56-58] Early studies suggested that the increases in extracellular Ca^{2+} activated proteolysis by activating phospholipase A_2 and increasing prostaglandin E_2 levels (a potent stimulator of proteolysis).[58,59] More recently, Baracos and associates[60] have shown that increases in extracellular Ca^{2+} increase skeletal muscle protein degradation, possibly by activating lysosomal thiol proteases, and that this increase in muscle proteolysis is independent of changes in prostaglandin E_2 levels.

Further work has confirmed the existence of a class of calcium-activated cytosolic thiol proteases, which have been termed the calcium-activated neutral proteases (CANPs). Studies employing immunochemical localization have reported association of CANP with myofibrillar Z-bands.[61] Treatment of isolated muscle with calcium ionophores has been shown to result in loss of Z-bands and myofibrillar alterations.[62–64] In vitro, CANP has also been shown to remove the Z-band protein α-actinin from isolated myofibrils,[65,66] which may explain the loss of Z-bands with increases in cytosolic Ca^{2+} in vivo.

Because of the similarities in the ultrastructural changes that occur with increases in cytosolic Ca^{2+} and eccentric exercise-induced muscle damage, several studies have suggested a role for the CANPs in this process. Furuno and associates[67] have reported that increased protein degradation by addition of Ca^{2+} or muscle injury activates muscle proteolysis by a nonlysosomal thiol protease, possibly the CANPs. Belcastro and associates[68] have observed a loss of 58 and 95 kDa protein bands on acrylamide gels of rat plantaris muscles after 1 hour of treadmill running, suggesting a loss of the Z-band proteins vimentin and α-actinin.[68] Recently, Belcastro[69] has observed an increase in both the u- and m-isoforms of the CANPs following level treadmill running in rats. Interestingly, myofibrils isolated from muscles following this exercise appeared to be more sensitive to proteolysis by the CANPs, suggesting possible covalent modification of the myofibrillar proteins with exercise and an increase in their affinity for CANP-dependent proteolysis.

Ubiquitin-Conjugating Degradative Pathway

A complex class of adenosine triphosphate (ATP)-dependent proteolytic enzymes has been characterized in several bacterial and mammalian cell lines.[70–72] The best characterized of these pathways involves the conjugation of the 8.5 kD molecular weight protein ubiquitin to abnormal, damaged, or short-lived proteins, which targets them for subsequent degradation. Compared to the lysosomal proteases, ubiquitin is thought to be a more selective protein degradative system. Ubiquitin-dependent proteolysis begins with the activation of ubiquitin by E_1, an enzyme that hydrolyzes ATP to form a reactive thiol with the C-terminal of ubiquitin. Ubiquitin is subsequently transferred to various cellular proteins. Substrates selected for proteolysis are conjugated to single or multiple ubiquitin chains that promote substrate hydrolysis by an ATPase-stimulated protease.[73]

Fagan and associates[71] were the first to provide clear evidence of the ATP-dependent ubiquitin proteolytic system in mammalian skeletal muscle extracts. Recent studies have described a large 1,500 kD multicatalytic protease called the proteasome, which has the capacity to degrade ubiquitin-protein conjugates or to degrade proteins in a manner independent of ubiquitin conjugation.[74,75] However, the functional roles of the ubiquitin-dependent and the ubiquitin-independent proteasomal degradative systems have not been delineated. Because the contractile proteins in skeletal muscle are selectively degraded in certain situations (such as disuse atrophy, starvation, exercise), the ubiquitin system, because of its targeting ability, may have a role in the exercise-induced degradation of myofibrillar proteins.

Using immunochemical techniques, Riley and associates[76] have reported higher levels of total ubiquitin in red rat skeletal muscle compared with that of white rats with the ratio of free to conjugated ubiquitin being similar. Also, using immunogold labeling, they showed localization of ubiquitin to the Z-band in both fiber types. In this report, they suggested that ubiquitin may be conjugated to α-actinin, a contractile protein component of the Z-band with an unusually short half-life considering its high molecular weight. Based on the immunochemical localization of ubiquitin to the myofibrillar Z-band, it is possible that this system is responsible for the selective degradation of contractile proteins following injury or inactivity and may be involved in protein degradation associated with contractile activity. As previously mentioned, Z-band damage and disintegration are prominent features of eccentric exercise-induced ultrastructural damage.

In a preliminary investigation, Riley and associates[77] have reported that rats exposed to 1 week of microgravity during space flight display a 26% increase in ubiquitin-protein conjugates in soleus muscle and a 40% increase in ubiquitin-protein conjugates in extensor digitorum longus muscle. More recently, Kasperek and Snider[78] have reported that total protein degradation from isolated rat soleus muscle is elevated 30 minutes after treadmill running to exhaustion (0% grade, 28 m/min) and that this elevated protein degradation was not inhibited in the presence of the lysosomal inhibitor chloroquine. They suggested that the elevated proteolytic activity following exercise was activated by a nonlysosomal pathway. These studies suggest that, possibly, ubiquitin-dependent systems are responsible for protein degradation in skeletal muscle as a result of changes in contractile activity.

Several recent studies have assessed the role of ubiquitin-dependent proteolysis in skeletal muscle during fasting and during glucocorticoid or denervation-induced atrophy in rats.[79-83] Furuno and associates[79] have reported that denervation-induced muscle atrophy is accompanied by a 2.5-fold increase in myofibrillar protein breakdown and that treatments which block lysosomal and Ca^{2+}-dependent proteolysis did not prevent this accelerated myofibrillar protein degradation in isolated rat muscle maintained at its resting length.[79] Medina and associates[80] have demonstrated that the expression of the mRNA for ubiquitin (polyubiquitin transcripts) increased twofold to fourfold after fasting or denervation and decreased to control levels following refeeding. These data suggest that myofibrillar protein degradation involves activation of an ATP-dependent ubiquitin-conjugating proteolytic pathway that may be responsible for the selective degradation of contractile proteins during fasting and denervation atrophy. In addition, measurement of ubiquitin-protein conjugates in muscle by solid-phase immunoassay revealed a 45% increase in conjugates following 48 hours of fasting and a 30% increase 3 days after denervation, respectively.[80] Recently, Tawa and associates[81,82] have shown that a protein-deficient diet in rats significantly decreased skeletal muscle proteolysis (by 30% to 45%) and that this decrease was specific to the reduction in ATP-dependent proteolysis. More recently, Wing and Goldberg[83] have indicated that short-term fasting (24 hours) in rats increases ATP-dependent skeletal muscle proteolysis and that surgical adrenalectomy eliminates this increase in proteolysis. In addition, administration of the glucocorticoid dexamethasone to fasted adrenalectomized animals restored the ATP-dependent proteolytic activity. Increased ATP-dependent proteolysis following dexamethasone administration was associated with increased expression of mRNA for ubiquitin, suggesting that glucocorticoids specifically activate myofibrillar protein degradation through the ubiquitin-ATP dependent proteolytic system.

The involvement of the lysosomal proteases as well as the CANPs in the activation of proteolysis following exercise has been documented. However, the role of the ubiquitin-dependent proteolytic system, if any, in response to acute exercise and muscle has yet to be determined.

Summary

The results of the studies previously discussed serve to document a coordinated series of metabolic changes that follow an acute bout of eccentric exercise and their relationship to alterations in nonspecific host defense mechanisms. The similarity of this coordinated response to the stereotypical "acute phase response" to infection has led to the hypothesis that an acute phase response is induced by exercise. The acute phase response may be involved in the metabolic adaptations to exercise and the remodeling processes that skeletal muscles undergo in response to exercise training.

This chapter has attempted to discuss the experimental evidence from human studies examining the changes in acute phase products and muscle protein turnover in association primarily with muscle-damaging activities. In addition, a discussion of the major proteolytic systems active in skeletal muscle has been presented to stimulate thinking about the role of these adaptive responses in situations of RSI. The similarities between the symptomatology of RSI and purely exercise-induced muscle injury have led to speculation that the initiating metabolic events may be the same. If, in fact, the initial damaging events in RSI are localized to skeletal muscle, then the changes in circulating leukocytes, creatine kinase activity, and cytokines may appear before the more characteristic signs and symptoms of these disorders are manifest. Exercise models of RSI would help identify the role of the acute phase response in this type of low-force, high-repetition activity early in the pathogenesis of these disorders.

The effects of muscle-damaging activity on skeletal muscle protein breakdown suggest that a necessary portion of the adaptive response to repeated activity is a generalized proteolysis, which is then followed by a net increase in skeletal muscle protein synthetic rates. It is possible that the repetitive nature of most activities or occupations that induce RSIs leads to a proteolytic response that is not necessarily followed by increased protein synthesis causing the failure of any normal or usual adaptive process.

References

1. Wolfe RR, Wolfe MH, Nadel ER, et al: Isotopic determination of amino acid-urea interactions in exercise in humans. *J Appl Physiol* 1984;56:221–229.
2. Meredith CN, Zackin MJ, Frontera WR, et al: Dietary protein requirements and body protein metabolism in endurance-trained men. *J Appl Physiol* 1989;66:2850–2856.
3. Frontera WR, Meredith CN, O'Reilly KP, et al: Strength conditioning in older men: Skeletal muscle hypertrophy and improved function. *J Appl Physiol* 1988;64:1038–1044.
4. Warhol MJ, Siegel AJ, Evans WJ, et al: Skeletal muscle injury and repair in marathon runners after competition. *Am J Pathol* 1985;118:331–339.
5. Evans WJ, Meredith CN, Cannon JG, et al: Metabolic changes following eccentric exercise in trained and untrained men. *J Appl Physiol* 1986;61:1864–1868.
6. Evans WJ, Cannon JG: The metabolic effects of exercise-induced muscle damage. *Exerc Sport Sci Rev* 1991;19:99–125.
7. Dinarello CA, Wolff SM: The role of interleukin-1 in disease. *N Engl J Med* 1993;328:106–113.
8. Fridén J, Seger J, Sjostrom M, et al: Adaptive response in human skeletal muscle subjected to prolonged eccentric training. *Int J Sports Med* 1983;4:177–183.
9. Newham DJ, McPhail G, Mills KR, et al: Ultrastructural changes after concentric and eccentric contractions of human muscle. *J Neur Sci* 1983;61:109–122.

10. Fielding RA, Meredith CN, O'Reilly KP, et al: Enhanced protein breakdown after eccentric exercise in young and older men. *J Appl Physiol* 1991;71:674–679.
11. Davies CT, White MJ: Muscle weakness following eccentric work in man. *Pflugers Arch* 1981;392:168–171.
12. O'Reilly KP, Warhol MJ, Fielding RA, et al: Eccentric exercise-induced muscle damage impairs muscle glycogen repletion. *J Appl Physiol* 1987;63:252–256.
13. Fielding RA, Manfredi TJ, Ding W, et al: Acute phase response in exercise: III. Neutrophil and IL-1 beta accumulation in skeletal muscle. *Am J Physiol* 1993;265:R166–R172.
14. Fielding R, Manfredi T, Ding W, et al: Prolonged alterations in skeletal muscle ultrastructure following eccentric exercise. *Clin Sci*, in press.
15. Rennie MJ, Edwards RH, Krywawych S, et al: Effect of exercise on protein turnover in man. *Clin Sci* 1981;61:627–639.
16. Wolfe RR, Goodenough RD, Wolfe MH, et al: Isotopic analysis of leucine and urea metabolism in exercising humans. *J Appl Physiol* 1982;52:458–466.
17. Kasperek GJ, Dohm GL, Snider RD: Activation of branched-chain keto acid dehydrogenase by exercise. *Am J Physiol* 1985;248:R166–R171.
18. Nawabi MD, Block KP, Chakrabarti MC, et al: Administration of endotoxin, tumor necrosis factor, or interleukin 1 to rats activates skeletal muscle branched-chain α-keto acid dehydrogenase. *J Clin Invest* 1990;85:256–263.
19. Devlin JT, Barlow J, Horton ES: Whole body and regional fuel metabolism during early postexercise recovery. *Am J Physiol* 1989;256:E167–E172.
20. Carraro F, Stuart CA, Hartl WH, et al: Effect of exercise and recovery on muscle protein synthesis in human subjects. *Am J Physiol* 1990;259:E470–E476.
21. Wong TS, Booth FW: Protein metabolism in rat gastrocnemius muscle after stimulated chronic concentric exercise. *J Appl Physiol* 1990;69:1709–1717.
22. Wong TS, Booth FW: Protein metabolism in rat tibialis anterior muscle after stimulated chronic eccentric exercise. *J Appl Physiol* 1990;69:1718–1724.
23. Yan Z, Biggs RB, Booth FW: Insulin-like growth factor immunoreactivity increases in muscle after acute eccentric contractions. *J Appl Physiol* 1993;74:410–414.
24. Colliander EB, Tesch PA: Responses to eccentric and concentric resistance training in females and males. *Acta Physiol Scand* 1991;141:149–156.
25. Tesch PA, Thorsson A, Colliander EB: Effects of eccentric and concentric resistance training on skeletal muscle substrates, enzyme activities and capillary supply. *Acta Physiol Scand* 1990;140:575–580.
26. Hather BM, Tesch PA, Buchanan P, et al: Influence of eccentric actions on skeletal muscle adaptations to resistance training. *Acta Physiol Scand* 1991;143:177–185.
27. Cannon JG, Kluger MJ: Endogenous pyrogen activity in human plasma after exercise. *Science* 1983;220:617–619.
28. Cannon JG, Evans WJ, Hughes VA, et al: Physiological mechanisms contributing to increased interleukin-1 secretion. *J Appl Physiol* 1986;61:1869–1874.
29. Baracos V, Rodemann HP, Dinarello CA, et al: Stimulation of muscle protein degradation and prostaglandin E_2 release by leukocytic pyrogen (interleukin-1): A mechanism for the increased degradation of muscle proteins during fever. *N Engl J Med* 1983;308:553–558.
30. Clowes GH Jr, George BC, Villee CA Jr, et al: Muscle proteolysis induced by a circulating peptide in patients with sepsis or trauma. *N Engl J Med* 1983;308:545–552.
31. Yang RD, Moldawer LL, Sakamoto A, et al: Leukocyte endogenous mediator alters protein dynamics in rats. *Metabolism* 1983;32:654–660.
32. Goldberg AL, Kettelhut IC, Furuno K, et al: Activation of protein breakdown and prostaglandin E_2 production in rat skeletal muscle in fever is signaled by a macrophage product distinct from interleukin-1 or other known monokines. *J Clin Invest* 1988;81:1378–1383.
33. Moldawer LL, Svaninger G, Gelin J, et al: Interleukin-1 and tumor necrosis factor do not regulate protein balance in skeletal muscle. *Am J Physiol* 1987;253:C766–C773.

34. Flores EA, Bistrian BR, Pomposelli JJ, et al: Infusion of tumor necrosis factor/cachectin promotes muscle catabolism in the rat: A synergistic effect with interleukin-1. *J Clin Invest* 1989;83:1614–1622.
35. Goodman MN: Tumor necrosis factor induces skeletal muscle protein breakdown in rats. *Am J Physiol* 1991;260:E727–E730.
36. Zamir O, Hasselgren PO, von Allmen D, et al: The effect of interleukin-1 alpha and the glucocorticoid receptor blocker RU 38486 on total and myofibrillar protein breakdown in skeletal muscle. *J Surg Res* 1991;50:579–583.
37. Fong Y, Moldawer LL, Marano M, et al: Cachectin/TNF of IL-1 alpha induces cachexia with redistribution of body proteins. *Am J Physiol* 1989;256:R659–R665.
38. Ballmer PE, McNurlan MA, Southorn BG, et al: Effects of human recombinant interleukin-1 beta on protein synthesis in rat tissues compared with a classical acute-phase reaction induced by turpentine: Rapid response of muscle to interleukin-1 beta. *Biochem J* 1991;279:683–688.
39. Cannon JG, Orencole SF, Fielding RA, et al: Acute phase response in exercise: Interaction of age and vitamin E on neutrophils and muscle enzyme release. *Am J Physiol* 1990;259:R1214–R1219.
40. Smith LL, McCammon M, Smith S, et al: White blood cell response to uphill walking and downhill jogging at similar metabolic loads. *Eur J Appl Physiol* 1989;58:833–837.
41. Babior BM, Kipnes RS, Curnutte JT: Biological defense mechanisms: The production by leukocytes of superoxide, a potential bactericidal agent. *J Clin Invest* 1973;52:741–744.
42. Smedly LA, Tonnesen MG, Sandhaus RA, et al: Neutrophil-mediated injury to endothelial cells: Enhancement by endotoxin and essential role of neutrophil elastase. *J Clin Invest* 1986;77:1233–1243.
43. Zerba E, Komorowski TE, Faulkner JA: Free radical injury to skeletal muscles of young, adult, and old mice. *Am J Physiol* 1990;258:C429–C435.
44. Colditz I, Zwahlen R, Dewald B, et al: In vivo inflammatory activity of neutrophil-activating factor, a novel chemotactic peptide derived from human monocytes. *Am J Pathol* 1989;134:755–760.
45. Young VR, Munro HN: Ntau-methylhistidine (3-methylhistidine) and muscle protein turnover: An overview. *Fed Proc* 1978;37:2291–2300.
46. Manfredi TG, Fielding RA, O'Reilly KP, et al: Plasma creatine kinase activity and exercise-induced muscle damage in older men. *Med Sci Sports Exerc* 1991;23:1028–1034.
47. Cannon JG, Fielding RA, Fiatarone MA, et al: Increased interleukin-1β in human skeletal muscle after exercise. *Am J Physiol* 1989;257:R451–455.
48. Cannon JG, Meydani SN, Fielding RA, et al: Acute phase response in exercise: II. Associations between vitamin E, cytokines, and muscle proteolysis. *Am J Physiol* 1991;260:R1235–R1240.
49. Fridén J, Sfakianos PN, Hargens AR: Muscle soreness and intramuscular fluid pressure: Comparison between eccentric and concentric load. *J Appl Physiol* 1986;61:2175–2179.
50. Carlson BM, Faulkner JA: The regeneration of skeletal muscle fibers following injury: A review. *Med Sci Sports Exerc* 1983;15:187–198.
51. Costill DL, Pascoe DD, Fink WJ, et al: Impaired muscle glycogen resynthesis after eccentric exercise. *J Appl Physiol* 1990;69:46–50.
52. Widrick JJ, Costill DL, McConell GK, et al: Time course of glycogen accumulation after eccentric exercise. *J Appl Physiol* 1992;72:1999–2004.
53. Vihko V, Salminen A, Rantamaki J: Exhaustive exercise, endurance training, and acid hydrolase activity in skeletal muscle. *J Appl Physiol* 1979;47:43–50.
54. Salminen A, Vihko V: Effects of age and prolonged running on proteolytic capacity in mouse cardiac and skeletal muscles. *Acta Physiol Scand* 1981;112:89–95.
55. Kasperek GJ, Conway GR, Krayeski DS, et al: A reexamination of the effect of exercise on rate of muscle protein degradation. *Am J Physiol* 1992;263:E1144–E1150.

56. Kameyama T, Etlinger JD: Calcium-dependent regulation of protein synthesis and degradation in muscle. *Nature* 1979;279:344–346.
57. Lewis SE, Anderson P, Goldspink DF: The effects of calcium on protein turnover in skeletal muscles of the rat. *Biochem J* 1982;204:257–264.
58. Rodemann HP, Waxman L, Goldberg AL: The stimulation of protein degradation in muscle by Ca^{2+} is mediated by prostaglandin E_2 and does not require the calcium-activated protease. *J Biol Chem* 1982;257:8716–8723.
59. Rodemann HP, Goldberg AL: Arachidonic acid, prostaglandin E_2 and F_2 alpha influence rates of protein turnover in skeletal and cardiac muscle. *J Biol Chem* 1982;257:1632–1638.
60. Baracos V, Greenberg RE, Goldberg AL: Influence of calcium and other divalent cations on protein turnover in rat skeletal muscle. *Am J Physiol* 1986;250:E702–E710.
61. Dayton WR, Schollmeyer JV: Immunocytochemical localization of a calcium-activated protease in skeletal muscle cells. *Exp Cell Res* 1981;136:423–433.
62. Leonard JP, Salpeter MM: Calcium-mediated myopathy at neuromuscular junctions of normal and dystrophic muscle. *Exp Neurol* 1982;76:121–138.
63. Rudge MF, Duncan CJ: Comparative studies on the role of calcium in triggering subcellular damage in cardiac muscle. *Comp Biochem Physiol* 1984;77:459–468.
64. Llados FT: Muscle damage induced by the ionophore A23187 can be prevented by prostaglandin inhibitors and leupeptin. *Experientia* 1985;41:1551–1552.
65. Goll DE, Dayton WR, Singh I, et al: Studies of the alpha-actinin/actin interaction in the Z-disk by using calpain. *J Biol Chem* 1991;266:8501–8510.
66. Reddy MK, Etlinger JD, Rabinowitz M, et al: Removal of Z-lines and alpha-actinin from isolated myofibrils by a calcium-activated neutral protease. *J Biol Chem* 1975;250:4278–4284.
67. Furuno K, Goldberg AL: The activation of protein degradation in muscle by Ca^{2+} or muscle injury does not involve a lysosomal mechanism. *Biochem J* 1986;237:859–864.
68. Belcastro AN, Parkhouse W, Dobson G, et al: Influence of exercise on cardiac and skeletal muscle myofibrillar proteins. *Mol Cell Biochem* 1988;83:27–36.
69. Belcastro AN: Skeletal muscle calcium-activated neutral protease (calpain) with exercise. *J Appl Physiol* 1993;74:1381–1386.
70. Jahngen JH, Haas AL, Ciechanover A, et al: The eye lens has an active ubiquitin-protein conjugation system. *J Biol Chem* 1986;261:13760–13767.
71. Fagan JM, Waxman L, Goldberg AL: Skeletal muscle and liver contain a soluble ATP+ubiquitin-dependent proteolytic system. *Biochem J* 1987;243:335–343.
72. Haas AL, Bright PM: The immunochemical detection and quantitation of intracellular ubiquitin-protein conjugates. *J Biol Chem* 1985;260:12464–12473.
73. Rechsteiner M: Natural substrates of the ubiquitin proteolytic pathway. *Cell* 1991;66:615–618.
74. Driscoll J, Goldberg AL: Skeletal muscle proteasome can degrade proteins in an ATP-dependent process that does not require ubiquitin. *Proc Natl Acad Sci USA* 1989;86:787-791.
75. Matthews W, Driscoll J, Tanaka K, et al: Involvement of the proteasome in various degradative processes in mammalian cells. *Proc Natl Acad Sci USA* 1989;86:2597–2601.
76. Riley DA, Bain JL, Ellis S, et al: Quantitation and immunocytochemical localization of ubiquitin conjugates within rat red and white skeletal muscles. *J Histochem Cytochem* 1988;36:621–632.
77. Riley DA, Bain JLW, Haas AL: Abstract: Increased ubiquitin conjugation of proteins during skeletal muscle atrophy. *J Cell Biol* 1986;103:401A.
78. Kasperek GJ, Snider RD: Total and myofibrillar protein degradation in isolated soleus muscles after exercise. *Am J Physiol* 1989;257:E1–E5.
79. Furuno K, Goodman MN, Goldberg AL: Role of different proteolytic systems in the degradation of muscle proteins during denervation atrophy. *J Biol Chem* 1990;265:8550–8557.

80. Medina R, Wing SS, Haas A, et al: Activation of the ubiquitin-ATP-dependent proteolytic system in skeletal muscle during fasting and denervation atrophy. *Biomed Biochim Acta* 1991;50:347–356.
81. Tawa NE Jr, Kettelhut IC, Goldberg AL: Dietary protein deficiency reduces lysosomal and nonlysosomal ATP-dependent proteolysis in muscle. *Am J Physiol* 1992;263:E326–E334.
82. Tawa NE Jr, Goldberg AL: Suppression of muscle protein turnover and amino acid degradation by dietary protein deficiency. *Am J Physiol* 1992;263:E317– E325.
83. Wing SS, Goldberg AL: Glucocorticoids activate the ATP-ubiquitin-dependent proteolytic system in skeletal muscle during fasting. *Am J Physiol* 1993;264:E668–E676.

Chapter 23
Mechanisms in the Initiation of Contraction-Induced Skeletal Muscle Injury

Robert B. Armstrong, PhD
Gordon L. Warren III, PhD
Dawn A. Lowe, PhD

Introduction

Contraction-induced skeletal muscle injury involves damage to subcellular components of muscle fibers (sarcomere level) and to associated connective tissue; it has been classified as type I skeletal muscle injury.[1] It results from exercise of muscles that are not conditioned for the particular intensity or duration of the activity. Whether or not type I skeletal muscle injury is a primary pathology in the repetitive motion disorders remains to be determined. Most data are compatible with a materials fatigue model for induction of the injury, which would predict that prolonged performance of relatively low stress contractions may result in muscle damage. There is mounting evidence that the damage plays a role in remodeling processes in muscles; under normal conditions the regeneration of injured muscle appears to be complete, with restoration of structure and improvements in function. However, in the presence of other muscle pathologies or predisposing conditions, recovery from contraction-induced injury may be impaired.

The obvious first question concerns the cause of contraction-induced injury. Hypotheses addressing the initiation of contraction-induced microinjury have been categorized as mechanical or metabolic.[2] There is evidence favoring both of these etiologies, although the mechanical hypothesis has the clearest experimental support. Factors involved in induction of contraction-induced injury will be discussed, followed by consideration of the site(s) of the initial lesions in the muscles.

Cause of Contraction-Induced Muscle Injury

In the context of repetitive motion disorders, it is appropriate to consider a materials fatigue model in discussing initiation of muscle microinjury. Figure 1 illustrates the model; the respective curves represent the numbers of contractions at a given level of stress required to induce materials failure. This model was recently discussed in some detail,[2] and presents three predictions. (1) When muscles perform contractions that generate high tensile stresses, relatively few contractile cycles will result in failure of some critical muscle component(s). The specific components that fail presumably constitute the site(s) of the ini-

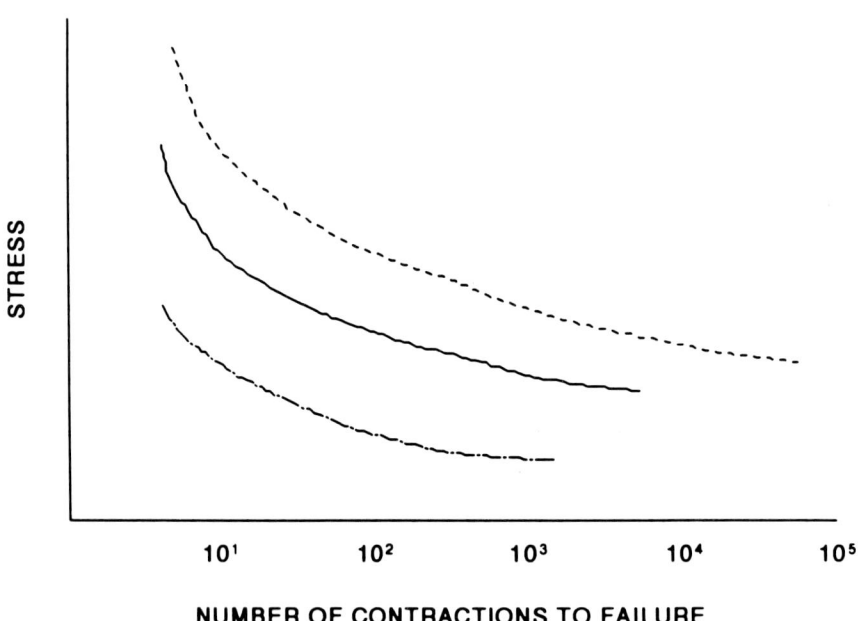

Fig. 1 Materials fatigue model for contraction-induced skeletal muscle injury. The solid curve represents the relationship for normal, healthy muscle; the dashed (**top**) line, for conditioned muscle (muscle trained with eccentric contractions); and the broken (**bottom**) line, for deconditioned muscle (muscle from subjects following bed rest, zero gravity conditions, or aging). The right limit for each curve represents the stress below which materials failure would not occur regardless of the number of contractile cycles.

tial lesions. When the muscle performs lower stress contractions, many contractile cycles must be completed before failure occurs. (2) There is a threshold stress, below which the muscle will not be injured irrespective of the number of contractile cycles (represented by the horizontal asymptote of each of the respective curves). (3) Conditioning the muscles (for example, exercise training with eccentric contractions) will shift the failure curve to the right, whereas deconditioning (for example, bed rest) will displace the curve to the left. Whereas most of the experimental work on muscle injury has used high force contractions (left portions of the curves), it seems probable that most repetitive motion injuries in the upper limb muscles result from relatively large numbers of contractions that generate lower stresses (right portions of the curves).

From studies on both animals and humans, it is clear that the magnitude of injury in muscles is directly related to the forces produced during the contractions.[3-5] Thus, eccentric contractions, in which the muscles are lengthened while active, produce the highest stresses and the greatest amount of injury. In the previous investigations on the relationship between force and injury, the separate contributions of lengthening velocity, length change, and initial length, all of which influence the forces produced during eccentric contractions, were not evaluated. The independent contributions of four mechanical factors (peak force, lengthening velocity, length change, and initial length) on injury in isolated rat soleus muscles were studied.[6] The data demonstrated that peak force is the primary factor in inducing damage as indicated by immediate reductions in maximal isometric tetanic force (P_o), although lengthening velocity also explains part of the variance.

The best test of the materials fatigue model in contraction-induced microinjury would be to determine the number of contractions to failure over a wide range of tensile stresses. This study has not been completed to date. However, there are a number of reports in the literature that can be interpreted to support the model. For example, Tiidus and Ianuzzo[5] found that both the forces produced by the muscles and the number of contractions were related to muscle soreness and enzyme release in human subjects. McCully and Faulkner[7] used an in situ mouse muscle preparation to study the relationship between the extent of injury from high force eccentric contractions and the duration of the exercise. They also found a linear relationship between injury and contraction number for ≤ 150 contractions, although with performance of 450 contractions, no further injury was observed. Similarly, Lieber and associates[8] reported a monotonic decrease in tension as a function of contraction number in rabbit tibialis anterior muscles performing eccentric contractions. After about 10 minutes of contractions, the eccentric forces approached an asymptote at approximately 40% of initial tension. The hypothesis that injury in an in vitro rat soleus muscle preparation would fit the materials fatigue model was tested.[9] When the muscles performed one through ten high-force (initial contraction produced 180% P_o) contractions, no significant declines in P_o immediately following the eccentric contractions occurred until after nine contractions. The sudden drop in P_o presumably resulted from materials fatigue of a critical force-producing or force-transmitting component of the muscle. More recent work using an in vivo mouse muscle injury model also supports the materials fatigue hypothesis. In this model, the foot of an anesthetized mouse is secured in a shoe affixed to a servomotor which is controlled by microcomputer. During percutaneous stimulation of the peroneal nerve the ankle undergoes plantar flexion so that the anterior crural muscles perform eccentric contractions. The tibialis anterior and extensor digitorum longus (EDL) muscles initially produce torques at the ankle during a 150-contraction protocol that average 2.07 times the maximal isometric tetanic torques (Fig. 2). The average torque progressively falls to an approximate asymptote of about 50% to 60% maximum by about the 50th contraction. However, individual muscles maintained initial torque levels for varying numbers of contractions before experiencing decreases. The P_o in isolated EDL muscles injured in this protocol has not recovered to baseline even after 14 days (Fig. 3).

The materials fatigue model of contraction-induced injury is based on materials science theory, so the implicit assumption is that the injury has a mechanical etiology. All studies support the important role of stress in induction of the pathology. However, the possibility that there is a metabolic component cannot be eliminated. Metabolic processes or products could affect the susceptibility of muscle structural components to stress. For example, Lieber and Fridén[10] have hypothesized that the greater injury observed in fast-twitch glycolytic (FG) fibers in their rabbit muscle injury model is caused by the relatively low oxidative capacity of the fibers. According to their hypothesis, these fibers fatigue during an eccentric contraction protocol. Because of their inability to maintain adenosine triphosphate (ATP) levels, they undergo rigor, and subsequent stretches of the stiff fibers result in mechanical disruption of force-producing or force-transmitting structures. Thus, in this hypothesis, there is a metabolic component in the susceptibility of the muscles to injury from high force eccentric exercise, even though the magnitude of injury would still be dic-

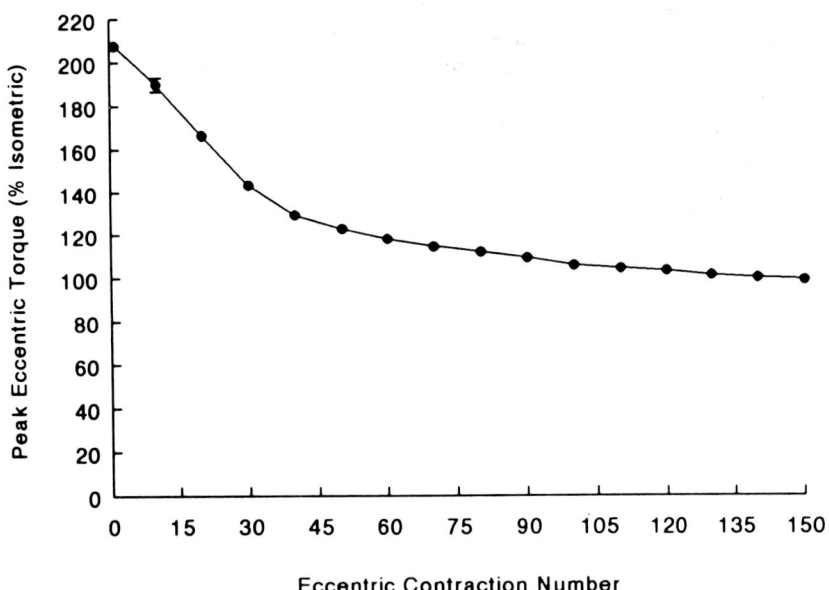

Fig. 2 Mean peak eccentric torques ± SEM (n = 65) as percent of maximal isometric torque produced by contraction of the anterior crural muscles at the ankle during stimulation of the peroneal nerve and plantar flexion of the ankle with a computer-controlled foot lever in anesthetized mice. Data were recorded every tenth contraction for 150 contractions. Although it is not apparent on the figure, individual muscles maintained initial peak torques for varying numbers of contractions, even though by the tenth contraction average torque had begun to decrease.

tated by the level of stress. In reference to the materials fatigue model (Fig. 1), a predisposing metabolic condition would effectively shift the failure curve to the left.

Two points may be made concerning their metabolic model. First, injury can be induced with eccentric contractions in the presence of normal muscle [ATP],[6] although admittedly whole muscle measurements may miss perturbations in high energy phosphate levels in small local regions that sustain damage. Second, the rapid adaptation in which resistance to injury is increased after only one conditioning bout of eccentric contractions[11] would seem to argue against the aerobic capacity of the muscle playing a primary role in susceptibility or resistance to damage. The time course of mitochondrial adaptation to exercise training is considerably longer.[12]

An alternative metabolic mechanism may also be proposed. Morgan[13] has hypothesized that injury from eccentric contractions results from sarcomere length inhomogeneities that develop during contractile activity. All sarcomeres in series are subjected to the same tensions during muscle contractions. "Weaker" sarcomeres are stretched farther than "stronger" sarcomeres, leading to reduced overlap of contractile filaments; i.e., weak sarcomeres are stretched onto the descending limb of the length-tension curve. Parallel elements at the level of the weak sarcomeres are then required to transmit more of the tension, leading to damage of these structures (plasmalemma, cytoskeleton). Although Morgan[13] did not discuss a metabolic influence, it seems possible that focal loss of energy balance could contribute to reductions in active

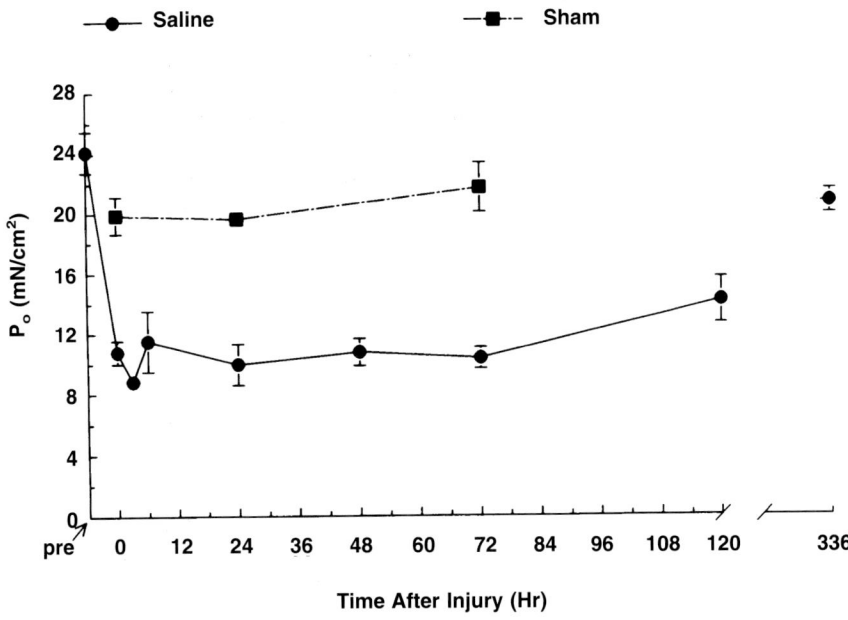

Fig. 3 Mean maximal isometric tetanic tensions (P_o) ± SEM (n = 4–6) for mouse EDL muscles that performed the eccentric contraction protocol described for Figure 2 or served as sham controls. P_o was measured in vitro in muscles isolated at different times between 0 hr and 14 days following the injury protocol.

force production in sarcomeres. Hence, a metabolic etiology could explain sarcomere length inhomogeneities and the resultant focal damage.

Whether or not there is a metabolic component in the etiology of the injury, the sarcomere inhomogeneity hypothesis is compatible with histologic data from a number of investigations, including those demonstrating the highly focal nature of the damage. Several studies have shown the injury is generally restricted to relatively small sections of some muscle fibers.[14–17] Containment of the injury within that focal region during later stages of the injury process (for example, during the phagocytic phase) is indicated by data from studies in which P_o has been followed during the postinjury period. Both human[18–20] and animal (Fig. 3) studies show that P_o is not reduced further from that observed immediately after the injury protocol during the phagocytic phase. Thus, contrary to some speculation, there does not appear to be an increase in the volume of involved tissue during the inflammatory or phagocytic period.[21] This is also supported by reports of the "walling off" of the lesions in the fibers[22,23] in other injury models, and the appearance of "plugs" that separate injured from normal sections of fibers in muscles that have performed eccentric contractions.[24]

Although muscle injury normally heals over time, there is evidence that continuous insults to the muscle result in chronic pathology. Hikida and associates[25] described the extensive damage that was evident in biopsies from the muscles of marathon runners both prior to and following a race competition. These observations suggest that continuous "overuse" of muscles can result in chronic muscle pathology.

Cellular Site of the Initial Lesion

The initial site of failure in the muscle fibers in contraction-induced injury is not known. In an effort to gain insight into this problem, we have performed studies to test various parts of the model shown in Figure 4, which is concerned with the early events in muscle injury. This model predicts that high tensile stresses produced during eccentric contractions damage contractile elements and/or structural elements in series (such as cytoskeletal proteins), contributing to the observed reductions in P_o. It also predicts that damage to the permeability barrier (plasmalemma, t-tubules) between the intracellular and extracellular spaces occurs, resulting in elevations in total muscle $[Ca^{2+}]$. As discussed earlier, sarcomere length inhomogeneities occurring during the contractions could explain disruption of parallel membrane components.[13] When the increases in total muscle $[Ca^{2+}]$ attain a threshold level, that is, when Ca^{2+} uptake by sarcoplasmic reticulum (SR) and mitochondria, Ca^{2+} binding by proteins, and Ca^{2+} extrusion by membrane pumps fail to counter influx of the ion through disruptions in the membranes, free cytosolic $[Ca^{2+}]$ rises. This leads to activation of Ca^{2+}-sensitive proteolytic and phospholipolytic pathways. Hence, the early events in the injury process are hypothesized to represent initial, Ca^{2+} overload, and autogenetic phases, all of which occur during the minutes or hours prior to invasion of the damaged tissue by inflammatory cells. Not shown in Figure 4 are the subsequent phagocytic and regenerative phases of the injury process that occur over days to weeks.

Experimental data generally support this model. As discussed in the preceding section on causes of contraction-induced injury, it has been demonstrated that the magnitude of injury is related to the peak forces produced during the exercise. There also is evidence of an early loss of integrity of the permeability barrier at specific sites in the injured fibers. Confocal laser scanning microscopy has shown that within the first several hours after performing high force eccentric contractions, discrete locations in the fibers swell, take up high molecular weight dextrans, lose normal t-tubular membrane structure as defined with membrane probes, and have elevated free cytosolic $[Ca^{2+}]$ (Fig. 5). Presumably the fibers lose cell membrane excitability in these swollen regions, although no differences were discernible in resting membrane potentials (from microelectrode measurements) between control and injured muscles.[26] There is vast literature on loss of intracellular enzymes and other proteins (such as myoglobin) into the circulation from injured muscles, but the latency between release from the cell and appearance in the blood prevent resolution of the precise time that the membranes are damaged. Immediately following downhill treadmill exercise in rats there are significant elevations of creatine kinase and lactate dehydrogenase activities in the plasma,[14] but because of the length of the exercise period (90 minutes), it is not possible to pinpoint the time of enzyme release from the injured muscles. In further support of the model (Fig. 4), studies show that within the first 2 hours following induction of injury in isolated mouse EDL muscles, there is an elevation in protein degradation.[27] Because the injury protocol and incubation were performed in vitro, the elevations in proteolysis presumably were caused by activation of proteolytic enzymes intrinsic to the muscle fibers. In this study, the rates of protein breakdown were not significantly related to the total $[Ca^{2+}]$ in the injured muscles. Two explanations for this are immediately apparent. First, proteolytic enzymes unrelated to Ca^{2+} were involved. Second, and in keeping with the model (Fig. 4), total $[Ca^{2+}]$ measurements probably do not provide accurate information about changes in free cytosolic $[Ca^{2+}]$ in the focal regions of damage

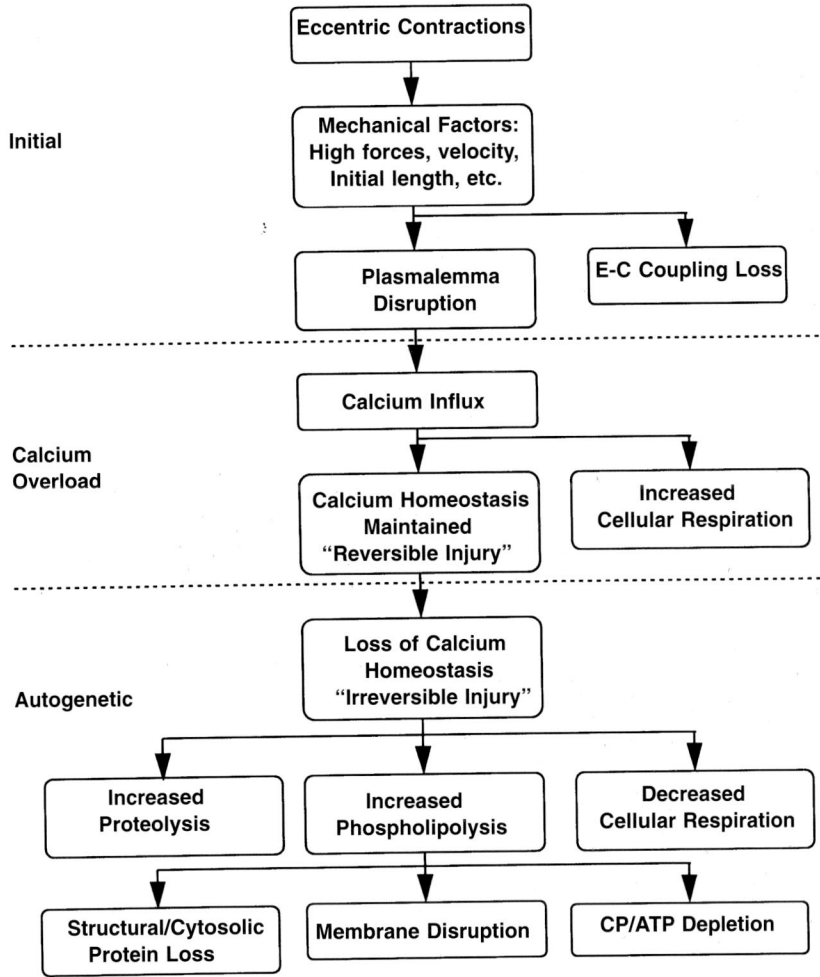

Fig. 4 Proposed theoretical model for the initiation and early stages of contraction-induced microinjury in skeletal muscle for the minutes to hours prior to invasion of the damaged tissue by inflammatory and phagocytic cells. This model is modified from that proposed earlier.[29]

in the muscles. As previously indicated,[24] focal regions in the injured muscles do show elevations in free cytosolic $[Ca^{2+}]$, but these lesions occupy a very small proportion of the total volume of the muscle.[24]

It is of interest to know which proteins in the muscle fibers are the first to be injured and/or degraded. Fridén and associates[28] recently reported that within 5 minutes of completion of eccentric contractions in rabbit EDL muscles there is a loss of the cytoskeletal protein desmin in some fibers. It is certainly possible that disruption of cytoskeleton from high tensile stresses (in long sarcomeres?) is the initial cellular event in the injury process. Disruption of cytoskeletal proteins could be responsible for the appearance of disarray in other cellular structures at both the light and electron microscopic levels. Disruption of banding patterns and Z-line disarray has been observed immediately after

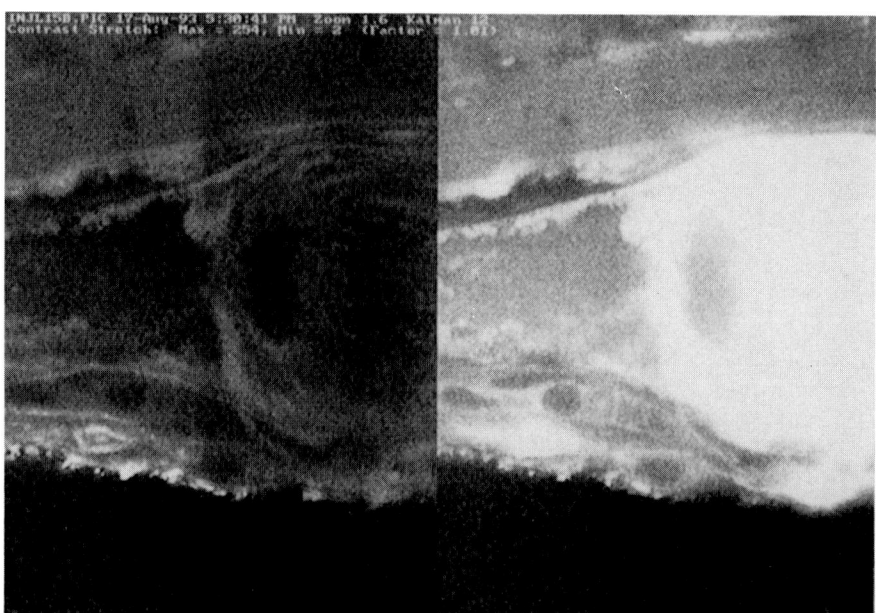
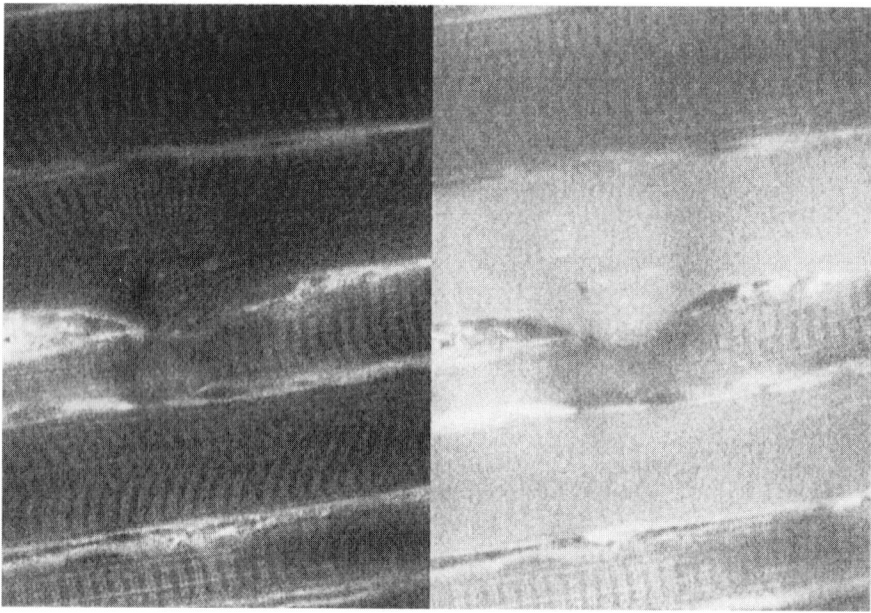

Fig. 5 A longitudinal optical section of two superfused mouse soleus muscle fibers simultaneously exposed to a membrane probe (DiOC$_{18}$) (**top**) and Texas Red–labeled dextran (MW 70,000) (**top right**) as viewed with a confocal laser scanning microscope. The fiber on the bottom has a swollen region that shows disruption of the normal transverse banding pattern and intense fluorescence from Texas Red, indicating failure of the permeability barrier. The photographs were taken within 2 hours following an eccentric contraction protocol. The swollen sections with intense Texas Red fluorescence were only observed in fibers that performed eccentric contractions; none were noted in muscles that performed isometric contractions or in controls. **Bottom left**, A longitudinal optical section of several superfused mouse soleus muscle fibers exposed to the probe and dextran (**bottom right**) described above as viewed with a confocal laser scanning microscope. This muscle also performed the eccentric contraction protocol. The second fiber from the top shows some swelling and disruption of banding pattern, whereas several of the other fibers display normal fluorescence patterns.

eccentric exercise prior to phagocyte invasion of the tissue in both in vivo and in vitro rodent models.[6,14]

Related to the question of which structures are first injured and/or degraded, it is of interest to know the cellular mechanism underlying the immediate and dramatic losses in contractile strength in muscles injured with eccentric contractions.[6,19,20] It is important to emphasize that these losses in strength are not explained by metabolic fatigue; the most obvious support for this contention is the fact that days are required for the muscle to recover (Fig. 3). Because of the appearance of disruptions in banding patterns, Z-lines, etc., in the muscles immediately after exercise, our assumption had been that damage to force producing and/or force transmitting structures was the explanation for the reductions in performance. However, a recent study[26] found that loss of excitation of the contractile apparatus explains a significant portion of the reductions in P_o. Mouse soleus muscles injured with eccentric contractions had reductions in P_o of about 43% compared with decreases of about 4% in muscles that performed isometric contractions. However, when the muscles then performed caffeine-induced contractions, there was no difference in force production between eccentric and isometric muscles after correcting for differences in initial P_o values; the eccentric contraction muscles in fact produced more force with the caffeine contractions than with electrical stimulation. What this suggests is that a significant proportion of the loss in P_o is due to failure to excite the SR to release Ca^{2+}, because caffeine directly stimulates SR Ca^{2+} release. To test whether the site of excitation failure was the plasmalemma, microelectrode measurements of resting membrane potential were made in muscles that completed an eccentric contraction injury protocol and in control muscles. We hypothesized that fibers in the injured muscles would show loss or attenuation of resting membrane potentials, which would support the contention that injury to the plasmalemma results in loss of the permeability barrier. However, no differences were observed between injured and control muscles. One explanation for this, as mentioned previously, is the focal nature of the damage in the fibers; it seems possible that because of the relatively small volume of injured tissue, it was not possible to demonstrate differences between groups. However, it is also possible that the site of the lesion is at the t-tubular level.[26]

Summary

Contraction-induced muscle microinjury fits a materials fatigue model, in which injury is caused by high stresses. According to this model, prolonged performance of suprathreshold stress contractions could result in damage to the muscles, and thus constitute a primary lesion in repetitive motion disorders; however, this possible etiology remains to be determined. One important characteristic of the injury is an immediate decrease in muscle performance, which continues over several weeks following the injury. The initial decline in muscle strength is partially explained by loss of excitation to the contractile apparatus. Muscles normally regenerate completely from this form of injury, and the pathology may serve as an important component in adaptation to overload.

Acknowledgments

The authors thank Mrs. Janene Kissinger and Mr. Todd Hoover for their help in preparing the manuscript.

References

1. Safran MR, Seaber AV, Garrett WE Jr: Warm-up and muscular injury prevention: An update. *Sports Medicine* 1989;8:239–249.
2. Armstrong RB, Warren GL, Warren JA: Mechanisms of exercise-induced muscle fibre injury. *Sports Medicine* 1991;12:184–207.
3. Katz B: The relation between force and speed in muscular contraction. *J Physiol* 1939;96:45–64.
4. McCully KK, Faulkner JA: Injury to skeletal muscle fibers of mice following lengthening contractions. *J Appl Physiol* 1985;59:119–126.
5. Tiidus PM, Ianuzzo CD: Effects of intensity and duration of muscular exercise on delayed soreness and serum enzyme activities. *Med Sci Sports Exerc* 1983;15:461–465.
6. Warren GL, Hayes DA, Lowe DA, et al: Mechanical factors in the initiation of eccentric contraction-induced injury in rat soleus muscle. *J Physiol* 1993;464:457–475.
7. McCully KK, Faulkner JA: Characteristics of lengthening contractions associated with injury to skeletal muscle fibers. *J Appl Physiol* 1986;61:293–299.
8. Lieber RL, Woodburn TM, Fridén J: Muscle damage induced by eccentric contractions of 25% strain. *J Appl Physiol* 1991;70:2498–2507.
9. Warren GL, Hayes DA, Lowe DA, et al: Materials fatigue initiates eccentric contraction-induced injury in rat soleus muscle. *J Physiol* 1993;464:477–489.
10. Lieber RL, Fridén J: Selective damage of fast glycolytic muscle fibres with eccentric contraction of the rabbit tibialis anterior. *Acta Physiol Scand* 1988;133:587–588.
11. Schwane JA, Armstrong RB: Effect of training on skeletal muscle injury from downhill running in rats. *J Appl Physiol* 1983;55:969–975.
12. Saltin B, Gollnick PD: Skeletal muscle adaptability: Significance for metabolism and performance, in Peachey LD (ed): *Handbook of Physiology, Section 10, Skeletal Muscle.* Bethesda, MD, American Physiological Society, 1983, pp 555–631.
13. Morgan DL: New insights into the behavior of muscle during active lengthening. *Biophys J* 1990;57:209–221.
14. Armstrong RB, Ogilvie RW, Schwane JA: Eccentric exercise-induced injury to rat skeletal muscle. *J Appl Physiol* 1983;54:80–93.
15. Ogilvie RW, Armstrong RB, Baird KE, et al: Lesions in the rat soleus muscle following eccentrically-biased exercise. *Am J Anat* 1988;182:335–346.
16. Kuipers H, Drukker J, Frederik PM, et al: Muscle degeneration after exercise in rats. *Int J Sports Med* 1983;4:45–51.
17. Fridén J, Sjöström M, Ekblom B: Myofibrillar damage following intense eccentric exercise in man. *Int J Sports Med* 1983;4:170–176.
18. Clarkson PM, Nosaka K, Braun B: Muscle function after exercise-induced muscle damage and rapid adaptation. *Med Sci Sports Med* 1992;24:512–520.
19. Howell JN, Chleboun G, Conatser R: Muscle stiffness, strength loss, swelling and soreness following exercise-induced injury in humans. *J Physiol* 1993;464:183–196.
20. Davies CT, White MJ: Muscle weakness following eccentric work in man. *Pflügers Archiv* 1981;392:168–171.
21. Smith LL: Acute inflammation: The underlying mechanism in delayed onset muscle soreness. *Med Sci Sports Exerc* 1991;23:542–551.
22. Carpenter S, Karpati G: Segmental necrosis and its demarcation in experimental micropuncture injury of skeletal muscle fibers. *J Neuropathol Exper Neurol* 1989;48:154–170.
23. Papadimitriou JM, Robertson TA, Mitchell CA, et al: The process of new plasmalemma formation in focally injured skeletal muscle fibers. *J Struct Biol* 1990;103:124–134.
24. Warren GL, Lowe DA, Hayes DA, et al: Cell membrane damage in exercise-induced muscle fiber injury. *Med Sci Sports Exerc* 1994;26:S124.

25. Hikida RS, Staron RS, Hagerman FC, et al: Muscle fiber necrosis associated with human marathon runners. *J Neurol Sci* 1983;59:185–203.
26. Warren GL, Lowe DA, Hayes DA, et al: Excitation failure in eccentric contraction-induced injury of mouse soleus muscle. *J Physiol* 1993;468:487–499.
27. Lowe, DA, Warren GL, Armstrong RB: Protein degradation in mouse soleus and EDL muscle following eccentric contraction-induced injury. *Med Sci Sports Exerc* 1994;26:S123.
28. Fridén J, Thornell LE, Lieber R: Muscle cytoskeletal disruption occurs within the first 15 minutes of cyclic eccentric contraction. *Med Sci Sports Exerc* 1994;26:S26.
29. Armstrong RB, Warren GL, Warren JA: Mechanisms of exercise induced muscle fibre injury. *Sports Med* 1991;12:184–207.

Directions for Future Research

The precise role, if there is one, that skeletal muscles play in the etiology and pathology of repetitive strain injury (RSI) is not known. Basic studies and numerous models have provided sufficient data about the structure and function of skeletal muscle to support the conclusion that skeletal muscles dramatically remodel, given the appropriate stimulus. The ability to make educated statements regarding RSI thus comes from extrapolating experimental studies in these related areas.[1] For example, conditions in which muscular use increases, such as voluntary exercise, hypergravity, compensatory hypertrophy (where synergists are ablated), chronic stretch, and electric stimulation, demonstrate that, as muscle use increases, contractile properties slow. Therefore, if muscle slowing could be demonstrated in RSI, it would be reasonable to call RSI a model of increased use. Similar studies can be performed and the results compared to more established models in order to define more precisely the role of skeletal muscle in RSI. A number of other studies are necessary to probe more significant issues, many of which are listed below.

Define the acute and chronic injury mechanisms in skeletal muscle.

Much of the difficulty in answering questions regarding the role of muscle in RSI results from a lack of understanding of muscle injury mechanisms that occur in well-defined models, such as eccentric contraction in animals. A good deal of evidence suggests that the initial injury events in skeletal muscle have a biomechanical basis, but the muscle structures most vulnerable to the mechanical stresses and strains placed on the fibers must be defined. These definitions should include the structures responsible for force generation (eg, actin and myosin), structural support proteins such as desmin, (α-actinin, titin and nebulin, and the connecting structures that link the myofibrils to the extracellular matrix.

After the initial injury events, inflammatory cells invade skeletal muscle and there is evidence that inflammatory-mediated injury can actually exceed that caused by the initial insult. Some studies suggest that this inflammation is actually <u>required</u> for proper remodeling (and perhaps for protection against further injury). Thus, the role of inflammation in helping a muscle to recover from an "injury" stimulus must be defined and, if inflammation is suppressed, it must be determined whether the muscle still recovers fully. With regard to RSI, because mechanical injury and subsequent inflammation can occur to any tissue, including muscle, tendon, or bone, it must be determined which is the "weak link" that actually initiates the sequence of events known as RSI.

Adequate tissue perfusion is required for tissue health and it is possible that altered perfusion secondary to interstitial fluid volume increase could initiate events that lead to RSI. For example, evidence exists that altered tissue perfusion itself may be painful in patients with chronic trapezius myalgia.[2] Thus, the role that compromised tissue perfusion and intramuscular pressure play in causing or exacerbating RSI must be determined. Such studies have been performed in the context of muscle injury secondary to tourniquet ischemia and compartment syndrome and have been shown to impart severe damage to muscle structure and function.

Define the role, if any, of altered muscle fiber recruitment patterns in RSI.

A difficulty in studying RSI is that there does not exist an adequate animal model as we know it. This may be because RSI does not develop in animals or because animals do not demonstrate the same clinical signs. Altered recruitment patterns may play a role in RSI because muscle fibers are recruited in an orderly fashion from slow motor units to fast fatigable motor units, which insures that the most fatigable units are rarely activated. To address this issue, reliable methods for measuring recruitment patterns must be developed in human models. Electromyography (EMG) probably will not provide this information[3] because data cannot be resolved to the motor unit level. Additionally, because human muscles do not demonstrate extreme fiber type distribution differences,[4] the strategy used in animal studies (whereby predominantly "slow" muscles are compared to predominantly "fast" muscles[5]) will not suffice for human studies. Such studies will probably require development of noninvasive methods, such as spectroscopy, magnetic resonance imaging, or positron emission tomography. Such studies would help define the recruitment patterns in muscle that occur during tasks that result in RSI. Because recruitment patterns can be trained, it may be possible to retrain an individual in order to alter the muscle activation pattern and thus prevent injury. Incidentally, if muscle recruitment patterns are a major factor in causing RSI, there are currently no studies underway that directly address this problem. This brings up the need to develop physiologically relevant models of repetitive muscle injury studies.

Define the conditioning methods required to prevent muscle injury.

Once a muscle is injured during eccentric exercise, this provides protection against further eccentric injury. However, it is not clear the extent to which exercise in one mode (eg, isometric exercise) can prevent injury performed in another mode (eg, eccentric contraction). With regard to RSI, it is not clear whether conditioning exercises should be performed in a mode similar to that used in a particular occupation or whether any type of exercise that increases strength and/or endurance will carry over to RSI prevention.

The frequency with which exercise should take place is also unanswered with respect to RSI. It had been demonstrated that the frequency of exercise that is most effective in strengthening muscle depends on the exact nature of the exercise performed. In eccentric training, a rest period of 1 to 2 days is optimal for strengthening human muscle. However, it is not known whether this is the time required for muscle remodeling to occur or whether it is the time required for the recovery of voluntary motivation and muscle activation. This is partly due to a lack of information regarding the mechanism of muscle damage and the mechanism(s) of action of protective exercise. Specific structural changes do occur in muscle after training, but it is not clear which of these changes, if any, protect the muscle against further injury. Because the mechanism of injury prevention cannot be determined in established models, it clearly is not possible at this time to define how often, if ever, muscles should be exercised to prevent RSI.

Determine clinical indicators of muscle dysfunction.

Obviously, it is much easier to quantify tissue properties, but clinical symptoms are usually the reason an individual is seeking medical attention. We currently do not have the ability to interpret altered muscle histology in terms of clinical symptoms in a clearly defined case of RSI. This is partly because a good RSI model does not exist and partly because there is a poor understanding of the source of muscular pain in RSI. It is not even clear whether the sensation of pain is an accurate predictor of tissue pathology. Thus, future studies must determine whether there are clinical measurements that can accurately predict impending muscle injury. In addition, such measurements must be standardized so that a broad base of information can be generated.

Determine the factor(s) that limit recovery degree and rate.

Finally, once a clear understanding of damage mechanisms are obtained and an appropriate model developed, it should be possible to address the key questions as to which tissue and systemic factors limit recovery after RSI. Because regeneration in skeletal muscle after traumatic injury or injury induced by myotoxic agents is affected by metabolic load, satellite cell number, innervation, activity level, and number of degeneration/regeneration cycles, it is reasonable to expect that these factors could also be involved in recovery from RSI.

References

1. Newham DJ: The consequences of eccentric contractions and their relationship to delayed onset muscle pain. *Eur J Appl Physiol* 1988;57:353–359.
2. Larsson SE, Ålund M, Cai H, et al: Chronic pain after soft-tissue injury of the cervical spine: Trapezius muscle blood flow and electromyography at static loads and fatigue. *Pain* 1994;57:173–180.
3. Jørgensen K, Fallentin N, Krogh-Lund C, et al: Electromyography and fatigue during prolonged, low-level static contractions. *Eur J Appl Physiol* 1988;57:316–321.
4. Edgerton VR, Smith JL, Simpson DR: Muscle fiber type populations of human leg muscles. *Histochem J* 1975;7:259–266.
5. Walmsley B, Hodgson JA, Burke RE: Forces produced by medial gastrocnemius and soleus muscles during locomotion in freely moving cats. *J Neurophysiol* 1978;41:1203–1216.

Section 5

Pathophysiology: Nerve

Section Editor:
Mary Ann Ruda, PhD

Lars B. Dahlin, MD, PhD
Göran Lundborg, MD, PhD
Ernst M. Noah, MD
Mary Ann Ruda, PhD

Donald A. Simone, PhD
Julia K. Terzis,
 MD, PhD, FRCS(C)

Overview

Injury to a nerve may represent an important component to the etiology of repetitive motion syndromes. The nerves carry pain messages from the site of peripheral tissue damage and thus are responsible for the noxious inputs that reach the central nervous system. Alternatively, injury to the nerve itself can be the source of the pain related to repetitve motion syndrome. If the nerve injury persists, the resultant pain may lead to central changes that occur in the neuronal circuitry that subserves nociception. These central changes may cause the patient to experience pain even after the injury itself has resolved following appropriate medical treatment. The chapters in this section will discuss important issues related to the role played by nerves in the repetitive motion syndrome.

Julia K. Terzis, MD, PhD, FRCS(C), and Ernst M. Noah, MD, lay the groundwork for a discussion of the role of the nerves in the upper extremity in repetitive motion syndromes. Their chapter presents the morphologic components that are the basis for nerve function. The anatomy of the upper extremity is presented in detail such that the unique aspects of the median, ulnar, axillary, and radial nerves are discussed individually. They also present information on the anatomic locations where the nerves are most vulnerable to compression, such as the cervical spine, brachial plexus, and other sites along the course of the nerve as it travels to its peripheral termination site. They end their chapter with a discussion of the types of potential nerve injuries such as compression injury with its subcomponents of ischemia, metabolic imbalance, and mechanical trauma.

Göran Lundborg, MD, PhD, and Lars B. Dahlin, MD, PhD, discuss the pathophysiology of nerve compression. Nerve injury may result from either acute trauma or chronic compression. Each situation has unique attributes and shares some common components. The authors address the multifactorial nature of the compression injury where the local microanatomy and topography of fascicles contribute differentially to the syndrome. The mechanical aspects of the compression injury are discussed in detail, especially with respect to data acheived from research in humans.

Donald A. Simone, PhD, addresses the peripheral neural mechanisms of muscle pain due to repetitive motion and inflammation. The classes of peripheral nociceptors are described in detail. Results of intraneural microstimulation and microneurography techniques in humans are used to characterize electrophysiologic responses of muscle nociceptors in humans. Muscle pain sensation is that of a "cramp" that is evoked by either group III or group IV afferent fibers. Repetitive motion may work through sensitization or spontaneous activity in these two groups of fibers.

Mary Ann Ruda, PhD, discusses alterations in gene expression in response to nerve injury. Using in situ hybridization and ribonucleic acid (RNA) blot analysis it is possible to determine the molecular response to nerve injury as reflected in induction or repression of individual gene expression. When the neuronal response to nerve cut is compared to that in a nerve constriction injury model, both appear to result in similar regulation of several peptide genes and transcription factor genes. The comparable changes seen after total nerve transection and constriction injury suggest that the stimuli evoking these alterations in gene expression are similar in both cases.

Chapter 24

Anatomy and Morphology of Upper Extremity Nerves and Frequent Sites of Compression

Julia K. Terzis, MD, PhD, FRCS(C)
Ernst M. Noah, MD

Introduction

One possible etiology of repetitive strain injury is an entrapment of peripheral nerves. A cumulative trauma injury caused by the overuse of muscle tendon units leads to inflammation, which is followed by pain and edema. The prevalence of repetitive strain injury is high among certain occupations, such as manufacturing assemblers, meat cutters, textile mill workers, and other workers who perform high-speed repetitive tasks for long, uninterrupted periods.

Rapid, repetitive, and forceful movements, particularly if they are associated with heavy static load or tensed postures, may lead to localized muscle fatigue or even ischemic and metabolic changes. The affected muscles and tendons are more subject to microtears and inflammatory changes that result in pain and impaired muscle function. These inflamed or thickened muscles or tendons and tendon sheaths might also compress adjacent peripheral nerves, resulting subsequently in a compression ischemic injury of the nerve.[1–4] Such situations may occur especially when a nerve passes through a fibrous or fibroosseous tunnel or under a constricting fibrous band, fascial or bony edge, or blood vessels.

Although the cumulative trauma in these performances is held responsible for the injury, anatomic features in the upper limb that are related to nerve entrapments have to be considered. The goal of this chapter is to give an overview of the macroscopic and microscopic morphology of peripheral nerves in the upper limb as well as to show sites for possible nerve entrapment.

Morphology of Peripheral Nerves

The peripheral nervous system is a complex composite structure of axons within their supportive cells, the Schwann cells, the Schwann cells' associated connective tissue sheaths, and the end organs these processes supply. The central nervous system receives incoming signals from the periphery through incoming or afferent fibers, the cell bodies of which are located in the dorsal root ganglion, and send impulses through outgoing or efferent motor fibers originating within the ventral horn of the spinal cord (Fig. 1).

The neurons interface with one another by multiple dendritic synapses.[5] Each neuron generally sends a single axon to the periphery. The axon is bounded by

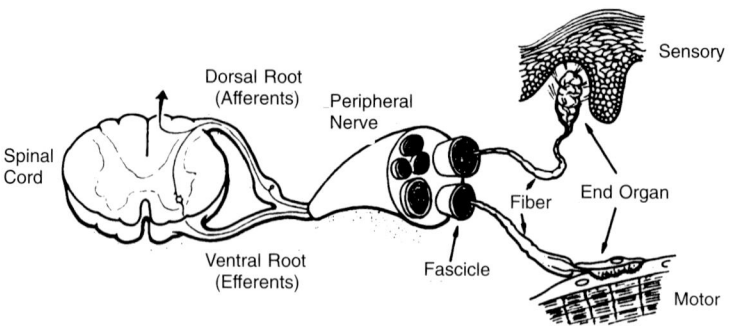

Fig. 1 Diagrammatic depiction of a peripheral nerve with its central and peripheral connections. (Reproduced with permission from Terzis JK, Smith KL (eds): *The Peripheral Nerve: Structure, Function and Reconstruction.* New York, NY, Raven Press, 1990, p 2.)

the trilaminar axolemma, which, with the help of a sodium-potassium-ATPase (adenosine triphosphatase) pump, maintains a resting electrical potential of about -70 mV by altering the intra- and extracellular concentration of monovalent ions.[6] The electrochemical gradient endows the neuron and axon with the property of excitability by depolarization of its membrane.

All axons are ensheathed by Schwann cells, which produce myelin. The Schwann cells appear with or slightly ahead of the axons.[7] Initially, each Schwann cell has multiple bundles of immature axons within its cytoplasm.[8] For those axons destined to remain unmyelinated (50% to 80% of the average nerve fiber population),[9] groups of eight to 15 axons eventually come to lie within individual enfoldings of the Schwann cell membrane.[10] In axons that become myelinated, the invaginating Schwann cell lays down many layers of specialized cell membrane by spiraling around the axon perimeter (Fig. 2).

The myelin sheath is a proteophospholipid multilayered spiral of compacted apposed cell membranes, which have extruded the Schwann cell cytoplasm from within.[11] The myelin insulation divides the axon into short regions (nodes of Ranvier; 1 to 2 mm), which are capable of depolarization, and longer regions (internodes of 16 to 19mm), which are unable to generate an action potential. Conduction proceeds by sequential activation of successive nodes without depolarization of the intervening internode. Bundles of these axons make up the spinal roots (dorsal and ventral), which join just distal to the sensory ganglion to form the appropriate spinal nerves. Nerve fibers, efferent or afferent, travel in bundles, termed fascicles, that are bound by supportive connective tissue, the perineurium (Fig. 3).

Within the fascicle, nerve fibers are packed in a mucopolysaccharide ground substance supported by the endoneurium, which consists of longitudinally oriented collagen fibrils and reticulum fibers.[12,13] The next level of organization is the perineurium, which is the connective tissue condensation around individual nerve fascicles. The perineurium consists of an inner layer of lamellated squamous-like cells and an outer layer of collagen fibers condensed into a lattice of longitudinal, circumferential, and oblique bundles.[12,14] In this way, the perineurium furnishes a strong support for the enclosed neural tissue and contributes to the tensile strength of the peripheral nerve. The perineurium is a spe-

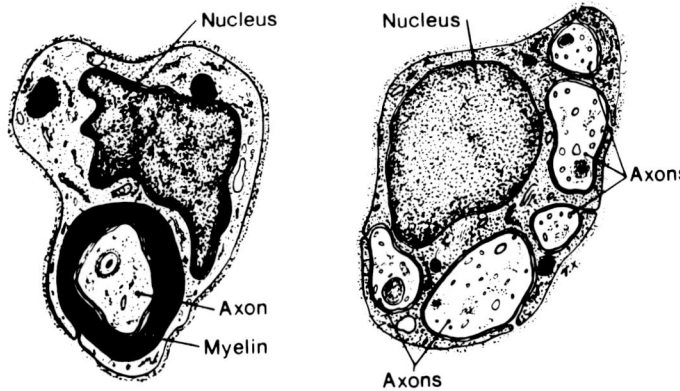

Fig. 2 Schematic drawing of a cross section of a myelinated (**left**) and an unmyelinated (**right**) nerve fiber. Note that there are numerous axons within the Schwann cell envelope in the unmyelinated fiber, whereas only one Schwann cell is associated with the myelinated axon. (Reproduced with permission from Millesi H, Terzis JK: Nonenclature in peripheral nerve surgery, in Terzis JK (ed): *Microreconstruction of Nerve Injuries*. Philadelphia, PA, WB Saunders, 1987, p 5.)

cialized structure that also serves as a diffusion barrier similar to the pia arachnoid in the central nervous system.[5]

The final supportive ensheathment of the peripheral nerve is the epineurium, a loose sheath that consists of the perifascicular and interfascicular connective tissue around and between the nerve fascicles. Its outer layers are continuous with the mesoneurium, the suspensory mesentery of the peripheral nerve, which arises from the areolar connective tissue of the underlying fascia. The innermost layers come in close apposition with the perineurium.[15]

Four basic patterns of intraneural architecture can be recognized. Peripheral nerves that contain one large fascicle are termed monofascicular. Those that contain a few fascicles are considered oligofascicular, and the term polyfascicular signifies multiple fascicles in one nerve segment.

As signal conduction requires a high energy mechanism, there is a specific vascular system supplying the nerve. Blood vessels of various diameters originating from adjacent vessels enter the nerve via the mesoneurium in a segmental pattern.[16] As these nutrient vessels reach the epineurium, they ramify within the epineurium and supply an internal plexus through ascending and descending branches.[17] Blood vessels transverse the perineurium connecting the vascular network of the epineurium with that of the endoneurium.[16] The endoneurial endothelial cells are connected to each other by tight junction and prevent the extravasation of proteins within the endoneurial space. These vessels, together with the perineurium, form the blood-nerve barrier.[5]

Anatomy of the Nerves of the Upper Extremity

The Brachial Plexus

Supraclavicular Part The brachial plexus (Fig. 4) is formed by the ventral rami of the spinal nerves of C5 to T1, and it is situated in the posterior triangle of the neck between the scalenus anterior and medius muscles. Emerging from the scalenus gap, the nerve fibers are joined together to form the primary

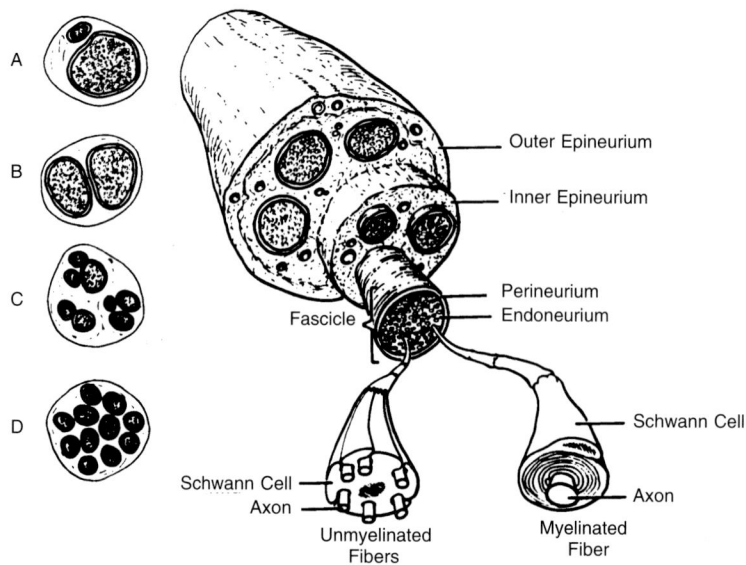

Fig. 3 Schematic drawing of peripheral nerve architecture. The connective tissue elements are described in the text. Note the inner and outer epineurial sheath. On the left, basic patterns of intraneural fascicular composition are demonstrated: **(A)** monofascicular, **(B)** oligofascicular, **(C)** polyfascicular pattern with distinct fascicular grouping and **(D)** without definitive fascicular arrangement. (Adapted with permission from Terzis JK, Smith KL (eds): *The Peripheral Nerve: Structure, Function and Reconstruction.* New York, NY, Raven Press, 1990, p 16.)

trunks. The roots of C5 and C6 unite to form the upper trunk, root C7 continues as the middle trunk, and the roots of C8 and T1 form the lower trunk. Subsequently, the nerve trunks divide into an anterior branch, which carries fibers to the flexor side of the upper limb, and a posterior branch, which supplies the extensor muscles of the extremity.[18]

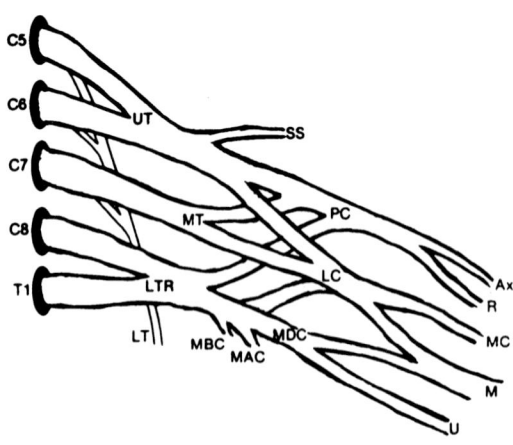

Fig. 4 Schematic drawing of the human brachial plexus. UT = upper trunk; MT = middle trunk; LTR = lower trunk; LT = long thoracic; SS = suprascapular; PC = posterior cord; LC = lateral cord; MDC = medial cord; MBC = medial brachii cutaneous; MAC = medial antebrachii cutaneous; Ax = axillary; R = radial; MC = musculocutaneous; M = median; and U = ulnar nerves. (Reproduced with permission from Terzis JK, Smith KL (eds): *The Peripheral Nerve: Structure, Function and Reconstruction.* New York, NY, Raven Press, 1990, p 16.)

In most cases, this division is localized in the supraclavicular part of the plexus. Direct muscular branches from this supraclavicular part are the dorsal scapular nerve (C5; rhomboid and levator scapula muscles), suprascapular nerve (C5,6; supra- and infraspinatus muscles), long thoracic nerve (C5-7; serratus anterior muscle) and the nerve to the subclavius muscle (C5,6).

Infraclavicular Part Surrounded by a fascia from the deep cervical fascia, the anterior branches of the upper and middle trunk form the lateral cord (C5-7) and the anterior branches of the lower trunk form the medial cord (C8,T1). All dorsal branches unite to form the posterior cord (C5-T1). According to their names, these cords are organized around the axillary artery in the axillary sheath and supply the shoulder with short branches and the distal limb with long branches. In this infraclavicular part of the brachial plexus, the basic organization into ventral flexor branches and dorsal extensor branches may be used to describe the different nerves.

The ventral short branches to the shoulder are the medial (C8,T1; medial cord) and lateral pectoral nerve (C5-7; lateral cord) to the pectoralis major and minor muscles. The dorsal short branches arise from the posterior cord. The subscapular nerve (C5-7) supplies the subscapularis muscle and usually the teres major muscle. The thoracodorsal nerve (C6-8) passes through the axilla to supply the latissimus dorsi muscle and occasionally the teres major muscle.

The ventral long branches of the infraclavicular part arise from the lateral and medial cord. The musculocutaneous nerve (C5-7) arises from the lateral cord, gives a branch to the coracobrachialis muscle; descends beneath the biceps brachii muscle and on the brachialis muscle, thereby innervating all the flexors of the arm; and terminates as the lateral antebrachial cutaneous nerve at the radial side of the forearm.

From the medial cord, the medial brachial cutaneous nerve (T1) arises to supply the medial skin of the arm from the axilla to the elbow; it is assisted by the intercostobrachialis nerve (T2). The medial antebrachial cutaneous nerve (C8,T1) courses at the medial side of the axillary artery and innervates the skin at the medial flexor side of the forearm (anterior branch) and the upper two-thirds of the ulnar side of the forearm (posterior branch). The posterior cord (C5-T1) gives off the nerves for the extensor muscles of the arm, and after supplying the posterior muscles of the shoulder it divides into the axillary nerve and the radial nerve.

The Median Nerve

The median nerve supplies most of the flexors of the forearm and hand as well as the skin of the wrist, the thenar eminence, the palm of the hand, and the volar side of the radial three and one-half fingers. It has a lateral root from the lateral cord (C6,7) and a medial root from the medial cord (C8,T1), which unite around the distal part of the axillary artery lateral to the vessel. In the middle of the arm, the median nerve crosses the brachial artery to reach its medial side. It passes across the elbow joint, giving an articular branch to the capsule, beneath the aponeurosis of the biceps brachii muscle, and in front of the insertion of the brachialis muscle. The nerve enters the forearm between the two heads of the pronator muscle. The nerve traverses between the superficial head of the pronator teres, which arises from the medial epicondyle and supracondylar ridge of the humerus (humeral head) and the deep head, which arises from the medial aspect of the coronoid process of the ulna (ulnar head). Fibrous bands at the dorsal surface of the superficial head are found in approximately 50% of anatomic specimens. In 40% of specimens, a fibrous band dorsal to the nerve arising from either a part of the deep ulnar head or directly from the coronoid process is found.[19] The nerve continues on the posterior surface of the flexor digitorum superficialis muscle and lies on the flexor digitorum profundus muscle. Muscular branches innervate the pronator teres, flexor carpi radialis, and the flexor digitorum superficialis. After passing through the pronator muscle, the median nerve gives rise to the anterior interosseous nerve, which supplies the flexor pollicis longus, the flexor digitorum profundus, and the pronator quadratus muscles.

A short distance before entering the carpal tunnel, the palmar cutaneous branch exits on the radial side of the median nerve to supply the skin of the lateral part of the palm. The main part of the median nerve passes through the carpal tunnel lateral to the tendon of the flexor pollicis longus muscle, and spreads out in three common palmar digital nerves, small branches to the lumbrical muscles I, II, (III), and terminates in the proper palmar digital nerves, which supply the skin of the palmar side of three and one-half fingers on the radial side.

The Ulnar Nerve

The ulnar nerve supplies the ulnar flexors at the forearm and hand and the skin of the ulnar side of the hand and the ulnar fingers. It arises from the medial cord of the infraclavicular part of the brachial plexus (C8,T1). It leaves the axilla at the medial side of the artery, passes through the medial brachial intermuscular septum into the extensor compartment of the arm, and courses down behind the medial epicondyle of the humerus below the tendinous arch between the humeral and ulnar heads of the flexor carpi ulnaris muscle. After it innervates this muscle it descends behind this muscle distally and eventually it comes to be adjacent to the ulnar artery. Another muscular branch innervates the ulnar part of the flexor digitorum profundus muscle. Proximal to the flexor retinaculum, the dorsal cutaneous branch of the ulnar nerve exits to supply the skin of the ulnar side of the dorsum of the hand and terminates in the dorsal digital nerves to supply the one and one-half ulnar fingers.

The main part of the nerve divides at the flexor retinaculum into a superficial and a deep branch. On the flexor retinaculum, the nerve passes the ulnar canal (Guyon's canal), which is formed on the lateral side by the pisiform bone and on the medial side by the hamulus of the hamate bone at the hypothenar eminence.

The superficial branch of the ulnar nerve descends into the palm of the hand on the ulnar side of the superficial arch innervating the palmaris brevis muscle and terminates into the proper palmar digital nerves to supply the ulnar one and one-half digits.

The deep branch of the ulnar nerve accompanies the deep palmar branch of the ulnar artery between the abductor digiti minimi and the flexor digiti minimi muscles and pierces the opponens digiti minimi. It innervates these muscles, all palmar and all dorsal interossei muscles, the third and fourth lumbricals, the adductor pollicis, and usually the deep head of the short flexor of the thumb. It also gives articular branches to the carpal joint.

The Axillary Nerve

The axillary nerve (C5,6) separates from the posterior cord and passes through the quadrangular space behind the humerus. It innervates the teres minor muscle and the deltoid muscle. Its cutaneous fibers form the superior lateral brachial cutaneous nerve and supply an area of skin above the deltoid muscle.

The Radial Nerve

The radial nerve supplies the extensor muscles of the arm and forearm and the skin at the dorsal side of the arm and the posterior side of the dorsum of the hand. It arises from the posterior cord, descends behind the axillary and brachial arteries, and passes posterior with the deep brachial artery between the long and medial heads of the triceps muscle. Then it curves around the humerus, lying in the spiral groove for the radial nerve (radial canal), and enters the flexor compartment in the elbow through the lateral intermuscular septum. At the axilla, the radial nerve forms the branches that innervate the three heads of the triceps muscle and the anconeus muscle. In the axilla, the nerve gives off the posterior brachial cutaneous nerve to the lateral side of the arm. In the radial canal, the inferior brachial cutaneous nerve separates to supply the skin of the dorsolateral part of the arm, and the posterior antebrachial cutaneous nerve arises to supply the skin of the dorsal side of the forearm.

After piercing the lateral intermuscular septum, the nerve lies between the brachialis and biceps tendons. Anterior to the humeroradial joint it enters the radial tunnel, a defined anatomic region. The tunnel is barely 5 cm long, begins proximally at the level of the capitellum of the humerus, and continues to the end of the supinator muscle. The tunnel is bounded medially by the brachialis muscle and anterolaterally by the brachioradialis muscle and the extensor carpi radialis longus muscle. In this proximal portion of the tunnel, the radial nerve innervates the adjacent muscles and gives branches to the periosteum of the lateral epicondyle and the capsule of the radiohumeral joint, including the annular ligament. At this level, the nerve divides into the superficial branch and the deep branch. The branches are still adjacent to each other and lie in fatty tissue. Slightly more distal, the nerves come in contact with the extensor carpi radialis brevis muscle. Distal to the origin of the muscle, the nerves lie in close relation to the neck of the radius and are crossed by a leash of vessels from the radial recurrent artery. Somewhere at this point the branches separate.[20]

The superficial branch of the radial nerve, a sensory nerve, descends under cover of the brachioradialis muscle on the lateral side of the radial artery. Proximal to the wrist it passes dorsally under the tendon of the brachioradialis muscle and winds around the lateral surface of the radial bone onto the extensor side to supply the dorsum of the hand (snuffbox) and the fingers with its 4-5 dorsal digital nerves. At the dorsum, there is a communicating branch with the ulnar nerve.

The deep branch of the radial nerve curves around the lateral side of the neck of the radius and pierces the supinator muscle to enter the posterior compartment of the forearm. With its terminal branch, the posterior interosseous nerve passes the extensor pollicis longus muscle onto the dorsal side of the interosseous membrane adjacent to the posterior interosseous artery. Muscular branches separate to innervate the extensor carpi radialis brevis, supinator, extensor digitorum, extensor digiti minimi, extensor carpi ulnaris, abductor pollicis longus, extensor pollicis brevis et longus, and the extensor indicis muscles. The nerve ramifies at the wrist joint.

Anatomic Mousetraps for Peripheral Nerves

Nerve compressions affect peripheral nerves at the anatomic locations where the nerves are most vulnerable, which are usually deep fibrous bands or tendinous or muscular arches. Understanding of these sites and knowledge of the anatomic pathways of nerves are obviously important in the evaluation of any neuropathy.

The Cervical Spine

As the spinal nerve passes through the intervertebral foramina, it might be compressed by any factor that decreases the diameter of the spinal foramen or stretches the roots. Most commonly, compression is caused by degenerated disks and diseased intervertebral joints. However, this compression might be aggravated by working in hyperextended positions for long periods or by repeated flexion of the neck (for example, by painters, cash register operators, and dental surgeons).[21] It was reported in 1993 that young dancers who perform headbanging suffer from syndromes similar to whiplash injuries.[22]

The Brachial Plexus

The brachial plexus could be irritated by such anatomic variations as a congenital cervical rib, an axillary arch, or even an accessory muscle (eg, the chondroepitrochlear muscle).[23] More often, the nerves of the brachial plexus are compressed as they pass through the scalenus gap. Numbness and pain can occur in the distal upper extremity, especially when the extremity is thrown back and the hand is raised (Fig. 5).[24] These syndromes (Outline 1) might be associated with occupations that require frequent reaching above the shoulder, prolonged carrying of heavy loads, or even wearing a knapsack.[25] Affected occupations include automobile repair mechanics, overhead assemblers, stockroom and shipping workers and grinders.[24]

Isolated lesions of individual nerves of the brachial plexus may occur due to occupational overuse, but are more significant in athletes.[26] In rare cases, shoulder pain may be related to an entrapment of the suprascapular nerve. There are three sites at which the suprascapular nerve might be injured: at its origin at Erb's point; at the suprascapular notch beneath the transverse scapular ligament; or at the spinoglenoid notch, the point at which the nerve passes around the scapular spine to enter the infraspinous fossa.[27] Lesions are reported in overhead workers, volleyball players, pitchers, dancers, and individuals involved in any of a variety of activities that require repeated wide excursions of the scapula.[21,28–31]

The long thoracic nerve might be stretched or damaged by its course through the scalenus medius muscle. Shah and Stefaniwsky[32] reported a young paraplegic man who frequently used a trapeze to mobilize himself in bed. After 4 months of repetitive body elevation, he suffered a winging scapula caused by nerve compression. Electrophysiologic studies of the long thoracic nerve revealed an increased nerve conduction time. Other case reports describe sports-related injuries.[33–36]

Cahill and Palmer[37] described the quadrilateral space syndrome, in which the axillary nerve is entrapped when it passes through the quadrilateral space, resulting in deltoid weakness with decreased shoulder abduction. Other cases of chronically irritated axillary nerves have been described.[38,39]

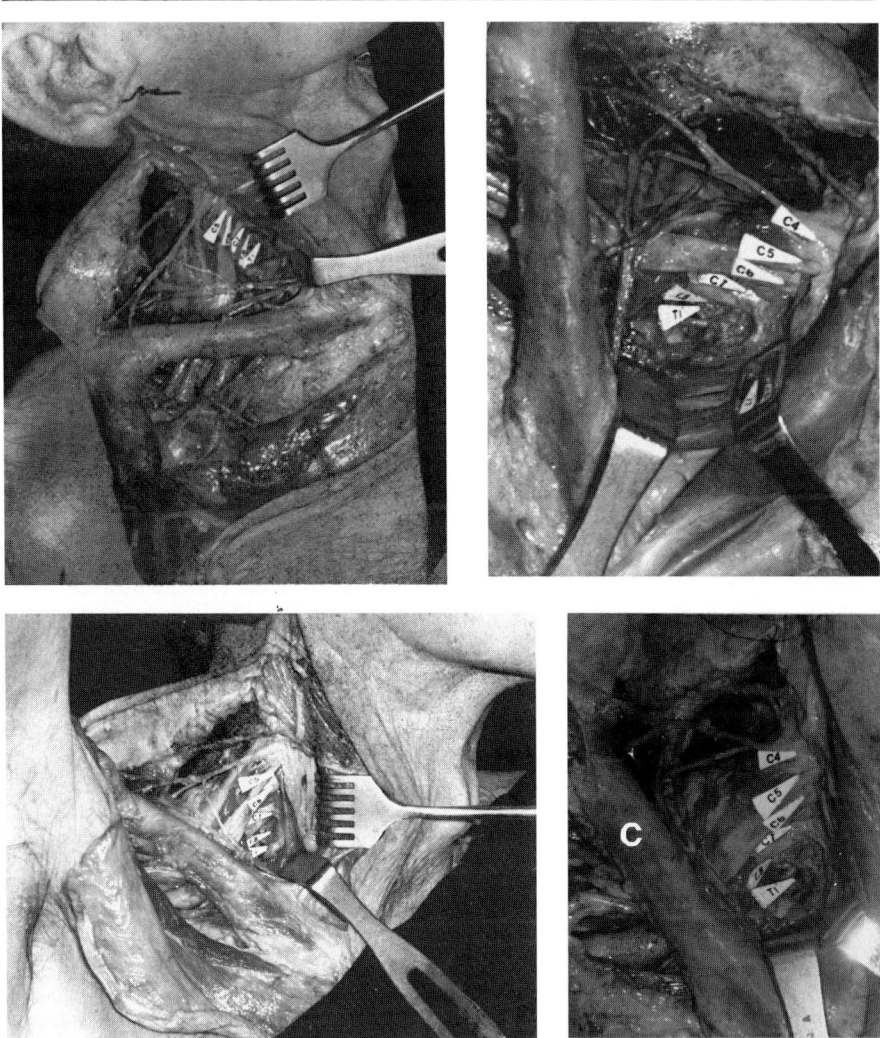

Fig. 5 Dissection of the brachial plexus in the anatomic position **(top left** and **top right)**. Note the impingement of the nerve trunks between the clavicle **(C)** and the first rib when arm is elevated **(bottom left** and **bottom right)**.

Outline 1 Neurologic symptoms of thoracic outlet syndrome

Neck pain

Paresthesia in ulnar side of hand

Intrinsic muscle weakness

In the axilla, the musculocutaneous nerve is vulnerable when piercing the coracobrachialis muscle. Proximal entrapments of the musculocutaneous nerve after exercise have been described; these entrapments might have been related to hypertrophy of the coracobrachialis muscle.[40,41] Sensory neuropathies can be caused by compression of the cutaneous branch of the musculocutaneous nerve under the aponeurosis or the tendon of the biceps brachii muscle. Felsenthal and associates[42] described nerve damage after acute compression due to heavy packing loaded the elbow or after exercise with hyperextension of the elbow.[40] Extensive repetitive supination, such as that used for inserting screws, might also lead to reduced nerve conduction.[43]

The Median Nerve

In a manner similar to the cutaneous branch of the musculocutaneous nerve, the median nerve might be affected by the aponeurosis of the biceps brachii tendon. Cases of an accessory bicipital aponeurosis, some originating from a third head of the biceps brachii muscle (Fig. 6) have been reported. Flexing the elbow compresses the median nerve.[44]

On its way down the arm, the median nerve might be affected by the "Ligament of Struthers."[45] In rare cases, this accessory ligament arises from the tip of a supracondylar bony spur to the medial epicondyle of the humerus, compressing the passing median nerve, especially in lateral rotation.[46] Care must be taken to avoid mistaking this ligament for the "Arcade of Struthers."

In the elbow, the median nerve passes between the two heads of the pronator teres muscle and under the edge of the flexor digitorum superficialis (Fig. 7). The nerve can be entrapped by either structure.[47] This pronator teres syndrome often presents as repetitive strain injury in athletes and in such workers as carpenters, mechanics, and writers.[4,48]

At the level of the pronator teres, the anterior interosseous nerve separates from the median nerve. This pure motor branch supplies the radial half of the flexor digitorum profundus, the flexor pollicis longus, and the pronator quadra-

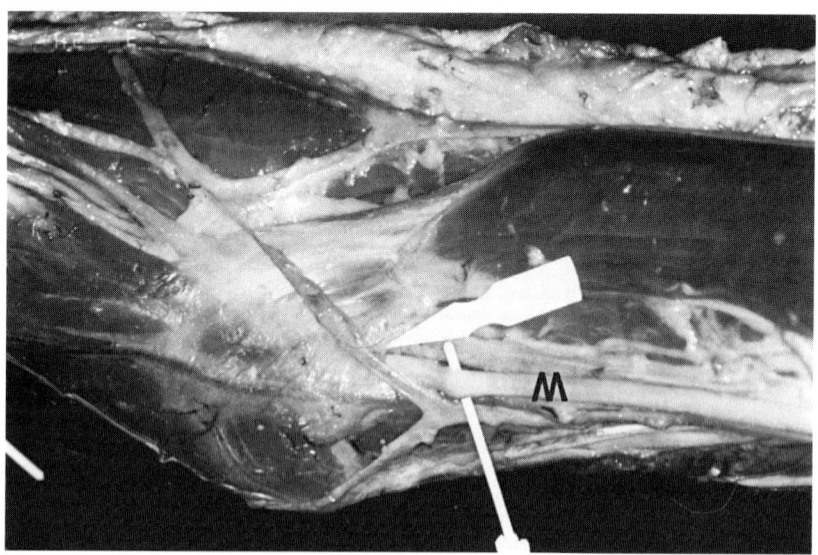

Fig. 6 Anterior aspect of the right arm-elbow region. The median nerve (M) can be compressed under the bicipital aponeurosis (arrow) of the biceps brachii muscle.

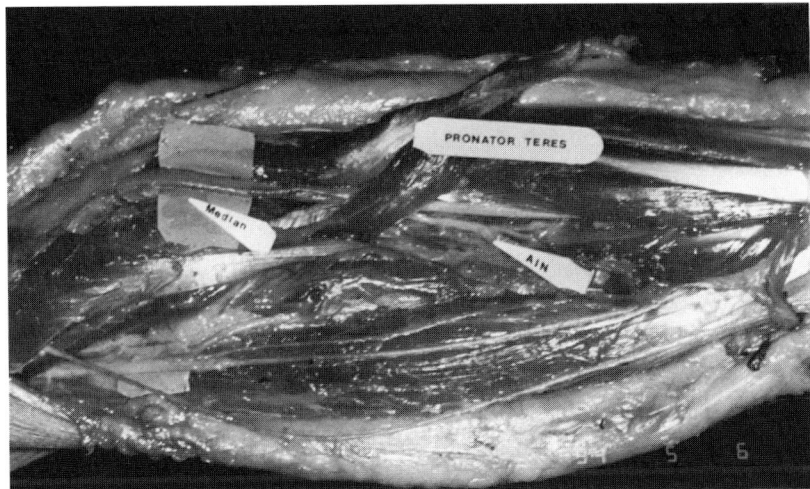

Fig. 7 Dissection of the left proximal forearm. The median nerve is shown entering the two heads of the pronator teres muscle. The pronator teres muscle has been freed from its insertion.

tus muscles. Injury to the nerve (Outline 2) could be related to an overuse of the pronator muscle.[48,49]

The Martin-Gruber type of communication between the median and ulnar nerves has to be remembered in connection with the anterior interosseous syndrome (Outline 3) or Kiloh Nevin Syndrome, described by Kiloh and Nevin[50] in 1952. In this not too infrequent anatomic variation, motor fibers to the intrinsic muscle of the hand travel with the median nerve until they are below the elbow. There, they exit to cross either from the main trunk or from the anterior interosseous nerve to the ulnar nerve. If an injury to the anterior interosseous nerve occurs before the nerve fibers cross to the ulnar nerve, the clinical picture of this lesion includes paralysis of hand muscles.[49]

Entrapment of the median nerve beneath the flexor retinaculum of the carpal tunnel is the most common entrapment neuropathy (Fig. 8).[21,46] The increase of pressure inside the carpal tunnel compresses the median nerve between the flexor tendons or the synovia and the overlying firm ligament.[51] Symptoms may be associated with different movements, such as extreme wrist movements of flexion or extension or forceful finger flexion while the wrist is held in flexion (milking cows). In addition, the median nerve might be squeezed by external pressure.[4] The carpal tunnel syndrome is most common in persons working in jobs that require use of handheld vibrating tools, repetitive wrist motion, and/or forced hand movements as performed by cashiers, assembly

Outline 2 Neurologic symptoms of pronator syndrome

Abnormal sensibility in volar thumb, index, and middle fingers

Finger flexor weakness

Proximal forearm pain

Outline 3 Muscles involved in anterior interosseous syndrome

Flexor digitorum profundus (radial half)

Flexor pollicis longus

Pronator quadratus

---

workers, grinders, typists, key-punch operators, seamstresses and cutters, musicians, packers, and bricklayers.[52]

The Ulnar Nerve

The ulnar nerve might be compressed by anatomic variations in the axilla as noted by Spinner and associates.[23] As the nerve passes from the anterior compartment of the brachium into the posterior compartment by penetrating the medial intermuscular septum, it might be impinged by the Arcade of Struthers. This arcade is formed by a thickening of the deep investing fascia of the arm, the superficial muscular fibers of the medial head of the triceps muscle, and the attachment of the internal brachial ligament and the medial intermuscular septum.[53] It was found to be present in 70% of 20 limbs studied by Kane and associates.[54] Care has to be taken to incise the structures, especially after an anterior transposition of the nerve.[55]

Ulnar nerve compression at the elbow is the second most common entrapment neuropathy.[56] The nerve might be affected as it lies in the condylar groove behind the medial epicondyle or as it enters the body of the flexor carpi ulnaris muscle[46] (Fig. 9). This cubital tunnel is formed by the medial edge of the trochlea, the medial epicondylar ridge, and the medial ligament of the elbow joint.

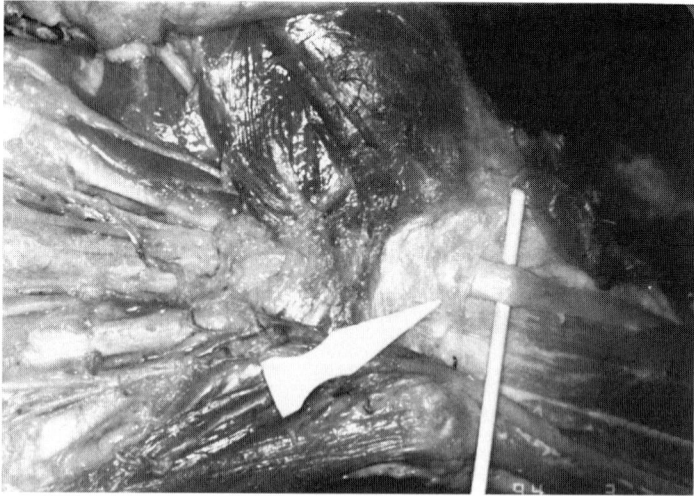

Fig. 8 Anatomic dissection showing the median nerve (elevated by probe) as it enters the flexor retinaculum (arrow) and the carpal tunnel.

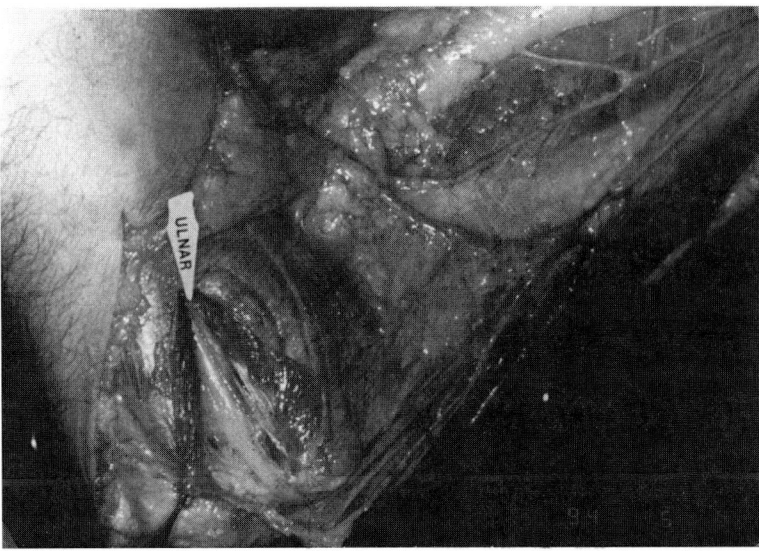

Fig. 9 Dissection of the ulnar nerve in the cubital tunnel. Note the nerve entering the two heads of the flexor carpi ulnaris muscle (arrow), a frequent site of compression.

The roof is formed by the triangular ligament stretching from the epicondyle to the olecranon.[57]

Cadaveric studies showed that flexion of the elbow lengthens the distance from the olecranon to the epicondyle by 5 mm. Meanwhile, the diameter of the cubital tunnel is reduced and the pressure rises.[58] In this position, the nerve is vulnerable to repeated minor trauma. During flexion, the ulnar nerve elongates an average of 4.7 mm, and it has been reported that the medial head of the triceps muscle can push the nerve 7 mm medially as the elbow flexes.[59] This traction might occur by repeated movement, and as a result of chronic irritation, or the gliding of the nerve around the elbow may be restricted by edema, inflammation, and subsequent scar formation.[46] In these cases, any activity that elevates and flexes the extremity, for example, painting, hammering, and shoveling, aggravates the symptoms.

Muscular adaptive changes that appear in overhand athletics include hypertrophy of the triceps and the flexor carpi ulnaris muscles; this hypertrophy might compress the cubital tunnel, leading to a progressive compressive neuropathy.

In addition, the ulnar nerve might be affected by external pressure as reported in drivers,[60] or it might be affected by leaning on the elbow during prolonged gambling.[61] The ulnar nerve enters the forearm, passing between the humeral and ulnar heads of the flexor carpi ulnaris muscle. The deep aponeurosis connecting both heads has been implicated in the pathogenesis of ulnar nerve entrapment (Fig. 9).[62,63]

Ulnar nerve entrapment at the wrist is possible when it passes through the canal of Guyon. It may be compressed by the pisohamate ligament or the superficial volar carpal ligament.[64] Compressive injuries might be related to a single traumatic incident or to repeated trauma, such as using a hammer or working at an occupation that involves heavy gripping.[46] The deep branch of the ulnar nerve can be compressed by recurrent occupational pressure, such as that in pizza cutters,[65] or during cycling.[66,67]

The Radial Nerve

Lesions of the radial nerve occur most commonly in the region of the spiral groove of the humerus. However, these are mostly related to fractures. Pressure injuries reported as "Saturday night palsy or bench palsy" are related to either sleep on the arm or to leaning the arm onto an edge, such as that of a bench, compressing the radial nerve.[21] Radial entrapment in the arm is rare compared to trauma-related palsy. Cases have been reported in which the radial nerve is compressed in the arm. This could be related to a fibrous arch from the lateral head of the triceps muscle,[68] to strenuous muscular activity,[69] or to a combination of both.[70] Continuous repetitive arm exercise combined with a sudden forceful contraction and stretch of the arm was found to cause a delayed upper arm radial palsy in three cases, and the author assumed that the nerve was damaged directly by muscle contraction.[71] Prolonged drumming in an orchestra has been held responsible for compression of the posterior brachial cutaneous nerve of the radial nerve at its course around the long head of the triceps muscle.[72]

Chronic pain on the lateral aspect of the elbow is commonly described as tennis elbow. Continuous controversy regarding etiology and treatment is related to this description. The numerous theories regarding the cause of the pain might be divided into two groups: lesions involving the fibrous and/or muscular structures of the lateral epicondyle and lesions related to the radial nerve. As a result of being frustrated by cases of intractable tennis elbow, several authors turned their attention to the radial nerve, especially its course through the radial tunnel.[20,73,74] Roles and Maudsley[75] first described the radial tunnel syndrome in 1972. They reported 36 patients, previously diagnosed as having a tennis elbow, who underwent surgical release of the radial nerve in the radial tunnel with good results. In an anatomic investigation. Fuss and Wurzl[73] showed that in extension of the elbow with the forearm in pronation and the wrist in flexion (tennis service), the tendinous edges of the supinator and extensor carpi radialis brevis compress the radial nerve. According to Lister and associates,[20] the radial tunnel is an anatomic area with four sides of potential compression: (1) fibrous bands in front of the radial head; (2) the leash of vessels from the radial recurrent artery; (3) sharp, tendinous margins of the extensor carpi radialis muscle; and (4) the arcade of Fröhse.

Roles and Maudsley[75] in 1972, followed by Lister and associates[20] in 1979 showed the entity of compression of the radial nerve within the radial tunnel. In the radial tunnel syndrome, there may be a spectrum of complaints including pain, paresthesia, and weakness, which should be distinguished from the posterior interosseous syndrome in which the problem is localized to a compression at the arcade of Fröhse (Fig. 10) and results in a purely motor deficit.[74]

The anatomic course of the posterior interosseous nerve as it pierces through the two heads of the supinator muscle makes it vulnerable to the compressive effects of local swelling. The proximal portion of the superficial head of the muscle may be partly or completely fibrous as it forms an inverted semicircular arch through which the nerve passes. Anatomic dissections have shown considerable variability in the thickness of this arch. In 70% of specimens, its medial aspect is membranous, whereas in the remaining 30% it is fibrous, forming the arcade of Fröhse.[76] The absence of this fibrous arch in fetuses suggests that it is developmental in nature, resulting from repeated rotatory movements of the forearm, although it causes the purely motor deficit in the posterior interosseous nerve syndrome (Outline 4).[76] Entrapment of the posterior interosseous nerve in this region results from forceful supination-pronation (Fig.

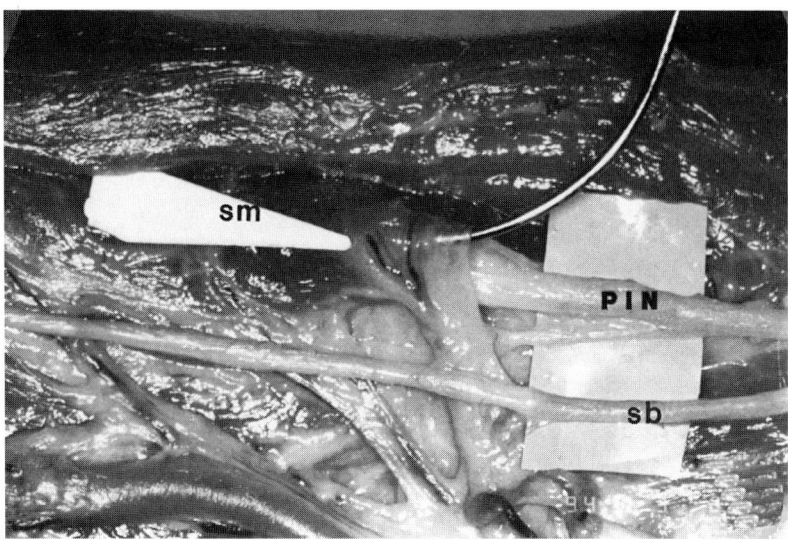

Fig. 10 The arcade of Fröhse at the lateral side of the proximal forearm. Note that the radial nerve has divided into the superficial branch (sb) and posterior interosseous nerve (PIN), which is piercing the fibrous band at the supinator muscle (sm).

11) of the arm or abrupt extension of the elbow, movements associated with tasks such as hammering, throwing, backhand tennis stroke, or conducting an orchestra.[4,77]

The superficial branch of the radial nerve may become entrapped in the forearm at the level of its passage between the brachioradialis muscle and the extensor carpi radialis longus tendon or when it pierces the superficial fascia.[78] Frequently the resulting paresthesia over the dorsal-radial aspect of the hand is related to occupations that require pronation-supination and/or hyperpronation of the forearm.[79]

Peripheral Nerve Injury

As a result of their vast experience in the treatment of patients with peripheral nerve injury, Seddon[80] and Sunderland[81] formulated schemes of classification of nerve injury, both of which correlate the pathophysiologic changes within

Outline 4 Muscles affected by posterior syndrome

Supinator

Extensor digitorum

Extensor digiti minimi

Extensor carpi ulnaris

Abductor pollicis longus

Extensor pollicis longus and brevis

Extensor indicis

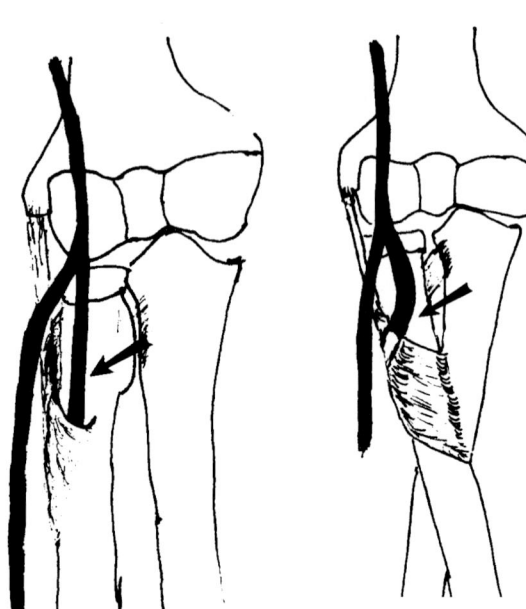

Fig. 11 Schematic drawing showing the posterior interosseous nerve (arrow) during supination **(left)** and pronation **(right)**.

the nerve with the clinical situation. Seddon[80] proposed three categories of nerve injuries. The first and mildest form of injury is neurapraxia, which simply means that the nerve is temporarily not conducting at the point of the lesion. Axon continuity is maintained, and nerve conduction proximal and distal to the lesion is preserved. Recovery is rapid, and impulse conduction is complete within weeks.[82-85] A more severe injury in which the axon is disrupted while the connective tissue remains intact is classified as axonotmesis. In this injury, the part of the axon distal to the lesion degenerates. Prognosis remains good because of the continuity of the supportive connective tissue.[82-85] The most severe injury occurs in the neurotmesis category of Seddon.[80] Complete anatomic severance of the peripheral nerve occurs, and no recovery is expected without surgical coaptation of the disrupted ends. Distal degeneration (Wallerian degeneration) as well as some degree of proximal degeneration occurs.[85]

The classification developed by Sunderland[81] considers the fascicular structure of peripheral nerves, and the categories are expanded to five degrees of nerve damage. First and second degree injuries are analogous to the neurapraxic and axonotmetic lesions in Seddon's classification. In the third degree injury, nerve fibers are severed along with their endoneurial covering, but the perineurium remains intact. Regeneration occurs, but the reinnervation of the target organs is haphazard as a result of intrafascicular mixing of growing axons. In the fourth degree injury, the perineurium is disrupted and the continuity of the nerve trunk is maintained by a intact epineurium. This is the lesion of a neuroma in continuity. The fifth degree injury denotes complete disruption of the nerve trunk.

Acute Compression Injury

Peripheral nerve injury resulting from external pressure can be experimentally produced by using a pneumatic tourniquet.[86] At levels of pressure as low as 30 mm Hg, Rydevik and associates[87] observed impaired venular flow, which is associated with increases of endoneurial fluid pressure and subsequent decreased nerve conduction velocity.[88] At pressures of 60 mm Hg, nerve fiber viability is endangered by creation of a local metabolic block, secondary to vascular occlusion, and on this level of pressure, mechanical structural deformation may be induced. At levels of compression of 90 mm Hg and higher, greater mechanical deformation of the axon and supportive structures leads to structural damage that may persist.[89]

According to this scheme, compression injuries are produced by three components: first, ischemia; second, a metabolic imbalance; and third, mechanical trauma. Ischemia is caused by venous obstruction, which results in congestion within the epineurial and perineurial vascular plexi.[90,91] With continued compression, the nerve becomes anoxic. At this point, a vicious circle starts because anoxia leads to dilatation of small vessels and capillaries, which results in leakage of proteins. Endoneurial edema follows, and the proliferation of fibroblasts further compromises the circulation and causes additional nerve damage.[92] Without adequate blood supply, the production of high-energy phosphates by oxidative phosphorylation is abandoned, which, in turn, leads to decreased efficiency of the axon transport mechanisms, the Na/K membrane pump, and the maintenance of the axon cell membrane.[93] Eventually, conduction and impulse transmission are lost.[94]

The next level of injury is caused by mechanical deformation. Higher compression results in the shearing of the Schwann cell. This shear damages the myelin, which then degenerates leaving an exposed area of axon. The involved Schwann cells become grossly swollen and their myelin lamellae separate from the cell bodies.[95] Because axon continuity is maintained, remyelination and return of full function will occur in these cases[96] if treatment is timely. Longer periods of compression with relatively higher pressure exerted over a small area of the affected peripheral nerve can produce a crushing injury, which creates a second, third, or even fourth degree lesion.

Chronic Compression Injury

The injury caused by low-grade chronic compression differs in etiology, histology, and clinical presentation from the acute compression injury. Histologic assessment suggests that chronic nerve compression is associated with myelin sheath asymmetry, epineurial fibrosis, perineurial thickening, and, in severe forms, endoneurial fibrosis.[81,97] To evaluate these changes, polyvinyl cuffs were placed around the sciatic nerve in rats or around the median nerve in monkeys with no initial compression.[97,98] No morphologic or electrophysiologic changes were apparent after 2 months. At 4 months, there was epineurial fibrosis and perineurial thickening, and at the ultrastructural level, paranodal swelling and segmental demyelination were observed. After 6 months, the inner epineurium evidenced fibrosis, the perineurial thickening was more pronounced, and the endoneurium was becoming fibrotic. The myelin sheath became progressively thinned, and the affected axons at the periphery of the fascicle demonstrated Wallerian degeneration. After 12 months of compression, all fascicles were affected uniformly. Attendant to the prolonged compression and intraneural proteinaceous edema from the loss of the blood-nerve barrier, fibroblasts eventually proliferate within the neural tissue rendering the nerve segment permanently scarred.

Repetitive Motion Injury

Minimal, if any, experimental work has been reported on the pathophysiologic changes in nerves that undergo high-speed repetitive movement. Although the morphologic changes have not been elucidated, it is assumed that repetitive motion injury of peripheral nerves is a multifactorial process. First, every joint movement exerts a longitudinal force on the passing nerves. Normal longitudinal excursion of nerves varies greatly from a maximum of 15.3 mm (average for the brachial plexus) to a minimum of 1.15 mm (average for digital nerves).[99,100] These excursions with additional physiological stretch are necessarily below the elastic limits of the peripheral nerve and permit normal joint range of motion. Especially in sports, because of hyperelasticity of the athlete or the force of the motion (pitcher), this normal range might be extended to the limits of the peripheral nerve, resulting in stretch injury. Also, a combination of flexion and extension, as in violin players, might stretch the nerve to its limit.

Second, mechanical damage caused by repetitive gliding through narrow canals, bony spears, or tendinous arches has to be considered. Postmortem histologic studies of the median nerve in the carpal tunnel revealed an increase in synovial density and arterial and venule proliferation in the epineurium and endoneurium. These areas corresponded to the area of the median nerve subject to mechanical stresses during flexion and extension.[101]

Third, an external compression by muscular hypertrophy, synovial thickening, tendinitis, and/or local edema might lead to a direct trauma or to ischemic periods in the nerve. When the pressure in the carpal tunnel was increased mechanically in an experiment, a graded loss of motor and sensory function similar to the changes in acute compression was seen.[102] It is interesting that hypertensive individuals noted a change in conduction at higher pressures than normotensive individuals. This supports the ischemic base of acute compression nerve injury.[102]

Fourth, biochemical factors have to be considered. In occupational acquired carpal tunnel syndrome, the local release of histamine followed by angioedema has been reported. Exposure to vibratory activity increased plasma histamine levels in the ipsilateral cubital vein with decrease of median nerve conduction.[103]

Systemic humeral factors may also predispose to repetitive injury neuropathy; for instance, pregnant women and women following gynecological surgery, especially hysterectomy and oophorectomy, are seen to have a higher incident of carpal tunnel syndrome.[104] Concomitant illness also needs to be considered. Several medical conditions are known to increase the vulnerability of nerves to mild compression. Foremost among these conditions is diabetes mellitus. Apart from their polyneuropathy, an increased incident of local compressive neuropathies is found in diabetic patients.[105] Compressive neuropathies are also associated with hypothyroidism, alcoholism, malnutrition, renal failure, and rheumatoid arthritis.[106–110] Also, a probably autosomal dominant genetic factor, which interferes with the metabolism of the Schwann cell, has been associated with local compressive neuropathies.[111,112]

References

1. Chaffin DB: Localized muscle fatigue: Definition and measurement. *J Occup Med* 1973;15:346–354.
2. Hagberg M: Local shoulder muscular strain: Symptoms and disorders. *J Hum Ergol* 1982;11:99–108.
3. Hagberg M: Occupational musculoskeletal stress and disorders of the neck and shoulder: A review of possible pathophysiology. *Int Arch Occup Environ Health* 1984;53:269–278.

4. Feldman RG, Goldman R, Keyserling WM: Classical syndromes in occupational medicine: Peripheral nerve entrapment syndromes and ergonomic factors. *Am J Ind Med* 1983;4:661–681.
5. Terzis JK, Smith KL (eds): *The Peripheral Nerve: Structure, Function and Reconstruction.* New York, NY, Raven Press, 1990.
6. Barchi RL: Excitation and conduction in nerve, in Sumner AJ (ed): *The Physiology of Peripheral Nerve Disease.* Philadelphia, PA, WB Saunders, 1980, pp 1–40.
7. Gamble HJ: Spinal and cranial nerve roots, in Landon DN (ed): *The Peripheral Nerve.* London, UK, Chapman & Hall, 1976, pp 330–354.
8. Dunn JS: Developing myelin in human peripheral nerve. *Scott Med J* 1970;15:108–117.
9. Ochoa J: The unmyelinated nerve fibre, in Landon DN (ed): *The Peripheral Nerve.* London, UK, Chapman & Hall, 1976, pp 106–158.
10. Thomas PK, Landon DN, King RHM: Diseases of the peripheral nerves, in Adams JH, Corsellis JAN, Duchen LW (eds): *Greenfield's Neuropathology,* ed 4. New York, NY, John Wiley & Sons, 1984, pp 807–920.
11. Geren BB: The formation from the Schwann cell surface of myelin in the peripheral nerves of chick embryos. *Exp Cell Res* 1954;7:558–562.
12. Thomas PK: The connective tissue of peripheral nerve: An electron microscope study. *J Anat* 1963;97:35–44.
13. Gamble HJ, Eames RA: An electron microscope study of the connective tissues of human peripheral nerve. *J Anat* 1964;98:655–663.
14. Thomas PK, Olsson Y: Microscopic anatomy and function of the connective tissue components of peripheral nerve, in Dyck PJ, Thomas PK, Lambert EH, et al (eds): *Peripheral Neuropathy,* ed 2. Philadelphia, PA, WB Saunders, 1984, vol 1, pp 97–120.
15. Sunderland S: The connective tissues of peripheral nerves. *Brain* 1965;88:841–854.
16. Lundborg G: The intrinsic vascularization of human peripheral nerves: Structural and functional aspects. *J Hand Surg* 1979;4A:34–41.
17. Bell MA, Weddell AG: A descriptive study of the blood vessels of the sciatic nerve in the rat, man and other mammals. *Brain* 1984;107:871–898.
18. Slingluff CL Jr, Terzis JK, Edgerton MT: The quantitative microanatomy of the brachial plexus in man: Reconstructive relevance, in Terzis JK (ed): *Microreconstruction of Nerve Injuries.* Philadelphia, PA, WB Saunders, 1987, pp 285–324.
19. Johnson RK, Spinner M, Shrewsbury MM: Median nerve entrapment syndrome in the proximal forearm. *J Hand Surg* 1979;4A:48–51.
20. Lister GD, Belsole RB, Kleinert HE: The radial tunnel syndrome. *J Hand Surg* 1979;4A:52–59.
21. Liveson JA (ed): *Peripheral Neurology: Case Studies in Electrodiagnosis,* ed 2. Philadelphia, PA, FA Davis Company, 1991, pp 19–59.
22. Kassirer MR, Manon N: Head banger's whiplash. *Clin J Pain* 1993;9:138–141.
23. Spinner RJ, Carmichael SW, Spinner M: Infraclavicular ulnar nerve entrapment due to a chondroepitrochlearis muscle. *J Hand Surg* 1991;16B:315–317.
24. Putz-Anderson V (ed): *Cumulative Trauma Disorders: A Manual for Musculoskeletal Diseases of the Upper Limbs.* London, UK, Taylor and Francis, 1988.
25. Guidotti TL: Occupational repetitive strain injury. *Am Family Phys* 1992;45:585–592.
26. Mendoza FX, Main WK, Main K: Peripheral nerve injuries of the shoulder in the athlete. *Clin Sports Med* 1990;9:331–342.
27. Mestdagh H, Drizenko A, Ghestem PH: Anatomical basis of suprascapular nerve syndrome. *Anat Clin* 1981;3:67–71.
28. Ferretti A, Cerullo G, Russo G: Suprascapular neuropathy in volleyball players. *J Bone Joint Surg* 1987;69A:260–263.
29. Kukowski B: Suprascapular nerve lesion as an occupational neuropathy in a semiprofessional dancer. *Arch Phys Med Rehabil* 1993;74:768–769.
30. Ringel SP, Treihaft M, Carry M, et al: Suprascapular neuropathy in pitchers. *Am J Sports Med* 1990;18:80–86.

31. Vastamäki M, Göransson H: Suprascapular nerve entrapment. *Clin Orthop* 1993; 297:135–143.
32. Shah K, Stefaniwsky L: Long thoracic nerve palsy: Case report. *Arch Phys Med Rehabil* 1982;63:585–586.
33. Bateman JE: Nerve injuries about the shoulder in sports. *J Bone Joint Surg* 1967;49A:785–792.
34. Goodman CE, Kenrick MM, Blum MV: Long thoracic nerve palsy: A follow-up study. *Arch Phys Med Rehabil* 1975;56:352–358.
35. Gregg JR, Labosky D, Harty M, et al: Serratus anterior paralysis in the young athlete. *J Bone Joint Surg* 1979;61A:825–832.
36. Woodhead AB III: Paralysis of the serratus anterior in a world class marksman: A case study. *Am J Sports Med* 1985;13:359–362.
37. Cahill BR, Palmer RE: Quadrilateral space syndrome. *J Hand Surg* 1983;8A:65–69.
38. Francel TJ, Dellon AL, Campbell JN: Quadrilateral space syndrome: Diagnosis and operative decompression technique. *Plast Reconst Surg* 1991;87:911–916.
39. McKowen HC, Voorhies RM: Axillary nerve entrapment in the quadrilateral space: Case report. *J Neurosurg* 1987;66:932–934.
40. Kim SM, Goodrich JA: Isolated proximal musculocutaneous nerve palsy: Case report. *Arch Phys Med Rehabil* 1984;65:735–736.
41. Pecina M, Bojanic I: Musculocutaneous nerve entrapment in the upper arm. *Int Orthop* 1993;17:232–234.
42. Felsenthal G, Mondell DL, Reischer MA, et al: Forearm pain secondary to compression syndrome of the lateral cutaneous nerve of the forearm. *Arch Phys Med Rehabil* 1984;65:139–141.
43. Bassett FH III, Nunley JA: Compression of the musculocutaneous nerve at the elbow. *J Bone Joint Surg* 1982;64A:1050–1052.
44. Spinner RJ, Carmichael SW, Spinner M: Partial median nerve entrapment in the distal arm because of an accessory bicipital aponeurosis. *J Hand Surg* 1991;16A: 236–244.
45. Al-Qattan MM, Husband JB: Median nerve compression by the supracondylar process: A case report. *J Hand Surg* 1991;16B:101–103.
46. Barrett DS, Donell ST: Entrapment neuropathies: 1. Upper limb. *Br J Hosp Med* 1991;46:94–98.
47. Kopell HP, Thompson WAL: Pronator Syndrome: A confirmed case and its diagnosis. *N Engl J Med* 1958;259:713–715.
48. Thompson JS, Phelps TH: Repetitive strain injuries: How to deal with "the epidemic of the 1990's." *Postgrad Med* 1990;88:143–149.
49. Spinner M: The anterior interosseous-nerve syndrome, with special attention to its variations. *J Bone Joint Surg* 1970;52A:84–94.
50. Kiloh LG, Nevin S: Isolated neuritis of the anterior interosseous nerve. *Br Med J* 1952;1:850–851.
51. Phalen GS: Reflections on 21 years' experience with the carpal-tunnel syndrome. *JAMA* 1970;212:1365–1367.
52. Wieslander G, Norback D, Gothe CJ, et al: Carpal tunnel syndrome (CTS) and exposure to vibration, repetitive wrist movements, and heavy manual work: A case-referent study. *Br J Ind Med* 1989;46:43–47.
53. Struthers J: On some points in the abnormal anatomy of the arm. *Br Foreign Med Chir Rev* 1854;14:170–179.
54. Kane E, Kaplan EB, Spinner M: Observations of the course of the ulnar nerve in the arm. *Ann Chir* 1973;27:487–496.
55. Al-Qattan MM, Murray KA: The arcade of Struthers: An anatomical study. *J Hand Surg* 1991;16A:311–314.
56. Clark CB: Cubital tunnel syndrome. *JAMA* 1979;241:801–802.
57. Feindel W, Stratford J: Cubital tunnel compression in tardy ulnar palsy. *Can Med Assoc J* 1958;78:351–353.
58. MacNicol MF: Extraneural pressures affecting the ulnar nerve at the elbow. *Hand* 1982;14:5–11.

59. Buehler MJ, Thayer DT: The elbow flexion test: A clinical test for the cubital tunnel syndrome. *Clin Orthop* 1988;233:213–216.
60. Abdel-Salam A, Eyres KS, Cleary J: Drivers' elbow: A cause of ulnar neuropathy. *J Hand Surg* 1991;16B:436–437.
61. Jarrell HR: Letter: Vegas neuropathy. *N Engl J Med* 1988;319:1487.
62. Amadio PC, Beckenbaugh RD: Entrapment of the ulnar nerve by the deep flexor-pronator aponeurosis. *J Hand Surg* 1986;11A:83–87.
63. Hang YS: Tardy ulnar neuritis in a little league baseball player. *Am J Sports Med* 1981;9:244–246.
64. Guyon F: Note sur une disposition anatomique propre à la face antérieure de la région du poignet et non encore décrite. *Bull Soc Anat Paris* 1861;6:184–186.
65. Jones HR Jr: Letter: Pizza cutter's palsy. *N Engl J Med* 1988;319:450.
66. Russell WR, Whitty CWM: Traumatic neuritis of the deep palmar branch of the ulnar nerve. *Lancet* 1947;1:828–829.
67. Smail DF: Handlebar palsy. *N Eng J Med* 1975;292:322.
68. Nakamichi K, Tachibana S: Radial nerve entrapment by the lateral head of the triceps. *J Hand Surg* 1991;16A:748–750.
69. Mitsunaga MM, Nakano K: High radial nerve palsy following strenuous muscular activity: A case report. *Clin Orthop* 1988;234:39–42.
70. Lotem M, Fried A, Levy M, et al: Radial palsy following muscular effort: A nerve compression syndrome possibly related to a fibrous arch of the lateral head of the triceps. *J Bone Joint Surg* 1971;53B:500–506.
71. Streib E: Upper arm radial nerve palsy after muscular effort: Report of three cases. *Neurology* 1992;42:1632–1634.
72. Makin GJ, Brown WF: Entrapment of the posterior cutaneous nerve of the arm. *Neurology* 1985;35:1677–1678.
73. Fuss FK, Wurzl GH: Radial nerve entrapment at the elbow: Surgical anatomy. *J Hand Surg* 1991;16A:742–747.
74. Posner MA: Compressive neuropathies of the median and radial nerves at the elbow. *Clin Sports Med* 1990;9:343–363.
75. Roles NC, Maudsley RH: Radial tunnel syndrome: Resistant tennis elbow as a nerve entrapment. *J Bone Joint Surg* 1972;54B:499–508.
76. Spinner M: The arcade of Fröhse and its relationship to posterior interosseous nerve paralysis. *J Bone Joint Surg* 1968;50B:809–812.
77. Spaans F: Occupational nerve lesions, in Vinken PJ, Bruyn GW (eds): *Handbook of Clinical Neurology: Diseases of Nerves Part 1*. Amsterdam, North-Holland Publishing, 1970, vol 7, pp 326–343.
78. Spindler HA, Dellon AL: Nerve conduction studies in the superficial radial nerve entrapment syndrome. *Muscle Nerve* 1990;13:1–5.
79. Dellon AL, Mackinnon SE: Radial sensory nerve entrapment in the forearm. *J Hand Surg* 1986;11A:199–205.
80. Seddon HJ: Three types of nerve injury. *Brain* 1943;66:237–288.
81. Sunderland S (ed): *Nerves and Nerve Injuries*, ed 1. Baltimore, MD, Williams & Wilkins, 1968.
82. Castaldo JE, Ochoa JL: Mechanical injury of peripheral nerves: Fine structure and dysfunction. *Clin Plast Surg* 1984;11:9–16.
83. Horn KL, Crumley RL: The physiology of nerve injury and repair. *Otolaryngol Clin N Am* 1984;17:321–333.
84. Spencer PS: Morphology of the injured peripheral nerve, in Daniel RK, Terzis JK (eds): *Reconstructive Microsurgery*. Boston, MA, Little Brown & Co, 1977, pp 342–349.
85. Simpson JA: Nerve injuries, general aspects, in Vinken PJ, Bruyn GW (eds): *Handbook of Clinical Neurology, Diseases of Nerves Part 1*. Amsterdam, North-Holland Publishing, 1970, pp 244–256.
86. Rudge P: Tourniquet paralysis with prolonged conduction block: An electrophysiological study. *J Bone Joint Surg* 1974;56B:716–720.
87. Rydevik B, Lundborg G, Bagge U: Effects of graded compression on intraneural blood flow: An in vivo study on rabbit tibial nerve. *J Hand Surg* 1981;6A:3–12.

88. Hargens AR, Romine JS, Sipe JC, et al: Peripheral nerve-conduction block by high muscle-compartment pressure. *J Bone Joint Surg* 1979;61A:192–200.
89. Lundborg G, Gelberman RH, Minteer-Convery M, et al: Median nerve compression in the carpal tunnel: Functional response to experimentally induced controlled pressure. *J Hand Surg* 1982;7A:252–259.
90. Eversmann WW Jr: Entrapment and compression neuropathies, in Green DP (ed): *Operative Hand Surgery,* ed 2. New York, NY, Churchill Livingstone, 1988, vol 2, pp 1423–1478.
91. Lundborg G: Ischemic nerve injury: Experimental studies on intraneural microvascular pathophysiology and nerve function in a limb subjected to temporary circulatory arrest. *Scand J Plast Reconstr Surg* 1970;6(suppl):3–113.
92. Sunderland S: The nerve lesion in the carpal tunnel syndrome. *J Neurol Neurosurg Psych* 1976;39:615–626.
93. Eversmann WW Jr, Ritsick JA: Intraoperative changes in motor nerve conduction latency in carpal tunnel syndrome. *J Hand Surg* 1978;3A:77–81.
94. Landon DN, Hall S: The myelinated nerve fibre, in Landon DN (ed): *The Peripheral Nerve.* London, UK, Chapman & Hall, 1976, pp 1–105.
95. Ochoa J, Fowler TJ, Gilliatt RW: Anatomical changes in peripheral nerves compressed by a pneumatic tourniquet. *J Anat* 1972, 113:433–455.
96. Trojaborg W: Rate of recovery in motor and sensory fibres of the radial nerve: Clinical and electrophysiological aspects. *J Neurol Neurosurg Psych* 1970;33:625–638.
97. Mackinnon SE, Dellon AL, Hudson AR, et al: Chronic nerve compression: An experimental model in the rat. *Ann Plast Surg* 1984;13:112–120.
98. Mackinnon SE, Dellon AL, Hudson AR, et al: A primate model for chronic nerve compression. *J Reconstr Microsurg* 1985;1:185–195.
99. Wilgis EF, Murphy R: The significance of longitudinal excursion in peripheral nerves. *Hand Clin* 1986;2:761–766.
100. McLellan DL: Letter: Longitudinal sliding of median nerve during hand movements: A contributory factor in entrapment neuropathy? *Lancet* 1975;1:633–634.
101. Armstrong TJ, Castelli WA, Evans FG, et al: Some histological changes in carpal tunnel contents and their biomechanical implications. *J Occup Med* 1984;26:197–201.
102. Szabo R: Pathophysiology of nerve entrapment syndromes. Cumulative Trauma Symposium. San Francisco, CA, 1986.
103. Wener MH, Metzger WJ, Simon RA: Occupationally acquired vibratory angioedema with secondary carpal tunnel syndrome. *Ann Intern Med* 1983;98:44–46.
104. Cannon LJ, Bernacki EJ, Walter SD: Personal and occupational factors associated with carpal tunnel syndrome. *J Occup Med* 1981;23:255–258.
105. Mulder DW, Lambert EH, Bastron JA, et al: The neuropathies associated with diabetes mellitus: A clinical and electromyographic study of 103 unselected diabetic patients. *Neurology* 1961;11:275–284.
106. Denny-Brown D: Neurological conditions resulting from prolonged and severe dietary (case reports in prisoners of war, and general review) restriction. *Medicine* 1947;26:41–113.
107. Marmor L, Lawrence JF, Dubois EL: Posterior interosseous nerve palsy due to rheumatoid arthritis. *J Bone Joint Surg* 1967;49A:381–383.
108. Marshall SC, Murray WR: Deep radial nerve palsy associated with rheumatoid arthritis. *Clin Orthop* 1974;103:157–162.
109. Millender LH, Nalebuff EA, Holdsworths DE: Posterior interosseous nerve syndrome secondary to rheumatoid synovitis. *J Bone Joint Surg* 1973;55A:753.
110. Preswick G, Jeremy D: Subclinical polyneuropathy in renal insufficiency. *Lancet* 1964;2:731–732.
111. Davies DM: Recurrent peripheral-nerve palsies in a family. *Lancet* 1954;2:266–268.
112. Mayer RF, Gracia-Mullin R: Hereditary neuropathy manifested by pressure palsies: A Schwann cell disorder? *Trans Am Neurol Assoc* 1968;93:238–240.

Chapter 25

Pathophysiology of Nerve Compression

Göran Lundborg, MD, PhD
Lars B. Dahlin, MD, PhD

Introduction

Compression injuries to peripheral nerves may occur as a result of acute trauma or chronic compression. The functional disorder induced by compression may vary from slight paresthesia and/or motor weakness to complete sensory loss and/or muscle paralysis. The character of the lesion is based on many factors, such as the magnitude and duration of the compressive trauma, the status of the patient (eg, existence of concomitant diseases such as diabetes mellitus), and the local structure of the nerve. The peripheral nerve trunk is a well-vascularized and anatomically complex structure, and compression, irritation, or stretching may initiate an inflammatory response in and around the nerve trunk with subsequent swelling and impaired vascular supply. Nerve trunks are mobile, gliding structures, and swelling of the epineurium or formation of an inflammatory reaction may impair or inhibit such gliding. A vicious circle may easily be induced in which swelling, inflammation, and impaired microcirculation combined with restricted gliding and microstretching injuries may lead to further events and, ultimately, to nerve fiber dysfunction (Fig. 1). Especially with repetitive motion, such a situation is quite plausible at anatomic locations where the nerve trunk is normally passing through a tight compartment.

The effects of compression on a nerve trunk depend on many factors, such as the local microanatomy and topography of fascicles. The connective tissue layers of a nerve trunk have a protective effect when the nerve is subjected to compression. Several small fascicles embedded in a large amount of epineurium are, therefore, less vulnerable to compression than large fascicles in a small amount of epineurium (Fig. 2). The amount of connective tissue is also more pronounced in superficial nerves and in nerve segments close to joints, probably because of the extra protection required.

There are clinical signs and symptoms induced by nerve compression from trauma. A good knowledge of the basic biologic reactions of the nerve trunk after trauma is necessary in order to understand these signs and symptoms. The purpose of this chapter is to provide a basic understanding of the clinical signs and symptoms of nerve compression secondary to repetitive motion.

Peripheral Nerve Structure and Function

The Axon

The functional units of a nerve trunk, the axons, represent extended peripheral extensions from the respective nerve cell bodies in the anterior horn of the spinal cord (motor neuron) or in the dorsal root ganglion (sensory neuron) (Fig.

382 Pathophysiology: Nerve

ACUTE EFFECTS **CHRONIC EFFECTS**

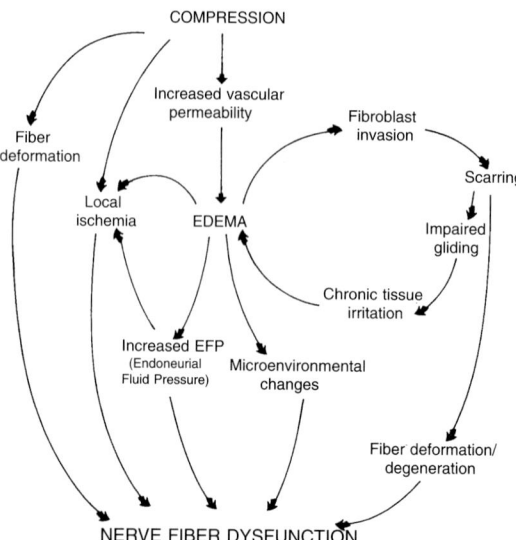

Fig. 1 Schematic drawing of the vicious circle that may be induced by compression of the peripheral nerve trunk. (Reproduced with permission from Lundborg G (ed): *Nerve Injury and Repair*. New York, NY, Churchill Livingstone, 1988, p 64.)

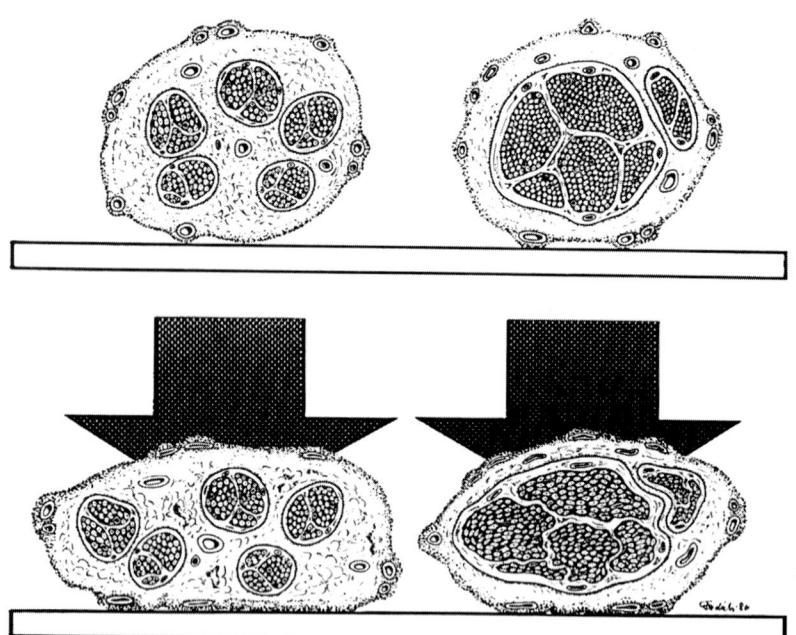

Fig. 2 Protective effects of the epineurium where a nerve is subjected to mechanical trauma. Several small fascicles embedded in a large amount of epineurium (**left**) are less vulnerable to transection injuries and compression than large fascicles in a small amount of epineurium (**right**). (Adapted with permission from Lundborg G (ed): *Nerve Injury and Repair*. New York, NY, Churchill Livingstone, 1988, p 65.)

3). The axons, together with surrounding Schwann cells, constitute nerve fibers. The fibers are of two basic ultrastructural types, myelinated and nonmyelinated (Fig. 4). In myelinated fibers, the axons are surrounded by single Schwann cells that are arranged longitudinally around the axon. Nonmyelinated axons, on the other hand, are located in a large number in the cytoplasm of a surrounding Schwann cell.

Three groups of nerve fibers have been defined[1] based on their dimensions. The largest myelinated somatic afferent or efferent fiber belongs to group A, which also has the highest conduction velocity. Group A can be further subdivided into three subgroups according to nerve fiber diameter: A-α (diameter 15 to 20 µm), A-β (diameter 8 to 15 µm), and A-δ (2 to 5 µm). Group B contains myelinated autonomic and preganglionic fibers. Within group C (diameter 0.1 to 1 µm) are the thinnest, nonmyelinated visceral and somatic afferent pain fibers, which have the lowest conduction velocities, as well as postganglionic autonomic efferent fibers. Although the A-α fibers represent efferent motor fibers, the A-β fibers have been associated with touch and the A-δ with sharp pricking pain and temperature. Burning pain has been referred to the thin, nonmyelinated C-fibers.[2]

Axonal Transport

Because of the extended anatomy of the neuron, there is a need for an efficient communication system (axonal transport) between various parts of the nerve cell. The distances between nerve cells are remarkable. The length of an axon can be 10 to 15,000 times the diameter of the nerve cell body.

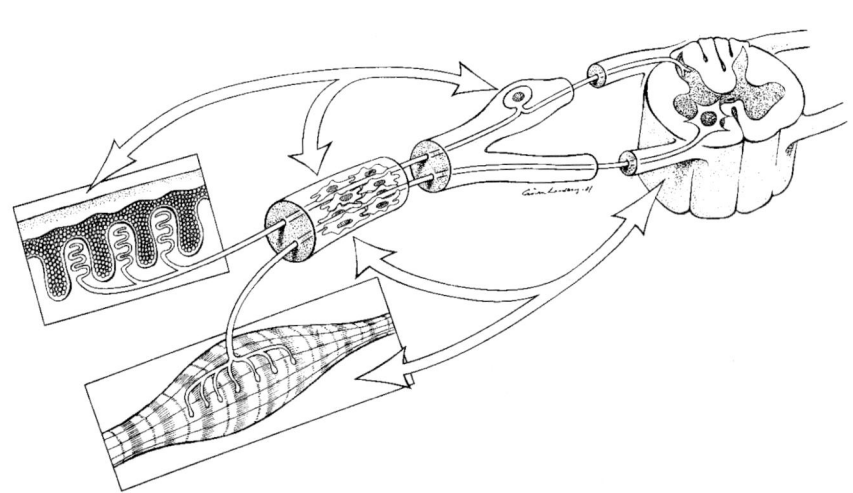

Fig. 3 Schematic drawing of the interaction between the nerve cells bodies, the nonneuronal-cells in the nerve trunk, and the targets in the peripheral nervous system. The nerve cell bodies depend on constant supply of information from the periphery. The targets, the nonneuronal cells, and the end organs are under a trophic influence from the nerve cell bodies. (Reproduced with permission from Lundborg G (ed): Nerve Injury and Repair. New York, NY, Churchill Livingstone, 1988, p 2.)

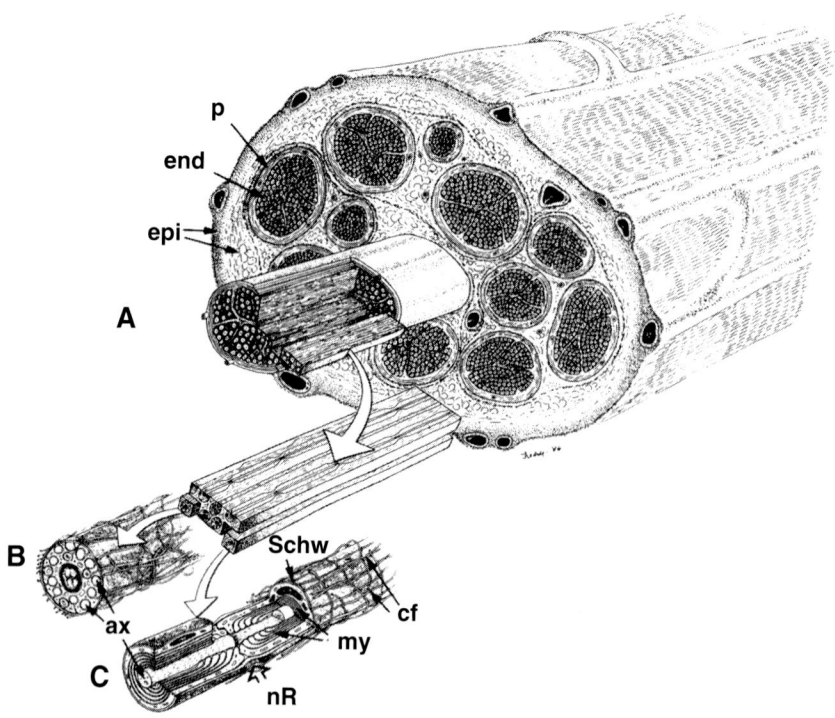

Fig. 4 The microanatomy of the peripheral trunk. **A,** The nerve trunk consists of fascicles surrounded by the perineurium (p) and embedded in loose connective tissue, the epineurium (epi). The connective tissue inside the fascicles is called endoneurium (end). Nonmyelinated nerve fibers are shown in **B**, where the axons (ax) are located in troughs in the cytoplasm of the Schwann cells (Schw). **C,** Myelinated nerve fibers consist of the axon around which single Schwann cells are wrapped, thereby creating the myelin sheath. The space between two single Schwann cells in a myelinated (my) nerve fiber creates the node of Ranvier (nR). Collagen fibers (cf) surround individual nerve fibers. (Reproduced with permission from Lundborg G (ed): *Nerve Injury and Repair.* New York, NY, Churchill Livingstone, 1988, p 33.)

Most substances necessary for the membrane integrity of the axon and the nerve terminal are synthesized in the nerve cell body. Such essential products are constantly transported from the nerve cell body to the periphery (anterograde transport) and from the periphery to the nerve cell body (retrograde transport). The latter is for disposal of materials and transport of trophic and tropic factors. Axonal transport carries several neuron components, such as organelles (for example, mitochondria), membranous vesicles, lipids, and a great amount of various proteins. Two phases of anterograde axonal transport have been identified.[3–5] There is slow axonal transport (0.1 to 30 mm/day) with two different components (slow component b [Scb] and slow component a [Sca]) involving cytoskeletal elements, such as subunits of microtubules and neurofilaments and axoplasmic matrix (eg, actin).[6–10] Fast axonal transport (up to 410 mm/day) involves various enzymes, transmitter substance vesicles, glycoproteins, and lipids.[4,11–17]

Retrograde transport (up to 300 mm/day) carries material from the periphery to the nerve cell body, and it has a dual function.[18–27] Neurotrophic substances, synthesized by peripheral target structures, are taken up by peripheral nerve terminals and transported by retrograde axonal transport to the central nerve cell bodies to maintain their survival and viability.[28] Material that is not needed in the periphery is transported back to the nerve cell body, and as much as 70% of the material transported in the anterograde direction is transported back to the cell body.[22] Anterograde and retrograde axonal transport are energy dependent.

Microanatomy of the Nerve Trunk

The nerve fibers are collected in bundles called fascicles, which often are organized in groups of four or five (Fig. 4). The perineurium is a mechanically strong membrane that consists of up to 15 lamellae, which are composed of flattened cells possessing basement membranes on both sides of each cell.[29-34]

The fascicles are embedded in a loose epineurial tissue called the epineurium (Fig. 4). The amount of epineurial tissue may vary with level and location of the nerve trunk. The epineurium has a protective function and also contains numerous microvessels.

Intraneural Microvascular System

Nerve fibers depend on a continuous supply of oxygen for their normal function. This nutritional support is provided by a rich intraneural microvascular network in all layers of the nerve (Fig. 5). The nerve trunk receives a segmental vascular supply along its course. The segmental vessels usually approach the nerve in a coiled manner, which enables an adaptation to the physiologic excursion of the nerve trunks. The epineurial vessels divide into ascending and descending branches; they also form numerous collaterals with vessels in the

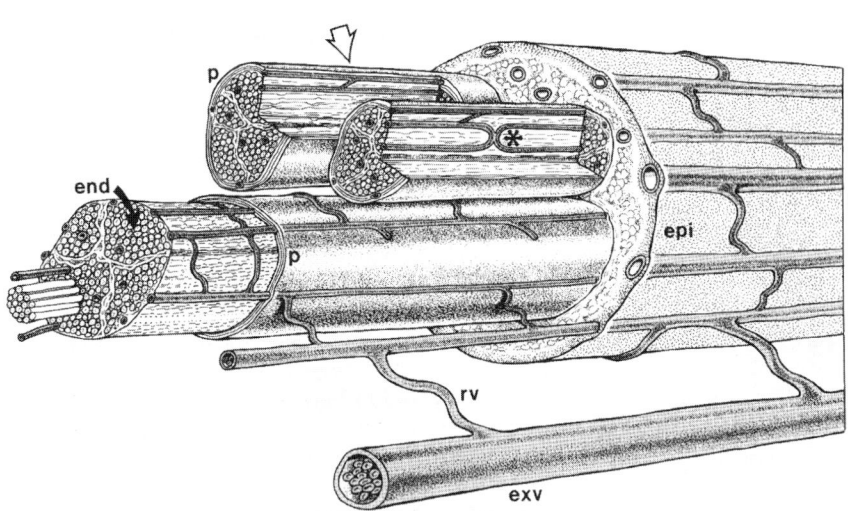

Fig. 5 Schematic drawing of the intraneural microcirculation in a peripheral nerve trunk. Vascular plexa in all layers of the nerve (endoneurium [end], perineurium [p], and epineurium [epi]) are fed via region feeding vessels (rv) from the extrinsic vessels (exv). Note the oblique course of vessels penetrating the perineurium (arrow) and the intrafascicular "double loop formation" (*). (Reproduced with permission from Lundborg G (ed): *Nerve Injury and Repair*. New York, NY, Churchill Livingstone, 1988, p 43.)

perineurial layer and in the endoneurium inside the fascicles. At their passage through the perineurium, these vessels often pierce the innermost lamella at an oblique angle (Fig. 5).[35-37] At this point, the penetrating vessels are easily closed as a result of increased intrafascicular pressure.[37-41]

Intraneural Diffusion Barriers

The vessels located in the epineurium respond to injury with a rapid increase in permeability, which results in edema and an inflammatory response, with invasion of macrophages (M Kanje, L Stenberg, A Ahlin, et al, personal communication). The extent and location of the edema depends on the severity of the injury.[36,37,42,43] In contrast to the epineurial vessels, the endoneurial vessels normally do not allow extravasation of proteins, thereby constituting a blood-nerve barrier analogous to the blood-brain barrier.[42,44] A slight trauma to a nerve, such as ischemia of short duration or low pressure compression, may cause an epineurial edema, whereas the endoneurial vascular bed is unaffected.[43]

The perineurial sheath can act as a diffusion barrier against several substances, including albumin.[37,45-48] The blood-nerve barrier together with the perineurial diffusion barrier regulate the environment inside the fascicles. The perineurial diffusion barrier prevents an epineurial edema from reaching the nerve fibers in the endoneurium. This barrier function has been shown to work both from the epineurium and in the opposite direction.[49] Therefore, if there is an endoneurial edema, the proteins cannot easily be drained outward through the perineurium, and a closed compartment syndrome in miniature may be induced.[2,39]

Endoneurial Fluid Pressure

Inside the fascicles, there is normally a slightly positive interstitial tissue fluid pressure (EFP), which has been estimated in rat sciatic nerves to be about 1.5 ± 0.7 mm Hg.[50] Because corresponding values of surrounding tissues are slightly negative (subcutaneous tissue -4.7 ± 0.8 mm Hg[51] and muscle -2 ± 2 mm Hg[52]), there may be an outwardly directed net pressure gradient over the perineurium of about 3 to 5 mm Hg. This gradient helps to give the fascicles a normal mechanical stiffness. This positive intrafascicular pressure is probably caused by several factors, among which one could be the hypertonicity of endoneurial fluid electrolytes as compared to serum electrolytes.[53]

Peripheral Nerve Excursions

On the outside of the nerve trunk there is a conjunctiva-like adventitia, which allows a great deal of motion of the nerve trunk. Also, in deeper layers of the nerve, there are gliding layers that allow the fascicles to slide in relation to surrounding intraneural tissues.[54] Peripheral nerves, therefore, are not rigidly fixed to their surrounding tissues. When an extremity moves, the nerves slide longitudinally in their beds over several millimeters. For instance, the total excursion of the brachial plexus during full abduction-adduction of the shoulder has been found to be around 15 mm.[55] The corresponding values for the median and ulnar nerves just proximal to the elbow are 7.3 and 9.8 mm, respectively, during full elbow flexion/extension. Proximal to the carpal tunnel, the excursions of the same nerves were found by Wilgis and Murphy[55] to be 14.5 mm and 13.8 mm, respectively. Millesi and associates[54] have studied the stress and strain phenomena in peripheral nerves as well as the movement of the median nerve against the retinaculum flexorum. The median nerve moves up to 9.6 mm against the retinaculum flexorum in wrist flexion and it moves to a slight degree in wrist extension. The nerve also moves with finger movements.[54] There also are movements within a peripheral nerve with flexion and extension. The median nerve has to slack down by 14.9% in order to adjust to full flexion and the corresponding 4.3% for full extension.[56] Nerve segments with branches are also much stiffer than segments of a nerve in which no branches are leaving the nerve.[57] Constraining effects on a nerve may also vary in relationship to the specific nerve and the anatomic site. This is important in peripheral nerves in which excursion is impaired because of perineurial fibrosis.

The pathophysiologic events in chronic nerve irritation or compression may to a great extent be explained by restriction of normal peripheral nerve excursion. When, during movements of an extremity, a nerve trunk is fixed to surrounding tissues by edema, inflammation, or subsequent fibrosis, the inhibition of the nerve's ability to glide may induce microscopic stretching lesions, edema, inflammation, and further fibrosis. Thereby, a vicious circle may be set up (Fig. 1).

Classification of Nerve Compression Injuries

Nerve lesions may originate from mechanical trauma, such as compression, vibration, stretching, and severance, or chemical, thermal, or ischemic trauma. For classification of nerve injuries, structural changes in the nerve trunk must be considered as well as functional consequences.

Metabolic Conduction Block

Inhibition of intraneural microcirculation, eg, by compression, may induce a local metabolic conduction block. A well-known example of such a metabolic block is the numbness of the foot when the peroneal nerve is compressed by one leg crossing over the other at knee level. A metabolic conduction block is also induced by an inflated tourniquet around the upper arm. Such a metabolic block, caused by local arrest of intraneural microcirculation, is immediately reversible when the pressure is removed. If the compression is extended, there may be edema in the fascicles and an increase in endoneurial fluid pressure that can compromise endoneurial capillary flow for some time.

Neurapraxia (Sunderland Lesion I)

With compression at a higher magnitude, a local conduction block, lasting for weeks or months, may be induced before it is spontaneously reversed. Seddon[58,59] gave the name neurapraxia to blocks of this type, which are based on local damage to the myelin sheath with preserved axonal continuity. Neurapraxia often includes motor paralysis while some sensory and sympathetic functions may be spared; this sparing is confined to thin fibers that are less vulnerable to compression.[60] Examples of neurapraxia include Saturday night palsy, which is a radial nerve lesion in the upper arm, or tourniquet paralysis, which occasionally is seen after inflation to too high a pressure of a tourniquet around the upper arm.[2]

Axonotmesis (Sunderland Lesion II)

A severe traction or crush injury may damage the axons to such an extent that their continuity is broken, although the endoneurial tubes (chain of Schwann cells together with their basal lamina) are still intact. In such cases, regeneration of the axons is required to restore functional recovery; however, because the preserved endoneurial tubes offer correctly oriented pathways, the growing axons end up at correct peripheral targets.

Neurotmesis (Sunderland Lesion III–V)

An even more severe injury than the axonotmesis is neurotmesis (Sunderland III–V), which includes the loss of continuity of some or all of the remaining connective tissue components of the peripheral nerve trunk, such as the endoneurial tubes (Sunderland III), perineurium (Sunderland IV), or epineurium (Sunderland V). The term neurotmesis also includes lesions in which, although the nerve appears to have its continuity preserved, it is totally disorganized over a longer distance. Such lesions require surgical repair and axonal growth over the repair site across the scar. The mechanisms of such restoration of function are beyond the scope of this chapter.

Effects of Nerve Compression

Mechanical Aspects

The tissues beneath a compressing device, eg, an inflated tourniquet, are deformed, and there is a pressure gradient pushing compressed tissue toward noncompressed areas. This pressure gradient is always greatest at the edges of the compressed segment, where compression may induce severe lesions to muscle as well as nerve structures. It has been suggested that the shear forces may be the mechanism by which the pressure gradient leads to injury of intraneural blood vessels, whereas the injury to the nerve fibers is probably related to the longitudinal displacement itself.[2,61,62] Studies on the tissue fluid pressure distribution beneath a pneumatic tourniquet applied to human cadaver limbs have verified a pronounced tissue fluid pressure gradient under the edges of the cuff.[63,64] In this context, it is important to lower the inflation pressure, and such lowering can be done by using wide cuffs and limb-shaped cuffs.[65] There are good reasons to believe that iterated and repeated compression may further increase the damage induced to soft tissues underlying the compression device.

Low Pressure Compression

When pressure of low magnitude is applied to a nerve trunk, the only response is impaired microvascular flow. In animal experiments, the first sign of impaired microcirculation during compression is reduced blood flow in epineurial venules, which occurs at about 20 to 30 mm Hg of compression.[66] This venular flow impairment may cause retrograde flow of the capillary circulation in the endoneurial space, which may lead to nerve fiber dysfunction caused by oxygen depletion. In addition, the endothelial cells of the endoneurial capillaries may suffer from oxygen depletion, thereby increasing the permeability and leading to endoneurial edema and a closed compartment syndrome in miniature. It has been demonstrated that after compression at a magnitude of 30 to 80 mm Hg for 2 to 4 hours, the endoneurial fluid pressure may be increased to more than three times the baseline value.[39] With higher pressure, all blood flow in the nerve may come to a complete standstill, as has been shown in animal experiments in which 60 to 80 mm Hg was sufficient to induce intraneural ischemia.[66] However, it has been shown in humans that the critical pressure level depends on the blood pressure.[67]

The permeability of epineurial vessels already is increased at a compression level of 50 mm Hg. It has been shown that such an edema did not spread to the endoneurial space because of the diffusion barrier located in the perineurium. At higher pressure levels, there also was an increase in the permeability of endoneurial vessels, with maximal leakage of protein at the edges of the compressed nerve segment.[43]

Axonal transport is impaired by local compression.[68] This impairment probably is caused by deformation of fibers as well as diminished nutritional supply resulting from obliteration of intraneural microvessels. Compression of the rabbit vagus nerve at 20 mm Hg for 2 hours did not result in block of fast axonal transport, whereas a pressure of 30 mm Hg for 2 hours induced a complete or partial block of intra-axonally transported proteins at the site of compression; this block is reversible within 24 hours.[27,69-72] However, if the duration was extended to 8 hours, there was even an inhibition of fast transport at 20 mm Hg and of slow transport at 30 mm Hg.[72] Retrograde transport can also be inhibited by compression, and it is reasonable to believe that a similar mechanism is involved. Pressures of 20, 30, and 200 mm Hg induce a graded inhibition of the retrograde transport;[27] this inhibition will induce biochemical and morphologic changes in the nerve cell bodies. Such changes may consist of a decrease in nuclear volume density and total cell profile area, an increased eccentricity of the nucleus, dispersion of Nissl substance, and a change of tubulin transport.[73-75] Even functional change, measured as an increased regenerative capacity of the neuron, has been found after acute and chronic nerve compression.[76,77]

Compression may affect nerve fibers differently, depending on location and fiber size. The effect of compression on nerve fibers differs according to fiber size—with larger fibers most susceptible to pressure.[1,60,78-81] It was recently demonstrated that thinner myelinated fibers were more susceptible to oxygen deprivation than thicker ones.[60] The nonmyelinated fibers are very resistant to compression and a very high pressure (> 400 mm Hg) is needed to affect those fibers. Such compression can also change the conduction properties of the nonmyelinated fibers to sympathetic activity, which may be important in the understanding of pain in these conditions.[82,83]

Double Crush and Reversed Double Crush Syndromes

As indicated by previous statements, comparative low pressure may interfere with anterograde axonal transport and could thus interfere with the provision to the distal axon and axolemma constituents of cytoskeletal elements as well as of transmitter substances required for synaptic function. The results are important for understanding the pathophysiology of the so-called double crush syndrome, entrapment of the same nerve structure occurring simultaneously at two different levels. This phenomenon, first described by Upton and McComas,[84] may help to explain combined entrapments of separate nerve trunks at several levels as well as the coexistence of distal compression neuropathy and cervical neuropathy. It may also help to explain failures sometimes seen after, for instance, median nerve decompression in cases of clinically apparent carpal tunnel syndromes. In such cases, there may be simultaneous entrapment of median nerve fibers at the elbow, the thoracic outlet, or cervical root levels. The observations that the blockage of fast axonal transport by compression is relatively more impaired in animals with experimental diabetes may have important clinical implications.[85]

There may be reasons to speculate also about the existence of a reversed double crush syndrome; ie, the distal entrapment of peripheral nerve might contribute to induction of an entrapment neuropathy of the same nerve at a more proximal level.[74] Distal compression neuropathies may sometimes appear with symptoms typical of radiculopathy; however, these symptoms may sometimes disappear following a distal decompression.[86] The biologic basis of such a reversed phenomenon may be the observed inhibition of retrograde axonal transport,[27] which induces changes in the nerve cell bodies.[73] This inhibition leads to a change in anterograde transport of cytoskeletal components such as tubulin,[75] thereby making more proximal parts of the neuron more vulnerable to trauma.

Effects of Compression on Human Nerves

Human nerves may be subjected to compression in many situations. Acute nerve compression injury is usually seen in association with blunt trauma, fractures in the upper arm, or pressure from a tourniquet inflated to a high pressure level.[2] Depending on the severity of the lesion, these injuries fall within any of the classifications given above (metabolic conduction block, neurapraxia, axonotmesis, or neurotmesis). Severe nerve compression lesions also may be seen when a peripheral nerve is locally compressed in an extremity of an individual who is intoxicated or in deep sleep. Usually those lesions fall within the category of neurapraxia, and spontaneous recovery may be expected after weeks to months. There are many types of chronic nerve compression injuries. In principle, nerve trunks may be compressed at any level where they pass through a tight anatomic compartment. However, the most common entrapment is the carpal tunnel syndrome, and the second most common entrapment is ulnar nerve compression at the elbow level. With repetitive motion, a tight condition is exaggerated by swollen muscles and edematous nerves with subsequent inflammation. In addition, the nerve sometimes passes beneath a sharp fascia edge. The pathophysiology behind the signs and symptoms elicited is basically the same as seen in experimental animals. With increasing insight into pathophysiology of nerve compression, it usually is possible to correlate the clinical symptoms to structural and/or functional changes in the nerve trunk.

When a traumatic cuff is inflated to suprasystolic pressure, the hand usually becomes completely anesthetic after 20 to 25 minutes. More than 60 years ago, Lewis and associates[87] concluded that the anesthesia occurred at the same rate with a cuff pressure of 150 mm Hg as at a pressure of 300 mm Hg. This observation was taken as an indication that ischemia of the compressed segment, rather than the mechanical changes induced, was the underlying cause of the loss of nerve function in the situation (metabolic conduction block). The same authors also used special clamps to apply a pressure of 60 to 70 mm Hg directly over the radial or median nerves in the forearm. They found that pressure level was sufficient to induce a local conduction block.

More recent human experiments have been carried out to address the question of critical pressure levels for peripheral nerve viability. These experiments are based on the work of Gelberman and associates,[88] who monitored tissue fluid pressure in the carpal canals of normal volunteers and of patients with carpal tunnel syndrome. In patients with symptoms of median nerve compression at the wrist, there was an average intracarpal canal tissue fluid pressure of 32 mm Hg as compared to an average level of 2.5 mm Hg in control subjects. The pressure levels increased with wrist flexion, as in Phalen's sign, and with wrist extension. Based on these data, a model was developed to study the effect of various levels of induced controlled intracarpal pressure on the sensory and motor function of the median nerve.[89] The tissue fluid pressure inside the canal was continuously monitored by a wick catheter at the same time as a piece of moulded rubber was pressed against the palmar aspect of the wrist. Thereby a localized controlled pressure could be applied to the median nerve, and various tests on motor and sensory function of the nerve could be carried out.

Critical Pressure Levels

A tissue fluid pressure of 30 mm Hg in the carpal canal was required to induce slight paresthesia in median innervated fingers. When the local pressure was increased to 50 to 60 mm Hg or more, complete blockage of motor and sensory conduction occurred. The amplitude of the sensory axon potential decreased rapidly, and the motor axon potential generally disappeared 10 to 30 minutes after disappearance of sensory nerve axon potential. When various pressure levels were tested, it was concluded that 50 mm Hg represented the lower critical pressure at which the function of a nerve fiber was actually jeopardized in normotensive patients.

It seemed as if ischemia rather than mechanical decompression *per se* was the actual cause of the disappearance of nerve conduction. This fact was evident in combined experiments in which a conduction block in the median nerve at the wrist level was first induced by a local external compression of 60 mm Hg (Fig. 6). Forty-five minutes after the disappearance of sensory function, a tourniquet was inflated around the upper arm to raise the suprasystolic pressure. Then, the local pressure on the median nerve at the wrist was released. Function did not recover because the ischemia in the previously compressed nerve segment was sustained by the inflated cuff around the upper arm. With deflation of the tourniquet, sensory and motor function in the median nerve at the wrist were rapidly restored.

Experiments carried out on hypertensive patients gave additional evidence of the significance of ischemia in nerve compression syndromes.[67] When local pressure was applied to the median nerve in hypertensive patients, sensory conduction was not completely blocked until the pressure in the carpal canal reached 60 to 70 mm Hg, a threshold 20 mm Hg higher than the 40 to 50 mm Hg found in normotensive patients. It could be concluded that in both hypertensive and normotensive subjects, the tissue pressure level for nerve fiber viability was consistently 30 mm Hg below the diastolic pressure, and that the susceptibility of a nerve trunk to external pressure varies according to the blood pressure.

Carpal Tunnel Syndrome: A Model for Nerve Compression Injury

Carpal tunnel syndrome represents a useful model for a nerve compression injury with reference to clinical signs and symptoms that reflect defined pathophysiologic events in the nerve. The carpal canal is a tight compartment that contains, in addition to the median nerve, nine flexor tendons, all of which are

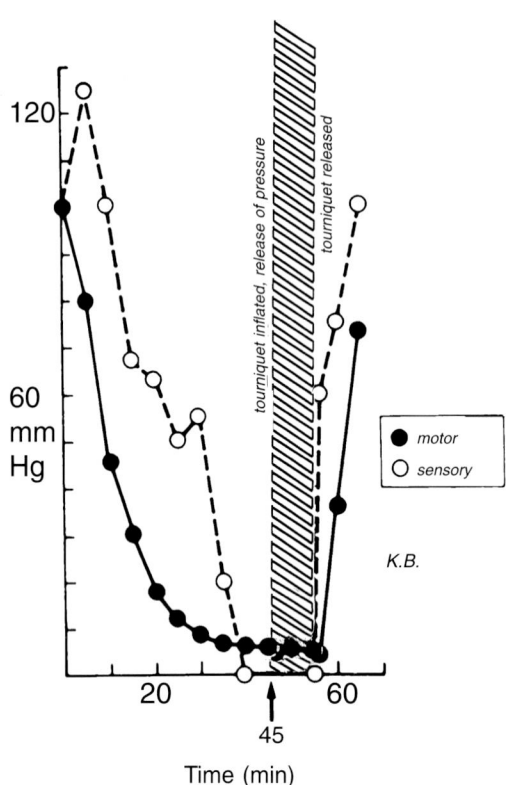

Fig. 6 Experiment in which an external pressure of 60 mm Hg was applied to the carpal canals of human volunteers. The action potential amplitude of the motor, sensory response was measured. The sensory response disappeared 40 minutes after application of localized pressure to the median nerve; 5 minutes later a tourniquet around the upper arm was inflated to 250 mm Hg, and the local pressure at the wrist level was released. The sensory response remained absent. Because the release of pressure on the median nerve was not followed by functional recovery as long as ischemia was induced by the tourniquet pressure, the result indicates that the local conduction block in the median nerve was caused by ischemia, not mechanical pressure. A rapid recovery of the responses was seen when the tourniquet was released. (Reproduced with permission from Lundborg G, Gelberman RH, Minteer-Convery M, et al: Median nerve compression in the carpal tunnel: Functional response to experimentally induced controlled pressure. *J Hand Surg* 1982;7A:252–259.)

surrounded by a loose paratenon. Any process that increases the volume of the contents or decreases the volume of the canal itself may lead to increased tissue pressure in the carpal canal. The symptoms induced by such a pressure increase may vary from nocturnal paresthesia to constant sensory impairment, pain, and atrophy of the thenar.

Early carpal tunnel syndrome is characterized by nocturnal periods of paresthesia and numbness in the median-innervated fingers, usually with complete relief of the symptoms during daytime. The mean pressure of 30 mm Hg monitored in the carpal canals of patients with carpal tunnel syndrome[88] corresponds to the critical pressure for impairment of intraneural venular blood flow[66] and of axonal transport[68–72] observed in animal experiments and to the data obtained from nerve compression experiments in humans. The symptoms, based on a metabolic problem caused by dysfunction of the microvessels, usually occur late at night as revealed by serial overnight recordings of intracarpal canal pressure in carpal tunnel syndrome patients.[90] At that time, the systolic blood pressure is probably much decreased, tissue fluid has been redistributed due to the horizontal position, the muscle pump is out, and the wrists may have been flexed for some time during sleep. These factors all contribute to the median nerve compression and symptoms. The symptoms are immediately reversible, which is characteristic of a metabolic block.

In an intermediate stage of carpal tunnel syndrome, the paresthesia in the hand may also occur during daytime, the dexterity in the hand is much impaired, and there may be a weak abductor pollicis brevis muscle. At this point there is a mixed lesion in which some fibers suffer from a local metabolic disorder and others suffer from a neurapraxia. Surgical decompression at this stage leads to complete relief of some symptoms, but those fibers that suffer from neurapraxia may need weeks or months to completely recover.

In a more advanced stage, where sensibility of the hand is permanently impaired and muscle atrophy may occur, there again is a mixed lesion, which is characterized by metabolic block, neurapraxia, and axonotmesis. Decompression may immediately reverse symptoms because of a metabolic problem. The neurapractic lesion may need a longer time to recover, and when axonotmesis occurs, axons have to regenerate if function in those fibers is ever to recover.

Repetitive Motion

The possible relation of carpal tunnel syndrome to occupational factors is a very controversial subject. This chapter does not discuss this topic because it is covered elsewhere in this volume. For information regarding the impact of occupation and job tasks on the prevalence of carpal tunnel syndrome, the interested reader is advised to read a recent review by Hagberg and associates.[91] The relative contribution of vibration exposure to the hand is supported by studies that show an increased prevalence of carpal tunnel syndrome and other nerve entrapments in workers exposed to vibration.[92,93]

However, it appears that the carpal tunnel is not an ideal anatomic construction for the grips and manipulative tasks required in modern society. The carpal ligament is basically a pulley structure analogous to the fibrous annular ligaments of the flexor tendon sheaths of the fingers, which are constructed to resist a tendency to volar displacement of the flexor tendons with finger flexion and wrist flexion. In such situations, the flexor tendons are pressed against the carpal ligament, creating a very difficult situation for the median nerve, which is located between the tendons and the ligament. In addition, the loose tenosynovium surrounding the flexor tendons may be irritated by edema and inflammation that occur with extended use of the fingers in forceful grip functions. The combination of iterated finger movements under load and flexed wrist over an extended period of time is far from an ideal situation for the median nerve in the carpal tunnel, although the possibility cannot be excluded that evolution has provided humans with a median nerve that resists such provocation. However, recent data on the conduction properties in nerves during repetitive cyclic compression of the nerve indicate that the cyclic loading itself does not play an important role in this context.[94]

References

1. Erlanger J, Gasser HS (eds): *Electrical Signs of Nervous Activity*. Philadelphia, PA, University of Pennsylvania Press, 1937.
2. Lundborg G (ed): *Nerve Injury and Repair*. Edinburgh, Churchill Livingstone, 1988.
3. Grafstein B, Forman DS: Intracellular transport in neurons. *Physiol Rev* 1980;60:1167–1283.
4. Weiss DG: General properties of axoplasmic transport, in Weiss DG, Gorio A (eds): *Axoplasmic Transport in Physiology and Pathology*. Berlin, Germany, Springer-Verlag, 1982, pp 1–14.
5. Vallee RB, Bloom GS: Mechanisms of fast and slow axonal transport. *Annu Rev Neurosci* 1991;14:59–92.
6. Black MM, Lasek RJ: Slow components of axonal transport: Two cytoskeletal networks. *J Cell Biol* 1980;86:616–623.

7. Brady ST, Lasek RJ. The slow components of axonal transport movements, composition and organization, in Weiss DG (ed): *Axoplasmic Transport*. Berlin, Germany, Springer-Verlag, 1982, pp 206–217.
8. McLean WG, McKay AL, Sjöstrand J: Electrophoretic analysis of axonally transported proteins in rabbit vagus nerve. *J Neurobiol* 1983;14:227–236.
9. Lasek RJ, Garner JA, Brady ST: Axonal transport of the cytoplasmic matrix. *J Cell Biol* 1984;99:212S–221S.
10. Archer DR, Dahlin LB, McLean WG: Changes in slow axonal transport of tubulin induced by local application of colchicine to rabbit vagus nerve. *Acta Physiol Scand* 1994;150:57–65.
11. Dahlström A: Axoplasmic transport (with particular respect to adrenergic neurons). *Philos Trans R Soc Lond (Biol)* 1971;261:325–358.
12. Lasek RJ: Protein transport in neurons. *Int Rev Neurobiol* 1970;13:289–324.
13. Lubinska L: Axoplasmic streaming in regenerating and in normal nerve fibres. *Progr Brain Res* 1964;13:1–71.
14. Griffin JW, Price DL, Drachman DB, et al: Incorporation of axonally transported glycoproteins into axolemma during nerve regeneration. *J Cell Biol* 1981;88:205–214.
15. Ochs S: Axoplasmic transport, in Tower D, Brady RO (eds): *The Nervous System: Volume 1. The Basic Neurosciences*. New York, NY, Raven Press, 1975, pp 137–146.
16. Sjöstrand J, McLean WG, Frizell M: The application of axonal transport studies to peripheral nerve problems, in Omer GE Jr, Spinner M (eds): *Management of Peripheral Nerve Problems*. Philadelphia, PA, WB Saunders, 1980, pp 917–927.
17. Brady ST: Microtubules and the mechanism of fast axonal transport, in Weiss DG (ed): *Axoplasmic Transport*. Berlin, Germany, Springer-Verlag, 1982, pp 301–306.
18. Ochs S: Characteristics, a model for fast axoplasmic transport in nerve. *J Neurobiol* 1971;2:331–345.
19. Lubinska L: On axoplasmic flow. *Int Rev Neurobiol* 1975;17:241–296.
20. Bisby MA: Orthograde and retrograde axonal transport of labeled protein in motoneurons. *Exp Neurol* 1976;50:628–640.
21. Bisby MA: Retrograde axonal transport, in Hertz L, Fedoroff S (eds): *Advances in Cellular Neurobiology*. New York, NY, Academic Press, 1980, vol 1, pp 69–117.
22. Bisby MA: Functions of retrograde axonal transport. *Fed Proc* 1982;41:2307–2311.
23. Kristensson K, Sjöstrand J: Retrograde transport of protein tracer in the rabbit hypoglossal nerve during regeneration. *Brain Res* 1972;45:175–181.
24. Kristensson K, Olsson Y: Retrograde transport of horseradish peroxidase in transected axons: 3. Entry into injured axons, subsequent localization in perikaryon. *Brain Res* 1976;115:201–213.
25. De Vito JL, Clausing KW, Smith OA: Uptake, transport of horseradish peroxidase by cut end of the vagus nerve. *Brain Res* 1974;82:269–271.
26. Olsson TP, Forsberg I, Kristensson K: Uptake and retrograde axonal transport of horseradish peroxidase in regenerating facial motor neurons of the mouse. *J Neurocytol* 1978;7:323–336.
27. Dahlin LB, Sjöstrand J, McLean WG: Graded inhibition of retrograde axonal transport by compression of rabbit vagus nerve. *J Neurol Sci* 1986;76:221–230.
28. Varon S, Adler R: Nerve growth factors and control of nerve growth. *Curr Top Dev Biol* 1980;16:207–252.
29. Thomas PK: The connective tissue of peripheral nerve: An electron microscope study. *J Anat* 1963;97:35–44.
30. Thomas PK: The cellular response to nerve injury: 1. The cellular outgrowth from the distal stump of transected nerve. *J Anat* 1966;100:287–303.
31. Shanthaveerappa TR, Bourne GH: The perineural epithelium of sympathetic nerves and ganglia and its relation to the pia arachnoid of the central nervous system and perineural epithelium of the peripheral nervous system. *Z Zellforsch* 1964;61:742–753.

32. Shanthaveerappa TR, Bourne GH: The effects of transection of the nerve trunk on the perineural epithelium with special reference to its role in nerve degeneration, regeneration. *Anat Rec* 1964;150:35–50.
33. Shanthaveerappa TR, Bourne GH: Perineural epithelium: A new concept of its role in the integrity of the peripheral nervous system. *Science* 1966;154:1464–1467.
34. Shanthaveerappa TR, Bourne GH: The "perineural epithelium", a metabolically active, continuous, protoplasmic cell barrier surrounding peripheral nerve fasciculi. *J Anat* 1962;96:527–537.
35. Lundborg G, Brånemark P-I: Microvascular structure and function of peripheral nerves: Vital microscopic studies of the tibial nerve in the rabbit. *Adv Microcirc* 1968;1:66–88.
36. Lundborg G: Ischemic nerve injury: Experimental studies on intraneural microvascular pathophysiology and nerve function in a limb subjected to temporary circulatory arrest. *Scand J Plast Reconstr Surg* 1970;6(suppl):3–113.
37. Lundborg G: Structure and function of the intraneural microvessels as related to trauma, edema formation and nerve function. *J Bone Joint Surg* 1975;57A:938–948.
38. Lundborg G: The intrinsic vascularization of human peripheral nerves: Structural and functional aspects. *J Hand Surg* 1979;4A:34–41.
39. Lundborg G, Myers R, Powell H: Nerve compression injury and increased endoneurial fluid pressure: "Miniature compartment syndrome." *Neurol Neurosurg Psychiatry* 1983;46:1119–1124.
40. Bell MA, Weddell AG: A morphometric study of intrafascicular vessels of mammalian sciatic nerve. *Muscle Nerve* 1984;7:524–534.
41. Bell MA, Weddell AG: A descriptive study of the blood vessels of the sciatic nerve in the rat, man and other mammals. *Brain* 1984;107:871–898.
42. Olsson Y, Kristensson K: Permeability of blood vessels and connective tissue sheaths in the peripheral nervous system to exogenous proteins. *Acta Neuropathol* 1971;5(suppl 5):61–69.
43. Rydevik B, Lundborg G: Permeability of intraneural microvessels and perineurium following acute, graded experimental nerve compression. *Scand J Plast Reconstr Surg* 1977;11:179–187.
44. Waksman BH: Experimental study of diphtheritic polyneuritis in the rabbit and guinea pig: III. The blood-nerve barrier in the rabbit. *J Neuropath Exp Neurol* 1961;20:35–77.
45. Olsson Y: Studies on vascular permeability in peripheral nerves: 1. Distribution of circulating fluorescent serum albumin in normal, crushed and sectioned rat sciatic nerve. *Acta Neuropathol* 1966;7:1–15.
46. Martin KH: Untersuchungen über die perineurale Diffusionsbarriere an gefriergetrockneten Nerven. *Zeitschrift der Zellforsch* 1964;64:404–428.
47. Söderfeldt B, Olsson Y, Kristensson K: The perineurium as a diffusion barrier to protein tracers in human peripheral nerve. *Acta Neuropathol* 1973;25:120–126.
48. Thomas PK, Olsson Y: Microscopic anatomy and function of the connective tissue components of peripheral nerve, in Dyck PJ, Thomas PK, Lambert EH, et al (eds): *Peripheral Neuropathy*, ed 2. Philadelphia, PA, WB Saunders, 1973, vol 1, pp 97–120.
49. Lundborg G, Nordborg C, Rydevik B, et al: The effect of ischemia on the permeability of the perineurium to protein tracers in rabbit tibial nerve. *Acta Neurol Scand* 1973;49:287–294.
50. Myers RR, Costello ML, Powell HC: Increased endoneurial fluid pressure in galactose neuropathy. *Muscle Nerve* 1979;2:299–303.
51. Chen HI, Granger HJ, Taylor AE: Interaction of capillary, interstitial, and lymphatic forces in the canine hindpaw. *Circ Res* 1976;39:245–254.
52. Hargens AR, Akeson WH, Mubarak SJ, et al: Fluid balance within the canine anterolateral compartment and its relationship to compartment syndromes. *J Bone Joint Surg* 1978;60A:499–505.

53. Myers RR, Heckman HM, Powell HC: Endoneurial fluid is hypertonic: Results of microanalysis and its significance in neuropathy. *J Neuropathol Exp Neurol* 1983;42:217–224.
54. Millesi H, Zöch G, Rath T: The gliding apparatus of peripheral nerve and its clinical significance. *Ann Chir Main Memb Super* 1990;9:87–97.
55. Wilgis EF, Murphy R: The significance of longitudinal excursion in peripheral nerves. *Hand Clin* 1986;2:761–766.
56. Zöch G, Reihsner R, Beer R: Stress and strain in peripheral nerves. *Neuroorthopaedics* 1991;10:371–382.
57. Zöch G: Über die Anpassung die Peripheren Nerven an die Bewegungen der Extremitäten durch Gleiten und Dehnung: Untersuchungen am Nervus medianus. *Acta Chir Austria* 1992;96(suppl):1–16.
58. Seddon HJ: Three types of nerve injury. *Brain* 1943;66:237–288.
59. Seddon H (ed): *Surgical Disorders of The Peripheral Nerves*, ed 2. Edinburgh, Churchill Livingstone, 1975.
60. Dahlin LB, Shyu BC, Danielsen N, et al: Effects of nerve compression or ischaemia on conduction properties of myelinated and non-myelinated nerve fibres: An experimental study in the rabbit common peroneal nerve. *Acta Physiol Scand* 1989;136:97–105.
61. Rydevik B, Lundborg G, Skalak D: Biomechanics of peripheral nerves, in Nordin M, Frankel VF (eds): *Basic Biomechanics of the Musculoskeletal System*, ed 2. Philadelphia, PA, Lea & Febiger, 1989, pp 75–87.
62. Ochoa J, Fowler TJ, Gilliatt RW: Anatomical changes in peripheral nerves compressed by a pneumatic tourniquet. *J Anat* 1972;113:433–455.
63. Hargens AR, McClure AG, Skyhar MJ, et al: Local compression patterns beneath pneumatic tourniquets applied to arms and thighs of human cadavera. *J Orthop Res* 1987;5:247–252.
64. Crenshaw AG, Hargens AR, Gershuni DH, et al: Wide tourniquet cuffs more effective at lower inflation pressures. *Acta Orthop Scand* 1988;59:447–451.
65. Pedowitz RA: *Tourniquet-Induced Neuromuscular Injury: Experimental Studies on Effects of Pneumatic Tourniquet Compression and Ischemia in the Rabbit, and Assessment of Clinical Techniques for Facilitating the Use of Lower Tourniquet Inflation Pressures*. Göteborg, Sweden, Göteborg University, 1991. Thesis.
66. Rydevik B, Lundborg G, Bagge U: Effects of graded compression on intraneural blood flow. An in vivo study on rabbit tibial nerve. *J Hand Surg* 1981;6A:3–12.
67. Szabo RM, Gelberman RH, Williamson RV, et al: Effects of increased systemic blood pressure on the tissue fluid pressure threshold of peripheral nerve. *J Orthop Res* 1983;1:172–178.
68. Dahlin LB: *Nerve Compression and Axonal Transport*. Göteborg, Sweden, Göteborg University, 1986. Thesis.
69. Rydevik B, McLean WG, Sjöstrand J, et al: Blockage of axonal transport induced by acute, graded compression of the rabbit vagus nerve. *J Neurol Neurosurg Psychiatry* 1980;43:690–698.
70. Dahlin LB, Danielsen N, McLean WG, et al: Abstract: Critical pressure level for impairment of fast axonal transport during experimental compression of rabbit vagus nerve. *J Physiol* 1982;325:84P.
71. Dahlin LB, Rydevik B, McLean WG, et al: Changes in fast axonal transport during experimental nerve compression at low pressures. *Exp Neurol* 1984;84:29–36.
72. Dahlin LB, McLean WG: Effects of graded experimental compression on slow and fast axonal transport in rabbit vagus nerve. *J Neurol Sci* 1986;72:19–30.
73. Dahlin LB, Nordborg C, Lundborg G: Morphologic changes in nerve cell bodies induced by experimental graded nerve compression. *Exp Neurol* 1987;95:611–621.
74. Dahlin LB, Lundborg G: The neuron and its response to peripheral nerve compression. *J Hand Surg* 1990;15B:5–10.
75. Dahlin LB, Archer DR, McLean WG: Axonal transport and morphological changes following nerve compression: An experimental study in the rabbit vagus nerve. *J Hand Surg* 1993;18B:106–110.

76. Dahlin LB, Kanje M: Conditioning effect induced by chronic nerve compression: An experimental study of the sciatic and tibial nerves of rats. *Scand J Plast Reconstr Surg Hand Surg* 1992;26:37–41.
77. Dahlin LB, Thambert C: Acute nerve compression at low pressures has a conditioning lesion effect on rat sciatic nerves. *Acta Orthop Scand* 1993;64:479–481.
78. Gasser HS, Erlanger J: The role of fiber size in the establishment of a nerve block by pressure or cocaine. *Am J Physiol* 1929;88:581–591.
79. Fowler TJ, Danta G, Gilliatt RW: Recovery of nerve conduction after a pneumatic tourniquet: Observations on the hind-limb of the baboon. *J Neurol Neurosurg Psychiatr* 1972;35:638–647.
80. Hargens AR, Romine JS, Sipe JC, et al: Peripheral nerve-conduction block by high muscle-compartment pressure. *J Bone Joint Surg* 1979;61A:192–200.
81. Ochoa J: Nerve fiber pathology in acute, chronic compression, in Omer GE Jr, Spinner M (eds): *Management of Peripheral Nerve Problems*. Philadelphia, PA, WB Saunders, 1980, pp 487–501.
82. Shyu BC, Olausson B, Huang KH, et al: Effects of sympathetic stimulation on C-fibre responses in rabbits. *Acta Physiol Scand* 1989;137:73–84.
83. Shyu BC, Danielsen N, Andersson SA, et al: Effects of sympathetic stimulation on C-fibre response after peripheral nerve compression: An experimental study in the rabbit common peroneal nerve. *Acta Physiol Scand* 1990;140:237–243.
84. Upton AR, McComas AJ: The double crush in nerve entrapment syndromes. *Lancet* 1973;2:359–362.
85. Dahlin LB, Archer DR, McLean WG: Treatment with an aldose reductase inhibitor can reduce the susceptibility of fast axonal transport following nerve compression in the streptozotocin-diabetic rat. *Diabetologia* 1987;30:414–418.
86. Carroll RE, Hurst LC: The relationship of thoracic outlet syndrome and carpal tunnel syndrome. *Clin Orthop* 1982;164:149–153.
87. Lewis T, Pickering GW, Rothschild P: Centripetal paralysis arising out of arrested bloodflow to the limb, including notes on a form of tingling. *Heart* 1931;16:1–32.
88. Gelberman RH, Hergenroeder PT, Hargens AR, et al: The carpal tunnel syndrome: A study of carpal canal pressures. *J Bone Joint Surg* 1981;63A:380–383.
89. Lundborg G, Gelberman RH, Minteer-Convery M, et al: Median nerve compression in the carpal tunnel: Functional response to experimentally induced controlled pressure. *J Hand Surg* 1982;7A:252–259.
90. Luchetti R, Schoenhuber R, Alfarano M, et al: Serial overnight recordings of intracarpal canal pressure in carpal tunnel syndrome patients with and without wrist splinting. *J Hand Surg* 1994;19B:35–37.
91. Hagberg M, Morgenstern H, Kelsh M: Impact of occupations and job tasks on the prevalence of carpal tunnel syndrome. *Scand J Work Environ Health* 1992;18:337–345.
92. Armstrong TJ, Fine LJ, Radwin RG, et al: Ergonomics and the effects of vibration in hand-intensive work. *Scand J Work Environ Health* 1987;13:286–289.
93. Cannon LJ, Bernacki EJ, Walter SD: Personal and occupational factors associated with carpal tunnel syndrome. *J Occup Med* 1981;23:255–258.
94. Szabo RM, Sharkey NA: Response of peripheral nerve to cyclic compression in a laboratory rat model. *J Orthop Res* 1993;11:828–833.

Chapter 26

Gene Regulation in the Dorsal Root Ganglion in Normal and Pathologic Situations

Mary Ann Ruda, PhD

Neurons of the dorsal root ganglion (DRG) represent the first stage in the transmission of information from the periphery to higher centers of the neuraxis. They innervate target structures of the skin, muscle, and viscera with distinct receptors specifically designed to detect changes in the environment. For example, unencapsulated free nerve endings are activated by noxious forms of stimulation while the encapsulated Pacinian corpuscles respond to vibrating stimuli. DRG neurons represent a diverse population of cells. They have been subdivided using criteria such as conduction velocity of their axon, cell body size, and neurochemical content. These further characterizations of dorsal root ganglion neurons provide a basis for delineating the function of the different subpopulations of DRG neurons.

Over the past several years, our laboratory and others have been studying the DRG as a model system of neuronal function. We have endeavored to characterize it in its constitutive state as well as after persistent noxious stimulation of the periphery or in models of nerve injury. The studies reviewed in this chapter use molecular approaches to identify alterations in gene expression in individual DRG neurons in response to cutting of the sciatic nerve or constriction injury of the sciatic nerve. Cutting a nerve represents a massive injury to all the DRG neurons that contribute axons to the nerve. At the time of the cut, a massive neuronal barrage occurs at the level of the spinal cord. Additionally, nerve cut prevents the retrograde transport of tissue factors such as growth factors from the periphery back to the DRG cell bodies that depend on them to signal biologic responses.[1]

The chronic constriction injury model[2] mimics pain sensations that are characteristic of many clinical chronic pain syndromes. The hyperalgesia, spontaneous pain, and cold allodynia that are characteristic of the injured limb are probably due to axonal damage caused by swelling of the nerve at the site of constriction. Electron microscopic data revealed destruction of most Aβ and Aδ fibers and a varying number of C-fibers distal to the injury site.[3–5] The entire complement of axons in the sciatic nerve may thus contribute to the altered sensations revealed on behavioral testing.[2,6]

In order to further characterize the DRG responses to nerve injury, we have combined these experimental approaches with an animal model that alters the pool of neurons that are present in the DRG. Capsaicin is a neurotoxin that, when administered neonatally, destroys a subpopulation of DRG neurons which are mainly small cells with unmyelinated axons.[7,8] Many of these cells function as nociceptors.[9] Thus, study of the response of DRG neurons to nerve injury in neonatal capsaicin-treated rats further characterizes the class of cells that exhibit either induction or repression of neuropeptide genes.[10,11] For the purpose of illustration, observations on three genes that encode the peptides calcitonin gene-related peptide (CGRP), somatostatin (SOM), and neuropeptide Y (NPY) will be discussed in detail. These three genes were selected because they represent different cell sized subpopulations of DRG neurons and have different constitutive levels of mRNA expression.

Experimental Approach

As part of the experimental design, Sprague-Dawley rats of both sexes received a single subcutaneous injection of capsaicin (50 mg/kg, Sigma) or vehicle (10:10:80 v/v Tween 80:ethanol:saline) on postnatal day 2. At 8 weeks of age, the sciatic nerve on one side was cut and a 1-cm portion removed to prevent reconnection. The animals were killed 7 days after nerve cut and perfused with 4% paraformaldehyde in 0.1 M phosphate buffer (pH 7.4).[12] A second group of male rats received constriction of the sciatic nerve, had their level of hyperalgesia behaviorally assessed, and were killed between 1 and 42 days later.[13] The L4 and L5 DRGs were postfixed overnight, cryoprotected in 30% sucrose, and cut on a cryostat at 15 µm. The sections were thaw-mounted onto Vectabond-coated slides and stored at −80°C. In situ hybridization histochemistry was performed as previously described[12] using oligonucleotide probes complementary to mRNAs encoding CGRP, SOM, and NPY. The probes were labeled with terminal deoxynucleotidyl transferase and ^{35}S-dATP to a specific activity of 5 to 10×10^8 cpm/µg.

For quantification, the number of labeled neurons in the L5 DRG ipsilateral and contralateral to the nerve cut was determined. Because it was difficult to discern the nucleolus in many small neurons, measurements were made of neurons with a visible nucleus in every third 15-µm thick section. This strategy eliminated the likelihood of examining the same neuron twice because the separation distance between sections was greater than the size of the neurons labeled in this study. The neuronal cross-sectional area was determined using a computer-based image analysis system (Image 1.41, NIH). Neurons were arbitrarily divided into three size categories: small cells with a cross-sectional area of less then 1,000 µm^2, medium cells with a size range of 1,000 to 2,000 µm^2, and large cells with a cross-sectional area greater than 2,000 µm^2.

For RNA blot analysis, the ipsilateral or contralateral L4 and L5 DRG of six to eight animals were pooled and additional L4 and L5 DRG from naive animals were collected. The RNA was extracted as previously described.[14] Total RNA was electrophoresed through a denaturing agarose gel and blotted to a nylon membrane. The filters were hybridized with the same probes used for in situ hybridization but were labeled with ^{32}P-dATP and terminal deoxynucleotidyltransferase to a specific activity of at least 10^9 CPM/µg. Cyclophilin mRNA expression was used to standardize lane loading for the purpose of quantification using the Molecular Dynamics PhosphoImager system.

Observations

In the L5 DRG of vehicle-treated rats contralateral to the sciatic nerve cut, numerous cells expressing CGRP mRNA were revealed by in situ hybridization histochemistry (Fig. 1A). The density of label varied between individual neu-

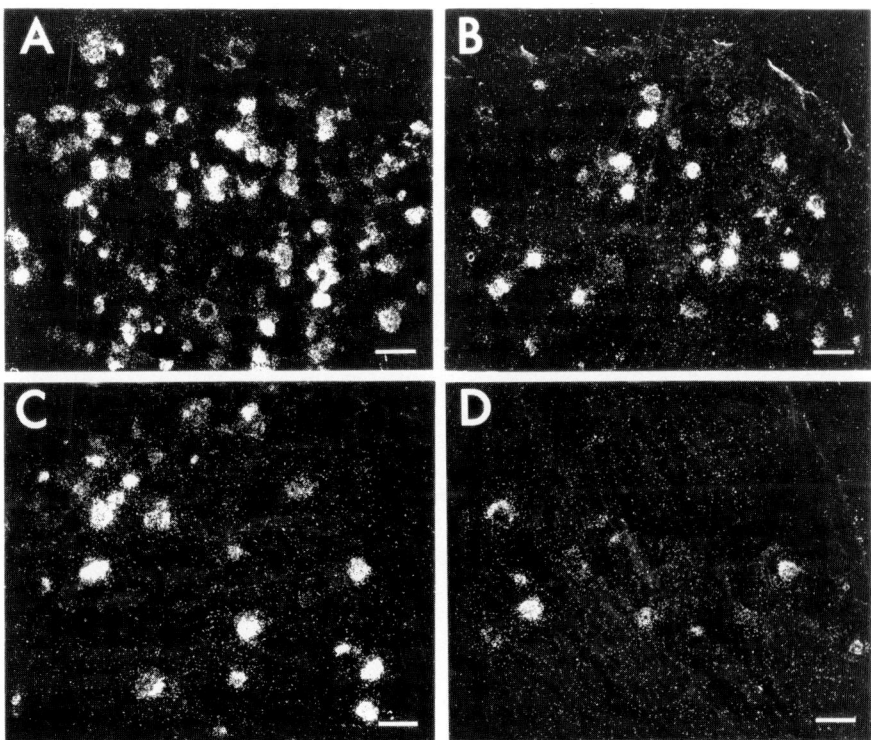

Fig. 1 In situ hybridization histochemistry of the L5 DRG after sciatic nerve cut using an ^{35}S-labeled oligonucleotide probe complimentary to CGRP mRNA. **A** and **B,** Tissue sections of the DRG of vehicle-treated rats. **C** and **D,** Tissue section from neonatal capsaicin-treated rats. **A** and **C,** contralateral to the axotomy. **B** and **D,** ipsilateral to the axotomy. The high constitutive level of mRNA expression for CGRP is attenuated after axotomy, resulting in a 54% reduction in the number of labeled neurons (compare **A** and **B**). Neonatal capsaicin-treated rats exhibited a reduced number of neurons expressing CGRP mRNA both constitutively (**C**) and after axotomy (**D**). Scale bar represents 100 µm. (Adapted with permission from Noguchi K, De León M, Nahin RL, et al: Quantification of axotomy-induced alterations of neuropeptide mRNA's in dorsal root ganglion neurons with special reference to neuropeptide Y mRNA and the effects of neonatal capsaicin treatment. *J Neurosci Res* 1993;35:54–66.)

rons that represented 37.8% of the neurons in the L5 DRG. The cross-sectional area of the labeled neurons ranged from approximately 500 µm² to 2,500µm², although the greatest number of cells had a cross-sectional area under 1,000 µm².

A clear diminution of neurons expressing CGRP mRNA was apparent 7 days after sciatic nerve cut (Fig. 1B). The nerve cut resulted in a 54% loss of neurons with detectable CGRP mRNA expression. The variable density of label over individual neurons was comparable to that seen in the constitutive state. The loss of cells with detectable levels of mRNA expression occurred across the entire spectrum of sizes although the small cells (< 1,000 µm² cross-sectional area) seemed to be disproportionately affected.

Neonatal capsaicin treatment resulted in a 37% reduction in the number of DRG neurons expressing CGRP mRNA. The small DRG neurons appeared to have the greatest reduction in number (Fig. 1C). Likewise, after sciatic nerve cut, the number of detectable neurons was further reduced by 53%, a percent reduction comparable to that found in vehicle-treated rats. Similarly, if one compares the percent change on the axotomized side of vehicle-treated and capsaicin-treated rats, the 36% change is comparable to that observed when the contralateral DRG of each group is compared.

SOM mRNA was constitutively expressed in a small subpopulation (10.6%) of the neurons in the L5 DRG of vehicle-treated rats (Fig. 2A). The intensity of label was variable in individual neurons which were exclusively small-sized cells with a cross-sectional area of 500 to 1,000 µm². Sciatic nerve cut reduced detectable SOM mRNA expression in L5 cells by 54% (Fig. 2B). The neurons expressing SOM mRNA were particularly susceptible to loss by neonatal capsaicin treatment (Fig. 2C). The capsaicin-treated rats had a 83% reduction in SOM cell number resulting in few labeled neurons in the DRG (Fig. 2C). After sciatic nerve cut, a few neurons expressing SOM mRNA could still be detected (Fig. 2D), but given the overall reduction after capsaicin treatment it would be difficult to determine the relevance of any further loss of expression after nerve cut.

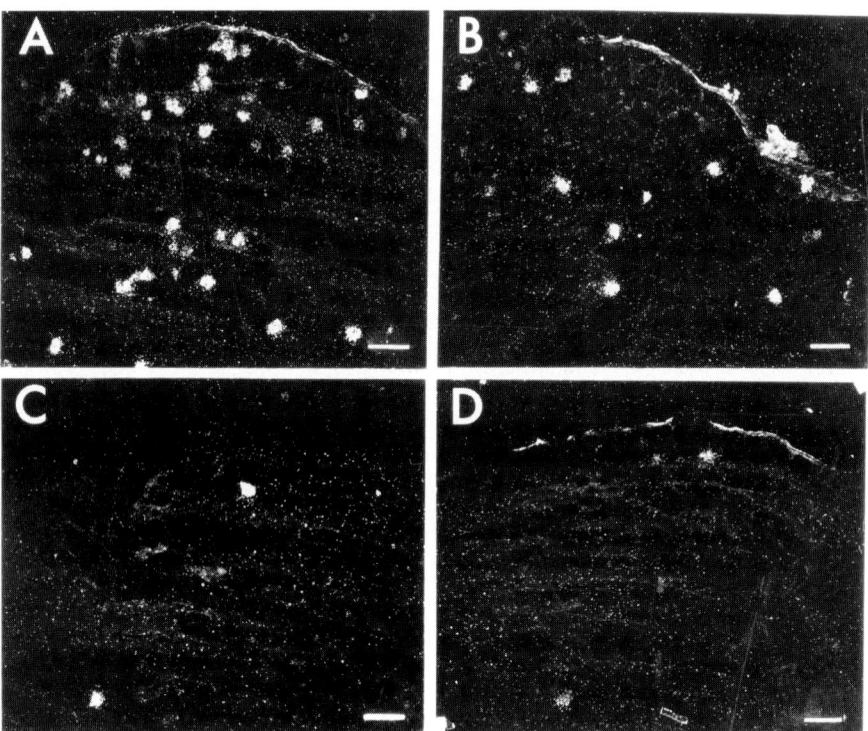

Fig. 2 In situ hybridization histochemistry of the L5 DRG after sciatic nerve cut using an ³⁵S-labeled oligonucleotide probe complimentary to SOM mRNA. **A** and **B,** tissue sections from DRG of vehicle-treated rats. **C** and **D,** tissue sections of DRG of neonatal capsaicin-treated rats. **A** and **C,** contralateral to the axotomy. **B** and **D,** ipsilateral to the axotomy. The constitutive level of mRNA expression for SOM is attenuated after axotomy, resulting in a 54% reduction in the number of labeled neurons in control rats. Almost all the DRG neurons expressing SOM mRNA are capsaicin-sensitive (compare **A** and **C**) resulting in few neurons expressing SOM mRNA in the DRG ipsilateral (**D**) and contralateral (**C**) to sciatic nerve cut. Scale bar represents 100 µm. (Adapted with permission from Noguchi K, De León M, Nahin RL, et al: Quantification of axotomy-induced alterations of neuropeptide mRNA's in dorsal root ganglion neurons with special reference to neuropeptide Y mRNA and the effects of neonatal capsaicin treatment. *J Neurosci Res* 1993;35:54–66.)

Expression of NPY mRNA could not be constitutively detected in DRG of either vehicle-treated (Fig. 3A) or capsaicin-treated rats on the side contralateral to sciatic nerve cut. Cutting of the sciatic nerve, however, dramatically induced neuronal NPY mRNA expression (Fig. 3B). After axotomy 24.4% of the L5 DRG neurons expressed NPY mRNA (Table 1). The labeled neurons had cross-sectional areas ranging from 500 µm² to greater than 2,500 µm². However, most labeled cells were larger than 1,500 µm². In neonatal capsaicin-treated rats, sciatic nerve cut resulted in an induction of NPY mRNA in the DRG (Fig. 3C) that was only slightly reduced (10%) from that observed in vehicle treated rats.

Analysis of mRNA for six neuropeptides and GAP43 in the chronic constriction injury model has recently been described.[13] As related to the peptides discussed in this review, changes in CGRP and NPY mRNA expression were detailed. Following a timecourse of 1 to 42 days (Fig. 4) the maximum reduction in CGRP mRNA expression occurred between 7 and 14 days after the constriction injury. At these timepoints the changes in mRNA expression ranged

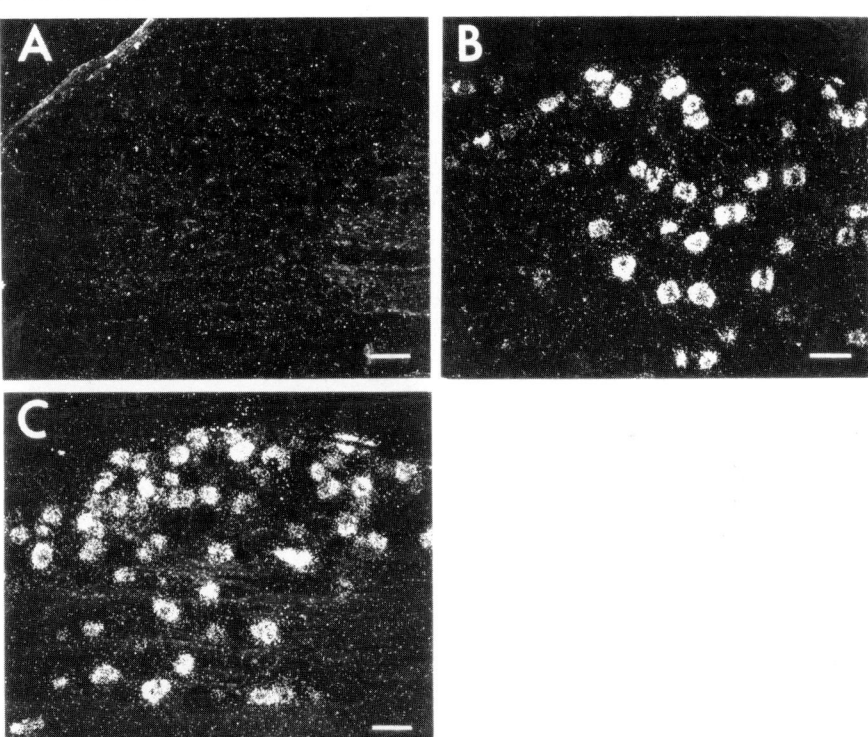

Fig. 3 In situ hybridization histochemistry of the L5 DRG after sciatic nerve cut using an ³⁵S-labeled oligonucleotide probe complimentary to NPY mRNA. Tissue sections of DRG contralateral to the axotomy of vehicle-treated rats (**A**) showed no detectable NPY mRNA expression. In contrast, DRG sections ipsilateral to axotomy (**B**) exhibited an aggregation of silver grains overlying many neuronal cell bodies, indicating intense labeling for NPY mRNAs. Neonatal capsaicin-treated rats following axotomy exhibited an intense labeling for NPY mRNA (**C**) that was comparable in number of labeled neurons to that of vehicle-treated litter mates. Scale bars represent 100 µm. (Adapted with permission from Noguchi K, De León M, Nahin RL, et al: Quantification of axotomy-induced alterations of neuropeptide mRNA's in dorsal root ganglion neurons with special reference to neuropeptide Y mRNA and the effects of neonatal capsaicin treatment. *J Neurosci Res* 1993;35:54–66.)

Table 1 Percentages of DRG* neurons expressing VIP, GAL, or NPY mRNAs following peripheral axotomy†

Treatment	VIP	GAL	NPY
Contra	0%	0.4% (4/1,008)	0%
Axotomy	19.9% (203/1,022)	33.7% (339/1,005)	24.4% (248/1,015)
Capsaicin + axotomy	12.6% (139/1,107)	24.7% (288/1,168)	21.9% (236/1,080)

* DRG, Dorsal root ganglion
† Numbers in each column indicate the percentage of DRG neurons expressing neuropeptide Y (NPY), vasoactive intestinal polypeptide (VIP), galanin (GAL), calcitonin gene-related peptide (CGRP), or somatostatin (SOM) mRNA. The animals were treated with either vehicle or capsaicin at neonatal day 2. Counts were made from over 1,000 neurons in the L5 DRG contralateral (Contra) and ipsilateral to sciatic nerve cut (axotomy). (Adapted with permission from Noguchi K, Dubner R, De León M, et al: Axotomy induces preprotachykinin gene expression in asubpopulation of dorsal root ganglion neurons. *J Neurosci Res* 1994;37:596–603.)

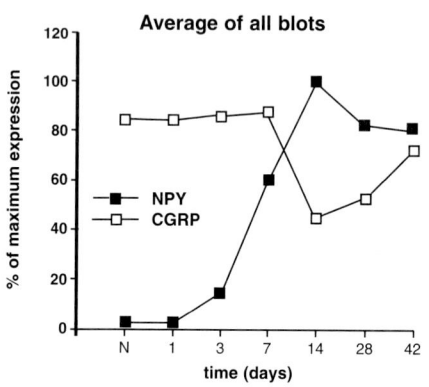

Fig. 4 Line graphs illustrating the effects of constriction injury on calcitonin gene-related peptide (CGRP) (open squares) and neuropeptide Y (NPY) (filled squares) mRNA levels. Graphs represent the average of three different RNA blots. The data are based on PhosphorImage (Molecular Dynamics) analysis of RNA blots standardized for RNA loading with cyclophilin mRNA. Time refers to the postoperative day at which animals were killed. Because no difference was found between RNA from naive or contralateral DRG (analysis of variance), RNA from naive (N) DRG was used for comparison. (Adapted with permission from Nahin RL, Ren K, De León M, et al: Primary sensory neurons exhibit altered gene expression in a rat model of neuropathic pain. *Pain* 1994;58:95–108.)

from 30% to 75%. By 42 days after injury, CGRP mRNA expression returned to approach the baseline constitutive level. The cells responsible for this reduction included small-, medium-, and large-sized DRG neurons, the same size groups that are found to constitutively express CGRP mRNA. On the contralateral side, 40% of the DRG neurons express CGRP mRNA, while at 14 days after constriction injury, only 30% of the L5 ipsilateral DRG neurons are labeled. This change represents a reduction of at least 25% of DRG neurons with detectable levels of CGRP mRNA after constriction injury.

Following constriction injury, NPY mRNA expression is induced by 3 days after injury and the induction persists through 42 days (Fig. 4). The neurons responsible for this induction are mainly the largest sized DRG neurons and represent 20% of the L5 DRG neurons.

Conclusion

In comparing the changes in gene expression that occur after axotomy and in the chronic constriction injury model, one is struck by the similarities. In both cases, the genes encoding the neuropeptides substance P (SP), CGRP, and SOM are repressed while those encoding NPY, vasoactive intestinal polypeptide (VIP), and galanin (GAL) are induced.[12,13,15] Other studies have shown that this change in gene expression results in altered peptide production. The differences in the two animal models occur in terms of the time of onset and duration of the alteration of gene expression. Axotomy typically exhibits a more rapid onset while constriction injury takes several days to show detectable changes in these peptide gene mRNAs. The different timecourse may reflect the fact that axotomy is an instantaneous injury while an initial minor nerve compression develops over time into a greater injury response. Because the peptide genes induced after axotomy are likely to be involved in axonal sprouting and regeneration, the induction of these same peptide genes after compression injury suggests that they provide a similar function in both types of injury. Similarly, the peptide genes repressed after injury are likely involved in normal sensory transmission, which is severed after nerve injury.

The chronic constriction injury model is a useful animal model of neuropathic pain. Similarities may exist between the nature of the nerve injury in this model with that in the repetitive motion syndrome where nerve compression may contribute to the painful state. If nerve compression is found to be a contributing factor in the repetitive motion syndrome (eg, carpal tunnel syndrome), it is likely that the changes in mRNA expression noted in the animal model also occur in humans with a compression injury. The striking changes in gene expression seen in dorsal root ganglion neurons may reflect the molecular basis for painful peripheral neuropathy.

References

1. Lindsay RM, Harmar AJ: Nerve growth factor regulates expression of neuropeptide genes in adult sensory neurons. *Nature* (Lond) 1989;337:362–364.
2. Bennett GJ, Xie YK: A peripheral mononeuropathy in rat that produced disorders of pain sensation like those seen in man. *Pain* 1988;33:87–107.
3. Basbaum AI, Gautron M, Jazat F, et al: The spectrum of fiber loss in a model of neuropathic pain in the rat: An electron microscopic study. *Pain* 1991;47:359–367.
4. Carlton SM, Dougherty PM, Pover CM, et al: Neuroma formation and numbers of axons in a rat model of experimental peripheral neuropathy. *Neurosci Lett* 1991;131:88–92.
5. Pover CM, Dougherty PM, Carlton SM, et al: Abstract: Correlation of axonal numbers and behavioral symptoms in rat experimental neuropathy model. *Soc Neurosci* 1992;22:56.
6. Attal N, Jazat F, Kayser V, et al: Further evidence for "pain related" behaviours in a model of unilateral peripheral mononeuropathy. *Pain* 1990;41:235–251.
7. Buck SH, Burks TF: The neuropharmacology of capsaicin: Review of some recent observations. *Pharmacol Rev* 1986;38:179–226.
8. Jancsó G, Kiraly E, Jancsö-Gäbor A: Pharmacologically induced selective degeneration of chemosensitive primary sensory neurons. *Nature* 1977;270:741–743.
9. Cervero F, Shouenborg J, Sjolund BH, et al: Cutaneous inputs to dorsal horn neurones in adult rats treated at birth with capsaicin. *Brain Res* 1984;301:47–57.
10. Hammond DL, Ruda MA: Developmental alterations in thermal nociceptive threshold and the distribution of immunoreactive calcitonin gene-related peptide and substance P after neonatal administration of capsaicin in the rat. *Neurosci Lett* 1989;97:57–62.
11. Hylden JL, Noguchi K, Ruda MA: Neonatal capsaicin treatment attenuates spinal Fos activation and dynorphin gene expression following peripheral tissue inflammation and hyperalgesia. *J Neurosci* 1992;12:1716–1725.
12. Noguchi K, De León M, Nahin RL, et al: Quantification of axotomy-induced alteration of neuropeptide mRNAs in dorsal root ganglion neurons with special ref-

erence to neuropeptide Y mRNA and the effects of neonatal capsaicin treatment. *J Neurosci Res* 1993;35:54–66.
13. Nahin RL, Ren K, De León M, et al: Primary sensory neurons exhibit altered gene expression in a rat model of neuropathic pain. *Pain* 1994;58:95–108.
14. De León M, Welcher AA, Suter U, et al: Identification of transcriptionally regulated genes after sciatic nerve injury. *J Neurosci Res* 1991;29:437–448.
15. Noguchi K, Dubner R, De León M, et al: Axotomy induces preprotachykinin gene expression in a subpopulation of dorsal root ganglion neurons. *J Neurosci Res* 1994;37:596–603.

Chapter 27

Peripheral Neural Mechanisms of Muscle Pain Resulting From Repetitive Motion and Inflammation

Donald A. Simone, PhD

Introduction

Repetitive motion disorders often involve injury to deep tissues that results in inflammation and a variety of painful syndromes. The painful syndromes may be characterized by ongoing spontaneous pain, referred pain, and deep hyperalgesia (enhanced sensitivity to pain), depending on the severity of injury and the tissues involved. Hyperalgesia, or deep tenderness, can be so severe that innocuous pressure or movement evokes pain. Although pain syndromes of deep origin are relatively common and can be crippling, the underlying neural mechanisms remain poorly understood. In recent years, however, significant progress has been made in defining the neural mechanisms that contribute to pain and hyperalgesia following injury to deep tissues. Electrophysiologic studies of animals and humans, as well as human psychophysical studies, have increased understanding of the neural apparatus that subserves deep pain, particularly muscle pain. In this chapter, some of the psychophysical attributes of deep pain will be described, followed by an overview of the peripheral neural mechanisms contributing to deep pain and hyperalgesia. This review will focus primarily on muscle pain because most psychophysical and electrophysiologic studies of humans have been done in this area.

Deep Pain Sensation: Subjective Quality and Localization

Pain produced by injury to deep structures has characteristic qualities of being dull, poorly localized, and referred to distant tissues.[1] One method of producing muscle pain experimentally is by intramuscular injection of algesic substances, such as hypertonic saline. In early psychophysical studies of muscle pain, it was found that hypertonic saline (6%) evoked aching pain at the site of injection and deep pain, which was referred away from the injection.[2] Subsequent studies revealed that intramuscular injection of hypertonic saline into paravertebral or distal limb muscles produced, in addition to pain, deep tenderness to palpation at the site of injection as well as within the region of referred pain.[3] Injections of hypertonic saline into interspinous ligaments also produced referred deep tenderness within the dermatome of the injected tissue.[4] Although these early qualitative studies introduced the general characteristics of deep pain (subjective quality, poor localization, and referral), relationships between the intensity of the stimulus and the quality, magnitude, and duration of pain, as well as the area of deep hyperalgesia, have only recently begun to be investigated.[5]

Psychophysical Scaling of Deep Pain and Hyperalgesia

A new model of muscle pain has recently been developed in which intramuscular injection of capsaicin, the pungent ingredient of hot chili pepper, is used. When injected into the medial or lateral gastrocnemius-soleus muscle, capsaicin produced immediate pain characterized as cramping. The pain was well localized initially, but gradually radiated within an area several centimeters in diameter surrounding the injection site. The pain was most intense during the first 30 seconds after injection, and gradually decreased during the next 5 to 15 minutes. Referred pain was not experienced. The appearance of referred pain may be related to the volume of the injected stimulus. In the studies in which hypertonic saline was used, a volume of 0.3 to 0.5 ml was usually injected. In the studies in which capsaicin was used, doses of 0.1 to 100 µg were administered in a volume of 10 µl. The larger volume of hypertonic saline would be expected to excite a larger number of nociceptors (pain receptors) than the smaller volume of capsaicin, and this may be a critical factor in the appearance of referred pain.

Using a direct scaling method for magnitude estimation, it was found that humans can accurately scale the magnitude of muscle pain. Figure 1, *left*, shows that the peak magnitude of pain produced by capsaicin is dose-dependent and increased monotonically with capsaicin dose. Capsaicin also produced a dose-dependent area of deep hyperalgesia surrounding the injection (Fig. 1, *right*). Within this area innocuous pressure evoked a sensation of pain. These psychophysical studies suggest that muscle pain usually is described as cramp-like, and that humans can scale the magnitude of muscle (cramping) pain. Furthermore, it is suggested that the area of deep hyperalgesia is directly related to the intensity of the pain-producing stimulus.

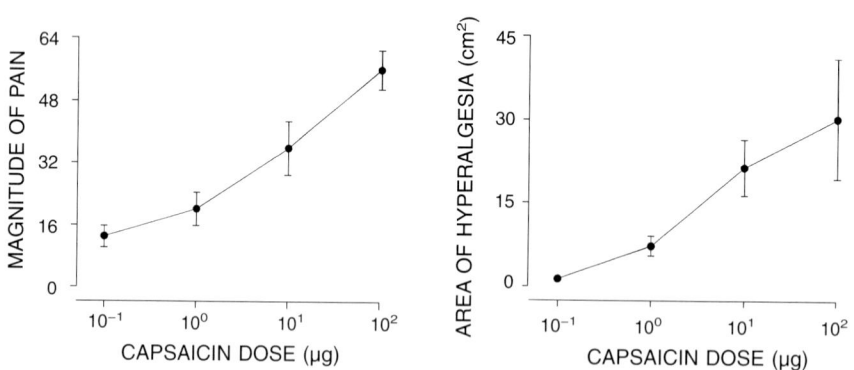

Fig. 1 Left, Mean (± SEM) peak magnitude of pain evoked by intramuscular injection of capsaicin (0.1 to 100 µg in 10 µl) for 10 subjects. Each subject received one injection of each dose into the gastrocnemius-soleus muscles. **Right,** Mean area (± SEM) of deep hyperalgesia produced by intramuscular injection of 0.1 to 100 µg capsaicin. The area of hyperalgesia was determined after the pain from capsaicin subsided using a blunt probe (3-mm diameter).

Peripheral Neural Mechanisms of Muscle Pain: Animal Studies

A nociceptor is defined as a sensory receptive ending that is excited by noxious or intense forms of stimulation. Activity of nociceptors is transmitted centrally by slowly conducting afferent nerve fibers. These slowly conducting afferent fibers are thinly myelinated (A-δ) and unmyelinated (C) fibers.[6,7] These fibers are referred to as group III and group IV afferents, respectively.[8] Group III fibers have conduction velocities of 2.5 to 30 m/sec, whereas the conduction velocity of group IV fibers is less than 2.5 m/sec. Electrophysiologic recordings from single muscle afferent nerve fibers in animals suggest that like cutaneous pain, muscle pain is mediated by slowly conducting afferents. Although most studies have been done on nerves that supply muscles of the hindlimb, there is no reason to suspect differences in pain mechanisms between the upper and lower extremities. Activity of single group III muscle afferents in cats was first reported by Paintal.[9] Although some afferents were excited by innocuous mechanical stimulation, others required noxious stimulation, including intense pressure and injection of hypertonic saline. Reports of additional studies have indicated that group III and group IV afferents are excited by noxious mechanical, thermal, and chemical stimuli.[10-12] Mense and associates[13-20] provided the most detailed descriptions of the response properties of slowly conducting muscle afferents and have divided them into four categories: (1) low threshold pressure-sensitive receptors that may be involved in the sensation of innocuous deep pressure; (2) contraction-sensitive receptors that might be responsible for autonomic adjustments during work; (3) thermosensitive receptors that may have a role in thermoregulation or in thermoreception (sensation associated with changes in tissue temperature); and (4) nociceptors that encode and transmit intensity of pain.

An interesting property of nociceptors, including muscle nociceptors, is that of sensitization. Following injury or inflammation of muscle, slowly conducting afferents develop spontaneous activity and enhanced sensitivity to innocuous mechanical stimulation.[21,22] Sensitization during inflammation is probably caused by release from inflamed tissue of chemicals, including vasoactive substances, neuropeptides, and inflammatory mediators. It has been shown, for example, that nociceptors are excited by bradykinin, serotonin, and potassium ions.[12,13,23] Moreover, bradykinin lowers the mechanical threshold of nociceptors.[24] Ongoing spontaneous activity and sensitization of deep nociceptors probably represent at least part of the neurophysiologic correlates of deep hyperalgesia.

The animal studies described above suggest that activation of groups III and IV muscle afferents contributes to muscle pain sensation. However, activity of these afferents has never been correlated with any measures of behavior indicative of pain. Until recently, it was not known whether humans possess a similar neural apparatus that subserves muscle pain. Fortunately, sophisticated electrophysiologic techniques have provided the means to identify group III and group IV muscle afferents in humans and to determine the sensations evoked by their activation.

Peripheral Neural Mechanisms of Muscle Pain: Human Studies

Intraneural microstimulation (INMS) and microneurography[25] are techniques that allow direct stimulation of and electrophysiologic recording from identified primary afferent fibers. Microneurography has been used to define stimulus-response functions for cutaneous mechanoreceptors[26-28] and nociceptors.[29-32]

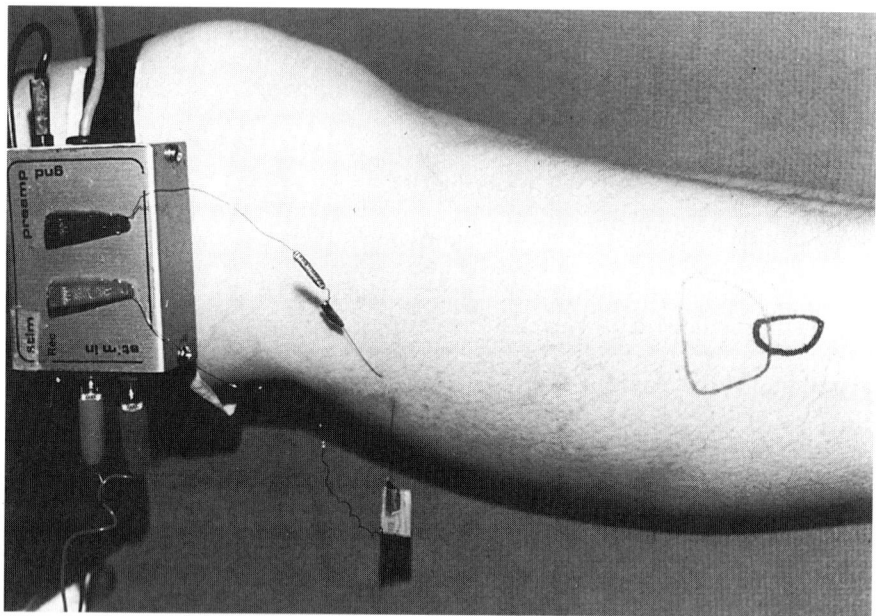

Fig. 2 Experimental setup for INMS and recording from single nociceptive muscle afferents. One electrode (lower) was inserted into the common peroneal nerve below the knee, and a second reference electrode (upper) was inserted into the skin. The larger pale circle represents the projected area of deep pain evoked during INMS (which was mapped by the subject) and the small dark circle represents the mechanical RF of a single group IV afferent. (Reproduced with permission from Simone DA, Machettini P, Caputi G, et al: Identification of muscle afferents subserving sensation of deep pain in humans. *J Neurophys* 1994;72:883–889.)

INMS has been used to stimulate identified mechanoreceptive[33–36] and nociceptive afferents[37] in order to determine elementary sensations evoked by their activation. It was found that activation of mechanoreceptive afferents evoked tactile sensations, whereas activation of nociceptive afferents evoked pain.

INMS and microneurography have recently been used to stimulate and record from slowly conducting skeletal muscle afferents.[38] Briefly, a tungsten microelectrode for stimulation and recording was inserted through the skin and into the common peroneal nerve at knee level. A second reference electrode was inserted into the skin a few centimeters away. Constant voltage of low intensity was passed through the electrode until it penetrated a nerve fascicle that innervated muscle. This was initially determined by the subject's subjective experience of sensation projected to deep tissue of the lower leg or by muscle twitching. Once the electrode was in a muscle fascicle, INMS was continued as the electrode was gently moved until the subject experienced a sensation of deep pain projected to muscle. The electrode was then switched to the recording mode, and innocuous and noxious pressure was applied in the vicinity of the projected painful field (PF) to search for mechanosensitive nociceptors. Once a nociceptor was identified and its receptive field (RF) mapped, conduction velocity was determined by stimulating the RF electrically via needle electrodes inserted into the RF and measuring conduction latency and distance between the stimulating and recording electrodes. The general setup for this procedure is shown in Figure 2, which also shows the projected field of pain during INMS at threshold for pain sensation and the RF of an identified nociceptor.

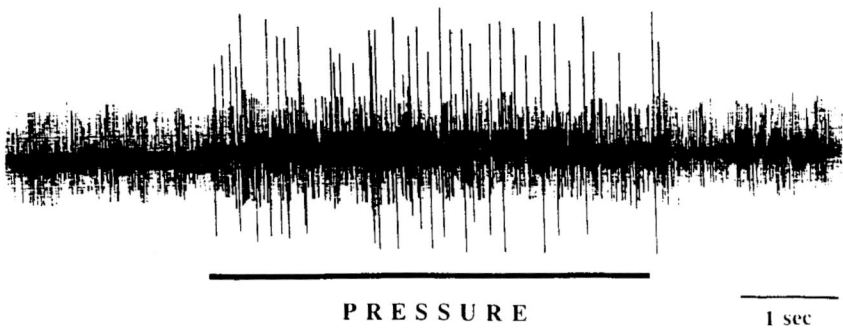

Fig. 3 Response of a group III afferent to sustained pressure applied to the skin overlying the receptive field. (Reproduced with permission from Simone DA, Machettini P, Caputi G, et al: Identification of muscle afferents subserving sensation of deep pain in humans. *J Neurophys* 1994;72: 883–889.)

During INMS of nociceptive muscle afferents (threshold intensity, frequency of 8 Hz, and train durations of 5 to 10 sec), pain projected to muscle was always described as cramping. The quality of pain was the same regardless of whether group III or group IV afferents were stimulated. These studies suggest that cramping pain may be the primary quality of pain from muscle. This differs from skin, in which activation of C nociceptors typically evokes a sensation of burning and A-δ nociceptors evoke sharp pricking pain. It appears that slowly conducting nociceptive afferents in muscle evoke only one type of pain sensation—that of a cramp.

The RF of mechanoreceptors with moderate to high receptor threshold usually was found within or adjacent to the PF evoked during INMS. Of 14 slowly conducting afferents (eight group III and six group IV), only one was spontaneously active (> 1 Hz). All were excited by pressure (Fig. 3), and evoked responses were slowly adapting. None were excited by innocuous stretching. RF areas for group III and group IV fibers, measured percutaneously, did not differ significantly and ranged from 0.36 to 7.96 cm^2.

Pain evoked during short trains of INMS was usually well localized and occupied a small area (0.32 to 20.35 cm^2) (Fig. 2). The areas of pain evoked during INMS of group III and group IV afferents did not differ significantly. Mean areas of painful PFs and mean areas of RFs of group III and group IV fibers did not differ from each other and are illustrated in Figure 4.

The finding that muscle pain evoked during INMS was well localized and never referred differs from classic psychophysical studies describing pain as being diffuse, referred, and not well localized. This difference probably is related to the relative numbers of nociceptive afferents excited. During INMS, it is presumed that a small number of fibers are stimulated, whereas many fibers are probably excited by an injection of 0.3 ml of hypertonic saline. The pain evoked during INMS was similar to that evoked by capsaicin. Again, in the psychophysical studies described above, the volume of capsaicin injected (10 μl) was very small and would be expected to activate a small number of afferents. This expectation is supported by the finding that diffuse and referred pain was produced by INMS of muscle afferents when the INMS intensity was sufficient to produce intense pain.[39]

Although INMS trains of short duration evoked a well-localized area of deep pain, long trains of INMS (at threshold intensity for pain sensation) resulted

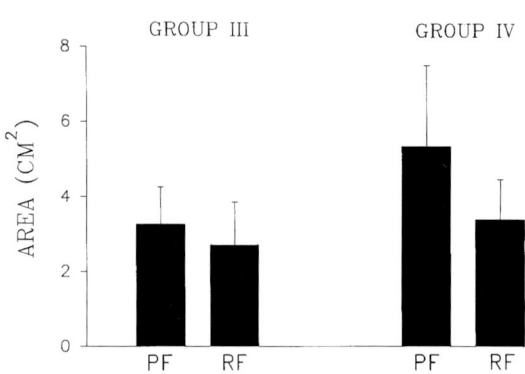

Fig. 4 Mean area (± SEMs) of projected painful field (PF) evoked during INMS of group III and group IV nociceptors and mean (± SEM) receptive field (RF) area of identified group III and group IV nociceptors.

in a gradual enlargement of the PF. This is similar to what happens following intramuscular injection of capsaicin. After approximately 30 sec, the pain begins to radiate and become diffuse and less localized. It is hypothesized that this phenomenon represents temporal summation, centrally. Thus, temporal summation may contribute to diffuseness of muscle pain observed in clinical pain syndromes.

Summary

Intraneural microstimulation and microneurography are powerful tools to investigate the peripheral neural apparatus that subserves deep pain. Preliminary results on response properties of muscle nociceptors in humans agree with and extend results in animals. The subjective quality of pain sensation in muscle appears to be that of cramping. It is not known whether pain from other tissues evokes different types of painful sensations. There is evidence from INMS and microneurography studies that pain projected to tendon is experienced as very sharp, pricking, and well localized.[38] Additional studies are needed to determine the quality of pain sensation associated with various types of deep tissues. This information could help in determining pathology associated with repetitive motion disorders as well as other painful syndromes.

Although it has been shown that muscle nociceptors in animals can become sensitized following injury or inflammation, it is unknown whether similar sensitization occurs for human muscle nociceptors. The techniques of INMS and microneurography should help in determining this information. For example, electrophysiologic recordings can be made from patients with painful disorders, including repetitive motion disorders, and characteristics of nociceptors observed directly. If it is known that certain disorders produce sensitization and hyperactivity of nociceptors, then the nociceptor itself would be a logical target for novel analgesics.

References

1. Lewis T (ed): *Pain.* New York, NY, The Macmillan Company, 1942.
2. Kellgren JH: Observations on referred pain arising from muscle. *Clin Sci* 1938;3: 175–190.
3. Feinstein B, Langton JNK, Jameson RM, et al: Experiments on pain referred from deep somatic tissues. *J Bone Joint Surg* 1954;36A:981–997.

4. Hockaday JM, Whitty CW: Patterns of referred pain in the normal subject. *Brain* 1967;90:481–496.
5. Simone DA, Caputi G, Marchettini P, et al: Cramping pain and deep hyperalgesia following intramuscular injection of capsaicin. *Soc Neurosci Abstr* 1992;18:134.
6. Erlanger J, Gasser HS: The compound nature of the action current of nerve as disclosed by the cathode ray oscillograph. *Am J Physiol* 1924;70:624–666
7. Erlanger J, Gasser HS: The action potential in fibers of slow conduction in spinal roots and somatic nerves. *Am J Physiol* 1930;92:43–82.
8. Lloyd DPC: Neuron patterns controlling transmission of ipsilateral hind limb reflexes in cat. *J Neurophysiol* 1943;6:293–315.
9. Paintal AS: Functional analysis of group III afferent fibres of mammalian muscles. *J Physiol* 1960;152:250–270.
10. Iggo A: Non-myelinated afferent fibres from mammalian skeletal muscle. *J Physiol* 1961;155:52P–53P.
11. Kniffki KD, Mense S, Schmidt RF: Responses of group IV afferent units from skeletal muscle to stretch, contraction and chemical stimulation. *Exp Brain Res* 1978;31:511–522.
12. Kumazawa T, Mizumura K: Thin-fibre receptors responding to mechanical, chemical and thermal stimulation in the skeletal muscle of the dog. *J Physiol (Lond)* 1977;273:179–194.
13. Fock S, Mense S: Excitatory effects of 5-hydroxytryptamine, histamine and potassium ions on muscular group IV afferent units: A comparison with bradykinin. *Brain Res* 1976;105:459–469.
14. Franz M, Mense S: Muscle receptors with group IV afferent fibres responding to application of bradykinin. *Brain Res* 1975;92:369–383.
15. Mense S: Nervous outflow from skeletal muscle following chemical noxious stimulation. *J Physiol (Lond)* 1977;267:75–88.
16. Mense S: Slowly conducting afferent fibers from deep tissues: Neurobiological properties and central nervous actions. *Progr Sensory Physiol* 1986;6:139–219.
17. Mense S: Structure-function relationships in identified afferent neurones. *Anat Embryol* 1990;181:1–17.
18. Mense S, Meyer H: Response properties of group III and IV receptors in the Achilles tendon of the cat. *Pflügers Arch* 1981;389(suppl):R25.
19. Mense S, Meyer H: Different types of slowly conducting afferent units in cat skeletal muscle and tendon. *J Physiol (Lond)* 1985;363:403–417.
20. Mense S, Stahnke M: Responses in muscle afferent fibres of slow conduction velocity to contractions and ischaemia in the cat. *J Physiol (Lond)* 1983;342:383–397.
21. Berberich P, Hoheisel U, Mense S: Effects of a carrageenan-induced myositis on the discharge properties of group III and IV muscle receptors in the cat. *J Neurophysiol* 1988;59:1395–1409.
22. Diehl B, Hoheisel U, Mense S: Histological and neurophysiological changes induced by carrageenan in skeletal muscle of cat and rat. *Agents Actions* 1988;25:210–213.
23. Kaufman MP, Iwamoto GA, Longhurst JC, et al: Effects of capsaicin and bradykinin on afferent fibers with endings in skeletal muscle. *Circ Res* 1982;50:133–139.
24. Mense S, Meyer H: Bradykinin-induced modulation of the response behaviour of different types of feline group III and IV muscle receptors. *J Physiol (Lond)* 1988;398:49–63.
25. Vallbo AB, Hagbarth KE: Activity from skin mechanoreceptors recorded percutaneously in awake human subjects. *Exp Neurol* 1968;21:270–289.
26. Macefield G, Gandevia SC, Burke D: Perceptual responses to microstimulation of single afferents innervating joints, muscles and skin of the human hand. *J Physiol (Lond)* 1990;429:113–129.
27. Nordin M, Hagbarth KE: Mechanoreceptive units in the human infra-orbital nerve. *Acta Physiol Scand* 1989;135:149–161.

28. Ribot-Ciscar E, Vedel JP, Roll JP: Vibration sensitivity of slowly and rapidly adapting cutaneous mechanoreceptors in the human foot and leg. *Neurosci Lett* 1989;104:130–135.
29. Ochoa J, Torebjork E: Sensations evoked by intraneural microstimulation of C nociceptor fibres in human skin nerves. *J Physiol (Lond)* 1989;415:583–599.
30. Torebjork HE: Afferent C units responding to mechanical, thermal and chemical stimuli in human non-glabrous skin. *Acta Physiol Scand* 1974;92:374–390.
31. Torebjork HE, Hallin RG: Identification of afferent C units in intact human skin nerves. *Brain Res* 1974;67:387–403.
32. Torebjork HE, LaMotte RH, Robinson CJ: Peripheral neural correlates of magnitude of cutaneous pain and hyperalgesia: Simultaneous recordings in humans of sensory judgments of pain and evoked responses in nociceptors with C-fibers. *J Neurophysiol* 1984;51:325–339.
33. Ochoa J, Torebjork E: Sensations evoked by intraneural microstimulation of single mechanoreceptor units innervating the human hand. *J Physiol (Lond)* 1983;342:633–654.
34. Torebjork HE, Ochoa JL: Specific sensations evoked by activity in single identified sensory units in man. *Acta Physiol Scand* 1980;110:445–447.
35. Vallbo, AB: Sensations evoked from the glabrous skin of the human hand by electrical stimulation of unitary mechanosensitive afferents. *Brain Res* 1981;215:359–363.
36. Vallbo AB, Olsson KA, Westberg KG, et al: Microstimulation of single tactile afferents from the human hand: Sensory attributes related to unit type and properties of receptive fields. *Brain* 1984;107:727–749.
37. Torebjork HE, Ochoa JL: New method to identify nociceptor units innervating glabrous skin of the human hand. *Exp Brain Res* 1990;81:509–514.
38. Simone DA, Machettini P, Caputi G, et al: Identification of muscle afferents subserving sensation of deep pain in humans. *J Neurophys* 1994;72:883–889.
39. Marchettini P, Cline M, Ochoa JL: Innervation territories for touch and pain afferents of single fascicles of the human ulnar nerve: Mapping through intraneural microrecording and microstimulation. *Brain* 1990;113:1491–1500.

Directions for Future Research

Develop, refine, and validate a compression model as related to mechanical issues.

Previous experimental models have demonstrated that the peripheral nerve undergoes a specific sequence of changes in response to the application of extrinsic pressure. Because of the nature of existing experimental compression models, however, the data that have been provided are not completely applicable to questions concerning cumulative trauma. Previous methods of experimental nerve compression have used static extrinsic pressure applied perpendicular to the longitudinal axis of nerve for relatively short periods of time. Pressures applied over longer periods of time have neither been controlled for the magnitude of applied pressure nor have they been cyclic in nature. A refined chronic compression model simulating the events that occur with repetitive upper extremity usage needs to be provided. The identification of specific metabolic and structural changes within nerve in response to interval applications of pressure applied in compression, tension, torsion and shear over extended periods of time would help explain the neural response to cumulative trauma.

Determine the clinical management of repetitive motion nerve injury.

Further studies are indicated to delineate basic guidelines for correct ergonomics at a given workstation. This could be done either through laboratory analysis of human kinetics using work simulation or studying energy consumption and the biomechanics of fatigue in an attempt to find the most energy-efficient methods of performing a given task. The first stage would be done in a laboratory setting. Later stages would make this model portable and capable of being taken into the workstations for field studies. Specific recommendations can be made using coherent models of what constitutes an ergonomically correct activity with classification systems. Special emphasis is needed to define nerve impairment in specific work environments.

Models should be developed that use various forms of treatments in prospective outcome studies which compare currently used treatment modalities to assess the long-term efficacy of treatment; for example, is nerve mobilization or immobilization the key to nonsurgical treatment of compressive neuropathy? If both methods are to be used, how are they to be employed to maximal advantage? To what point should nonsurgical management be allowed to continue before resorting to surgery, especially in workers' compensation cases? What is the role of nonsteroidal anti-inflammatory drugs in the management of repetitive strain nerve injury? Further evaluation of other modalities of nerve testing must be done to increase the sensitivity and specificity of nerve tests, especially with regard to unmyelinated nerve fibers, which may be responsible for the early symptoms. In addition, more sensitive methods of testing those populations at risk must be employed to reduce required sample size.

Explore changes in central neuronal function in repetitive motion syndrome.

Although the role of altered neuronal circuits in persistent pain states has recently received much attention, its relationship to repetitive motion syndrome is unknown. Central changes are thought to have a critical function in the persistence of pain after the obvious recovery from peripheral tissue damage. The continuing neuronal barrage that occurs following tissue injury can lead to excitotoxic events in neurons that may be related to N-Methyl-D-Aspartate (NMDA) receptor activation. Excitotoxity may result in neuronal cell death, altering the neuronal circuits that were programmed to handle pain messages.

Several factors are critical to determining the role of central changes in pain related to the repetitive motion syndrome. The time after onset of the syndrome for the occurrence of persistent pain as well as the impact of the age of the individual at pain onset should be determined. A thorough sensory evaluation is critical and requires standardized testing to determine the extent of neurologic damage. The progressive nature of the syndrome may exhibit a time difference in the loss of sensory submodalities.

Because of a potential relationship in neuronal plasticity following injury to that which occurs during normal neuronal development, parallels should be sought in the repetitive motion syndrome and development. Changes in neuronal phenotypic expression in the dorsal root ganglion have been identified in animal models of nerve injury and may play a role in altered sensations. The potential role of these changes in the repetitive motion syndrome are unknown but should be investigated to explain the persistent pain associated with this syndrome.

Characterize nerve damage in the repetitive motion syndrome.

With the assumption that an underlying cause of the pain associated with the repetitive motion syndrome is nerve injury, factors that contribute to the repair of damaged nerves should be investigated for possible treatment efficacy. Growth factors play a key role in axonal maintenance and guidance both in normal development and the response to nerve injury. Several families of growth factors have been isolated and localized to neurons and glial cells. Addition of growth factors, such as nerve growth factor, to a damaged nerve may help improve the progression of the nerve injury.

In addition to growth factors, many neurochemicals present in dorsal root ganglion neurons have been shown to be differentially regulated following nerve injury. Their role in the persistent pain associated with the syndrome needs to be addressed.

Characterize nociceptors in deep tissue.

One area that requires much more research is the characterization of nociceptors in deep tissues. Properties such as conduction velocity, types of stimuli that excite deep nociceptors, adaptation, and stimulus-response functions need to be further defined. While much work has been done in animals, little has been done in humans. Because pain and hyperalgesia may accompany repetitive motion disorders, it is important to know which types of nociceptors are excited during these painful conditions. It is equally important to determine whether nociceptors in deep tissues become sensitized in humans following tissue injury and inflammation and to determine the mediators involved. Understanding the biochemical mechanisms that lead to sensitization of nociceptors and accompanying hyperalgesia may lead to novel therapeutic approaches for deep pain.

Section 6

Clinical Issues

Section Editor:
Robert M. Szabo, MD

Peter C. Amadio, MD
Sidney J. Blair, MD, FACS
William F. Blair, MD
Terrence P. Glennon, MD
Barry Goldstein, MD, PhD
Jay Himmelstein, MD, MPH
Joseph P. Iannotti, MD, PhD
Craig L. Levitz, MD

Michael Madison, PhD
Robert P. Nirschl, MD, MS
Glenn Pransky, MD, MOccH
Joel M. Press, MD
Steven A. Stiens, MD
Robert M. Szabo, MD
Jeffrey L. Young, MD

Overview

The term repetitive motion disorder implies a presumptive etiology. To the clinician treating a patient with a painful upper extremity, this etiologic inference is of only minor relevance. In managing a patient, the clinician faces four tasks, three of them medical and one bureaucratic.

The first task is to make a diagnosis in which the injured tissue is identified and the nature and site-specific location of the injury is determined. There are many unresolved controversies in the area of diagnosis. The level of desired accuracy must be balanced with the increased costs of additional diagnostic studies. The clinical section of this book describes the generally accepted medical diagnostic categories, or "labels," that have been applied to patients with cumulative trauma disorders of the upper extremity. They are specific and imply a well-defined anatomic region affected by a well-defined pathologic process.

Once a diagnosis has been made, the contributing factors must then be evaluated. These include intrinsic factors (anatomic abnormalities, metabolic disorders) as well as extrinsic factors (the nature of the patient's job, as well as his or her avocations). Here too, data are sparse and interpretation difficult. Why do some workers in the same job suffer from a disorder, whereas other workers in the same job do not? How does the work environment interact with intrinsic risk factors? Does repetitive work simply accelerate a natural aging process; if so, should a limit be set to cumulative exposure? Can the risk factors be quantitated and ranked?

The third task the clinician faces is to select a treatment program. This may include acute intervention such as drugs, splinting, or surgery. With repetitive motion disorders, the prescribed rehabilitative program frequently includes stretching and muscle strengthening, alteration of tools and aerobic conditioning and other exercises. In this area, too, there are few comprehensive prospective studies, and reliable data are unavailable to guide the design of a program of treatment and rehabilitation.

Finally, the clinician may be required to make a determination as to whether the condition is "caused" by the job; this requirement is not a medical mandate, but rather a bureaucratic one. Such a determination is "medically" impossible. The job may constitute an environment that contributes to an increase in the propensity for a condition, but is not itself the cause of the condition. Nevertheless, we clinicians should be committed to improve our understanding of repetitive motion disorders so that we can help our patients cope with the medical and social issues that surround this modern plague.

Chapter 28
Carpel Tunnel Syndrome as a Work-Related Disorder

Robert M. Szabo, MD
Michael Madison, PhD

Introduction

Carpal tunnel syndrome (compression of the median nerve at the wrist) is the most common and best known of the compression neuropathies of the upper extremity. The syndrome is characterized by pain and paresthesias on the palmar-radial aspect of the hand, symptoms that are often worse at night and/or exacerbated by repetitive, forceful use of the hand.

Carpal tunnel syndrome commonly affects middle-aged people in the workplace. The extent to which the type of work contributes to this condition is controversial and of great interest with respect to prevention, treatment, and compensation. Some studies find little evidence supporting the concept of carpal tunnel syndrome as a work-related disorder,[1-5] whereas others propose that more than half of cases of carpal tunnel syndrome may be attributed to workplace factors.[6-8] Carpal tunnel syndrome is one of the most common diagnoses for workers' compensation claims in the United States, but in the rest of the world it is rarely considered to be a work-related disorder; in France, for example, it is not an allowable diagnosis for workers' compensation.

Diagnostic Issues

The first step in evaluating the industrial setting of carpal tunnel syndrome is to have an accurate diagnosis. Most epidemiologic studies, however, including the most widely cited ones, have relied on diagnostic criteria that we consider inadequate.

The term carpal tunnel syndrome refers to impairment of the median nerve and its branches in the hand that results in compression at the wrist. The syndrome is a final common pathway of a variety of local and systemic disorders; therefore it is both a diagnosis and a symptom of some other condition.[9] The presence of a deficit of the median nerve at the wrist is sufficient to diagnose carpal tunnel syndrome (as idiopathic carpal tunnel syndrome), and for epidemiologic studies may be adequate. However, the astute physician will continue diagnostic study in order to discover the underlying causes.

Chronic carpal tunnel syndrome can be classified into early, intermediate, and late.[10] Patients with early chronic carpal tunnel syndrome have intermittent pain and paresthesias in the distribution of the median nerve; it is worse at night or following specific activities. Sensory latencies are more often prolonged than are motor latencies, and muscle abnormalities are absent on electromyographic testing. While gross morphologic changes in the nerve are absent, there is transient reversible epineural ischemia and impaired axonal transport.[11] Patients frequently respond to splinting, steroid injections into the carpal canal, or modification of precipitating activities.

In intermediate chronic carpal tunnel syndrome, paresthesias and numbness become more prevalent. Sensory threshold testing values are elevated, and distal motor latencies are increased. The persistent compromise of intraneural microcirculation, as well as epineural and intrafascicular edema, make a lasting response to conservative measures unlikely. Carpal tunnel release is indicated for definitive treatment. Sectioning the transverse carpal ligament increases the anterior-posterior dimensions of the carpal canal, thereby increasing the carpal canal volume and reducing interstitial pressure.[12]

Patients with advanced chronic carpal tunnel syndrome have permanent loss of sensory and motor function, as well as thenar muscle atrophy. Nerve conduction velocities are delayed, and distal sensory and motor latencies are prolonged. Fibrillation potentials are present on electromyographic testing of the thenar muscles. Long-standing endoneural edema will eventually cause fibrosis of the median nerve, as well as partial demyelination and axonal degeneration.

Demonstration of the nerve deficit is based on patient history, physical examination, and nerve conduction studies (Table 1). The history and the physical examination, which should include a variety of sensory tests and perhaps hand diagrams, rely on the patient's verbal reports of sensation or pain. In a motivated and honest patient, a combination of these tests may suffice to demonstrate the nerve deficit. However, if the case is clouded by workers' compensation issues, the patient's reports may be unreliable. This is not to say that the patient is malingering; rather, he or she may have a very low threshold for perceiving discomfort, and patients who are forewarned about carpal tunnel syndrome may subconsciously amplify minor discomforts until they are perceived as significant symptoms. For this reason, nerve conduction studies are essential to demonstrate the nerve deficit objectively. When properly used, these tests have sensitivity and specificity near 90%.[13] Unfortunately, most epidemiologic studies of carpal tunnel syndrome have not used nerve conduction studies to obtain a diagnosis, and it is therefore uncertain whether all cases were indeed carpal tunnel syndrome.

The interpretation of nerve conduction studies is hindered because many patients with carpal tunnel syndrome have systemic neuropathies. Thus a comparison of right to left hand, or median nerve to ulnar nerve, may fail to demonstrate a difference because the impairment affects all of these nerves. The incremental technique of Kimura[14] may allow localization of the median nerve deficit to the wrist. Repeated tests over a period of time can be useful in monitoring progression or recovery.

The circumstances under which tests are performed are critical. In many cases of carpal tunnel syndrome, particularly those that are work-related, symptoms appear only in response to a period of provocative activity (dynamic carpal tunnel syndrome).[15] If the patient is tested out of the context in which symptoms typically occur, false-negative results may be obtained. It is appropriate immediately prior to testing to have the patient simulate the activities that cause symptoms. White and associates[16] repeatedly performed vibrograms on a series of subjects with and without carpal tunnel syndrome. They found that vibrogram thresholds were lowest on Monday, rose steadily through the week to become highest on Friday, and then declined over the weekend. They also found that thresholds in female subjects were elevated during menses. On a

Table 1 Diagnostic Tests for Carpal Tunnel Syndrome

Test	How Performed	Condition Measured	Positive Result	Interpretation of Positive Result*
Phalen's test	Patient places elbows on table, forearms vertical, wrists flexed	Paresthesias in response to position	Numbness or tingling on radial-side digits within 60 sec	Probable CTS (sensitivity, 0.75; specificity, 0.47)
Percussion test (Tinel's)	Examiner lightly taps along median nerve at the wrist, proximal to distal	Site of nerve lesion	Tingling response in fingers at site of compression	Probable CTS if response is at the wrist (sensitivity, 0.60; specificity, 0.67)
Carpal tunnel compression test	Direct compression of median nerve by examiner	Paresthesias in response to pressure	Paresthesias within 30 sec	Probable CTS (sensitivity, 0.87; specificity, 0.90)
Hand diagram	Patient marks sites of pain or altered sensation on outline diagram of the hand	Patient's perception of site of nerve deficit	Signs on palmar side of radial digits without signs in palm	Probable CTS (sensitivity, 0.96; specificity, 0.73); negative predictive value of a negative test = 0.91
Hand-volume stress test	Measure hand volume by water displacement; repeat after 7-min stress test and 10-min rest	Hand volume	Hand volume increased by 10 ml or more	Probable dynamic CTS
Direct measurement of carpal tunnel pressure	Wick or infusion catheter is placed in carpal tunnel; pressure is measured	Hydrostatic pressure while resting and in response to position or stress	Resting pressure of 25 mm Hg or more (this value is variable and may not be valid in and of itself)	Hydrostatic compression at wrist is probable cause of CTS
Static two-point discrimination	Determine minimum separation of two points perceived as distinct when lightly touched on palmar surface of digit	Innervation density of slowly adapting fibers	Failure to discriminate points more than 6 mm apart	Advanced nerve dysfunction
Moving two-point discrimination	As above, but with points moving	Innervation density of quickly adapting fibers	Failure to discriminate points more than 5 mm apart	Advanced nerve dysfunction
Vibrometry	Vibrometer head is placed on palmar side of digit; amplitude at 120 Hz increased to threshold of perception; compare median and ulnar nerves in both hands	Threshold of quickly adapting fibers	Asymmetry with contralateral hand or between radial and ulnar digits	Probable CTS (sensitivity, 0.87)

Table 1 Diagnostic Tests for Carpal Tunnel Syndrome (cont.)

Test	How Performed	Condition Measured	Positive Result	Interpretation of Positive Result*
Semmes-Weinstein monofilament test	Monofilaments of increasing diameter touched to palmar side of digit until patient can tell which digit is untouched	Threshold of slowly adapting fibers	Value greater than 2.83 in radial digits	Median nerve impairment (sensitivity, 0.83)
Distal sensory latency and conduction velocity	Orthodromic stimulus and recording across wrist	Latency and conduction velocity of sensory fibers	Latency greater than 3.5 msec or asymmetry greater than 0.5 msec compared with contralateral hand	Probable CTS
Distal motor latency and conduction velocity	Orthodromic stimulus and recording across wrist	Latency and conduction velocity of motor fibers of median nerve	Latency greater than 4.5 msec or asymmetry greater than 1.0 msec	Probable CTS
Electromyography	Needle electrodes placed in muscle	Denervation of thenar muscles	Fibrillation potentials, sharp waves, increased insertional activity	Very advanced motor median nerve compression

(Adapted with permission from Szabo RM, Madison M: Carpal tunnel syndrome. *Orthop Clin North Am* 1992;23:105.)
*CTS = carpal tunnel syndrome.

daily basis, thresholds rose during the day. In these subjects, false results could be obtained depending on the timing of the vibrometry tests.

The accuracy required in the diagnosis of carpal tunnel syndrome depends on the purpose. If a patient is being considered for surgery, a very accurate diagnosis is needed. In surveillance of incidence of carpal tunnel syndrome in industry for purposes of monitoring public health, a more sensitive but less specific diagnostic method may suffice.[17]

Risk Factors

A 10% incidence of carpal tunnel syndrome in the workplace would be considered alarmingly high, but on the other hand, this would mean that 90% of workers are not afflicted. What factors determine whether or not a worker develops carpal tunnel syndrome? We propose to address this question by considering the interaction of intrinsic risk factors (various innate anatomic, physiologic, or behavioral characteristics of the worker) with extrinsic risk factors (job-related factors) that make a worker more likely to develop carpal tunnel syndrome. Several of the intrinsic and extrinsic risk factors that enter into this equation will be discussed briefly.

Intrinsic Risk Factors

Anatomic Variants Any anatomic variant that decreases the dimensions of the carpal tunnel or increases the volume of its contents may, by increasing compression on the median nerve, constitute a risk factor for carpal tunnel syndrome. Examples of such factors are malunited distal radius fracture, neuroma, lipoma, posttraumatic osteophyte, a persistent median artery, and an abnormal muscle belly. A palmaris longus can have its muscle belly reversed, acting as a space-occupying mass in the carpal tunnel.[18] Abnormally long lumbrical muscles,[19] anomalous muscle bellies of the flexor digitorum superficialis[20] and of the insertion of the palmaris longus, as well as a palmaris profundus[21] have been reported as causes of median nerve compression. Anomalous tendon slips from the flexor pollicis longus to the flexor digitorum profundus of the index finger can also be responsible for chronic tenosynovitis leading to carpal tunnel syndrome.[22] Hypertrophic tenosynovium is a common finding at surgery, and in the past was commonly attributed to tenosynovitis. However, recent histologic studies have shown a paucity of inflammatory elements, and the hypertrophy of the synovium seems to have some other, noninflammatory basis.[23,24] A recent report of significant amyloid deposits found on histologic examination of flexor tenosynovium in 89% of 149 patients with carpal tunnel syndrome suggests that this may be an important tenosynovial pathology in idiopathic carpal tunnel syndrome.[25]

Siegel and associates[26] found an abnormally proximal origin of the lumbrical muscles in 32% of 128 consecutive hands undergoing surgery for carpal tunnel syndrome. Of the patients who performed repetitive hand motions, 84% had an origin of the lumbricals more proximal than that found in a control group of cadaver hands. These findings suggest that hypertrophy of the lumbricals in relation to repetitive work may be a contributory factor to carpal tunnel syndrome in individuals with an anatomic predisposition based on proximal origins. Ditmars[27] divided the typical presentation of carpal tunnel syndrome into several common patterns, one of which he termed the lumbrical pattern. He found that patients with this pattern often had only borderline abnormality on nerve conduction studies, but tended to do well with open surgical release of the flexor retinaculum.

Nakamichi and Tachibana,[28] in a study of 128 patients with carpal tunnel syndrome, found that if a space-occupying lesion in the carpal tunnel was present (in 7 patients studied), the symptoms were always unilateral; when reduction in nerve conduction velocity was bilateral, an anatomic abnormality was not found.

A small or thick wrist has also been proposed as an intrinsic risk factor for carpal tunnel syndrome.[29]

Physiologic Variants Several conditions have been shown to be intrinsic risk factors for carpal tunnel syndrome, including diabetes, alcoholism, smoking, rheumatoid arthritis, obesity, pregnancy, eclampsia, myxedema, and hemodialysis. Edema is a common manifestation in these conditions, and the fat, swollen, edematous hand is an often-seen clinical presentation of carpal tunnel syndrome. The mechanisms whereby edema leads to impairment of the median nerve are unknown. Systemic neuropathy is another common feature of these risk factors. It is a frequent observation in nerve conduction studies that median nerve deficits are usually bilateral, even if use of the hands is asymmetric and symptoms are unilateral.[28,30–32] Increasing age is a risk factor for slowing of nerve conduction velocities and may contribute to the bilateral deficits found in workers.[32]

Nathan and Keniston[33] analyzed intrinsic and extrinsic risk factors for carpal tunnel syndrome in 3,429 hands on which nerve conduction studies were performed. They found that the physical condition of the individual accounted for most of the variation in median nerve conduction. Specifically, increased body mass index and a sedentary lifestyle were significant risk factors for slowing of nerve conduction and for carpal tunnel syndrome. Age and wrist geometry were of lesser importance, and job-related activities had only very minor predictive value for carpal tunnel syndrome. Wrist dimension as a risk factor accounts for 17% of carpal tunnel syndrome in regression analysis.[33]

Behavioral characteristics that reflect cultural factors in labor-management relations, litigation, and compensation in our society may play a role in the perception and reporting of symptoms of carpal tunnel syndrome. In a cross-sectional study, sensory conduction of the median nerve was measured in 101 Japanese furniture factory workers.[34] The prevalence of slowing in the Japanese workers was reported to be 17.8%, while the prevalence of carpal tunnel syndrome based only on symptoms was 2.5%; the prevalence of carpal tunnel syndrome confirmed by slowing was 2.0%. The prevalence of slowing in the Japanese workers was not significantly different from the prevalence of slowing in 316 American workers from four industries (22.0%),[34] but the prevalence of carpal tunnel syndrome symptoms and complaints was much lower in the Japanese. Japanese workers may have been less likely to complain about symptoms of carpal tunnel syndrome than their American counterparts because their culture stresses conformity, not confrontation.[35]

Extrinsic Risk Factors

Several features of manual work have been proposed as risk factors for development of carpal tunnel syndrome. These include flexion and extension of the wrist, forceful use of the hand, repetitive motion of the hand, and exposure to vibration. Workers whose job incorporates one or more of these actions are expected to have a higher prevalence of carpal tunnel syndrome than a similar group of workers, matched for intrinsic risk factors, whose jobs do not include these factors.

Position of the Hand Magnetic resonance imaging studies have shown that when the wrist is flexed the median nerve is compressed between the flexor digitorum tendons and the flexor retinaculum.[36] In cadaveric studies of median nerves, the region that lies within the carpal tunnel is flattened and fibrotic compared to more proximal or distal portions, which is interpreted as the result of a prolonged history of compression.[37] In addition to mechanical compression, the median nerve may also be subjected to hydrostatic compression with wrist flexion or extension, as has been shown by fluid pressure measurements in patients and in normal volunteers.[38–40]

Flexion and extension of the wrist and fingers are accompanied by sliding of both the flexor digitorum tendons and the median nerve within the carpal tunnel. We have observed in cadaver preparations that displacement of the median nerve is only about 40% of the displacement of the flexor tendons during simulated active finger flexion.[41] This implies that there are frictional interactions between the median nerve and flexor tendons that may be increased by pressure in the carpal tunnel. These frictional interactions may also cause stretching of the median nerve, so that traction is added to compression as a pathophysiologic variable.

Epidemiologic studies of occupational carpal tunnel syndrome have usually not isolated the issue of wrist or finger position from grip force and repetition. Motion analysis studies of sign language interpreters for the deaf[42] and grocery checkers[43] have shown that workers with symptoms had more frequent and more extensive flexion and extension than those without symptoms, suggesting that extreme flexion or extension may be an extrinsic risk factor. However, the chain of causality can also be read in the opposite direction; that is, median nerve impairment may interfere with proprioception, resulting in exaggerated motions. Minimizing wrist flexion and extension by redesign of tools has been the area in which ergonomic interventions have been most successful.

Forceful Use of the Hand When the wrist is flexed, increased grip force will correlate with increased tension in the flexor digitorum tendons, which in turn will cause increased pressure on the flexor retinaculum, which functions as a pulley for these tendons. Because the median nerve is located between the flexor tendons and the flexor retinaculum, the pressure on it also will increase (Fig. 1).[44] This scenario provides a plausible mechanism to relate forceful grip to compression of the median nerve.

Such a relationship, however, has not been well established in epidemiologic studies. Silverstein and associates[45] demonstrated a significant relationship between forceful use of the hand and symptoms in the wrist and hand, but the diagnosis was not specifically carpal tunnel syndrome and could have encompassed a variety of other conditions. In reviewing the published literature on work-related repetitive hand injuries, Hagberg and associates[6] concluded that forceful use of the hand appeared to be an extrinsic risk factor for carpal tunnel syndrome, but no specific compelling set of data was cited.

Repetitive Motion In the studies by Silverstein and associates,[45] workers in jobs involving repetitive motion were also found to be at increased risk for symptoms in the hand (again, carpal tunnel syndrome was not a specific diagnosis). Repetition also may be a risk factor in typing, in which neither high force nor extreme wrist flexion/extension are implicated as risk factors. However, Nathan and associates[5] found no relationship between exposure to keyboard work in hours per day and median nerve deficit.

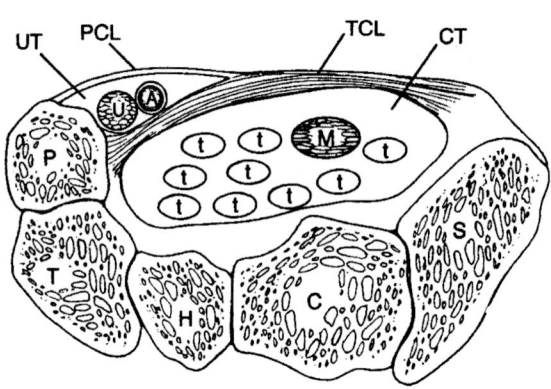

Fig. 1 Cross-section of the wrist, demonstrating the relationship of the carpal tunnel (CT) and the ulnar tunnel (UT). A, ulnar artery; C, capitate; H, hamate; M, median nerve; P, pisiform; PCL, palmar carpal ligament; S, scaphoid; t, flexor tendon; T, triquetrum; TCL, transverse carpal ligament; U, ulnar nerve. (Reproduced with permission from Szabo RM, Steinberg DR: Nerve entrapments of the wrist. J Am Acad Orthop Surg 1994;2:115–123.)

Several reports describe the hydrostatic pressure, measured with wick catheters, in the carpal canal of patients with carpal tunnel syndrome and in normal volunteers.[38–40] Resting pressure was higher in the patients with carpal tunnel syndrome; flexion or extension caused a pressure spike that was higher in these patients and was relieved when the hand was returned to the neutral position; surgical release of the transverse retinaculum altered the pressure behavior of the carpal canal so that it resembled that found in normal volunteers. Two of these studies demonstrated that repetitive motion of the wrist causes cyclic hydrostatic compression of the median nerve in the carpal tunnel.[39,40] Because motion of the hand and wrist causes transient increase in hydrostatic pressure in the carpal canal, we hypothesized that impulse loading of the median nerve may be a mechanism by which repetitive motion leads to carpal tunnel syndrome. This hypothesis was tested using an experimental setup in which cyclic compression could be applied to the tibial nerve of a rat. Approximately 20,000 cycles of pressure between 30 and 60 mm Hg, simulating a day's activity of an assembly line worker engaged in repetitive work, had the same effect on nerve conduction as constant compression at an intermediate pressure.[46] One might argue that the typical worker's injury differs by being chronic. However, on any given day the worker starts the day with an asymptomatic hand, and only after a certain amount of acute exposure do symptoms develop. It appears, therefore, that impulse loading is not a contributory factor to carpal tunnel syndrome.

Vibration Hand-arm vibration syndrome is a clinical condition of the hands characterized by vascular changes (Raynaud's phenomenon), sensorineural changes, and often sclerodactyly.[47] The digital nerves of the fingers are most affected, although the dysfunction may extend proximally. The median nerve tends to be more susceptible than the ulnar nerve.[48]

In contrast to carpal tunnel syndrome, the dose-response (exposure-prevalence) relationship between use of hand-held vibrating tools and occurrence of hand-arm vibration syndrome has been well established in epidemiologic studies.[47,49] In forestry workers, Miyashita and associates[50] found that there is a latency period, with symptoms typically not appearing until after 2,000 hours of exposure. Symptoms were present in more than 50% of workers with more than 8,000 hours of exposure. In the United States, hand-arm vibration syndrome appears to be under-diagnosed, or misdiagnosed as carpal tunnel syndrome. Miller and associates[51] reviewed workers' compensation claims for carpal tunnel syndrome in Minnesota and determined that 11% represented probable hand-arm vibration syndrome and an additional 8% possible hand-arm vibration syndrome.

Because hand-arm vibration syndrome and carpal tunnel syndrome have a number of symptoms in common (for example, nocturnal paresthesias and altered sensation in the fingers), their differentiation may be difficult, therefore requiring exacting nerve conduction studies and sensory testing. Release of the flexor retinaculum in a patient with hand-arm vibration syndrome is unlikely to improve the patient's condition. This situation is complicated by the fact that carpal tunnel syndrome and hand-arm vibration syndrome may coexist in a patient who uses vibrating tools.[52] In such individuals, transection of the flexor retinaculum may diminish nerve symptoms without significantly improving the vascular problems.[53]

The evaluation of occupational exposure to vibration as an extrinsic risk factor for carpal tunnel syndrome is complicated by the difficulties in distinguishing carpal tunnel syndrome from hand-arm vibration syndrome. Nonetheless, several epidemiologic studies appear to indicate that vibration is a risk factor for carpal tunnel syndrome.[52-55] It may function as a double crush phenomenon; that is, impairment of the median nerve in the fingers from vibration may lower its threshold for symptomatic reaction more proximally, in the wrist. In experimental animal studies, local vibration in the extremities has been shown to damage both myelinated and unmyelinated fibers.[56,57]

Interaction of Extrinsic Risk Factors Extrinsic risk factors typically do not exist in isolation, but rather are all represented to varying degrees in any given task. The interaction of these factors is not well worked out, but has been investigated in a few instances. For example, Hartung and associates[58] found that the force with which a vibrating tool is gripped greatly influences transmission of vibration to the hand. Silverstein and associates[45] found that in comparison to workers with low force-low repetition jobs, odds ratio for hand symptoms in workers with high force-low repetition jobs was 2.9; for workers in low force-high repetition jobs it was 5.5; and for high force-high repetition it was 15.[45] Although not specifically directed to carpal tunnel syndrome, these findings nonetheless suggest that extrinsic risk factors may interact in multiplicative rather than additive ways.

Role of Work in Carpal Tunnel Syndrome

When a worker develops a clinical case of carpal tunnel syndrome, this reflects the interaction of a set of intrinsic and extrinsic risk factors (as well as the influence of the psycho-social environment). There are both valid and arbitrary reasons for attempting to quantify the relative contributions of the intrinsic and extrinsic risk factors to the clinical case. The valid reasons are that by doing so one may, first of all, improve treatment and, second, identify jobs with an unusually high prevalence of carpal tunnel syndrome, institute interventions designed to reduce this prevalence (for example, ergonomic tinkering, task diversification), and evaluate the effectiveness of these interventions. The arbitrary reason is that in the United States (but not elsewhere) the physician may be required to determine whether the condition results from the job, and thus is covered by workers' compensation.

The methods used to quantify the role of work in the development of carpal tunnel syndrome are statistical ones based on studies of populations of workers. For example, the prevalence of carpal tunnel syndrome has been measured in various occupations: industrial workers with jobs of high force and high repetition (5.6%);[45] chain saw operators (25%);[59] meatcutters (15%);[8] poultry processors (20%);[60] frozen food workers (46%);[61] garment workers (6.8%);[62] and ski-manufacturer workers (34%).[63]

Cross-sectional studies of this type are very difficult to carry out, and the studies cited are flawed in one or more ways. Without analyzing each study, the recurrent problems can be summarized as follows: (1) Nonrigorous diagnosis: usually only a history of pain or paresthesia plus a positive physical examination are used for diagnosis of carpal tunnel syndrome; nerve conduction studies are seldom used. (2) Failure to determine whether the carpal tunnel syndrome symptoms began only after the worker started the job. (3) Failure to quantify exposure based on observation of the affected individuals. (4) Failure to measure background exposure: a full-time worker spends approximately 21% of the hours in a year on the job; exposure to extrinsic risk factors during the remaining 79% should also be measured. (5) Failure to measure intrinsic risk factors: usually age and gender are measured, but not other factors.

(6) Failure to account for selection bias; for example, affected workers who have moved into less-strenuous jobs.

A somewhat better type of study involves a case-referent analysis, in which affected workers are compared to a referent group matched for some intrinsic risk factors (usually age and gender) as well as matched in a contrasting way for extrinsic risk factors (exposure at work). This type of analysis permits the calculation of odds ratios. Examples incude the studies of Wieslander and associates[64] which compared 38 men operated on for carpal tunnel syndrome to two referents drawn from among other surgical cases (hospital referents) and two further referents from the population register and telephone directory, respectively (population referents), and the studies of Stetson and associates,[65] which compared 103 industrial workers with clinical symptoms suggestive of carpal tunnel syndrome to 137 asymptomatic workers. Case-referent investigations have some of the same difficulties as cross-sectional studies, such as nonrigorous diagnosis, failure to quantify off-work exposure, failure to account for intrinsic risk factors.

Nathan and Keniston[33] approached the question of quantifying the role of work in carpal tunnel syndrome in a different way. They grouped all patients from a variety of sources for whom they had nerve conduction studies as well as other data, and performed a stepwise regression analysis of combined intrinsic and extrinsic risk factors to assess their relative contributions to carpal tunnel syndrome. They determined that work-related factors accounted for less than one-eighth of the risk factors for carpal tunnel syndrome. Their sample encompassed patients with a broad range of jobs, and included some nonworking individuals. There may be specific jobs in which the contributions of work are greater. Nonetheless, their analysis is useful in establishing the relative importance of extrinsic risk factors in a general population.

Evaluation of a Clinical Case

For the sake of argument, suppose that the difficulties inherent in epidemiologic studies could be overcome and that a definitive analysis of a particular job is carried out in which the proportion of cases of carpal tunnel syndrome that are attributable to the exposure at work is precisely determined. While this type of information may be useful to an occupational safety officer, it would be of little value to the clinician treating an affected worker. This is because the epidemiologic data is statistical in nature, and there is no way to know how it might apply to a particular case. Even if a patient experiences symptoms only at work, an honest clinician is still unable to describe the extent to which the patient's carpal tunnel syndrome is related to the job. Quantitative understanding of intrinsic risk factors and their relationship to exposure to extrinsic factors at work is very imperfect. There is a fundamental incompatibility between the epidemiologic perspective and the clinician's perspective, with the result that even very compelling epidemiologic data is of only limited use to the clinician. Figure 2 shows a hypothetical relationship between prevalence of carpal tunnel syndrome and exposure to extrinsic risk factors. At best, epidemiologic data might define the odds ratios for carpal tunnel syndrome between two jobs and the odds ratios between these and a matched sample of nonworking individuals, but it can contribute little to analyzing the etiology of a specific case.

It is unfortunate that workers' compensation determinations must be made in individual clinical cases, where it is impossible to quantify the contribution of the job to the clinical problem. The proper arena for workers' compensa-

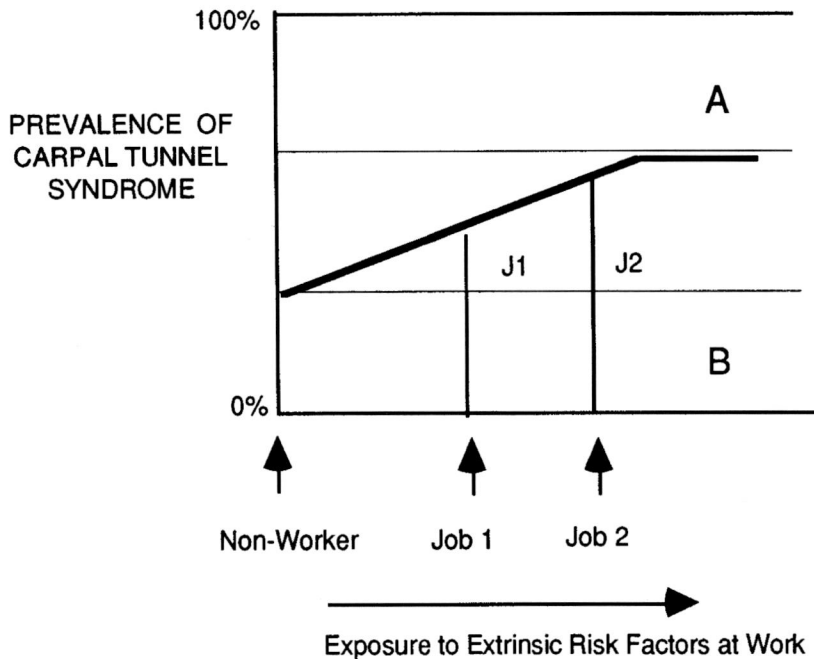

Fig. 2 Hypothetical relationship between prevalence of carpal tunnel syndrome and exposure to extrinsic risk factors. A, Many workers will never develop carpal tunnel syndrome, regardless of work exposure. B, Some workers will develop carpal tunnel syndrome even with no job exposure. Comparing two jobs (Job 1 and Job 2) with different extrinsic risk factors, the odds ratio for carpal tunnel syndrome in Job 2 compared to Job 1 is: B+J2/B+J1. However, the extent to which a particular case is job-related cannot be determined.

tion issues with regard to carpal tunnel syndrome and similar conditions is at the statistical level, where surveillance, intervention, and regulation can be carried out in a meaningful way.

Summary

With respect to carpal tunnel syndrome, workers with physically demanding jobs should undergo careful screening to disqualify those with unacceptable intrinsic risk factors, and a program of continuing physical conditioning should be required. In addition, it should be recognized that after 10 to 20 years, a worker should be transferred to a less demanding task. The belief that *any* worker can do *any* job until age 65, which is a premise of much workers' compensation policy and labor union rhetoric, is not realistic.

References

1. Schottland JR, Kirschberg GJ, Fillingim R, et al: Median nerve latencies in poultry processing workers: An approach to resolving the role of industrial "cumulative trauma" in the development of carpal tunnel syndrome. *J Occup Med* 1991;33:627–631.
2. Hadler NM: The roles of work and of working in disorders of the upper extremity. *Baillieres Clin Rheumat* 1989;3:121–141.

3. Hadler NM: Illness in the workplace: The challenge of musculoskeletal symptoms. *J Hand Surg* 1985;10A:451–456.
4. Nathan PA, Meadows KD, Doyle LS: Occupation as a risk factor for impaired sensory conduction of the median nerve at the carpal tunnel. *J Hand Surg* 1988;13B: 167–170.
5. Nathan PA, Keniston RC, Meadows KD: Keyboarding as a risk factor for carpal tunnel syndrome: Comparing clerical workers to managers in eight industries. *Orthop Trans* 1994;18:161.
6. Hagberg M, Morgenstern H, Kelsh M: Impact of occupations and job tasks on the prevalence of carpal tunnel syndrome. *Scand J Work Environ Health* 1992;18:337–345.
7. Occupational disease surveillance: Carpal tunnel syndrome. *MMWR* 1989;38:485–489.
8. Masear VR, Hayes JM, Hyde AG: An industrial cause of carpal tunnel syndrome. *J Hand Surg* 1986;11A:222–227.
9. Szabo RM, Madison M: Carpal tunnel syndrome. *Orthop Clin North Am* 1992;23: 103–109.
10. Gelberman RH, Rydevik BL, Pess GM, et al: Carpal tunnel syndrome: A scientific basis for clinical care. *Orthop Clin North Am* 1988;19:115–124.
11. Dahlin LB, Rydevik B: Pathophysiology of nerve compression, in Gelberman RH (ed): *Operative Nerve Repair and Reconstruction*. Philadelphia, PA, JB Lippincott, 1991, vol 2, pp 847–866.
12. Richman JA, Gelberman RH, Rydevik BL, et al: Carpal tunnel volume determination by magnetic resonance imaging three-dimensional reconstruction. *J Hand Surg* 1987;12A:712–717.
13. Jablecki CK, Andary MT, So YT, et al: Literature review of the usefulness of nerve conduction studies and electromyography for the evaluation of patients with carpal tunnel syndrome. *Muscle Nerve* 1993;16:1392–1414.
14. Kimura J: The carpal tunnel syndrome: Localization of conduction abnormalities within the distal segment of the median nerve. *Brain* 1979;102:619–635.
15. Braun RM, Davidson K, Doehr S: Provocative testing in the diagnosis of dynamic carpal tunnel syndrome. *J Hand Surg* 1989;14A:195–197.
16. White KM, Congleton JJ, Huchingson RD, et al: Vibrometry testing for carpal tunnel syndrome: A longitudinal study of daily variations. *Arch Phys Med Rehabil* 1994;75:25–28.
17. Katz JN, Larson MG, Fossel AH, et al: Validation of a surveillance case definition of carpal tunnel syndrome. *Am J Pub Health* 1991;81:189–193.
18. Brones MF, Wilgis EF: Anatomical variations of the palmaris longus, causing carpal tunnel syndrome: Case reports. *Plast Reconstr Surg* 1978;62:798–800.
19. Eriksen J: A case of carpal tunnel syndrome on the basis of an abnormally long lumbrical muscle. *Acta Orthop Scand* 1973;44:275–277.
20. Smith RJ: Anomalous muscle belly of the flexor digitorum superficialis causing carpal-tunnel syndrome: Report of a case. *J Bone Joint Surg* 1971;53A:1215–1216.
21. Dyreby JR, Engber WD: Palmaris profundus: Rare anomalous muscle. *J Hand Surg* 1982;7A:513–514.
22. Linburg RM, Comstock BE: Anomalous tendon slips from the flexor pollicis longus to the flexor digitorum profundus. *J Hand Surg* 1979;4A:79–83.
23. Schuind F, Ventura M, Pasteels JL: Idiopathic carpal tunnel syndrome: Histologic study of flexor tendon synovium. *J Hand Surg* 1990;15A:497–503.
24. Neal NC, McManners J, Stirling GA: Pathology of the flexor tendon sheath in the spontaneous carpal tunnel syndrome. *J Hand Surg* 1987;12B:229–232.
25. Badalamente MA, Sampson SP, Hurst LC, et al: Amyloid tenosynovial deposition in idiopathic carpal tunnel syndrome: A histologic, histochemical and ultrastructural study. *Orthop Trans* 1994;18:166.
26. Siegel DB, Kuzma GR, Eakins DF: The effects of anomalous origins of the lumbrical muscles in the etiology of idiopathic carpal tunnel syndrome. *American Societies for the Surgery of the Hand, Meeting Abstracts*. Kansas City, KS, American Society for the Surgery of the Hand, 1993, p 22.

27. Ditmars DM Jr: Patterns of carpal tunnel syndrome. *Hand Clin* 1993;9:241–252.
28. Nakamichi K, Tachibana S: Unilateral carpal tunnel syndrome and space-occupying lesions. *J Hand Surg* 1993;18B:748–749.
29. Bleeker ML, Bohlman M, Moreland R, et al: Carpal tunnel syndrome: Role of carpal canal size. *Neurology* 1985;35:1599–1604.
30. Loslever P, Ranaivosoa A: Biomechanical and epidemiological investigation of carpal tunnel syndrome at workplaces with high risk factors. *Ergonomics* 1993:36:537–555.
31. Lundborg G, Dahlin LB, Lundstrom R, et al: Vibrotactile function of the hand in compression and vibration-induced neuropathy: Sensibility index. A new measure. *Scand J Plast Reconstr Surg Hand Surg* 1992;26:275–279.
32. Nathan PA, Meadows KD, Doyle LS: Relationship of age and sex to sensory conduction of the median nerve at the carpal tunnel and association of slowed conduction with symptoms. *Muscle & Nerve* 1988;11:1149–1153.
33. Nathan PA, Keniston RC: Carpal tunnel syndrome and its relation to general physical condition. *Hand Clin* 1993;9:253–261.
34. Nathan PA, Takigawa K, Keniston RC, et al: Slowing of sensory conduction of the median nerve and carpal tunnel syndrome in Japanese and American industrial workers. *J Hand Surg* 1994;19B:30–34.
35. Nathan PA, Keniston RC, Myers LD, et al: Obesity as a risk factor for slowing of sensory conduction of the median nerve in industry: A cross-sectional and longitudinal study involving 429 workers. *J Occup Med* 1992;34:379–383.
36. Zeiss J, Skie M, Ebraheim N, et al: Anatomic relations between the median nerve and flexor tendons in the carpal tunnel: MR evaluation in normal volunteers. *AJR* 1989;153:533–536.
37. Armstrong TJ, Castelli WA, Evans FG, et al: Some histological changes in carpal tunnel contents and their biomechanical implications. *J Occup Med* 1984;26:197–201.
38. Thurston AJ, Krause BL: The possible role of vascular congestion in carpal tunnel syndrome. *J Hand Surg* 1988;13B:397–399.
39. Chaise F, Witvoët J: Measurement of carpal tunnel pressures in the idiopathic carpal tunnel syndrome without motor deficit. *Rev Chir Orthop* 1984;70:75–78.
40. Szabo RM, Chidgey LK: Stress carpal tunnel pressures in patients with carpal tunnel syndrome and normal patients. *J Hand Surg* 1989;14A:624–627.
41. Szabo RM, Bay BK, Sharkey NA, et al: Median nerve displacement through the carpal canal. *J Hand Surg* 1994;19A:901–906.
42. Feuerstein M, Fitzgerald TE: Biomechanical factors affecting upper extremity cumulative trauma disorders in sign language interpreters. *J Occup Med* 1992;34:257–264.
43. Harber P, Bloswick D, Beck J, et al: Supermarket checker motions and cumulative trauma risk. *J Occup Med* 1993;35:805–811.
44. Smith EM, Sonstegard DA, Anderson WH Jr: Carpal tunnel syndrome: Contribution of flexor tendons. *Arch Phys Med Rehab* 1977;58:379–385.
45. Silverstein BA, Fine LJ, Armstrong TJ: Occupational factors and carpal tunnel syndrome. *Am J Indus Med* 1987;11:343–358.
46. Szabo RM, Sharkey NA: Response of peripheral nerve to cyclic compression in a laboratory rat model. *J Orthop Res* 1993;11:828–833.
47. Nagata C, Yoshida H, Mirbod SM et al: Cutaneous signs (Raynaud's phenomenon, sclerodactylia, and edema of the hands) and hand-arm vibration exposure. *Int Arch Occup Environ Health* 1993;64:587–591.
48. Brismar T, Ekenvall L: Nerve conduction in the hands of vibration exposed workers. *Electroencephalogr Clin Neurophysiol* 1992;85:173–176.
49. Letz R, Cherniack MG, Gerr F, et al: A cross sectional epidemiological survey of shipyard workers exposed to hand-arm vibration. *Br J Indus Med* 1992;49:53–62.
50. Miyashita K, Shiomi S, Itoh N, et al: Epidemiological study of vibration syndrome in response to total hand-tool operating time. *Br J Ind Med* 1983;40:92–98.

51. Miller RF, Lohman WH, Maldonado G, et al: An epidemiologic study of carpal tunnel syndrome and hand-arm vibration syndrome in relation to vibration exposure. *J Hand Surg* 1994;19A:99–105.
52. Rosen I, Stromberg T, Lundborg G: Neurophysiological investigation of hands damaged by vibration: Comparison with idiopathic carpal tunnel syndrome. *Scand J Plast Reconstr Surg Hand Surg* 1993;27:209–216.
53. Hagberg M, Nystrom A, Zetterlund B: Recovery from symptoms after carpal tunnel syndrome surgery in males in relation to vibration exposure. *J Hand Surg* 1991;16A:66–71.
54. Ekenvall L, Nilsson BY, Gustavsson P: Temperature and vibration thresholds in vibration syndrome. *Br J Indus Med* 1986;43:825–829.
55. Wieslander G, Norback D, Gothe CJ, et al: Carpal tunnel syndrome (carpal tunnel syndrome) and exposure to vibration, repetitive wrist movements, and heavy manual work: A case-referent study. *Br J Indus Med* 1989;46:43–47.
56. Ho ST, Yu HS: Ultrastructural changes of the peripheral nerve induced by vibration: An experimental study. *Br J Indus Med* 1989;46:157–164.
57. Lundborg G, Dahlin, LB, Hansson HA, et al: Vibration exposure and peripheral nerve fiber damage. *J Hand Surg* 1990;15A:346–351.
58. Hartung E, Dupuis H, Scheffer M: Effects of grip and push forces on the acute response of the hand-arm system under vibrating conditions. *Int Arch Occup Environ Health* 1993;64:463–467.
59. Farkkila M, Pyykko I, Jantti V, et al: Forestry workers exposed to vibration: A neurological study. *Br J Ind Med* 1988;45:188–192.
60. Muffly-Elsey D, Flinn-Wagner S: Proposed screening tool for the detection of cumulative trauma disorders of the upper extremity. *J Hand Surg* 1987;12A:931–935.
61. Chiang HC, Chen SS, Yu HS, et al: The occurrence of carpal tunnel syndrome in frozen food factory employees. *Kao Hsiung I Hsueh Ko Hsueh Tsa Chih* 1990;6:73–80.
62. Punnett L, Robins JM, Wegman DH, et al: Soft tissue disorders of the upper limbs in female garment workers. *Scand J Work Environ Health* 1983;9:283–290.
63. Barnhart S, Demers PA, Miller M et al: Carpal tunnel syndrome among ski manufacturing workers. *Scand J Work Environ Health* 1991;17:46–52.
64. Wieslander G, Norback D, Gothe CJ, et al: Carpal tunnel syndrome (CTS) and exposure to vibration, repetitive wrist movements, and heavy manual work: A case-referent study. *Br J Ind Med* 1989;46:43–47.
65. Stetson DS, Silverstein BA, Keyserling WM, et al: Median sensory distal amplitude and latency: Comparisons between nonexposure managerial/professional employees and industrial workers. *Am J Ind Med* 1993;24:175–189.

Chapter 29

De Quervain's Disease and Tenosynovitis

Peter C. Amadio, MD

Introduction

De Quervain's disease, the other tendon entrapment syndromes, and the various forms of true or putative tenosynovitis of the hand and wrist are common repetitive motion disorders.[1-12] All are characterized by pain with motion of the affected tendon. The tendon and its sheath are often swollen or tender. In some instances, tendon motion may be completely impeded by this swelling. The diagnosis is made on the basis of physical examination; imaging studies and laboratory tests are rarely useful. There have been no population-based studies on the incidence of these conditions, but the reported experience of large referral practices suggests that they are all diseases of middle adulthood, with most patients ranging in age from 30 to 60 years.[2-5,13,14] Women are more frequently affected than men, with a ratio of 2:1 or 3:1.[2,3,5,13,15] Most common is de Quervain's disease, followed by trigger thumb, triggering of the middle and ring fingers, triggering of the other fingers, intersection syndrome, and syndromes of the flexor carpi radialis, extensor carpi ulnaris, and the finger and thumb extensors.[2,5,13]

De Quervain's disease in particular and tenosynovitis in general have been considered typical occupational overuse disorders for decades. Despite this common impression, the scientific foundation for the terminology (which suggests a component of inflammation) and for the conclusion that the disorders are work-related is remarkably shaky and circumstantial. Although epidemiologic studies of workers have shown that there is an increased risk of complaints of upper extremity symptoms with repetitive work, the clinical diagnosis in such reports is often characterized simply as "occupational cervicobrachial disorder" or "tenosynovitis." Thus, the clinical foundation for a specific diagnosis of tendon entrapment cannot be determined.[1,3,6,7,11,12,16-18] The term tenosynovitis was applied early, but the histopathology (in the absence of systemic inflammatory disease) typically shows peritendinous fibrosis without inflammation, fibrocartilaginous metaplasia of tendon sheath tissue, and occasional microcalcification within the sheath or tendon.[19-22] Because there is a lack of inflammation, the term tendon entrapment may be preferable in some cases to tenosynovitis, particularly for syndromes in which fibrosis and limited motion are the characteristic features.

This chapter will discuss the etiology, clinical diagnosis, and treatment of the common tendon entrapment syndromes of the hand and wrist. Features of epidemiology that relate to overuse, pathomechanics, and pathophysiology will be discussed in other chapters.

Tendon Entrapment Syndromes: Clinical Issues

All tendon entrapment syndromes are aggravated by movement and to some extent improved with rest. Splinting is a mainstay of treatment. Nonsteroidal anti-inflammatory drugs (NSAIDs) are often used in treatment, especially by primary-care providers, but there are few data to support the efficacy of this intervention. Steroid injection is commonly used as an alternative to surgery when activity modification, rest, and NSAIDs prove ineffective.[13–15,23–32] The literature supports the efficacy of both single and repeated steroid injections; however, frequently repeated steroid injections at a single site may be hazardous.[33] Surgical incision of the affected tendon sheath is nearly universally supported as the appropriate next step when all nonsurgical methods have failed.[2,4,5,13–15,20,27–29,31,34–37]

De Quervain's Disease

De Quervain's disease is the name commonly given to entrapment of the tendons of the extensor pollicis brevis (EPB) and abductor pollicis longus (APL) at the level of the extensor retinaculum.[20,38–40] The clinical evolution of this condition was reviewed by Finkelstein[20] and Leao.[41] The earliest clinical descriptions referred to the disease as a crepitant inflammation of the EPB and APL; the pathology (stenosis and fibrosis of the tendon sheath) were identified, and surgical release was recommended as the appropriate treatment by de Quervain in 1895. According to de Quervain, the disease was caused by overexertion from household duties. Finkelstein also concluded that the etiology of the disease was excessive housework; 16 of his 24 patients were women who worked in the home. Finkelstein described the classic diagnostic test: "If one places the thumb within the hand and holds it tightly with the other fingers, and then bends the hand severely in an ulnar direction, then an intense pain is experienced on the styloid process of the radius" (Fig. 1).

Subsequent authors have emphasized the common history of a recent change in activity level and have reported larger series,[4,36] but the message remains the same: most patients are women aged 30 to 60 years who are more likely to be involved in housework than factory work. An association with the care of infants in the first few months postpartum has been reported.[42] There have been no reports relating the incidence of de Quervain's disease to the frequency or intensity of repetitive work. In one large study in which the incidence of tenosynovitis in a factory setting was specifically reviewed, "no case fulfilling the criteria for de Quervain's disease was detected."[12]

Anatomy plays a critical role in both the diagnosis and treatment of de Quervain's disease (Fig. 2). The pain of de Quervain's disease is localized to the extensor retinaculum; ie, at the radial styloid. Similar but more distal pain may arise from the thumb carpometacarpal or scaphotrapezial joints. These joints may be painful during the Finkelstein test (Fig. 1), but the pain will not be located at the radial styloid. Intersection syndrome will cause a similar but more proximal and dorsal pain with the Finkelstein test.[43] Radial neuritis may also be aggravated by the Finkelstein test, but the pain will be located proximally and radially, where the nerve exits from beneath the brachioradialis. Radial neuritis is characterized further by hypoesthesia in the radial nerve distribution and a positive Tinel sign over the nerve, two phenomena not associated with uncomplicated de Quervain's disease.[44]

The anatomy of the APL and EPB has received considerable attention based on the theory that anatomic anomalies within the tendon sheath may predis-

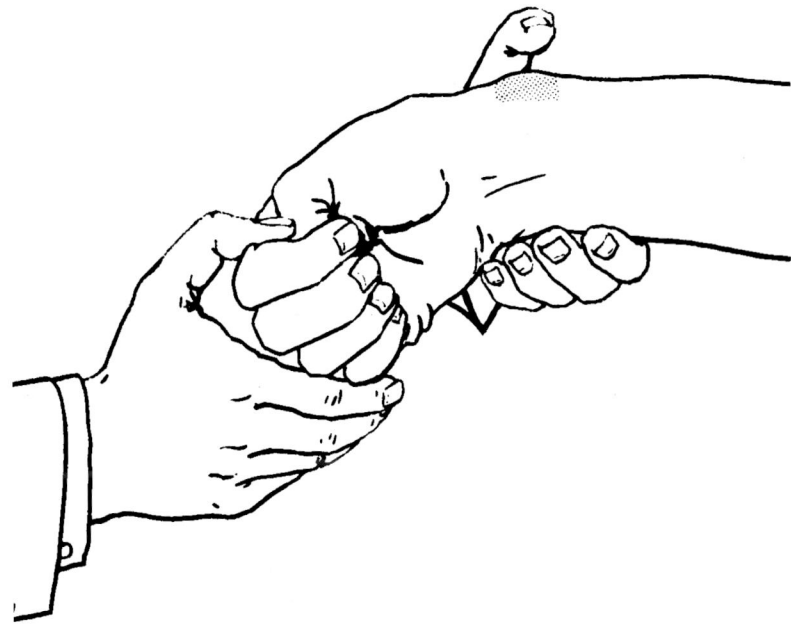

Fig 1 The Finkelstein test. (Reproduced with permission from the Mayo Foundation.)

pose to de Quervain's disease. Although anatomic texts may show a single sheath for AOL and EPB, and a single tendon for each, the EPB and APL most often have separate subsheaths, and the APL usually has more than one tendon.[45–48] These variations are not more common in patients with de Quervain's disease, but knowledge of these variations is useful: an unsuspecting surgeon might assume that an extra APL tendon is really the EPB and fail to release the real EPB subsheath. As Louis[49] has pointed out, some surgical failures may be caused by not releasing the EPB.

Early reports on the treatment of de Quervain's disease emphasized surgical release as the best treatment and generally reported favorable results.[50,51] Woods[50] titled his 1964 paper "A Plea for Early Operation," but other authors have been less sanguine. Arons[51] summarized these concerns in his report of 16 patients referred to him for reoperation. Complications in Arons' report included radial neuroma, tendon subluxation, painful longitudinal scarring, and depigmentation secondary to repeated steroid injections. Most of Arons' patients had multiple diagnoses, fibromyalgia being most common. Even in a series of 11 patients referred to Arons without treatment, six also had fibromyalgia. Arons[51] emphasized the importance of managing fibromyalgia with therapy and job modifications, not surgery. He also stressed the importance of zigzag skin incisions, which provide extensile exposure without the risk of a painful hypertrophy. Current surgical technique emphasizes this type of exposure, combined with careful identification and protection of all branches of the radial nerve and release of both the APL and EPB subsheaths. A dorsal sheath incision is preferred, to reduce the risk of painful dislocation of the tendons from within the released retinaculum with wrist flexion.[52–54]

Although most of the complications resulting from failure of surgical treatment of de Quervain's disease can be managed by completing a previously in-

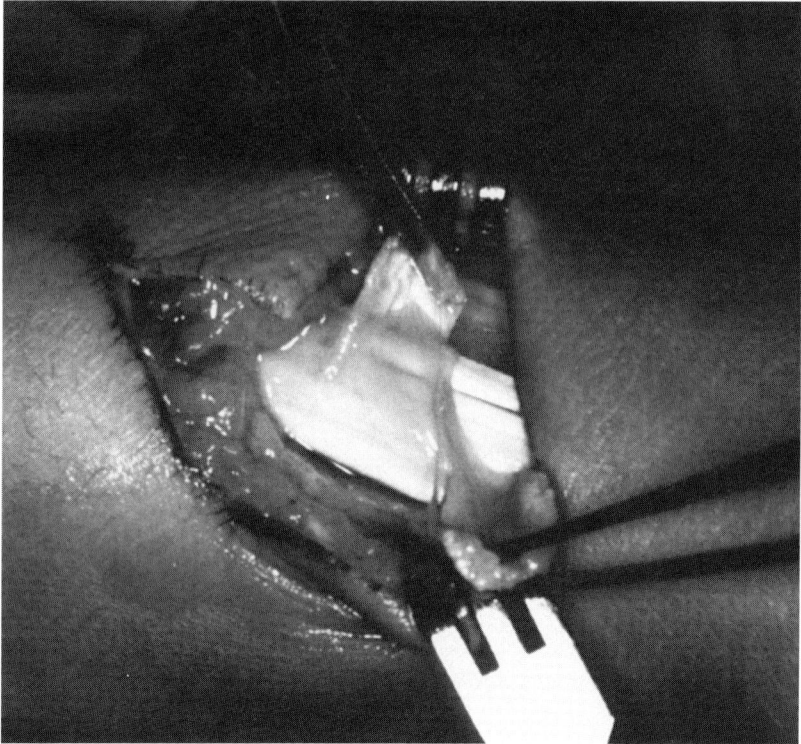

Fig. 2 Anatomy of de Quervain's disease. Note the multiple tendons of abductor pollicis.

complete release,[49] neurolysis of an adherent radial nerve,[51] or retinacular reconstruction for cases of painful tendon subluxation[52,53,55] (Fig. 3), awareness of these problems has prompted a new look at nonsurgical treatment. Lapidus, an early proponent of surgery,[5,35] later revised his opinion to recommend steroid injection as the main form of treatment.[31] Recently, Harvey and associates[27] reported that in a series of 79 patients, 80% were treated successfully with one or two injections of hydrocortisone acetate. Thus, the current trend seems to favor a more conservative course, with surgery being reserved for refractory cases.

Intersection Syndrome

An anatomic neighbor to de Quervain's disease is the extensor intersection syndrome, so called because of its location in the bursa at the intersection between the radial wrist extensor tendons and the APL and EPB muscle bellies in the distal dorsal forearm, 6 to 10 cm proximal to the wrist[43] (Fig. 4). Symptoms consist of local pain with wrist flexion and extension. Often there is a dramatic palpable or even audible leathery crepitus. Local swelling is commonly present. The syndrome is differentiated from de Quervain's disease by a more proximal and dorsal location. Thompson and associates[10] nicely summarized the early literature of the association of intersection syndrome with repetitive motion and report 419 cases over 8 years in a British automobile factory gearing up after World War II. As with de Quervain's disease, there is

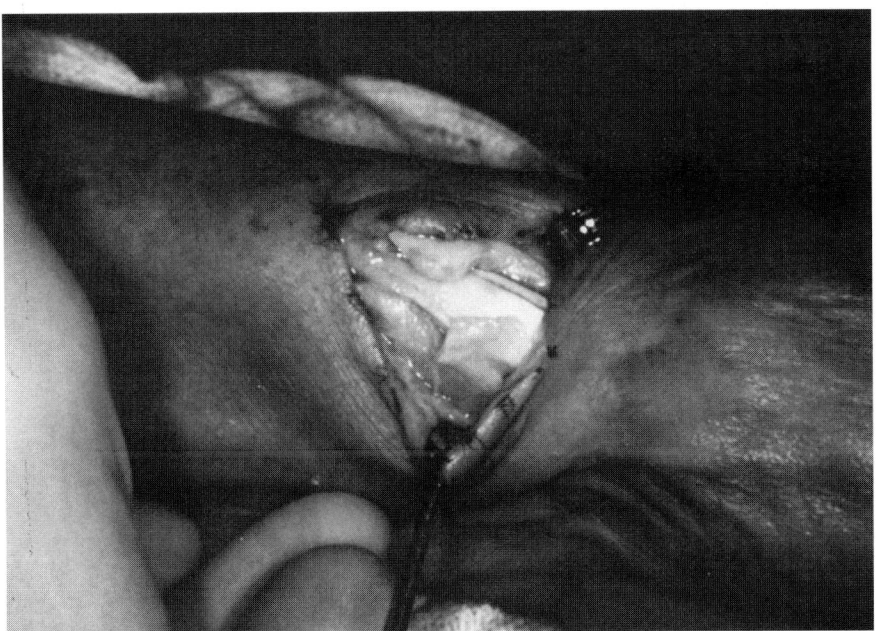

Fig. 3 Retinacular reconstruction. After a zigzag incision in the extensor retinaculum, dorsal and volar flaps are fashioned. These are then transposed and sutured to each other to recreate a lengthened retinacular sheath.

often a history of recent intensive activity; unlike de Quervain's disease, intersection syndrome is far more common in men than in women and most frequently occurs in workers in the manufacturing or construction industries whose jobs involve both heavy work and repetitive wrist motions.[10]

Compared with reports on the treatment of de Quervain's disease, almost all reports describe good results from rest and activity modification in the treatment of intersection syndrome; only five of 419 cases in the study by Thompson and associates were treated surgically.[10] My own experience has been similar; most cases respond to rest, activity modification, and steroid injection.

Refractory cases of intersection syndrome may require surgery. A local release of the bursa that lies between the wrist extensor tendons and the muscle bellies of APL and EPB is recommended.[10,56,57] The APL muscle often has a fibrous proximal edge, which can be excised. Good results from this surgery have been the rule, although the number of cases reported is small. Grundberg and Reagan[43] have pointed out that this proximal bursal swelling and tenderness may arise from a stenosing tenosynovitis in the space where the wrist extensors pass beneath the extensor retinaculum; they have released the retinaculum in this location instead, with similar good results.

Trigger Finger and Thumb

Trigger finger and thumb collectively represent roughly two thirds of all cases of tendon entrapment in most series.[2,4,5,30] Patients are somewhat older on average than those with other entrapment syndromes, with peak ages between 40 and 70. Women predominate at ratios of 2:1 or 3:1. History of a work in-

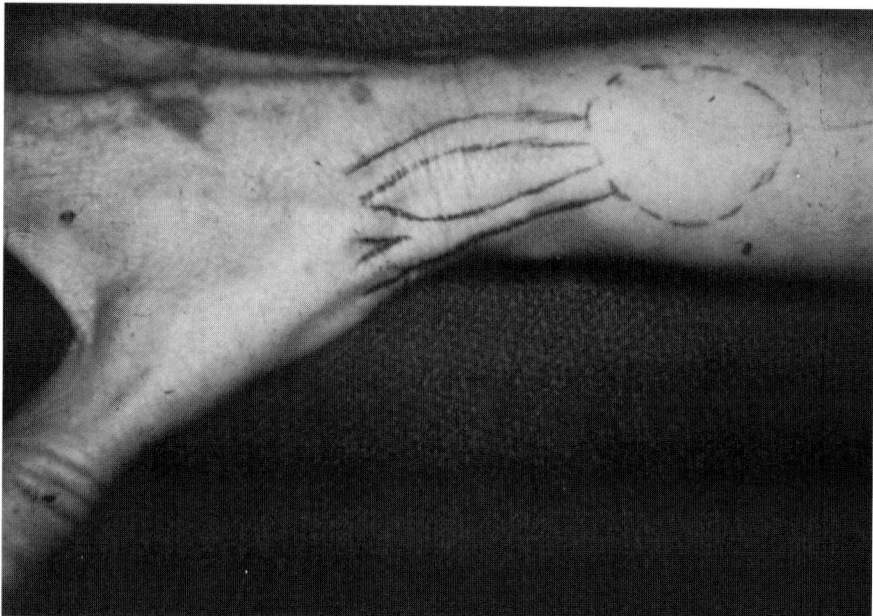

Fig. 4 Intersection syndrome. The area of pain is marked by the dotted circle. The tendons of the extensor pollicis brevis and abductor pollicis longus are also marked.

jury or work involving repetitive movement is infrequently implicated as a cause; most patients with trigger digits work in the home or are retired.[2,4,5,13,15,30]

Clinical findings in patients with trigger finger and thumb include pain, nodular enlargement of the tendon, and a characteristic clicking or locking with grip. The pathology typically includes thickening of the A1 pulley, with or without nodular tenosynovial thickening. The synovium may invade the tendon in severe cases. Hueston and Wilson[58] have suggested that the typical nodule represents a delamination of the normal spiral fibers of the flexor tendon, caused by tethering on a tight pulley, rather than by an actual growth or excrescence on the tendon.

Treatment of trigger finger and thumb has traditionally involved open surgical release.[2,4,5,59,60] Surgery is usually done under local anesthesia, through a small transverse or longitudinal incision over the offending A1 pulley. Care must be taken to avoid injury to the digital nerves, particularly in the thumb, where the radial digital nerve can be directly superficial to the pulley.[61] Hyperextension of the metacarpophalangeal joint, commonly performed to aid exposure, puts the nerve directly below the skin and thus in particular jeopardy.

Complications of trigger digit release are few, but recent reports have emphasized that persistent tenderness can be a problem in up to a third of cases. In the 1970s, steroid injection began to supplant open release as the initial treatment of choice.[31] Up to 90% of trigger digits can be successfully managed by one, two, or three injections.[13–15,23–30,32,45] Freiberg and associates[25] have suggested that digits with a discrete nodule in the tendon are more likely to respond to injection than those with more diffuse swelling. A recent controlled study has confirmed that it is the steroid, and not the local anesthetic or the mere volume of the injection, that is therapeutic.[30] Evans and associates[62] have shown that a program of differential tendon gliding exercises and extension splinting (Fig. 5) can also result in resolution of triggering, with good results in 73% of 35 patients so treated.

Other treatments have also been advised for trigger digits. Tanaka and associates[63] proposed percutaneous trigger digit release, but their results show little advantage over the results from open surgery. Because of the additional risks of inadvertent nerve or artery injury, this technique would appear to be of little advantage for most patients. Seradge and Kleinert[64] have suggested that a narrowing of the tendon, or reduction tenoplasty, be performed in preference to pulley release, particularly in cases where triggering persists even after A1 pulley release. Kapandji[65] has suggested that pulley reconstruction be considered in all cases, so as to retain the restraining and guiding function of the pulley.

Linburg Syndrome

In 1979 Linburg and Comstock[66] reported the clinical significance of anomalous fibrous or tendinous bands connecting the flexor pollicis longus and index profundus tendons in the distal forearm (Fig. 6). This anomaly, which restricts independent thumb flexion with the index finger extended, is present in roughly 15% of extremities. The clinical syndrome is much less common. The anomaly was postulated to cause symptoms in patients whose job or avocation required repetitive, simultaneous thumb flexion and index extension. The

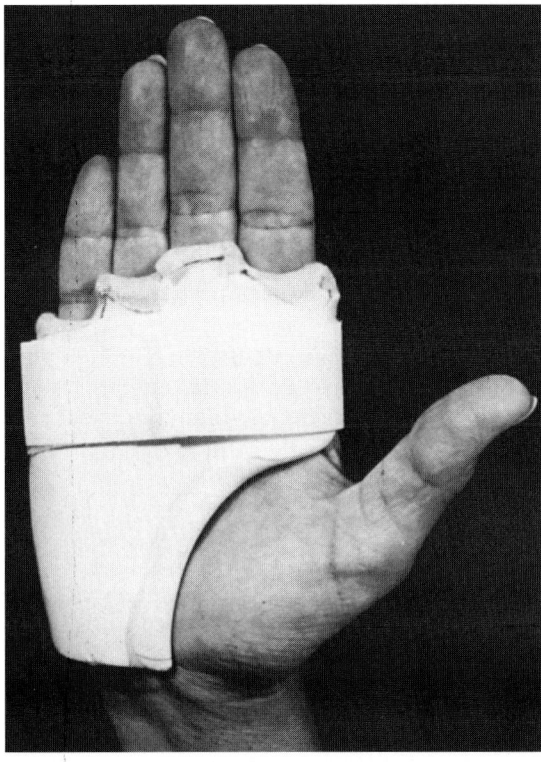

Fig. 5 The Evans splint blocks metacarpophalangeal joint flexion. It should be worn most of the day but should be removed occasionally for range-of-motion exercises.

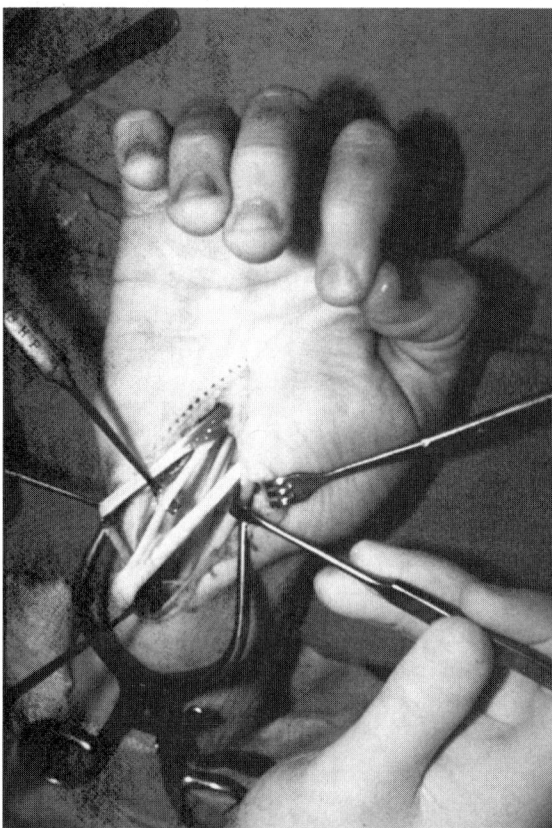

Fig. 6 Linburg syndrome. Note the Z-shaped tendon structure elevated. The top limb of the Z is the index profundus; the bottom limb is flexor pollicis. The cross limb represents the anomalous Linburg connection. Note the simultaneous flexion of the thumb and index fingers with traction on the cross limb. This patient had symptoms of carpal tunnel syndrome as well as painful finger movement. All symptoms were relieved by excision of this anomalous connection and carpal tunnel release.

most common symptom is aching pain in the forearm. Paresthesias in the median nerve distribution may also be present. Physical findings include tenderness in the volar distal forearm and a positive Linburg sign (pain with passive index finger extension with the thumb held actively flexed). Steroid injection was ineffective, but surgical release resulted in good clinical improvement in most cases.[37,66] In some patients, peritendinous fibrosis may mimic the clinical findings of Linburg syndrome; in such cases, tenolysis alone may be an effective treatment.

In some patients there seems to be an association between Linburg syndrome and carpal tunnel syndrome, as noted in Figure 6. Occasionally it may be possible to treat both problems by simply excising the Linburg connection and not releasing the flexor retinaculum.

Other Tendon Syndromes

Flexor Carpi Radialis

Entrapment of the flexor carpi radialis may occur in its sheath at the wrist.[34,67] Patients are typically middle-aged and female. The etiology relates primarily to arthritic changes at the scaphotrapezial joint; osteophytes from that joint may abrade the flexor carpi radialis, causing pain, synovitis, and occasionally tendon rupture. Most patients will respond to symptomatic management; those

Flexor Carpi Ulnaris

Pain on the volar ulnar side of the wrist, aggravated by wrist flexion, is the hallmark of flexor carpi ulnaris irritation. There is no sheath for entrapment, but the tendon can become painful at its insertion to the pisiform.[68,69] Often such symptoms are brought on by repetitive wrist flexion, particularly during sports activity, but occasionally at work as well. The literature on the condition is limited, but what there is suggests that rest is usually effective in controlling symptoms. When symptoms persist and are disabling, excision of the pisiform often brings relief, suggesting that at least some of the symptoms may be pisotriquetral as well.

Extensor Pollicis Longus

Entrapment of the extensor pollicis longus (EPL) has two main causes: deformity following Colles' fracture,[70] and repetitive wrist motion—the so-called "drummer boy's palsy."[71,72] This is the only entrapment syndrome in which rupture rather than triggering or locking is the rule. Pain with thumb extension is the first symptom; usually swelling and tenderness are noted at Lister's tubercle. After rupture occurs, loss of extension is the main symptom. Treatment in the early phase, before rupture, consists of rest and anti-inflammatory medication.[73] Early retinacular release and synovectomy may prevent rupture in some cases. After rupture has occurred, tendon transfer is necessary to restore active thumb extension.[74,75]

Extensor Digitorum

Entrapment of the finger extensor tendons has been reported, but it is rare.[76–79] Either the fourth (extensor digitorum communis and extensor indicis proprius)[76] or fifth (extensor digiti minimi) compartments[78] may be involved. The standard formula of steroid injection, followed by release if that is unsuccessful, seems appropriate management.

Extensor Carpi Ulnaris

Stenosing tenosynovitis of the extensor carpi ulnaris is uncommon.[80,81] It follows the typical pattern, occurring predominantly in middle-aged women, and has little reported connection with work. Symptoms are aggravated by ulnar deviation of the wrist. Often a mass can be palpated over the tendon at the level of the wrist. The differential diagnosis includes posttraumatic lateral subluxation of this tendon.[82] Localized tenosynovitis of the extensor carpi ulnaris can also be an early sign of rheumatoid arthritis, particularly in cases in which signs of inflammation, redness, and swelling are marked. Treatment consists of surgical release of the dorsal retinaculum (Fig. 7).[80,81] The anatomy of this tendon sheath deserves special attention. The floor of the tunnel through which the extensor carpi ulnaris passes at the wrist is the ulna. In addition to the overlying extensor retinaculum, there is a medial wall that lies deep to the retinaculum and restrains displacement of the tendon medial to the ulnar styloid. It is this wall that is injured in cases of painful posttraumatic subluxation of

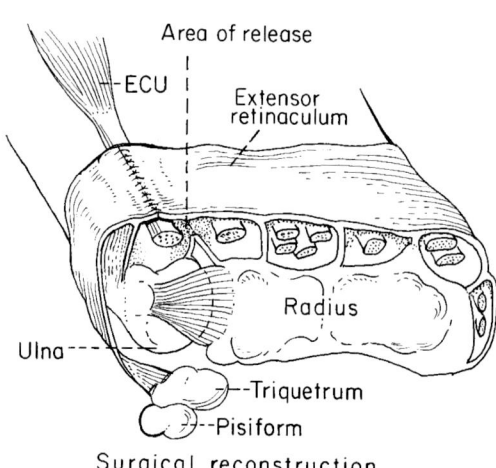

Fig. 7 Anatomy of the extensor carpi ulnaris (ECU). The incision and repair of the extensor retinaculum and the area of release for ECU stenosing tenosynovitis are shown. (Reproduced with permission from the Mayo Foundation.)

the tendon. This wall must not be damaged during release for entrapment. Instead, the release should include either the retinaculum alone or the retinaculum in combination with the lateral wall, which separates the extensor carpi ulnaris from the extensor digiti minimi. Hajj and Wood[80] recommend repairing the extensor retinaculum after releasing the lateral wall; Nachinolcar and Khanolkar[81] advise a simple release. Reported results of surgery are good. Steroid injection is reported to be effective in only a minority of cases.

Tendon Pain Without Entrapment

A syndrome of pain has been described at tendon insertions or along the path of tendons. Patients with this syndrome may have associated local swelling at the site of pain, but there are no signs or symptoms of entrapment.[1,3,6,8,11,12,16,17,83] Women are affected more frequently than men. These symptoms appear to increase in intensity in response to increased levels of repetitive work. However, Hadler[84,85] has shown that similar levels of repetitive work produce greatly different rates of reported symptoms in different populations, suggesting that other factors, perhaps cultural or socioeconomic, may be at least as important as repetition in determining whether patients consider themselves impaired in any way. Nathan and associates[86-88] have emphasized the role of body habitus, smoking, and other physical and cultural features of the patient in determining whether the patient considers repetitive activity disabling. It is not clear whether such symptoms represent a fibromyalgia or enthesopathy syndrome or a separate and different overuse pathology. Treatment has typically consisted of activity modification, NSAIDs, and physical measures. Surgery is usually unrewarding. Biopsy specimens of affected tissue typically show benign noninflammatory fibrous connective tissue.[10] Epidemics of such syndromes have been reported in many places around the world, with resolution often related as much to social as medical intervention. If there is an underlying lesion, its nature is not clear.

Summary

Tenosynovitis as a general term is a poor descriptor for the common problems that affect tendons in the hand and wrist. Many such problems fall into the general category of tendon entrapment syndromes. Tendon entrapment is most common in middle-aged women. The majority of tendon entrapment syndromes occur outside the workplace. Histologically, fibrocartilagenous metaplasia of tendon sheath and peritendinous fibrosis are more typical than acute or chronic inflammation. Symptoms of tendon entrapment are often aggravated by and may hinder work, and for this reason entrapment syndromes are often compensable under workers' compensation laws, but their cause is not clearly related to repetitive trauma in most cases. A second, much less common category includes intersection syndrome and some cases of de Quervain's disease and EPL entrapment in particular. These conditions do show frank inflammation and appear to be caused by repetitive work, and specific treatments, usually nonsurgical, are available. The third and perhaps largest group in the working population is the so-called nonspecific tenosynovitis, actually a loose term for any localized aching and tenderness near a tendon in the hand and wrist. Symptoms are common in those involved in repetitive work, but different populations with similar work levels may show different apparent rates of disease, suggesting that other factors may play a role. For this group, a specific anatomic lesion usually cannot be identified. Inflammation is usually not present histologically. Treatment is empiric, and both cultural and socioeconomic factors appear to play a major role.

References

1. Armstrong TJ, Foulke JA, Joseph BS, et al: Investigation of cumulative trauma disorders in a poultry processing plant. *Am Indust Hygiene Assoc J* 1982;43:103–116.
2. Fahey JJ, Bollinger JA: Trigger-finger in adults and children. *J Bone Joint Surg* 1954:36A:1200–1218.
3. Kurppa K, Viikari-Juntura E, Kuosma E, et al: Incidence of tenosynovitis or peritendinitis and epicondylitis in a meat-processing factory. *Scand J Work Environ Health* 1991;17:32–37.
4. Lapidus PW, Fenton R: Stenosing tenovaginitis at the wrist and fingers: Report of 423 cases in 369 patients with 354 operations. *Arch Surg* 1952;64:475–487.
5. Lipscomb PR: Chronic nonspecific tenosynovitis and peritendinitis. *Surg Clin North Am* 1944;24:780–797.
6. Luopajarvi T, Kuorinka I, Virolainen M, et al: Prevalence of tenosynovitis and other injuries of the upper extremities in repetitive work. *Scand J Work Environ Health* 1979;5(suppl 3):48–55.
7. Rosenthal EA: Tenosynovitis: Tendon and nerve entrapment. *Hand Clin* 1987;3:585–609.
8. Silverstein B, Fine L, Stetson D: Hand-wrist disorders among investment casting plant workers. *J Hand Surg* 1987;12A:838–844.
9. Tanaka S, Seligman P, Halperin W, et al: Use of workers' compensation claims data for surveillance of cumulative trauma disorders. *J Occup Med* 1988;30:488–492.
10. Thompson AR, Plewes LW, Shaw EG: Peritendinitis crepitans and simple tenosynovitis: A clinical study of 544 cases in industry. *Br J Industr Med* 1951;8:150–160.
11. Viikari-Juntura E: Neck and upper limb disorders among slaughterhouse workers: An epidemiologic and clinical study. *Scand J Work Environ Health* 1983;9:283–290.
12. Viikari-Juntura E: Tenosynovitis, peritendinitis and the tennis elbow syndrome. *Scand J Work Environ Health* 1984;10:443–449.
13. Newport ML, Lane LB, Stuchin SA: Treatment of trigger finger by steroid injection. *J Hand Surg* 1990;15A:748–750.
14. Otto N, Wehbe MA: Steroid injections for tenosynovitis in the hand. *Orthop Rev* 1986;15:290–293.

15. Rhoades CE, Gelberman RH, Manjarris JF: Stenosing tenosynovitis of the fingers and thumb: Results of a prospective trial of steroid injection and splinting. *Clin Orthop* 1984;190:236–238.
16. Armstrong TJ, Fine LJ, Goldstein SA, et al: Ergonomics considerations in hand and wrist tendinitis. *J Hand Surg* 1987;12A:830–837.
17. Kivi P: Rheumatic disorders of the upper limbs associated with repetitive occupational tasks in Finland in 1975–1979. *Scand J Rheum* 1984;13:101–107.
18. Semple C: Editorial: "Tenosynovitis." *J Hand Surg* 1986;11B:155–156.
19. Amadio PC, Frasca P, Hunter JM: Histology and scanning electron microscopy of flexor tendons in trigger fingers. *Trans Orthop Res Soc* 1982;7:345.
20. Finkelstein H: Stenosing tendovaginitis at the radial styloid process. *J Bone Joint Surg* 1930;12:509–540.
21. Howard NJ: Pathological changes induced in tendons through trauma and their accompanying clinical phenomena. *Am J Surg* 1941;51:689–706.
22. Meachim G, Roberts C: The histopathology of stenosing tendovaginitis. *J Pathol* 1969;98:187–192.
23. Anderson B, Kaye S: Treatment of flexor tenosynovitis of the hand ("trigger finger") with corticosteroids: A prospective study of the response to local injection. *Arch Intern Med* 1991;151:153–156.
24. Carlson CS Jr, Curtis RM: Steroid injection for flexor tenosynovitis. *J Hand Surg* 1984;9A:286–287.
25. Freiberg A, Mulholland RS, Levine R: Nonoperative treatment of trigger fingers and thumbs. *J Hand Surg* 1989;14A:553–558.
26. Gray RG, Kiem IM, Gottlieb NL: Intratendon sheath corticosteroid treatment of rheumatoid arthritis-associated and idiopathic hand flexor tenosynovitis. *Arthritis Rheum* 1978;21:92–96.
27. Harvey FJ, Harvey PM, Horsley MW: De Quervain's disease: Surgical or nonsurgical treatment. *J Hand Surg* 1990;15A:83–87.
28. Kolind-Sorensen V: Treatment of trigger fingers. *Acta Orthop Scand* 1970;41:428–432.
29. Kraemer BA, Young VL, Arfken C: Stenosing flexor tenosynovitis. *South Med J* 1990;83:806–811.
30. Lambert MA, Morton RJ, Sloan JP: Controlled study of the use of local steroid injection in the treatment of trigger finger and thumb. *J Hand Surg* 1992;17B:69–70.
31. Lapidus PW, Guidotti FP: Stenosing tenovaginitis of the wrist and fingers. *Clin Orthop* 1972;83:87–90.
32. Marks MR, Gunther SF: Efficacy of cortisone injection in treatment of trigger fingers and thumbs. *J Hand Surg* 1989;14A:722–727.
33. Fadale PD, Wiggins ME: Corticosteroid injections: Their use and abuse. *J Am Acad Orthop Surg* 1994;2:133–140.
34. Gazarian A, Foucher G: Tendinitis of the palmaris longus muscle: Apropos of 24 cases. *Ann Chir Main Memb Super* 1992;11:14–18.
35. Lapidus PW: Stenosing tenovaginitis. *Surg Clin North Am* 1953;33:1317–1347.
36. Lipscomb PR: Stenosing tenosynovitis at the radial styloid process (De Quervain's disease). *Ann Surg* 1951;134:110–115.
37. Lombardi RM, Wood MB, Linscheid RL: Symptomatic restrictive thumb-index flexor tenosynovitis: Incidence of musculotendinous anomalies and results of treatment. *J Hand Surg* 1988;13A:325–328.
38. Faithfull DK, Lamb DW: De Quervain's disease: A clinical review. *Hand* 1971;3:23–30.
39. Muckart RD: Stenosing tendovaginitis of abductor pollicis longus and extensor pollicis brevis at the radial styloid (De Quervain's disease). *Clin Orthop* 1964;33:201–208.
40. Strickland JW, Idler RS, Creighton JC: De Quervain's stenosing tenosynovitis. *Indiana Med* 1990;83:340–341.
41. Leao L: De Quervain's disease: A clinical and anatomical study. *J Bone Joint Surg* 1958;40A:1063–1070.

42. Schned ES: De Quervain tenosynovitis in pregnant and postpartum women. *Obstet Gynecol* 1986;68:411–414.
43. Grundberg AB, Reagan DS: Pathologic anatomy of the forearm: Intersection syndrome. *J Hand Surg* 1985;10A:299–302.
44. Dellon AL, Mackinnon SE: Radial sensory nerve entrapment in the forearm. *J Hand Surg* 1986;11A:199–205.
45. Jackson WT, Viegas SF, Coon TM, et al: Anatomical variations in the first extensor compartment of the wrist: A clinical and anatomical study. *J Bone Joint Surg* 1986;68A:923–926.
46. Leslie BM, Erickson WB Jr, Morehead JR: Incidence of a septum within the first dorsal compartment of the wrist. *J Hand Surg* 1990;15A:88–91.
47. Minamikawa Y, Peimer CA, Cox WL, et al: De Quervain's syndrome: Surgical and anatomical studies of the fibroosseous canal. *Orthopedics* 1991;14:545–549.
48. Strandell G: Variations of the anatomy in stenosing tenosynovitis at the radial styloid process. *Acta Chir Scand* 1957;113:234–240.
49. Louis DS: Incomplete release of the first dorsal compartment: A diagnostic test. *J Hand Surg* 1987;12A:87–88.
50. Woods TH: De Quervain's disease: A plea for early operation. A report on 40 cases. *Br J Surg* 1964;51:358–359.
51. Arons MS: De Quervain's release in working women: A report of failures, complications, and associated diagnoses. *J Hand Surg* 1987;12A:540–544.
52. McMahon M, Craig SM, Posner MA: Tendon subluxation after De Quervain's release: Treatment by brachioradialis tendon flap. *J Hand Surg* 1991;16A:30–32.
53. Alegado RB, Meals RA: An unusual complication following surgical treatment of de Quervain's disease. *J Hand Surg* 1979;4A:185–186.
54. White GM, Weiland AJ: Symptomatic palmar tendon subluxation after surgical release for De Quervain's disease: A case report. *J Hand Surg* 1984;9A:704–706.
55. Kapandji AI:. Enlargement plasty of the radio-styloid tunnel in the treatment of De Quervain tenosynovitis. *Ann Chir Main Memb Super* 1990;9:42–46.
56. Howard NJ: Peritendinitis crepitans: A muscle-effort syndrome. *J Bone Joint Surg* 1937;19:447–459.
57. Dobyns JH, Sim FH, Linscheid RL: Sports stress syndromes of the hand and wrist. *Am J Sports Med* 1978;6:236–254.
58. Hueston JT, Wilson WF: The aetiology of trigger finger explained on the basis of intratendinous architecture. *Hand* 1972;4:257–260.
59. Thorpe AP: Results of surgery for trigger finger. *J Hand Surg* 1988;13B:199–201.
60. Williams JG: Surgical management of traumatic non-infective tenosynovitis of the wrist extensors. *J Bone Joint Surg* 1977;59B:408–410.
61. Carrozzella J, Stern PJ, von Kuster LC: Transection of radial digital nerve of the thumb during trigger release. *J Hand Surg* 1989;14A:198–200.
62. Evans RB, Hunter JM, Burkhalter WE: Conservative management of the trigger finger: A new approach. *J Hand Therapy* 1988;1:59–68.
63. Tanaka J, Muraji M, Negoro H, et al: Subcutaneous release of trigger thumb and fingers in 210 fingers. *J Hand Surg* 1990;15B:463–465.
64. Seradge H, Kleinert HE: Reduction flexor tenoplasty: Treatment of stenosing flexor tenosynovitis distal to the first pulley. *J Hand Surg* 1981;6A:543–544.
65. Kapandji IA: Plastie D'agrandissement des poulies metacarpiennes. *Ann des de Chirurgie de la Main* 1983;2:281–282.
66. Linburg RM, Comstock BE: Anomalous tendon slips from the flexor pollicis longus to the flexor digitorum profundus. *J Hand Surg* 1979;4A:79–83.
67. Weeks PM: A cause of wrist pain: Non-specific tenosynovitis involving the flexor carpi radialis. *Plast Reconstr Surg* 1978;62:263–266.
68. Carroll RE, Coyle MP Jr: Dysfunction of the pisotriquetral joint: Treatment by excision of the pisiform. *J Hand Surg* 1985;10A:703–707.
69. Paley D, McMurtry RY, Cruickshank B: Pathologic conditions of the pisiform and pisotriquetral joint. *J Hand Surg* 1987;12A:110–119.

70. Mannerfelt L, Oetker R, Ostlund B, et al: Rupture of the extensor pollicis longus tendon after Colles fracture and by rheumatoid arthritis. *J Hand Surg* 1990;15B:49–50.
71. Dawson WJ: Sports-induced spontaneous rupture of the extensor pollicis longus tendon. *J Hand Surg* 1992;17A:457–458.
72. Zvijac JE, Janecki CJ, Supple KM: Non-traumatic spontaneous rupture of the extensor pollicis longus tendon. *Orthopedics* 1993;16:1347–1350.
73. De Smet L, Kinnen L: Impending rupture of the extensor pollicis longus tendon after an undisplaced fracture of the lower end of the radius. *Acta Orthop Belgica* 1987;53:512–513.
74. Chitnis SL, Evans DM: Tendon transfer to restore extension of the thumb using abductor pollicis longus. *J Hand Surg* 1993;18B:234–238.
75. Magnussen PA, Harvey FJ, Tonkin MA: Extensor indicis proprius transfer for rupture of the extensor pollicis longus tendon. *J Bone Joint Surg* 1990;72B:881–883.
76. Cusenz BJ, Hallock GG: Multiple anomalous tendons of the fourth dorsal compartment. *J Hand Surg* 1986;11A:263–264.
77. Fernandez Vazquez JM, Linscheid RL: Anomalous extensor muscles simulating dorsal wrist ganglion. *Clin Orthop* 1972;83:84–86.
78. Hooper G, McMaster MJ: Stenosing tenovaginitis affecting the tendon of extensor digiti minimi at the wrist. *Hand* 1979;11:299–301.
79. Ritter MA, Inglis AE: The extensor indicis proprius syndrome. *J Bone Joint Surg* 1969;51A:1645–1648.
80. Hajj AA, Wood MB: Stenosing tenosynovitis of the extensor carpi ulnaris. *J Hand Surg* 1986;11A:519–520.
81. Nachinolcar UG, Khanolkar KB: Stenosing tenovaginitis of extensor carpi ulnaris: Brief report. *J Bone Joint Surg* 1988;70B:842.
82. Burkhart SS, Wood MB, Linscheid RL: Posttraumatic recurrent subluxation of the extensor carpi ulnaris tendon. *J Hand Surg* 1982;7A:1–3.
83. Fry HJ: Overuse syndrome of the upper limb in musicians. *Med J Australia* 1986;144:182–183;185.
84. Hadler NM: Cumulative trauma disorders: An iatrogenic concept. *J Occup Med* 1990;32:38–41.
85. Hadler NM: Arm pain in the workplace: A small area analysis. *J Occup Med* 1992;34:113–119.
86. Nathan PA, Keniston RC: Carpal tunnel syndrome and its relation to general physical condition. *Hand Clinics* 1993;9:253–261.
87. Nathan PA, Keniston RC, Myers LD, et al: Obesity as a risk factor for slowing of sensory conduction of the median nerve in industry: A cross-sectional and longitudinal study involving 429 workers. *J Occup Med* 1992;34:379–383.
88. Nathan PA, Takigawa K, Keniston RC, et al: Slowing of sensory conduction of the median nerve and carpal tunnel syndrome in Japanese and American industrial workers. *J Hand Surg* 1994;19B:30–34.

Chapter 30
Rehabilitation of Repetitive Motion Disorders of the Wrist

Terrence P. Glennon, MD

Overview and Principles

The best results from rehabilitation programs are often achieved when the patient with an overuse syndrome is treated as an injured athlete, with use of a sports medicine approach to treat the injury. The general principles that guide the rehabilitation of overuse syndromes are delineated in Outline 1 as a series of eight phases.[1]

Range of motion exercises are often used to restore joint range of motion and soft-tissue extensibility. These exercises may be categorized as passive, active-assistive, or active. Specific techniques such as contract/relax stretching, which involves contraction of the shortened muscle unit until fatigue sets in, followed by passive stretching, have been demonstrated to be efficacious in increasing muscle length.[2]

Muscle strength and endurance can be enhanced by using a variety of strengthening regimens, ranging from the very simple to the very complex. Use of devices, such as elastic bands, or strengthening exercises, such as progressive resistance exercises or isometric exercises, have been shown to augment muscle strength. No single specific strengthening program seems to have any inherent advantage and the best type for an individual patient should be determined by the particular needs of that patient. For strengthening the muscles that move the wrist, a simple and practical sample piece of exercise equipment

Outline 1   Eight phases of rehabilitation of overuse syndromes

Phase I	Control the inflammatory process
Phase II	Control pain
Phase III	Restore joint range of motion and soft tissue extensibility
Phase IV	Improve muscular strength
Phase V	Improve muscular endurance
Phase VI	Develop activity-specific biomechanical skill patterns (coordination retraining)
Phase VII	Improve general fitness
Phase VIII	Establish maintenance programs

(Reproduced with permission from Saal JA: Rehabilitation of the injured athlete, in DeLisa JA, Currie DM, Gans GM, et al (eds): *Rehabilitation Medicine: Principles and Practice*. Philadelphia, PA, JB Lippincott, 1988, pp 840–864.)

is shown in Figure 1. This exercise uses materials that may be found around the home, and has the advantage of providing both concentric and eccentric exercise to both the forearm flexors and extensors. In addition, the exercise can be performed in a variety of positions, with the elbows flexed or extended, to target various muscle groups.[3]

Restoration of activity-specific training should occur prior to returning the individual to full activity. In overuse syndromes, this can be difficult because the activities must be performed over such a long period of time. However, the therapist or physician can observe the patient's technique to optimize the biomechanics. The balance between augmenting strength and endurance and exacerbating symptoms resulting from disorders such as tendinitis may be difficult to achieve, and should be monitored closely. This rehabilitation phase is hastened by avoidance of absolute immobilization, beyond that which is absolutely necessary, so as to avoid deconditioning of the involved muscles.[4]

Rehabilitation of Tendinitis at the Wrist

The prototypical tendinitis at the wrist is de Quervain's disease, which is stenosing tenosynovitis of the abductor pollicis longus and extensor pollicis brevis tendons. Other wrist tendons may be affected by tendinitis, including the extensor pollicis longus, extensor indicis proprius, extensor digiti minimi, extensor and flexor carpi ulnaris, flexor carpi radialis, or flexor digitorum. Reha-

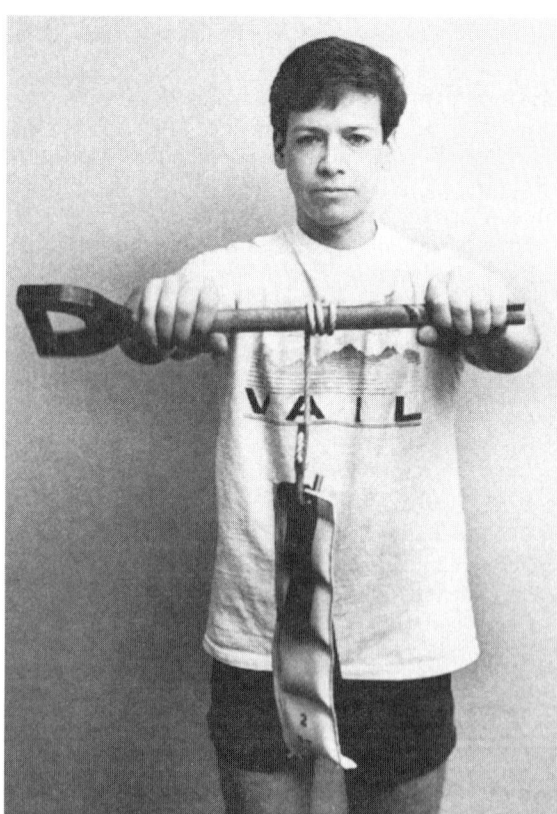

Fig. 1 Illustration of a basic wrist exercise using materials commonly available around the house. The patient rolls the dowel so that the weight is raised and lowered by taking up the rope. Both wrist flexors and wrist extensors can be strengthened concentrically and eccentrically using this exercise. (Reproduced with permission from Press JM, Wiesner SL: Prevention: Conditioning and orthotics. *Hand Clin* 1990;6:383–392).

bilitation is provided along a continuum, with acute treatment to control inflammation while limiting deconditioning of the involved muscles.[5]

Nonsurgical treatment is always attempted first. Surgical treatment is proposed after conservative management has failed, with the parameters of such a delineation usually described as persistence or progression of symptoms despite adequate nonsurgical intervention. Treatment programs consist of removal of the causative activity,[6] relative rest by immobilization, ice application, and anti-inflammatory medication. The first priority in treatment of tendinitis is to control inflammation, thereby controlling pain.[7] Medications used to accomplish this include oral nonsteroidal anti-inflammatory drugs (NSAIDs) or a local injection of a corticosteroid preparation. Topical agents have also been effective in reducing symptoms.[8]

While not specifically studied in the treatment of wrist tendinitis, ultrasound has been demonstrated in controlled, double-blind studies to be useful in improving pain scores, range of motion, and strength in patients with repetitive motion syndromes of the upper limb.[9] The results of studies on laser treatment are more variable, however, and have not demonstrated consistent efficacy in the treatment of such disorders.[9-12]

Splints are applied to immobilize the affected portion of the upper limb while leaving other joints free to move, minimizing the effects of immobility. The use of a thermoplastic orthosis will provide the patient with a custom fit.[13] Active range of motion of uninvolved joints, including sport- or job-specific activity that does not exacerbate the pain, should be continued, thus preventing weakness, contractures, and loss of coordination.

Mobility of the affected joints is maintained with active or active-assistive range of motion, within pain tolerance, and the patient is gradually weaned from the splint into a program of progressive range of motion and stretching. As pain becomes controlled, a more aggressive stretching program may be introduced to stretch the muscle, thus reducing the tension on the inflamed tendon. The contract/relax proprioceptive neuromuscular facilitation method of stretching may produce more effective stretching than simple static passive stretching.[2] An appropriate strengthening program is then introduced.

If surgery is required, postoperative rehabilitation should begin after 7 to 10 days and progress over 4 to 6 weeks.[5] Again, the goals of restoration of full range of motion and strength should be reached before return to full activity.

Rehabilitation of Nerve Entrapment at the Wrist

As with the treatment of tendinitis, initial nonsurgical treatment of nerve entrapments at the wrist is recommended. While the ulnar nerve may be entrapped at Guyon's canal, median neuropathy at the wrist, otherwise known as carpal tunnel syndrome, is by far the more common entrapment syndrome, and has been more closely associated with repetitive motion activities.[14] Conservative treatment has been more effective in milder cases of carpal tunnel syndrome.[15,16] Treatment consists of restriction of the offending activity, anti-inflammatory medication (corticosteroid injection or oral NSAIDs), and immobilization with orthotics, particularly at night in patients with nocturnal symptoms. Patients with more severe carpal tunnel syndrome, as evidenced by a longer duration of symptoms, thenar atrophy, or markedly prolonged nerve conduction parameters, do not tend to respond as well to conservative treatment; thus, surgical intervention is recommended.[15] Splinting is most effective if applied within 3 months of symptom onset.[17]

Strength assessments in patients following carpal tunnel release have demonstrated significant weakness up to 6 weeks after surgery.[18] Exercise programs produced improved strength in some movements at 3 weeks, though no significant difference in strength was noted in comparison to a group of patients who did not exercise.[19]

The osteopathic literature suggests methods of manipulation and stretching designed to stretch the transverse carpal ligament and dilate the canal, thus reducing carpal canal pressure. The study was a report of a single case, with improvement in nerve conduction parameters after 2 months of treatment. Stretching was performed by placing traction on the transverse carpal ligament as well as by hyperextension of the fingers to distend the canal by pulling the thicker, more proximal portions of the tendons into the canal.[20]

Rehabilitation of Muscular Overuse Syndrome at the Wrist

In addition to tendinitis and nerve entrapment, a third category of injury has been identified. Distinct from the more inclusive terms "repetitive strain injury" (RSI) or "cumulative trauma disorder" (CTD), the term "overuse syndrome,"[21,22] although it has been used as a more comprehensive term as well, has more recently been applied to a syndrome of regional muscular pain and tenderness, without evidence of inflammation.[23] Pathologic findings on muscle biopsy, including mitochondrial abnormalities, abnormal percentage of fiber types, and abnormal fiber diameters, were found.[24] These changes are analogous to those found in patients with fibromyalgia, suggesting the possibility that muscular overuse syndrome may be a regional version of this disorder.[21,25]

Symptoms of muscular overuse syndrome generally consist of pain beginning in a specific area, then spreading proximally and distally. Signs include tenderness of the intrinsic muscles and joint ligaments, as well as tenderness located proximal to the original site of pain.

As with the other syndromes, initial rehabilitation begins with removal or correction of the offending activity. Because inflammation has not been determined to play a role in this syndrome, anti-inflammatory medication is not particularly effective. The efficacy of other medications, particularly those used in fibromyalgia syndrome, such as tricyclic antidepressants, has not been investigated. Successful treatment has been documented with periods of absolute rest followed by judicious resumption of activity after correction of any errors in technique. The only prevention of recurrence may be absolute limits on certain activities.[26] Successful treatment of patients with this disorder is complicated by the paucity of corroborating evidence on routine clinical and laboratory evaluation, combined with the often-present psychologic components that accompany such complaints.

References

1. Saal JA: Rehabilitation of the injured athlete, in DeLisa JA, Currie DM, Gans GM, et al (eds): *Rehabilitation Medicine: Principles and Practice.* Philadelphia, PA, JB Lippincott, 1988, pp 840–864.
2. Tanigawa MC: Comparison of the hold-relax procedure and passive mobilization on increasing muscle length. *Phys Ther* 1972;52:725–35.
3. Press JM, Wiesner SL: Prevention: Conditioning and orthotics. *Hand Clin* 1990;6:383–392.
4. Rizzo TD Jr: Rehabilitation of hand and wrist injuries in sports. *Phys Med Rehab Clin North Am* 1994;5:115–131.

5. Stern PJ: Tendinitis, overuse syndromes, and tendon injuries. *Hand Clin* 1990;6:467–476.
6. Kiefhaber TR, Stern PJ: Upper extremity tendinitis and overuse syndromes in the athlete. *Clin Sports Med* 1992;11:39–55.
7. Pitner MA: Pathophysiology of overuse injuries in the hand and wrist. *Hand Clin* 1990;6:355–364.
8. Hochberg FH, Lavin P, Portney R, et al: Topical therapy of localized inflammation in musicians: A clinical evaluation of aspercreme versus placebo. *Med Probl Perform Art* 1988;3:9–14.
9. Binder A, Hodge G, Greenwood AM, et al: Is therapeutic ultrasound effective in treating soft tissue lesions? *Br Med J* 1985;290:512–514.
10. England S, Farrell AJ, Coppock JS, et al: Low power laser therapy of shoulder tendonitis. *Scand J Rheumatol* 1989;18:427–431.
11. Lundeberg T, Haker E, Thomas M: Effect of laser versus placebo in tennis elbow. *Scand J Rehab Med* 1987;19:135–138.
12. Vecchio P, Cave M, King V, et al: A double-blind study of the effectiveness of low level laser treatment of rotator cuff tendinitis. *Br J Rheumatol* 1993;32:740–742.
13. Prokop LL: Upper-extremity rehabilitation: Conditioning and orthotics for the athlete and performing artist. *Hand Clin* 1990;6:517–524.
14. Weinstein SM, Herring SA: Nerve problems and compartment syndromes in the hand, wrist, and forearm. *Clin Sports Med* 1992;11:161–188.
15. Gelberman RH, Aronson D, Weisman MH: Carpal-tunnel syndrome: Results of a prospective trial of steroid injection and splinting. *J Bone Joint Surg* 1980;62A:1181–1184.
16. Phalen GS: The carpal-tunnel syndrome: Seventeen years' experience in diagnosis and treatment of six hundred fifty-four hands. *J Bone Joint Surg* 1966;48A:211–228.
17. Kruger VL, Kraft GH, Deitz JC, et al: Carpal tunnel syndrome: Objective measures and splint use. *Arch Phys Med Rehabil* 1991;72:517–520.
18. Nathan PA, Meadows KD, Keniston RC: Rehabilitation of carpal tunnel surgery patients using a short surgical incision and an early program of physical therapy. *J Hand Surg* 1993;18A:1044–1050.
19. Groves EJ, Rider BA: A comparison of treatment approaches used after carpal tunnel release surgery. *Am J Occup Ther* 1989;43:398–402.
20. Sucher BM: Myofascial release of carpal tunnel syndrome. *J Am Osteopath Assoc* 1993;93:92–94,100–101.
21. Lederman RJ, Calabrese LH: Overuse syndromes in instrumentalists. *Med Probl Perform Art* 1986;1:7–11.
22. Goodman G, Staz S: Occupational therapy for musicians with upper extremity overuse syndrome: Patient perceptions regarding effectiveness of treatment. *Med Probl Perform Art* 1989;4:9–14.
23. Miller MH, Topliss DJ: Chronic upper limb pain syndrome (repetitive strain injury) in the Australian workforce: A systematic cross sectional rheumatological study of 229 patients. *J Rheumatol* 1988;15:1705–1712.
24. Dennett X, Fry HJ: Overuse syndrome: A muscle biopsy study. *Lancet* 1988;1:905–908.
25. Lederman RJ: AAEM minimonograph #43: Neuromuscular problems in the performing arts. *Muscle Nerve* 1994;17:569–577.
26. Fry HJ: Overuse syndrome of the upper limb in musicians. *Med J Aust* 1986;144:182–183,185.

Chapter 31
Cubital Tunnel Syndrome in the Work Environment

William F. Blair, MD

History

Cubital tunnel syndrome is defined by a specific set of symptoms and clinical findings associated with acquired pathophysiology of the ulnar nerve at or near the medial side of the elbow. Typical symptoms are numbness and paresthesias in the ring and small fingers, and clinical findings include reduced sensibility in these fingers, atrophy of the intrinsic muscles of the hand, and changes on electrophysiologic testing.

The syndrome was first proposed by Gowers in 1899, who recognized that prolonged elbow flexion could result in ulnar nerve palsy.[1] Knowledge of the anatomic basis for the compression was improved by Buzzard,[2] who described compression of the ulnar nerve between the two heads of the flexor carpi ulnaris muscle. General understanding of cubital tunnel syndrome has been improved by numerous original and review articles.[3,4]

The association between specific occupational activities and cubital tunnel syndrome has been widely recognized in industrial countries since the late 19th century. Spaans[5] in 1970 thoroughly reviewed the European literature and documented an association between ulnar neuropathy and the occupational activities of brass workers, crystal grinders, diamond cutters, enamelers, glass cutters, gold beaters, rollers, telegraphists, telephonists, locksmiths, mechanics, plumbers, stonecutters, and joiners. In the English literature, problems were cited in chess players,[6] telephonists,[7] and those in clerical occupations.[8]

More recently, Feldman and associates[9] emphasized the difference between repetitive elbow flexion and direct compression as causative factors of the syndrome. Frequent, repetitive elbow movements, as made by workers operating the handles of boring and punching machines, were described as problematic.[5] Massey and Riley[10] emphasized simultaneous elbow flexion-extension and forearm supination-pronation during occupational or athletic movements, such as holding rifles, shoveling, and throwing. Direct compression is presumably a result of chronically leaning on the elbows;[9] craftsmen and clerical personnel, for example, press their proximal forearms against a workbench to stabilize their hands while performing their tasks.[8,9] However, the relationship between occupationally based activities and cubital tunnel syndrome remains difficult to define. Dellon and associates[11] noted that in a population of 128 patients with cubital tunnel syndrome, 40% had jobs that entailed repetitive elbow motion. Perhaps because of the limited data available, the relationship between occupation and cubital tunnel syndrome may not be widely understood or appreciated. For example, in recent texts on cumulative trauma disorders, cubital tunnel syndrome is mentioned only briefly,[12,13] or not at all.[14]

Anatomy

The ulnar nerve enters the elbow region by passing through the medial intermuscular septum of the arm. It then descends distally and medially on the anterior surface of the medial head of the triceps muscle. The nerve passes into the ulnar groove on the dorsal aspect of the medial epicondyle, placing it within the cubital tunnel. This fibro-osseous tunnel, bordered medially by the elbow joint, can be conceptualized as having the following three parts: (1) the ulnar groove in the medial epicondyle; (2) a fascial arcade extending from the medial epicondyle to the olecranon and connecting the ulnar and humeral heads of the flexor carpi ulnaris muscle; and (3) the muscle bellies of the flexor carpi ulnaris (Fig. 1). In the cubital tunnel the ulnar nerve provides one articular branch to the elbow joint and, more distally, two branches to the flexor carpi ulnaris muscle. As the nerve leaves the cubital tunnel it passes between the flexor carpi ulnaris and flexor digitorum profundus muscles, coming to rest on the palmar surface of the latter.[15]

Superficial to the cubital tunnel, in the deep subcutaneous tissues of the medial side of the elbow, is the medial antebrachial cutaneous nerve. It passes obliquely from proximal and anterior to distal and posterior. This nerve or its branches are usually distal to the medial epicondyle.

When the elbow is moved from extension to flexion, the distance between the medial epicondyle and the olecranon increases, and the fascia that forms the roof of the cubital tunnel becomes taut. The cross-sectional geometry of the cubital tunnel changes from a relatively round configuration to that of a flattened triangle, narrowing the cross-sectional area by approximately 55%.[16]

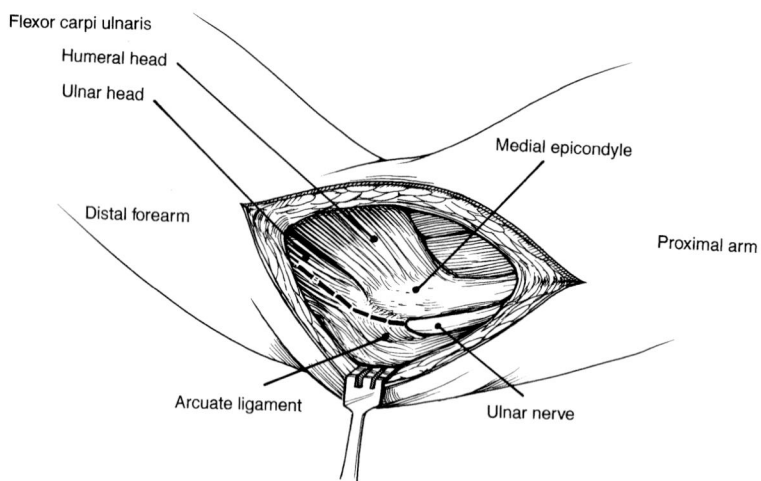

Fig. 1 The anatomy of the cubital tunnel. The ulnar nerve courses posterior to the medial epicondyle, under the medial fascial arcade and under a transverse fascial arch between the two heads of the flexor carpi ulnaris muscle. Above, exposure of the tunnel is achieved with a longitudinal incision that extends distally in the groove between the medial epicondyle and olecranon. (Reproduced with permissioin from Ferlic DC: In-situ decompression of the ulnar nerve at the elbow, in Gelberman RH (ed): *Operative Nerve Repair and Reconstruction.* Philadelphia, PA, JB Lippincott, 1991, vol 2, pp 1063–1067.)

The ulnar nerve also elongates by as much as 4.7 mm over a full range of elbow motion. Wrist extension, elbow flexion, and shoulder abduction can all combine to contribute to an increase in intraneural and extraneural pressure within the cubital tunnel that may be as much as six times higher than baseline, resting values.[17]

Normally, the median nerve tracks posteriorly and medially out of the depth of the groove as the elbow moves from extension to flexion. If the nerve is hypermobile it moves up and onto the medial epicondyle (Type A) or over and anterior to the epicondyle (Type B) at 90° of elbow flexion. Type A ulnar nerves occur in 12% of individuals, and Type B in 4%.[18]

Clinical Presentation

Cubital tunnel syndrome in the occupational environment usually begins insidiously, with activity-related paresthesias in the ring and small fingers and, occasionally, in the medial forearm. Sustained elbow flexion aggravates the symptoms, often awakening the patient at night.[19] With progression of the syndrome, the paresthesias become baseline, and sensory loss develops in the ulnar half of the ring finger and in all of the small finger. This can also be accompanied by pain on the medial aspect of the elbow and proximal forearm. Extrinsic and intrinsic muscle denervation also progresses gradually. Patients often do not appreciate early, low-grade losses of pinch and grip strength. With progression they notice hand fatigue, loss of dexterity, difficulty maintaining production rates, and job-related disability. They may also eventually notice intrinsic muscle atrophy; in some cases claw deformity of the ring and small fingers develops.

Individuals with Type A hypermobile ulnar nerves who perform repetitive motions will not be aware of the phenomenon. However, sometimes individuals with Type B hypermobile nerves, especially if it jumps or pops as it passes over the epicondyle, will perceive the phenomenon. It is usually described as intermittent, occurring with selected activities, associated with medial elbow and proximal forearm pain, and sometimes causing paresthesias to radiate to the medial side of the hand.

Although both sensory and motor changes occur concurrently in most patients, advanced sensory changes can occur without motor loss, and advanced motor changes can occur without apparent sensory deficit. These variations can be partially attributable to common anomalies in the innervation patterns of the ulnar nerve. Sensory branches passing from the ulnar to the median nerve in the palm may result in sensory deficits that are greater than those of the classic ulnar nerve distribution. Motor fibers from the median nerve in the palm to the third and fourth lumbricals may prevent clawing. The clinical presentation can be quite confusing in the presence of median to ulnar nerve communications in the forearm, with an incidence as high as 15%.[20]

Clinical Assessment

The evaluation of an employee with possible cubital tunnel syndrome preferably follows an established workplace-based protocol. The first priority in the assessment is obtaining a thorough medical history, one which includes questions that address the diagnosis of cubital tunnel syndrome directly. Taking the history should also include questions intended to rule out important disorders in the differential diagnosis. These disorders would include cervical root compression neuropathy, thoracic outlet syndrome, ulnar nerve compression at

Guyon's canal, and polyneuropathy with ulnar nerve involvement. The second priority is completion of a thorough physical examination that should include (1) inspection of the hand and forearm for muscle atrophy and the inside of the elbow for swelling or sudden dislocation of the nerve anteriorly during active elbow flexion; (2) direct palpation of the ulnar nerve in the cubital tunnel, palpation while moving the elbow through flexion and extension to detect subluxation of the ulnar nerve over the medial epicondyle, and gentle pressure to elicit tenderness in the cubital tunnel itself or in adjacent areas; (3) motor testing of the flexor digitorum profundus to the ring and small fingers and testing of the hand intrinsics;[21] (4) quantitation of strength with pinch meters and a five-step grip meter; (5) sensory examination that includes two-point discrimination and perhaps vibration testing; (6) a vascular examination with Allen's testing in the distal forearm; and (7) appropriate special tests, such as percussion to elicit a Tinel sign and the elbow flexion test.[22]

Palpation is an especially important part of the examination for cubital tunnel syndrome. A palpable mass in the cubital tunnel could indicate a fusiform, neuromatous enlargement of the ulnar nerve, or a mass occupying the tunnel, such as a ganglion cyst. Palpation for tenderness or a Tinel sign at locations other than the cubital tunnel should also be included because numerous, although unusual, causes of compression have been documented proximal and distal to the cubital tunnel itself. From proximally to distally, other locations of compression neuropathy are the supracondyloid process,[23] the arcade of Struthers,[24] snapping triceps muscles,[25] anconeus epitrochlearis muscles,[26] sub-anconeus muscles,[27] and deep flexor pronator aponeurosis.[28]

The diagnosis of very mild cubital tunnel syndrome remains a clinical diagnosis, although mild to more advanced syndromes are confirmed with electrophysiologic testing. This testing, which is best done by a qualified and experienced neurologist, can include a variety of parameters.[29] The more commonly used tests are motor conduction studies, sensory conduction studies, proximal segment motor latencies, amplitude changes in compound muscle action potentials and sensory nerve action potentials, and electromyography (EMG). The definition of cubital syndrome on the basis of absolute electrophysiologic values is of limited merit, as normal and abnormal values are technique and laboratory dependent. Also, electrophysiologic values must be interpreted in the clinical context because 65% of the population may have 10 to 20 m/s slowing across the elbow.[30]

The results of the clinical assessment have been used to develop algorithms to guide treatment based on either intensity of symptoms or mechanism of injury.[3,31] The classification system proposed by McGowan[32] in 1950 was widely used. It was comprised of three grades, based on the severity of motor deficit. The obvious limitation, as noted by Ferlic,[3] was that the sensory component of the syndrome was not included. Dellon[31] later proposed a modified three-stage classification system that included mild, moderate, and severe categories based on clinical changes with sensory, motor, and special testing. This classification system lacked specificity; in 1993 Dellon and associates[11] introduced an alternative ten-grade system that reflects increasing symptoms and progressive loss of sensory and motor function in advancing cubital tunnel syndrome (Table 1).

Treatment

Traditional strategies for treating cubital tunnel syndrome fall into either conservative or surgical categories. Conservative treatment is indicated in the intermittently or mildly symptomatic patient for whom the two-point discrimi-

Table 1 A numerical scale for grading cubital tunnel syndrome

Numeric score		Description of Impairment*
Sensory	Motor	
0	0	None
1		Paresthesis, intermittent
	2	Weakness, mild:
		pinch/grip
		Female: 10-14/26-39
		Male: 13-19/31-59
3		Abnormal threshold, mild vibration, or pressure
	4	Weakness, moderate:
		pinch/grip
		Female: 6-9/15-25
		Male: 6-12/15-30
5		Paresthesia, persistent
6		Abnormal 2PD: 5th finger $_s$2PD 7-10, $_m$2PD 4-6 mm
	7	Muscle wasting, mild (1-2/4)
8		Abnormal 2PD: 5th finger $_s$2PD ≥ 11, $_m$2PD ≥ 7 mm
9		Anesthesia
	10	Muscle wasting, severe (3-4/4)

*2PD, two-point discrimination; $_s$2PD, static two-point discrimination; $_m$2PD, moving two-point discrimination.
(Reproduced with the permission from Dellon AL, Hament W, Gittelshon A: Nonoperative management of cubital tunnel syndrome: An 8-year prospective study. *Neurology* 1993;43:1673–1677.)

nation is normal, there is no muscle atrophy, and electrical abnormalities are at most only slightly abnormal. Treatment should include education about the avoidance of direct pressure on the medial aspect of the elbow and avoidance of activities that result in repetitive or full flexion of the elbow. For patients bothered primarily by nighttime symptoms, a soft elbow pad can be worn in a reverse manner, to decrease inadvertent elbow flexion and, hopefully, nighttime symptoms. For patients with daytime and nighttime symptoms, a well-padded thermoplastic posterior splint, positioning the elbow at 45° of flexion, can be helpful. This lightweight, rigid splint can be worn during the day, night, or both, depending on the patient's willingness to comply with the treatment.

The surgical treatment of cubital tunnel syndrome was first described by Sargent[33] in 1922. Since that time there has been a proliferation of recommended surgical techniques. The established techniques fall into one of two categories, decompression or transposition, with the type of transposition being either subcutaneous or deep. The indications for surgery are an increased two-point discrimination value in the ulnar nerve distribution, intrinsic muscle atrophy, or painful dysesthesias that are unresponsive to conservation care. Surgery for decompression includes in situ decompression[34] (Fig. 2) or medical epicondylectomy[35] (Fig. 3). Surgery to achieve transposition includes anterior subcutaneous transposition,[36] anterior intramuscular transposition,[37] and deep submuscular transposition.[38] The relative efficacy of these and other surgical techniques was explored in an extensive literature analysis by Dellon.[31] One feature common to each of the surgeries is a medial approach to the elbow.

The medial antebrachial cutaneous nerve must be identified and protected during surgery. Injury to this nerve branch can result in paresthesias along the medial side of the elbow, and pain at the incision site and medial elbow. All of these symptoms can be misinterpreted as persistent cubital tunnel syndrome, can be a source of distress for the patient, and can interfere with plans to return to work.

The approach to treating cubital tunnel syndrome in the work environment, if job-related repetitive motion or compression to the medial aspect of the forearm and elbow are possibly contributing factors, must necessarily differ from the traditional approach. Treatment should be based in prevention. Preplacement screening for a history of paresthesias in the ulnar nerve distribution, cubitus valgus, or a subluxating ulnar nerve should help to reduce the incidence of cubital tunnel syndrome. Job rotations should be established in the workplace, especially when tasks require combined elbow flexion-extension and forearm pronation-supination. Surveillance programs and employee educational programs should facilitate the early recognition of this syndrome. With the onset of possible cubital tunnel syndrome, the symptoms should be carefully documented along with measures of sensibility, grip strength, and pinch strength. Work activities should be modified to avoid the aggravating factor, and the patient should be placed in either a reverse elbow pad or a static elbow splint for nighttime wear. If the symptoms resolve, a job change is warranted, and the examination should be carefully repeated to document resolution of symptoms and recovery of normal sensibility and strength. If the symptoms do not resolve, an electrophysiologic evaluation to include EMG and nerve conduction velocities (NCV) of the ulnar and median nerves is appropriate. If the studies are nega-

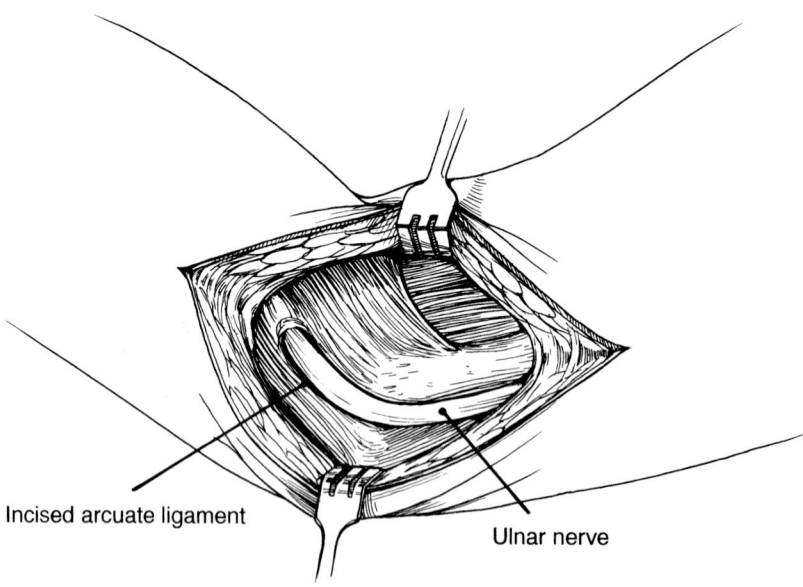

Fig. 2 In situ release of the ulnar nerve. The fascial arcade and arcuate ligament between the two heads of the flexor carpi ulnaris are released. (Reproduced with permission from Ferlic DC: In-situ decompression of the ulnar nerve at the elbow, in Gelberman RH (ed): *Operative Nerve Repair and Reconstruction.* Philadelphia, PA, JB Lippincott, 1991, vol 2, pp 1063–1067.)

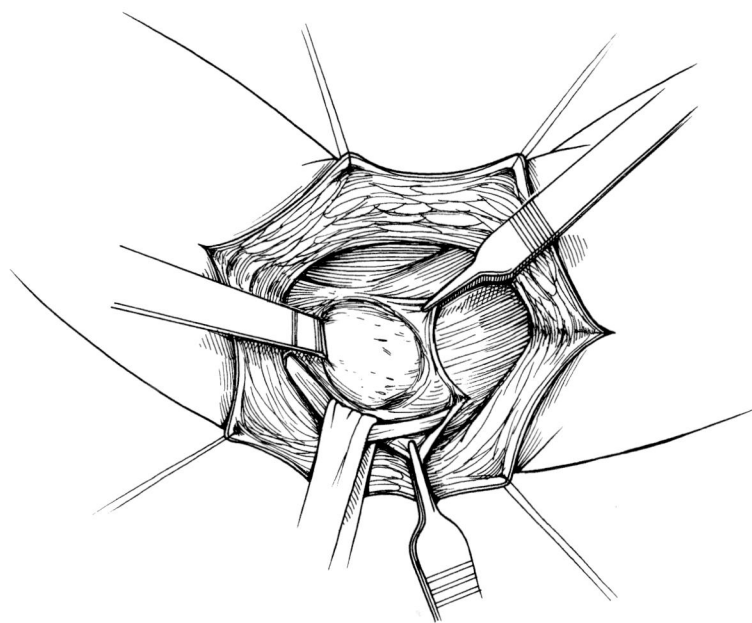

Fig. 3 Medial epicondylectomy for the treatment of cubital tunnel syndrome. Part of the flexor-pronator origin is mobilized anteriorly and the periosteum posteriorly prior to performing the osteotomy. (Reproduced with permission from Heithoff SJ, Millender LH: Medial epicondylectomy, in Gelberman RH (ed): *Operative Nerve Repair and Reconstruction.* Philadelphia, PA, JB Lippincott, 1991, vol 2, pp 1087–1096.)

tive, continued observation and clinical follow-up are appropriate. If EMG and NCV studies are positive and the symptoms beyond minimal in nature, early surgical treatment should be recommended. Surgical treatment is inappropriate in the presence of normal EMGs and NCVs. Although the relative efficacy of specific operations remains controversial, it is widely agreed that surgery done early has a better prognosis than surgery done late.

The rate of return to work after cubital tunnel surgery is variable. Both the ability and willingness of patients to return to their previous employment is highly important. If an operation has truly corrected the anatomic predisposition to developing cubital tunnel syndrome, and the patient's job does not require direct compression on a nerve that was transposed or left in situ, a return to the previous place of employment and job is a reasonable and safe goal.

Outcomes

To assess the value of either conservative or surgical care in the treatment of cubital tunnel syndrome, it is helpful to first understand its natural history. Eisen and Danon,[39] in 1974, addressed this clinical issue by first defining cubital tunnel syndrome using electromyographic criteria. They then compared EMG and NCV findings in 30 patients with mild cubital tunnel syndrome to those of 48 control patients. In the cubital tunnel syndrome group, the motor conduction velocity across the elbow was 46.8 m/s, whereas it was 53.2 m/s in controls, a statistically significant difference. The motor latency was 3.4 m/s in the cubital tunnel syndrome patients, and 3.0 m/s in the controls, also significant. The most important finding, however, was that 90% of the patients improved at a mean follow-up of 22 months. Yet it is not clear that the improvement represented natural history alone because the report did not specifically state that the study group was not treated conservatively.

Conservative treatment was subsequently addressed by Dimond and Lister.[40] They treated 42 patients in a posterior elbow splint, with the elbow flexed and the wrist supported. At an average follow-up of 8.7 months, 86% of the patients were improved. The value of this study is difficult to assess because it was not prospective, specific entrance criteria were not presented, and some of the follow-ups were of short duration.

The most conclusive findings to date concerning the nonsurgical management of cubital tunnel syndrome were presented by Dellon and associates.[11] They prospectively assessed the results of conservative treatment in 128 patients, 121 (94%) of whom were available for follow-up. Forty-three of the patients had bilateral cubital tunnel syndrome. Follow-up information was available for 164 patients with cubital tunnel syndrome, at a mean follow-up of 58.6 months. A numerical grading scale based on symptoms, sensory changes, and motor loss was developed. Using a Kaplan-Meier life-table analysis, survival curves (with survival defined as not having an operation) were calculated. With a numerical score of 1 for a very mild cubital tunnel syndrome, 21% had surgery; with scores of 2, 3, or 4 for a mild syndrome, 33% had surgery; and with numerical scores of 5, 6, or 7 for a moderate syndrome, 62% had surgery. Patients with higher scores in this study were indicated primarily for surgical treatment. To state these results from a different perspective, patients who had a very mild cubital tunnel syndrome and who were undergoing conservative care had a 79% chance of not progressing to indications for surgical treatment. It should be recognized that this study did not factor out work relatedness in the analysis, and might not be applicable to cubital tunnel syndrome derived in the work environment.

The results of surgical treatment for cubital tunnel syndrome are most difficult to determine when reviewing selected articles describing specific operations. This concept was well developed by Dellon[31] in his comprehensive review of 50 published reports on more than 2,000 patients treated for cubital tunnel syndrome. He concluded that "there are at present no statistically significant guidelines based on prospective randomized studies for choosing one operation over another." His analysis does support surgical treatment in the early stages of the syndrome because any of the surgical techniques yielded 90% excellent results in this group. Although Dellon went on to recommend anterior submuscular transposition with a flexor slide, he did not claim that this recommendation was based on the results of higher quality clinical research. In summary, surgery for the very early stages of cubital tunnel syndrome provides results that are superior to surgery done for later stages, and the choice of a specific operation is based on surgeons' bias, which is usually derived from surgical training, anecdotal experience, and knowledge of the notably limited clinical research.

The assessment of the results of treatment of cubital tunnel syndrome in the work environment presents a special problem and might not be possible at present. One aspect of the dilemma is that the diagnosis of cubital tunnel syndrome in the work environment is at times difficult to make. Although some employees present with a straightforward description of their syndrome, others present in the context of other repetitive motion disorders or acquired medical conditions. The description of the symptoms can be more complex because of coexistent loci of discomfort and because of symptom amplification in some workers, presumably for a variety of reasons. Similarly coexisting conditions can confound the physical examination. Other disorders involving the medial cord of the plexus proximal to the ulnar nerve itself or distally may contribute to decreased sensibility, and other conditions may predictably decrease performance on either extrinsic or intrinsic motor testing. Furthermore, a patient's participation in the measured aspects of the physical examination require cognition and volition. Intentional or unintentional nonoptimum performance can significantly confound the examination; therefore, the examination must include a reliability measure. In summary, from a practical perspective, the clinical assessment and the confirmation of the diagnosis of cubital tunnel syndrome is often very difficult in workers experiencing occupational exposures. Often the clinician must depend quite heavily on the results of electrophysiologic testing, but it must be kept in mind that 65% of the normal population may have decreased conduction velocities across the elbow and that this finding is a function of increasing age.[30] The tendency to overinterpret electrophysiologic findings when diagnosing, staging, and especially when indicating surgical treatment, must be avoided.

Previous publications on both the conservative and surgical care of patients with cubital tunnel syndrome have not factored out employment variables, including occupation or work-related elbow functions. This leaves the discussion of assessment and treatment, protocols, the specifics of conservative or surgical care of patients involved in repetitive elbow motions, and guidelines for return to work anecdotal at best. However, this awareness provides a significant basis for participation in future clinical investigations by American industry, government, and clinical research centers.

References

1. Gowers WR, Taylor J (eds): *A Manual of Diseases of the Nervous System*, ed 3. London, UK, Churchill Livingstone, 1899.
2. Buzzard EF: Some varieties of traumatic and toxic ulnar neuritis. *Lancet* 1922;1: 317–319.
3. Ferlic DC: Clinical assessment and conservative treatment of cubital tunnel syndrome, in Gelberman RH (ed): *Operative Nerve Repair and Reconstruction*. Philadelphia, PA, JB Lippincott, 1991, vol 2, pp 1055–1061.
4. Sunderland S (ed): *Nerves and Nerve Injuries*. Baltimore, MD, Williams & Wilkins, 1968, pp 736–780.
5. Spaans F: Occupational nerve lesions, in Vinken PJ, Bruyn GW (eds): *Handbook of Clinical Neurology*. Amsterdam, The Netherlands, North-Holland Publishing, 1970, vol 7, pp 326–343.
6. Collins RT (ed): *A Manual of Neurology and Psychiatry in Occupational Medicine*. New York, NY, Grune and Stratton, 1961.
7. Richards RL: Traumatic ulnar neuritis: The results of anterior transposition of the ulnar nerve. *Edinb Med J* 1945;52:14–21.
8. Malabar FL: Ulnar nerve, in Kopell HP, Thompson WAL (eds): *Peripheral Entrapment Neuropathies*, ed 2. Huntington, NY, Robert E. Krieger Publishing Co, 1976, pp 127–134.
9. Feldman RG, Goldman R, Keyserling WM: Classical syndromes in occupational medicine: Peripheral nerve entrapment syndromes and ergonomic factors. *Am J Ind Med* 1983;4:661–681.
10. Massey EW, Riley TL: Nontraumatic mononeuropathies: A review. *Milit Med* 1981; 146:30–36.

11. Dellon AL, Hament W, Gittelshon A: Nonoperative management of cubital tunnel syndrome: An 8-year prospective study. *Neurology* 1993;43:1673–1677.
12. Harter BT: Indications for surgery in work-related compression neuropathies of the upper extremity, in Kasdan ML (ed): *Occupational Medicine: Occupational Hand Injuries*. Philadelphia, PA, Hanley and Belfus, 1989, vol 4, pp 489–491.
13. Putz-Anderson V (ed): *Cumulative Trauma Disorders: A Manual for Musculoskeletal Diseases of the Upper Limbs*. London, UK, Taylor and Francis, 1988, pp 15–20.
14. Isernhagen SJ: Ergonomics and cumulative trauma, in Isernhagen SJ (ed): *Work Injury: Management and Prevention*. Rockville, MD, Aspen Publishers, 1988, pp 54–64.
15. Siegel DB, Gelberman RH: Ulnar nerve: Applied anatomy and operative exposure, in Gelberman RH (ed): *Operative Nerve Repair and Reconstruction*. Philadelphia, PA, JB Lippincott, 1991, vol 1, pp 413–424.
16. Apfelberg DB, Larson SJ: Dynamic anatomy of the ulnar nerve at the elbow. *Plast Reconstr Surg* 1973;51:76–81.
17. Pechan J, Julis I: The pressure measurement in the ulnar nerve: A contribution to the pathophysiology of the cubital tunnel syndrome. *J Biomech* 1975;8:75–79.
18. Childress HM: Recurrent ulnar-nerve dislocation at the elbow. *Clin Orthop Rel Res* 1975;108:168–173.
19. Spinner M, Linscheid RL: Nerve entrapment syndromes, in Morrey BF (ed): *The Elbow and Its Disorders*. Philadelphia, PA, WB Saunders, 1985, pp 691–712.
20. Kaplan EB, Spinner M: Normal and anomalous innervation patterns in the upper extremity, in Omer GE Jr, Spinner M (eds): *Management of Peripheral Nerve Problems*. Philadelphia, PA, WB Saunders, 1980, pp 75–99.
21. Blair WF: Motor testing, in Gelberman RH (ed): *Operative Nerve Repair and Reconstruction*. Philadelphia, PA, JB Lippincott, 1991, vol 1, pp 159–170.
22. Buehler MJ, Thayer DT: The elbow flexion text: A clinical test for the cubital tunnel syndrome. *Clin Orthop Rel Res* 1988;233:213–216.
23. Fragiadakis EG, Lamb DW: An unusual case of ulnar nerve compression. *Hand* 1970;2:14–16.
24. Spinner M (ed): *Injuries of the Major Branches of Peripheral Nerves of the Forearm*, ed 2. Philadelphia, PA, WB Saunders, 1978, pp 159–227.
25. Hayashi Y, Kojima T, Kohno T: A case of cubital tunnel syndrome caused by the snapping of the medial head of the triceps brachii muscle. *J Hand Surg* 1984;9A:96–99.
26. Dahners LE, Wood FM: Anconeus epitrochlearis, a rare cause of cubital tunnel syndrome: A case report. *J Hand Surg* 1984;9A:579–580.
27. Sucher E, Herness D: Cubital canal syndrome due to subanconeus muscle. *J Hand Surg* 1986;11B:460–462.
28. Amadio PC, Beckenbaugh RD: Entrapment of the ulnar nerve by the deep flexor-pronator aponeurosis. *J Hand Surg* 1986;11A:83–87.
29. Kincaid JC: AAEE minimonograph: 31. The electrodiagnosis of ulnar neuropathy at the elbow. *Muscle Nerve* 1988;11:1005–1015.
30. Tackmann W, Vogel P, Kaeser HE, et al: Sensitivity and localizing significance of motor and sensory electroneurographic parameters in the diagnosis of ulnar nerve lesions at the elbow: A reappraisal. *J Neurol* 1984;231:204–211.
31. Dellon AL: Review of treatment results for ulnar nerve entrapment at the elbow. *J Hand Surg* 1989;14A:688–700.
32. McGowan AJ: The results of transposition of the ulnar nerve for traumatic ulnar neuritis. *J Bone Joint Surg* 1950;32B:293–301.
33. Sargent P: Discussion of 'some varieties of traumatic and toxic ulnar neuritis.' *Lancet* 1922;1:325–326.
34. Ferlic DC: In-situ decompression of the ulnar nerve at the elbow, in Gelberman RH (ed): *Operative Nerve Repair and Reconstruction*. Philadelphia, PA, JB Lippincott, 1991, vol 2, pp 1063–1067.

35. Heithoff SJ, Millender LH: Medial epicondylectomy, in Gelberman RH (ed): *Operative Nerve Repair and Reconstruction*. Philadelphia, PA, JB Lippincott, 1991, vol 2, pp 1087–1096.
36. Eaton RG: Anterior subcutaneous transposition, in Gelberman RH (ed): *Operative Nerve Repair and Reconstruction*. Philadelphia, PA, JB Lippincott, 1991, vol 2, pp 1077–1085.
37. Kleinman WB: Anterior intramuscular transposition, in Gelberman RH (ed): *Operative Nerve Repair and Reconstruction*. Philadelphia, PA, JB Lippincott, 1991, vol 2, pp 1069–1076.
38. Leffert RD: Anterior submuscular transposition of the ulnar nerves by the Learmonth technique. *J Hand Surg* 1982;7A:147–155.
39. Eisen A, Danon J: The mild cubital tunnel syndrome: Its natural history and indications for surgical intervention. *Neurol* 1974;24:608–613.
40. Dimond ML, Lister GD: Cubital tunnel syndrome treated by long-arm splintage. *J Hand Surg* 1985;10A:430.

Chapter 32

Tennis Elbow Tendinosis: Pathoanatomy, Nonsurgical and Surgical Management

Robert P. Nirschl, MD, MS

Introduction

The medically recorded historical aspects of tennis elbow date at least to 1873.[1] The understanding of tennis elbow has advanced significantly in recent years. This advancement has been aided immeasurably by current surgical experience, which is dedicated to identification of the pathoanatomy. The prior lack of understanding is articulated well by Bernhang,[2] who cites multiple and confusing diagnostic considerations.

Nomenclature and Pathoanatomy

The modern era of histologic evaluation was initiated with Goldie's report.[3] Coonrad and Hooper[4] expanded the concepts of pathoanatomic identification. Although Cyriax[5] speculated that the extensor brevis was the key area in lateral tennis elbow, the report of Nirschl and Pettrone[6] finally clarified location and histologic patterns. A companion report by Nirschl and Pettrone[7] expanded the informational base concerning medial tennis elbow.

The histologic evaluation of tennis elbow tendinosis identifies a noninflammatory response in the tendon. This histopathology has been named angiofibroblastic tendinosis and is likely the result of a degenerative and avascular process.[8] The histologic appearance is characterized by disorganized immature collagen formation in association with immature fibroblastic and vascular elements. In view of the histopathology, such terms as epicondylitis and tendinitis are misnomers (Fig. 1).

The gross pathologic presentation of surgical specimens of medial and lateral elbow tendinosis reveals a grayish edematous friable material. The location of tendinosis is classically in the extensor carpi radialis brevis (ECRB) tendon (100% in my series) and additionally in the extensor communis (EC) tendon (35%) laterally and in the pronator teres (PT) and the flexor carpi radialis (FCR) tendons (95%) medially.[8] Twenty percent of patients with lateral elbow tendinosis have associated bony exostosis at the lateral epicondyle. Patients treated surgically for medial elbow tendinosis also have associated clinical symptoms of ulnar nerve neurapraxia—60% in our 1980 study[7] and 24% in our 1995 report[9] (RP Nirschl, unpublished data).

Etiology and Other Factors

Tennis elbow tendinosis issues are varied, but the majority of factors are focused on age, systemic factors, and repetitive overuse. The male:female ratio

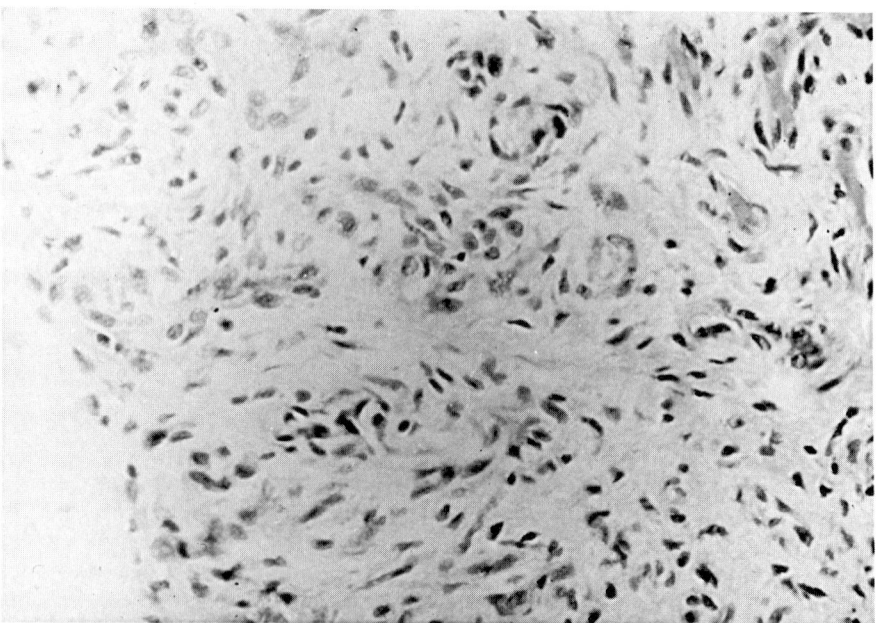

Fig. 1 Photomicrograph of angiofibroblastic tendinosis. These changes consist of disorganized and immature vascular and fibroblastic elements without evidence of inflammatory cells. The pathologic process is likely degenerative and may be initiated by anoxic events.

has been essentially equal. The usual range is 30 to 55 years, with a median of 42.5 years.[8-10] Highly active forearm activity, such as competitive tennis, may result in involvement in younger age groups (a 12-year-old competitive tennis player being the youngest in my experience).

Systemic Factors (Mesenchymal Syndrome)

Observation has identified an important subset of patients who present with elbow tendinosis. This subset (approximately 15% of patients) presents with multiple areas of tendon abnormality, including combination problems of shoulder tendinosis, medial and lateral elbow tendinosis, neurapraxia of ulnar and median nerves (carpal tunnel syndrome), trigger fingers, and de Quervain's syndrome (all often bilateral). I have termed this clinical presentation mesenchymal syndrome[11] and have theorized that a systemic factor (perhaps an alteration of the cross-linkage of collagen) exists. An important subset of the mesenchymal syndrome may include estrogen-deficient women because this subset is often associated with premature (ie, before 35 years) hysterectomy and low estrogen levels.

Repetitive Overuse

The majority of elbow tendinosis patients have a clear association with repetitive overuse of the dominant arm secondary to performance activities (eg, activities related to sports, occupation, and performing arts).[8,10,12] Common activities include racquet and throwing sports, occupational computer keyboard use, hand shaking (politicians), and manual activities (dentistry, carpentry, electrical work, etc). Elbow tendinosis is common in the musical performing arts (piano, string instruments, drums). In addition, a broader pathoanatomy of inflammatory myositis may be present in injuries to musicians.

It is theorized that multiple repetition overuse (often eccentric loading, especially in racquet sports) results in tension loading with secondary anoxic and degenerative consequences ("heart attack of tendon"). It is further theorized that those patients with mesenchymal syndrome have a preexistent vulnerability which makes them highly susceptible to overuse exposure.

Incidence

The incidence of elbow tendinosis varies depending on etiologic exposure, both hereditary and environmental. A study of adult tennis players revealed that 50% of this sport-specific group will experience symptoms of elbow tendinosis during their playing years.[8] Lateral elbow tendinosis is five times more common than medial elbow tendinosis in this overall series (Fig. 2). Posterior elbow tendinosis (triceps) also occurs on occasion, but it is most likely to occur in association with olecranon fossa chondromalacia (most commonly seen in competitive baseball pitchers and javelin throwers).

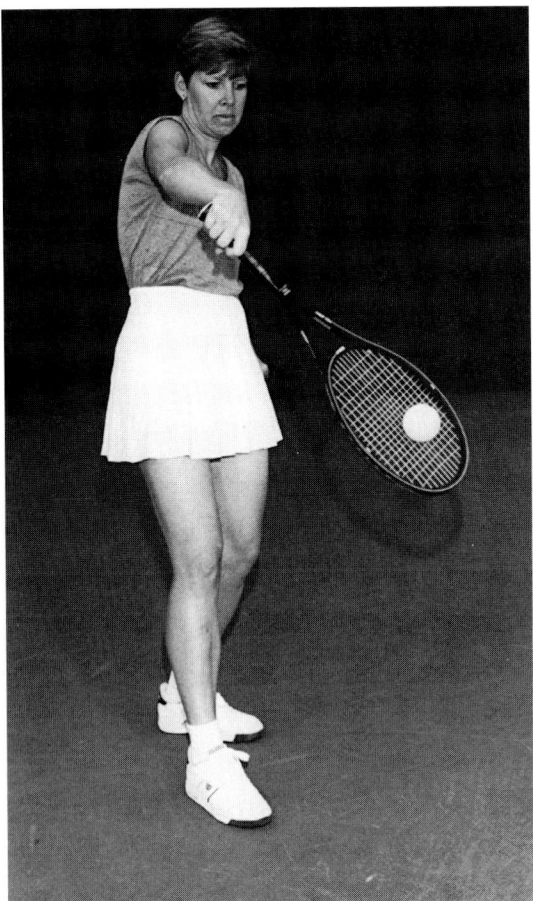

Fig. 2 Performance technique as etiologic factor. Poor performance technique in occupation, sports, or performing arts likely plays an important role in injury-producing overuse. The illustrated poor tennis backhand increases the potential for overuse of the relatively small and weak forearm wrist extensors. (Reproduced with permission from Nirschl R, Sobel J: *Arm Care*. Arlington, VA, Medical Sports Publishing, in press.)

Associated Myositis

My clinical observations support the consideration of an associated muscular problem in a minority of cases of medial and lateral elbow tendinosis. This clinical presentation most commonly involves the extensor muscle groups, particularly in computer keyboard operators and musicians (eg, those who play piano or use a bow with a string instrument). The symptoms are more diffuse with tenderness over the muscle mass (usually wrist extensors) in contradistinction to the more classic presentation of tenderness and provocative stress testing at the tendon origin. It is theorized that muscle overuse, especially in association with fine finger movement, results in a form of inflammatory myositis.

Radial Nerve Neurapraxia

It has been widely circulated, especially among hand surgeons, that compression and malfunction of the posterior interosseous branch of the radial nerve is a major contributor to the etiology of lateral elbow tendinosis.[13,14] In my experience, this malady is rare. The symptoms, like those associated with extensor muscle myositis, are more diffuse in the muscle mass. Provocation with forearm supination is more common. In my opinion, confirmation by electromyography is mandatory to confirm the diagnosis. Of the nearly 1,000 surgical cases of elbow tendinosis in my personal series, only two cases of objectively identifiable radial nerve neurapraxia have been noted.

Clinical Presentation

The typical presentation of lateral elbow tendinosis is a history of increased wrist extensor activity related to gradual onset of pain over the origin of the ECRB tendon and proximal forearm extensor muscle mass.

Palpable tenderness over the ECRB tendon origin is classic. Less tenderness by palpation may be noted over the origin of the finger extensor tendon (the EC tendon). Provocative signs include pain with manual wrist and finger extension stress testing with the elbow flexed and extended. Finger extension pain resulting from provocation suggests involvement in the EC tendon. Pain at the ECRB origin is also common with provocative pronation stress testing. Radiographs may reveal bony exostosis at the lateral epicondyle in 20% of cases.

The onset of medial elbow tendinosis is similar to that of lateral elbow tendinosis. Wrist flexor and pronation activity results in pain in the common flexor origin close to the medial epicondyle. Medial tendinosis pain is exaggerated by provocative stress testing (eg, wrist flexion and forearm pronation). Associated ulnar nerve problems may include a positive Tinel sign at the zone 3 level of the medial epicondylar groove.

Nonsurgical Treatment Program

The treatment protocol for tennis elbow tendinosis follows a pattern utilized at our institution for the past 15 years.[15,16] The basics of treatment fall into two broad categories, namely, comfort and cure. The comfort aspect of the program usually progresses in 1 to 2 weeks to a point where the curative aspect of the program can be implemented. The key to the curative aspect of the program resides in rehabilitative exercise.[16] The goals of rehabilitation are to revascularize and recollagenize tendinosis tissue, as well as to restore strength, endurance, and flexibility. It should be noted that the entire extremity, including the shoulder and upper back, is often weak, and the exercise programs must be dedicated to all these regions. On average, the rehabilitative process takes 4 months. The program is initiated in our sports medicine rehabilitation facility (usually two times per week for 3 weeks) and proceeds thereafter to a home exercise program with occasional reevaluation as needed.

As a companion to the rehabilitation program, control of overuse is always appropriate, particularly on return to performance activities such as occupation, performing arts, or sports. The intensity, duration, and frequency of activity is relatively easy to alter. Beneficial technique and equipment changes may be more difficult to accomplish but should always be addressed. Froimson's report[17] introduced into the literature the concept of muscular constraint as an aid in pain relief. I expanded the concept and introduced the term counterforce.[18] Biomechanical analysis[19] supports the overwhelming clinical observations[8,17] of pain improvement by use of the counterforce concept. My current opinion is that brace design should offer full tension control across the entire brace width and that even muscular balance should be maintained (Figs. 3 and 4).

Surgical Indications

The ultimate decision for surgery is made by the patient, depending on the magnitude of symptoms and the alteration in quality of life. The indications for surgical intervention include unacceptable pain with decreased function fol-

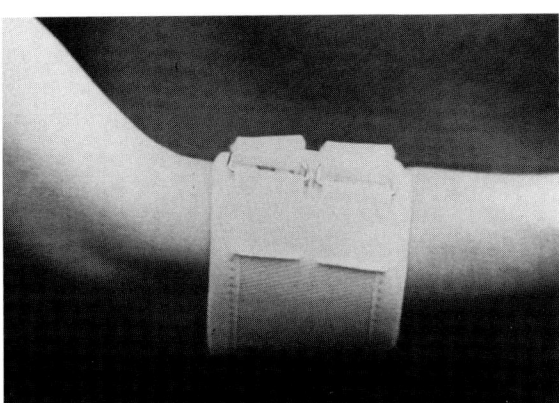

Fig. 3 Lateral elbow counterforce brace. The wide brace design allows full tension control and maintains balanced muscular function. It is also effective in pain control. (Reproduced with permission from Nirschl RP: Elbow tendinosis/tennis elbow. Clin Sports Med 1992;11:851–870.)

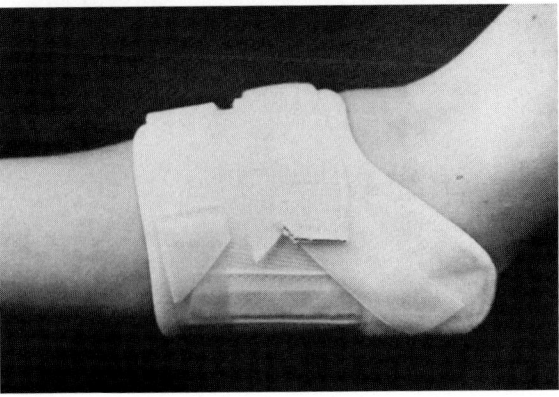

Fig. 4 Medial elbow counterforce brace. The wide brace design allows full tension control and maintains balanced muscular function. It is also effective in pain control. (Reproduced with permission from Nirschl RP: Elbow tendinosis/tennis elbow. Clin Sports Med 1992;11:851–870.)

lowing an appropriate rehabilitation program. Pain is usually present even with light activities of daily living. It should be noted that a quality rehabilitation program requires active patient participation and usually takes 4 months. In general, people rarely seek surgical solutions before having symptoms for 1 year. In our original surgical series, the average time from the onset of symptoms to surgical intervention was over 2 years (Outline 1).[6,7]

Certain patients have been identified who are at risk of experiencing an unfavorable result with rehabilitative management and are, therefore, more likely to require surgical intervention (Outline 2). These patients include those who with the incidences of iatrogenic atrophy changes of cortisone injections (80%), symptoms initiated by direct trauma (20%), the presence of lateral epicondyle exostosis (20%) or a history of mesenchymal syndrome (eg, widespread tendinosis involving the shoulders, elbows, and wrists—75%).[12] Despite the increased potential for unsuccessful conservative management in these patients, it is still worthwhile to initiate a quality conservative rehabilitation approach for a period of 4 to 6 weeks. Failure of progressive improvement suggests the need for a surgical intervention and the patient has been educated for the postoperative period.

History of Surgical Procedures

The surgical management of medial and lateral tennis elbow tendinosis has undergone great change. Hohmann[20] in Germany initiated surgical concepts. His approach was to release the extensor aponeurosis, but identification of pathologic change was lacking. A variation of Hohmann's approach was introduced by Bosworth[21] and included resection of the orbicular ligament. Garden[22] introduced another variation by lengthening the extensor brevis tendon distally. Other reports increased confusion and introduced other approaches, such as

Outline 1 Surgical indications

Failure of a quality rehabilitation program
   3 or 4 months of supervised resistance exercise
   Properly sequenced exercises
   Quality effort by patient

Persistent pain generally lasting more than 1 year
   Requiring a change in sports or occupational activity
   Persisting with activities of daily living
   Rest pain (Note: Rule out other potential factors for rest pain, including malignancy)

Requirement of high activity level

Outline 2 Predictors for increased rehabilitation failure

Iatrogenic atrophy from multiple cortisone injections

Initiation of symptoms by direct trauma

Mesenchymal syndrome (history of widespread tendinosis)

Presence of epicondylar bony exostosis

local denervation,[23] radial nerve decompression,[13] and removal of gunsight spurs from the distal humerus.[24] All of the above reports have several common elements, including failure to accurately identify the pathoanatomy and inconsistent results concerning pain control and functional strength return.

The modern era of surgical intervention was initiated by a dedication to understanding the true pathoanatomy of tennis elbow tendinosis; a surgical approach directed to the pathologic alteration was then developed. This process was first reported by Goldie,[3] advanced by Coonrad and Hooper,[4] and clarified by Nirschl and Pettrone[6] for lateral elbow and for medial elbow.[7] The basics of the modern surgical approach are not dedicated to tension release of largely normal tendons (eg, extensor aponeurosis or conjoined tendon laterally and common flexor origin medially) but to resection of the pathologic angiofibroblastic tendinosis tissue, which in large part resides in the ECRB and PT/FCR complex of the lateral elbow and medial elbow, respectively.

Surgical Principles

The surgical management of tennis elbow, as noted, has undergone significant change. The key to modern surgical technique is identification and removal of the pathologic tissue (angiofibroblastic tendinosis). In contrast to previous techniques, normal tendon origins are not released. It is emphasized again that the goal of surgery is not tendon release but an actual identification and removal of the painful pathologic angiofibroblastic tendinosis tissue. Further clarification of this important principle may best be presented in the form of a question. Who would release an Achilles tendon from its insertion in the treatment of Achilles tendinosis? The author's surgical approach for lateral and medial elbow tendon exposure is depicted in Figures 5 and 6.

Reasons for Failed Surgery

My experience with salvage procedures is now quite extensive concerning failed medial and lateral elbow tendinosis surgery. The overwhelming reason for the lack of primary surgical success is failure to address the tendinosis pathoanatomy (eg, the tendinosis pathology has not been resected). The failed surgical intervention is always a form of tendon release. On the lateral side, the finger extensors have been released; and on the medial side, the common flexor origin is released. Salvage surgery is dedicated to reidentifying and excising the true pathoanatomy. Iatrogenic surgical harm is also commonplace. On the lateral side, this includes the failure of finger extensor reattachment, posterolateral elbow instability secondary to lateral collateral ligament disruption, and scar entrapment in the area of the radial head. On the medial side, valgus instability, ulnar nerve neurapraxic symptoms, and neuroma causalgia of the medial antebrachial cutaneous nerve are typical iatrogenic problems. The most common problem both medially and laterally is, however, failure to achieve the presurgical goals of pain relief and functional improvement. Typical failure mechanisms are summarized in Outlines 3 and 4.

Medial Tendinosis Surgery and the Ulnar Nerve

There is a major statistical relationship between those surgical patients who have medial tendinosis and those with ulnar nerve symptoms of our original reported series. Sixty percent of patients undergoing medial tennis elbow surgery also had ulnar nerve neurapraxia symptoms.[7] The study of Ollivierre and

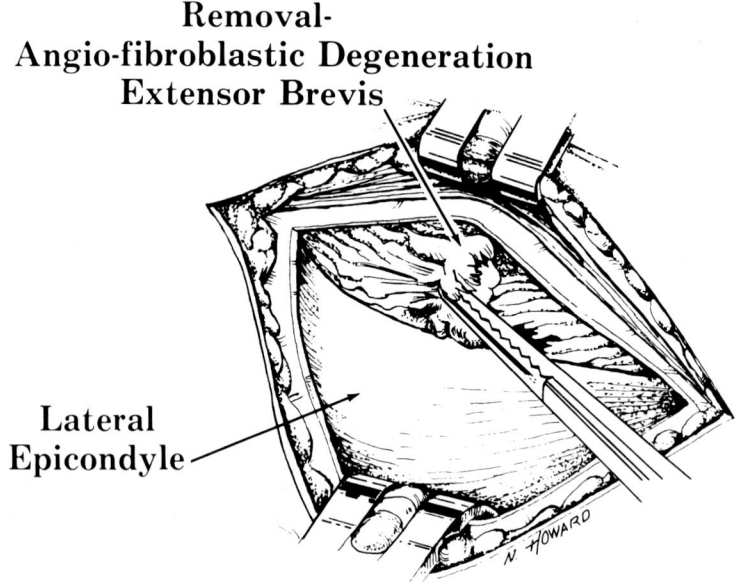

Fig. 5 Surgical treatment of lateral tennis elbow tendinosis. (Reproduced with permission from Nirschl RP: Elbow tendinosis/tennis elbow. *Clin Sports Med* 1992;11:851–870.)

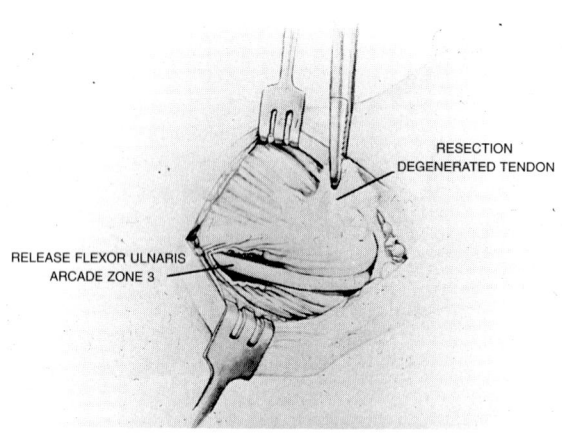

Fig. 6 Surgical treatment of medial tennis elbow tendinosis. (Adapted with permission from Nirschl RP: Elbow tendinosis/tennis elbow. *Clin Sports Med* 1992;11:851–870.)

Nirschl[9] reported an incidence of 24%. It is theorized that tendinosis damage to segments of the common flexor origin compromises the medial epicondylar groove, especially distal at the flexor ulnaris arcade. To further clarify this relationship, the medial epicondylar groove has been divided into three zones: zone 1 proximal to the medial epicondylar, zone 2 at the medial epicondyle, and zone 3 distal to the medial epicondyle (Fig. 7).[8,25] The majority of ulnar nerve symptoms are the result of compression in zone 3. Decompression of this zone by release of the flexor ulnaris arcade will generally resolve the symp-

Outline 3 Failed lateral elbow surgery

Failure to address tendinosis pathology
  Tendon release of extensor aponeurosis when pathology is in extensor brevis

Iatrogenic harm
  Failure of extensor aponeurosis reattachment
  Posterolateral elbow instability secondary to disruption of lateral collateral ligament
  Scar impingement about radial head

Wrong diagnosis
  Secondary agenda gains (payment expectations from legal or workers' compensation activity evidenced by retained symptoms)

Outline 4 Failed medial elbow surgery

Failure to address tendinosis pathology
  Release of common flexor origin without resection of pathoanatomy

Iatrogenic harm (valgus instability)
  Failure of reattachment of common flexor origin
  Distortion of ulnar collateral ligament

Iatrogenic harm
  Causalgic neuroma medial antebrachial cutaneous nerve

Ulnar nerve
  Failure to address compression of nerve at initial surgery
  Postsurgical iatrogenic scar about nerve

Wrong diagnosis
  Secondary agenda gains

---

toms. Compression from osteophytic spurs, loose bodies, or rheumatoid synovitis can also occur in zone 2, and compression in zone 1 may be caused by a tight medial intermuscular septum.

Anterior transfer of the ulnar nerve is occasionally indicated, primarily when ulnar nerve symptoms are related to tension. Indications include the following: (1) nerve subluxation or dislocation from the epicondylar groove; (2) skeletal valgus; (3) dynamic valgus ligamentous instability; and (4) necessity of surgical exposure to the medial elbow compartment.[8,25] When ulnar nerve transfer is indicated, my preference is an anterolateral subcuticular position supported by a medially based buttress fashioned from the fascia of the common flexor origin to maintain nerve position. The keys to ulnar nerve transfer success are relaxed angles in zones 1 and 3 while avoiding iatrogenic surgical scar entrapment.

Postsurgical Protocol

The postsurgical protocols for lateral and medial elbow are similar (Table 1). The elbow is protected at 90° for 1 week in a lightweight elbow immobilizer. The immobilizer allows active use of the wrist, hand, and shoulder as the patient's tolerance permits. The immobilizer is removed for active and active-assisted range-of-motion exercise starting on postsurgical day 3 but is worn at

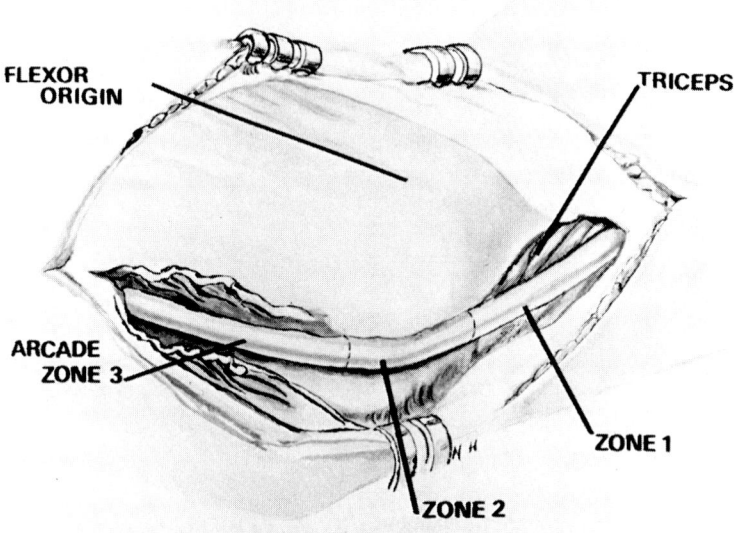

Fig. 7 Medial epicondylar groove in the ulnar nerve zones. (Adapted with permission from Nirschl RP: Elbow tendinosis/tennis elbow. Clin Sports Med 1992;11:851–870.)

other times for up to 1 week. Most patients tolerate normal activities of daily living without significant restriction by day 10. Rehabilitative exercises, as described concerning nonsurgical treatment, commence 3 weeks following surgery. A counterforce elbow brace is worn during rehabilitative exercises as well as during higher forearm activity (including a return to sport). Although full racquet and throwing sport competitive activity is not recommended until full strength returns, modified sport technique patterns are often initiated 6 to 8 weeks after lateral elbow surgery, and 10 to 12 weeks following medial elbow surgery. Full pain-free functional strength and thus clearance for competitive sports play and full occupational activity is typically restored by 6 months, provided that a quality postoperative rehabilitative exercise program has been adhered to.

Results of Surgery

Surgical results with the technique of accurate pathoanatomic identification and resection have been highly consistent and rewarding. Overall improvement with restoration to a level of activity that existed prior to the onset of symptoms has been observed in 90% of patients. Significant relief of pain for activities of daily living has been observed in 97% of patients. This statistical success, initially reported in 1979,[6] has been maintained in both medial and lateral tendinosis surgery. It is emphasized that a positive result is enhanced by quality rehabilitation following surgery. A number of variables may play a role in the small percentage of patients who have poor results with the current surgical technique. These variables include the presence of multiple pathologic issues beyond tendinosis (eg, associated nerve or ligament injury and osteoarthritis),

Table 1 Tennis elbow postsurgical protocol

Days 1 to 7	Ice 3 to 4 times per day for 20 minutes at a time Medication: Anti-inflammatory or pain medications as per physician's instructions Maintain full shoulder motion with active ranging several times per day
Days 1 to 3	Keep elbow bandaged and in an immobilizer at all times
Day 2	Start ranging fingers and wrist for 2 minutes, 3 to 5 times per day
Day 3	May shower; remove bandage and gently range elbow in shower; cleanse wound with alcohol
Days 3 to 6	Wear immobilizer except while showering and gently limbering the elbow
Days 7 to 17	Continue elbow ranging activities with bending and straightening motions (90% of normal motion by day 17 is usual); continue active motion of shoulder, wrist, and fingers; add active pronation and supination; may use arm for light activity only; immobilizer is used for protection only; leave immobilizer off most of the time
Days 17 to 21	Begin tennis elbow exercise program without weights; begin squeezing a foam ball; use counterforce brace when exercising
Day 21	Include resistance exercises in tennis elbow exercise program; increase use of arm to include normal activities of daily living
6 to 8 weeks	Begin modified return to sport activity following lateral tennis elbow surgery
10 to 12 weeks	Begin modified return to sport activity following medial tennis elbow surgery
6 months	Return to competitive play or usual occupation

(Adapted with permission from the Virginia Sportsmedicine Institute and the Nirschl Orthopedic Sportsmedicine Clinic, Arlington, VA.)

the emotional aspects of pain, occasional reparative tissue that remains unhealthy, and secondary gain issues such as the hidden agenda of some patients with workers' compensation.

Discussion

The basic premise for consistent success in treating elbow tendinosis is to recognize the pathoanatomy and implement treatment that has the capacity to transform an unhealthy pathologic area to healthy tissue. The conservative program, as presented, is basic to all tendinosis (cumulative overuse) problems. My success in the nonsurgical treatment program is 90% in patients previously untreated. This success is somewhat predicated on patient activity level, and it might be noted that the patient population at our institution is highly active. Patients who have had prior treatment focused on comfort (especially with iatrogenic damage secondary to multiple cortisone injections) have less success with the conservative effort. However, this approach is still worth pursuing if a meaningful rehabilitative effort has not been previously attempted. Those patients who have unacceptable pain and a compromised activity level in spite of a quality rehabilitative effort can usually benefit from surgical intervention. The goal of surgery is not tendon release but an actual identification and removal of the painful pathologic, angiofibroblastic tendinosis tissue.

References

1. Runge F: Zur Genese und Behandlung des Schreibekrampfes. *Berl Clin Wnschr* 1873;10:245–248.
2. Bernhang AM: The many causes of tennis elbow. *NY State J Med* 1979;79:1363–1366.
3. Goldie I: Epicondylitis lateralis humeri: A pathogenetical study. *ACTA Chir Scand Suppl* 1964;339:7–119.
4. Coonrad RW, Hooper WR: Tennis elbow: Its course, natural history, conservative and surgical management. *J Bone Joint Surg* 1973;55A:1177–1182.
5. Cyriax JH: The pathology and treatment of tennis elbow. *J Bone Joint Surg* 1936;18:921–940.
6. Nirschl RP, Pettrone FA: Tennis elbow: The surgical treatment of lateral epicondylitis. *J Bone Joint Surg* 1979;61A:832–839.
7. Nirschl RP, Pettrone F: Medial tennis elbow: Surgical treatment. *Orthop Trans* 1980;4:298–299.
8. Nirschl RP: Elbow tendinosis/tennis elbow. *Clin Sportsmed* 1992;11:851–870.
9. Gruchow HW, Pelletier D: An epidemiologic study of tennis elbow: Incidence, recurrence, and effectiveness of prevention strategies. *Am J Sports Med* 1979;7:234–238.
10. Priest JD, Braden V, Gerberich SG: The elbow and tennis: Part I. An analysis of players with and without pain. *Phys Sports Med* 1980;8:80–91.
11. Nirschl RP: Mesenchymal syndrome. *VA Med Mon* 1969;96:659–662.
12. Dulany R: Tennis strokes, in Pettrone FA (ed): *American Academy of Orthopaedic Surgeons: Symposium on Upper Extremity Injuries in Athletes*. St. Louis, MO, CV Mosby, 1986, pp 47–58.
13. Roles NC, Maudsley RH: Radial tunnel syndrome: Resistant tennis elbow as a nerve entrapment. *J Bone Joint Surg* 1972;54B:499–508.
14. Von Rossum J, Buruma OJS, Kamphuisen HAC, et al: Tennis elbow: A radial tunnel syndrome? *J Bone Joint Surg* 1978;60B:197–198.
15. Nirschl RP, Sobel J: Conservative treatment of tennis elbow. *Phys Sports Med* 1981;9:42–54.
16. O'Connor FG, Sobel JR, Nirschl RP: Five-step treatment for overuse injuries. *Phys Sports Med* 1992;20:128–142.
17. Froimson AI: Treatment of tennis elbow with forearm support band. *J Bone Joint Surg* 1971;53A:183–184.
18. Nirschl RP: Good tennis is good medicine. *Phys Sportsmed* 1973;1:27–36.
19. Groppel JL, Nirschl RP: A mechanical and electromyographical analysis of the effects of various joint counterforce braces on the tennis player. *Am J Sports Med* 1986;14:195–200.
20. Hohmann G: Das Wesen und die Behandlung des Sogenannten Tennisellenbogens. *Muncener Med Wochenschrift* 1933;80:250–252.
21. Bosworth DM: Surgical treatment of tennis elbow: A follow-up study. *J Bone Joint Surg* 1965;47A:1533–1536.
22. Garden RS: Tennis elbow. *J Bone Joint Surg* 1961;43B:100–106.
23. Kaplan EB: Treatment of tennis elbow (epicondylitis) by denervation. *J Bone Joint Surg* 1959;41A:147–151.
24. Begg RE: Epicondylitis or tennis elbow: Frequent finding of gunsight type spur in lateral epicondyle of distal humerus. *Orthop Rev* 1980;9:33–42.
25. Nirschl RP: Muscle and tendon trauma: Tennis elbow, in Morrey BF (ed): *The Elbow and Its Disorders*. Philadelphia, PA, WB Saunders, 1985, pp 481–496.

Chapter 33
Rehabilitation of Repetitive Trauma at the Elbow

Joel M. Press, MD
Jeffrey L. Young, MD

Lateral Epicondylitis

Repetitive overload injuries at the elbow are caused by repetitive microtrauma and the subsequent biomechanical alterations that ensue. Stated simply, these injuries reflect an inability of the tissues to adapt to the repetitive tensile loads they face. The theoretical mechanism behind this failure is the presence of either an "absolute" overload (ie, too much stress) on normal structures or a "relative" overload (ie, normal stress) placed on weak or inflexible structures.[1,2] On the microscopic level, the result is connective tissue failure or abnormal cellular matrix formation;[2] on the macroscopic level, it is organ alteration. Clinically, this may present in the form of overt tissue damage or tissue injury with tears or extensive scarring, or, more commonly, it may manifest itself subclinically, but detectably, as muscle inflexibility or weakness. Alterations in the tissue overloads, although subclinical, can be readily seen and evaluated by magnetic resonance imaging (MRI).[3] This tissue damage creates biomechanical deficits and decreases biomechanical efficiency by altering normal motion or force couple activity. This process occurs over time with a variable but often prolonged prodromal time. During this process, the injured worker develops adaptations in local and distant aspects of the kinetic chain to try to compensate for the injury, the overloads, and the biomechanical deficits.[2,4]

The elbow joint does not act in isolation but rather is an integral component of the upper extremity kinetic chain. Events and forces occurring either at the shoulder or the hand will ultimately involve the elbow as well. The ability of the elbow to precisely and painlessly shorten or lengthen the upper limb is contingent not only on the integrity of the elbow joint proper, but also on the spine and the sternoclavicular, acromioclavicular, scapulothoracic, and glenohumeral joints. Inability to comfortably lean or bend forward because of lumbar spine-based restrictions necessitates greater elbow extension when reaching downward or forward. Loss of cervicothoracic flexion and rotation requires greater elbow flexion to keep finer manual work in the center of one's field of vision. Acromioclavicular or sternoclavicular joint pain limits the weightbearing tolerance of the "strut" from which the upper limb is suspended, thereby reducing loads one can dynamically or isometrically support at varying degrees of elbow flexion. Scapulothoracic dyskinesis and cervicothoracic kyphosis may lead to rotator cuff impingement and glenohumeral joint-based pain, which will also reduce upper limb weightbearing. Finally, capsular restrictions and loss of internal/external rotation at the shoulder may induce compensatory increases in the amount of forearm pronation/supination employed during repetitive tasks. The same process applies to regions distal to the elbow; loss of wrist extension necessitates greater elbow extension to elevate an object held in the hand to the same height. Thus, when analyzing the injured worker's source of elbow pain, looking beyond the elbow is critical. Furthermore, any successful elbow rehabilitation program must address deficits in the scapular stabilizer muscles, cervicothoracic extensor muscles, and muscles about the glenohumeral joint. Finally, proper posture, with the head centered over the shoulders, decreases the activity of the stabilizing muscles of the shoulder and neck and prevents these muscles from fatiguing. Fatigue would lead to new substitution patterns and more musculotendinous overload.

Proper functioning of the elbow allows the hand to be positioned in space and provides a stabilizing role for power production and performance of work and sports activities.[5] Although most activities of daily living require between 30° and 140° of flexion and between 50° of pronation and 50° of supination, the articular orientation of the joint allows for approximately 150° of flexion, 75° of pronation, and 85° of supination for an arc of forearm rotation averaging 160° to 170°.[6,7] These motions, which are integral to proper elbow rehabilitation, occur at the ulnar humeral, radiohumeral, and proximal and distal radioulnar joints. Restriction in motion or laxity at any of these joints because of ligamentous, capsular, or musculotendinous factors needs to be assessed properly in the rehabilitation process.[8] As can be inferred from the preceding paragraph, restrictions in motion elsewhere along the kinetic chain can change activities from those that are performed in the usual range of joint motion to those performed at extremes or limits of permissible joint motion, with accompanying increases in musculotendinous stress as well.

Lateral epicondylitis typically occurs in the workplace. It is found in individuals who use video display terminals and need to stabilize their upper extremities proximally at the shoulder and elbow to allow rapid interphalangeal flexion and extension for keyboard activity. Wrist extension overload is common, often complicated by the tenodesis action of the wrist extensors on finger flexion. Medical technicians who in the process of drawing and agitating blood samples repeatedly extend, pronate, and supinate the wrist comprises another group based in the hospital industry who present with this problem. The pathophysiology of lateral epicondylitis or chronic tendinosis at the elbow is well described by Nirschl.[9] Histologic patterns from biopsy studies reveal a degenerative process with angiofibroblastic tendinosis and only a few, if any, inflammatory cells. The pathology of the degenerative process occurs over time rather than from a single event.

Patients with lateral epicondylitis have tenderness, with associated swelling, over the lateral epicondylar region and pain with resisted wrist extension that may extend distally into the forearm. Weakness of grip strength, because of the loss of tenodesis, is common. Flexing the elbow while holding objects in the hand with the forearm pronated may also induce pain. However, it is overload of the wrist extensors rather than the brachioradialis that is occurring. The tissues injured are usually the extensor carpi radialis brevis tendon and, to a lesser degree, the extensor digitorum communis.[10]

Medial epicondylitis, or overload injuries to the flexor-pronator muscles, develops secondarily to repeated insults to the relevant muscle groups followed by inadequate healing time, and thereby leads to subsequent muscle tears, fibrosis, and elbow flexion contractures, with upwards of 15° of extension loss.[5,9] Complete rupture of the flexor muscle mass is rare. Clinically, patients present with pain, tenderness, and swelling radial to the medial epicondyle, with resisted wrist flexion and pronation activities increasing the symptoms.[11] Patients who require repetitive flexion and pronation activities in the workplace or at home (eg, performing assembly line work, turning a screwdriver, or shaking baby bottles) are most susceptible.

Treatment for both medial and lateral epicondylitis incorporates similar principles of rehabilitation. The specific phases and concepts of rehabilitation are discussed in reference to lateral epicondylitis, the more common clinical entity.

Acute Phase

Initial treatment at the acute phase focuses on control of inflammation, relief of pain, and patient education. Often no true inflammatory process is active, yet pain perception due to nocioceptive fiber activation still occurs. A decrease in abusive activity to the injured structures is in order, although absolute rest is usually counterproductive and can increase random cross-linking of collagen fibers while tissue repair is under way. On rare occasions in the highly acute phase, the use of a cock-up wrist splint may be helpful for a few days to rest the extensor musculature. It is extremely important to identify activities that the person is involved with at home or recreationally that exacerbate the condition. Bathing and lifting young children, cooking on a stovetop with iron cookware, and carrying a heavy attache case can all produce wrist extensor muscle overload. Cryotherapy, elevation, medications, and therapeutic modalities may be instituted to minimize any harmful excesses of inflammatory exudation, hemorrhage, and diminished oxygen perfusion.[8,9] Cryotherapy can include local ice massage for 10- to 15-minute intervals three to five times daily during the acute period. Cold compression dressings are commercially available and easily used. Anti-inflammatory medications may be helpful regarding inflammation and exudation, but in the absence of overt inflammatory cells they probably help because of their general analgesic properties. Therapeutic modalities can be quite helpful in decreasing pain either via endorphin pathways or gate-control theories of pain relief.[12] Therapeutic modalities include high-voltage electric nerve and muscle stimulation, interferential treatment, and transcutaneous electric nerve stimulation.[13,14] Iontophoresis and phonophoresis effects on lateral epicondylitis are debated.[15–19] Ultrasound, a deep-heating modality, does not appear to be efficacious in lateral epicondylitis.[11] Regardless of which type of therapeutic modality is employed, a passive, modality-oriented approach should be used only as an adjunct for the patient to be able to tolerate a more aggressive, active therapy program and is not advocated for more than a few therapy sessions.[20]

Patient education early in the rehabilitation process can allow the patient to avoid actions that exacerbate the symptoms as well as learn what activities or actions to avoid in the future to prevent injury recurrence. Offending activities include shaking hands, picking up a coffee cup, needlework, and turning a key. Using ratchet or power-driven tools also reduces the amount of forceful pronation/supination needed to turn screws or flexion/extension necessary to drive nails.

Recovery Phase

Restoration of normal tissue function occurs following proper anatomic healing. Symptom resolution alone is inadequate. During the recovery phase, after pain has started to subside and inflammation is under control, the focus is on enhancing the proliferative invasion of vascular elements and fibroblasts and proper collagen deposition and maturation.[9,21] This time frame is usually within 1 to 2 weeks for lateral epicondylitis. Prolonged immobilization adversely influences the orientation and mechanical properties of periarticular soft tissue.[22] Promotion of healing followed by aggressive strengthening and elimination of biomechanical deficits then prevents further tissue overload and recurrent symptoms and pathology.

As the acute symptoms diminish, the therapeutic exercise program becomes the focus with the initial goal of restoring full pain-free flexibility. Specific attention is given to the wrist and finger extensors and supinators. In more chronic cases, biomechanical deficits of extensor inflexibility are noted, often up to a 10° to 15° lack of passive wrist flexion, as compared with the asymptomatic side.[19] To improve wrist flexion mobility, which is often limited by the tight extensor musculature, the wrist extensors are placed on passive stretch with the elbow extended (Fig. 1). Myofascial release techniques and joint mobilizations may be useful at this stage, along with deep-heating modalities to improve collagen extensibility and muscle reeducation.[23,24] As flexibility starts to approach normal levels, strength training is initiated. At first, multiple angle isometrics within the pain-free range, focusing on the wrist extensors, are begun. The patient next progresses to limited motion arcs at submaximal intensity, and then to maximal intensity isometrics in the shortened, middle, and lengthened positions.[21,25] Isometric exercises are helpful early in the acute phase of rehabilitation because they can effectively decrease swelling (through the pumping action of the muscle), they do not irritate the joint because there is no motion, they prevent neural dissociation (the muscle contractions stimulate the mechanoreceptors system),[26,27] and they prevent further atrophy of muscle.

A progressive resistance program is then incorporated that may include free weights (Fig. 2). Strengthening of the muscles of pronation and supination can be accomplished using a weighted rod (Fig. 3). Weights are increased as guided by tolerance. The use of isokinetic devices may be helpful for the determination of strength imbalances; however, strengthening and endurance training at higher velocities are not as relevant in the injured worker with repetitive stress injury at the elbow, and no real-life tasks are performed isokinetically.[26,28,29]

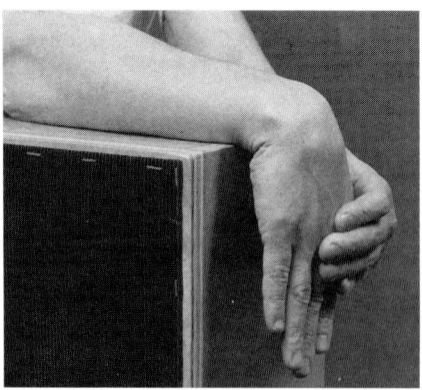 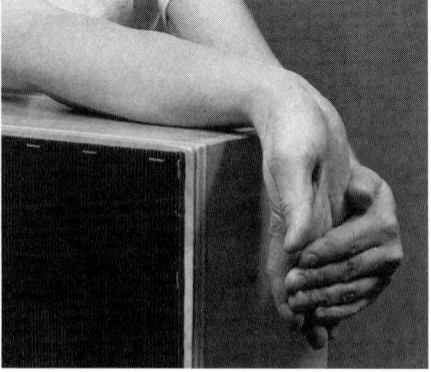

Fig. 1 Passive stretching of the wrist extensors with the contralateral hand. (Reproduced with permission from Wiesner SL: Rehabilitation of elbow injuries in sports. *Phys Clin Rehab North Am* 1994;5:81–113.)

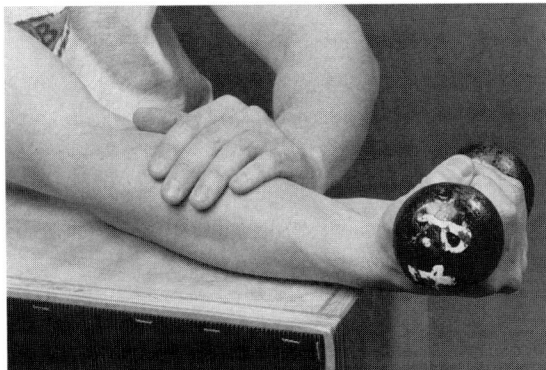

Fig. 2 Strengthening of the wrist flexors with free weights. (Reproduced with permission from Wiesner SL: Rehabilitation of elbow injuries in sports. *Phys Clin Rehab North Am* 1994;5: 81–113.)

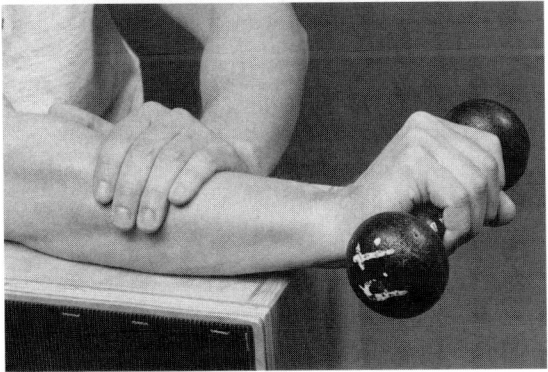

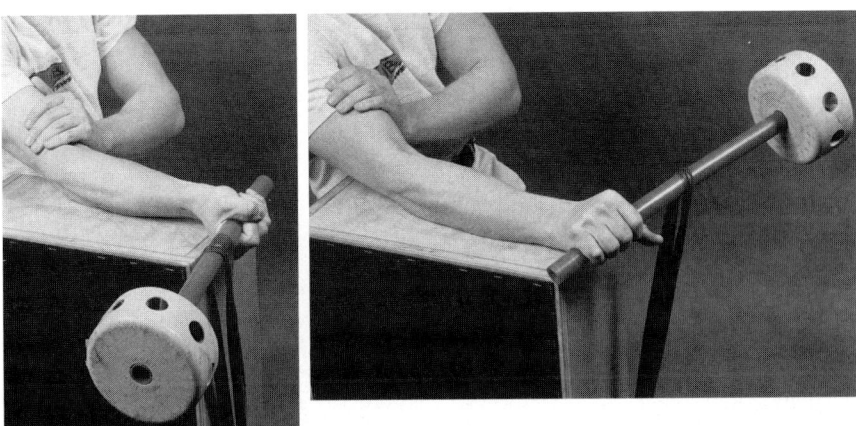

Fig. 3 Strengthening of the wrist pronators and supinators with a weighted object. (Reproduced with permission from Wiesner SL: Rehabilitation of elbow injuries in sports. *Phys Clin Rehab North Am* 1994;5:81–113.)

Triceps strengthening may be helpful because as supination becomes more forceful, the biceps brachii become more activated and the triceps become more important in maintaining a stable angle of elbow flexion.[30]

As guided by symptoms, more complex concentric-eccentric strengthening and endurance routines are initiated through the use of a wrist roll (Fig. 4) and resistive tubing (Fig. 5).[31] Eccentric training is a critical component of the rehabilitation program because often the overload injury at the elbow occurs because of chronic eccentric stress on the wrist extensors, as is the case with extensive keyboard use. Furthermore, eccentric exercises create less compressive force across a joint and may offer greater tendon loading.[26] Proprioceptive neuromuscular facilitation techniques to upgrade functional patterns, including push-ups, partial weightbearing, and weight shifts, are also initiated at this time.[32] Liberal icing following exercise may be beneficial to control the inflammatory process.

During the recovery phase, anatomic and functional deficits along the kinetic chain must be addressed for complete rehabilitation. Attention needs to be directed specifically at any biomechanical limitations relating to the cervical, shoulder, and scapular stabilizing muscle functions. The cervical region and shoulder girdle provide a proximal base of support for elbow placement in space. Therefore, the effects of agonist-antagonist imbalances, which may involve limited cervical mobility, internal shoulder rotation inflexibility, and weakness of the posterior shoulder and scapular stabilizer muscles, transfer into abnormal compensatory overload patterns at the elbow.[33-35] For these reasons, scapular muscle strengthening, cervicothoracic extension training, and posture upgrading (eg, chest out, chin tucked positioning) are critical components of a complete elbow rehabilitation program.

General body conditioning is another important component in the recovery phase of elbow rehabilitation. Advantages include (1) central and peripheral aerobics providing increased regional perfusion; (2) neurophysiologic synergy and overflow providing neurologic stimulus to injured tissue; (3) minimization

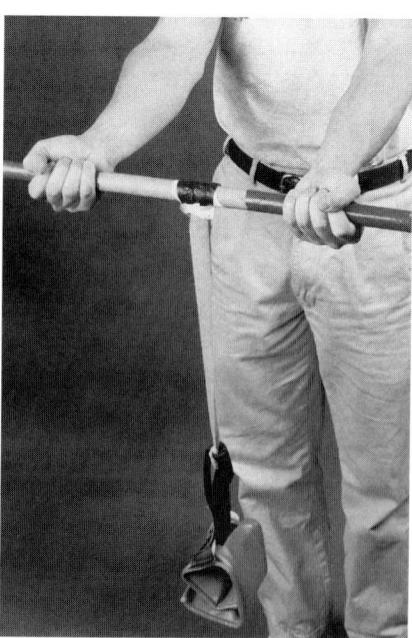
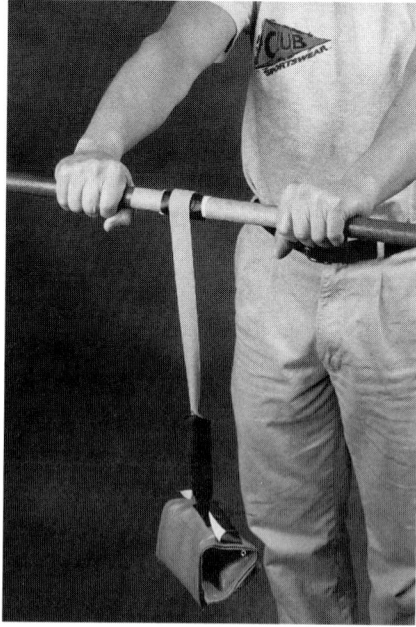

Fig. 4 Concentric and eccentric strengthening is accomplished by raising and lowering weights supported by a rope to a bar. (Reproduced with permission from Wiesner SL: Rehabilitation of elbow injuries in sports. *Phys Clin Rehab North Am* 1994;5:81–113.)

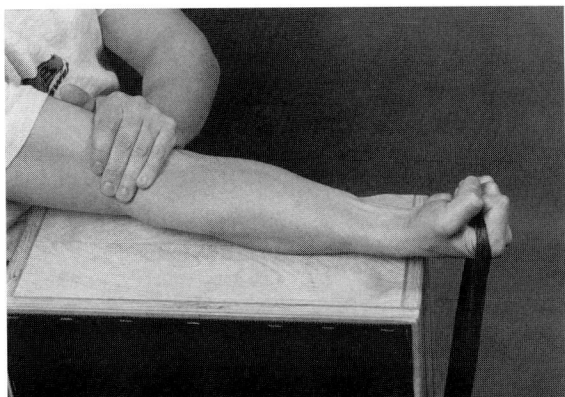
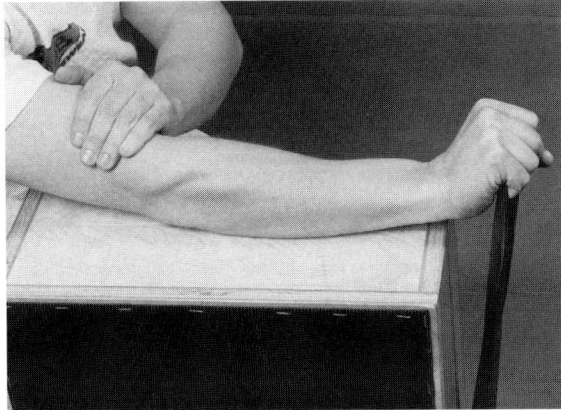

Fig. 5 Wrist flexor strengthening with the use of rubber tubing. To accomplish eccentric strengthening also, the wrist is slowly lowered back to a neutral position from full wrist flexion. (Reproduced with permission from Wiesner SL: Rehabilitation of elbow injuries in sports. *Phys Clin Rehab North Am* 1994;5:81–113.)

of weakness of adjacent uninjured tissue in the kinetic chain; and (4) minimization of negative psychologic effects.[9] It is important to recognize that the more the "general" conditioning exercise resembles the ultimate task, the more transferable the benefits of the conditioning exercise become. Therefore, an upper body ergometer is only useful for cardiovascular conditioning, but is also much more specific to upper body work than is aerobic training by running, bicycling, or stairclimbers.

Maintenance Phase

Critical to the proper rehabilitation of any injured structure is a proper regimen of flexibility and strengthening exercises to prevent a recurrence of injury. Regular eccentric strengthening of the elbow extensors and maintenance of elbow flexion-extension and pronation-supination flexibility are important. Work site evaluations by trained personnel may give tremendous insight into ergonomic interventions that can greatly decrease upper extremity repetitive stress injuries. For example, the height at which arms are held relative to the body has considerable impact on local and central circulatory and metabolic responses. In their classic work, Astrand and associates[36] investigated the energy costs of hammering nails at bench level into a wall at head level and overhead into the ceiling. Although oxygen uptake for the three tasks was similar, working at progressively increasing degrees of humeral elevation resulted in greater heart rate, blood pressure, and ventilatory responses and greater blood lactate accumulation. In a worker who already has injured muscle and has pain in the forearms, working at increased angles of elevation could conceivably contribute to greater increases in forearm intracompartmental pressures, relative hypoperfusion of previously injured tissues, and pain. From a work output standpoint, it was discovered that, while the carpenters were able to maintain the same hammer stroke rate under the three conditions, the number of nails driven in per minute decreased with arm elevation, implying that individual strikes became less powerful or less accurate. Thus, the argument could be made that it would be in the best interests of both worker and employer to ensure the proper ergonomic setting and to modify an employee's work setting. Emphasis on proper posture to maintain stability in the cervicothoracic spine and shoulder girdle is also essential.

If abnormal forces at the elbow cannot be controlled with adequate exercise or proper ergonomic modifications, control of force loads with bracing can be effective. Counterforce braces at the elbow can control intrinsic overload of the elbow by constraining key muscle groups while maintaining muscle balance.[9] Elbow counterforce bracing has been noted by Burton[37] and Groppel and Nirschl[38] to decrease elbow angular acceleration and decrease electromyographic activity.

Corticosteroid Injection

Local injection of corticosteroid may be considered in a patient who has failed aggressive rehabilitation after approximately 3 or 4 weeks. When used, an injection of corticosteroid often combined with a local anesthetic should be injected not into the tendon itself but at the point of maximal tenderness, which is commonly below the extensor brevis origin in the triangular recess formed by the medial slope of the lateral condyle and the brevis tendon.[29] Following injection, the patient is advised to avoid strenuous activities with the forearm for 2 weeks.[19] Most importantly, the use of injections should be only one component of a comprehensive rehabilitation program, and the injections should be spaced at least 1 month apart, with no more than three injections being administered in the same region within a 1-year period.[39-41] Some clinical reports have noted that patients who have had several corticosteroid injections are significantly more difficult to rehabilitate.[26] Furthermore, when encountering "recalcitrant" cases of conservatively treated lateral epicondylitis, the clinician must always consider two other issues: (1) surgery may be necessary, or (2) an incorrect initial diagnosis was made (eg, failure to recognize posterior interosseus nerve entrapment, cervical radiculopathy).

Surgical Considerations

Lateral Epicondylitis Surgical intervention is a consideration in the rehabilitation of repetitive stress injuries to the elbow. In lateral epicondylitis, clinical indications for surgical selection include a failed quality rehabilitative program; altered quality of life; constant pain or rest pain; objective changes recorded by laboratory testing or imaging (eg, radiographs, arthrogram, MRI, sonogram); persistent weakness, atrophy, and dysfunction; and inability to return to work.[21] Preferred surgical approaches are beyond the scope of this chapter and can be referenced elsewhere.[19,21,42]

Medial Epicondylitis Surgical concepts of medial epicondylitis are the same as those for the lateral side. In addition, ulnar nerve dysfunction may be an associated problem, and surgical treatment may be required to resolve this difficulty as well.[9] Medial collateral ligament attrition or rupture has also been observed on occasion, and surgical repair or reconstruction may be indicated in these circumstances.[9]

Cubital Tunnel Syndrome

Cubital tunnel syndrome or ulnar neuropathy at the elbow is usually caused by an overload injury from repetitive tension, compression, or friction, the latter condition being the result of repetitive subluxation of the ulnar nerve across the medial epicondyle. This is the most common site of ulnar nerve entrapment in the upper limb. The ulnar nerve itself is a dynamic structure. It undergoes change throughout the arc of flexion of the elbow.[43] Apfelberg and Larson[44] have shown that it both elongates and is moved medially by the medial head of the triceps through elbow flexion. Hence, the tethering of the nerve by scar tissue interferes with its normal longitudinal and transverse mobility during elbow flexion and adversely affects function. Furthermore, the volume in the cubital tunnel is reduced with elbow flexion.[45] Ulnar intraneural pressure increases with elbow flexion and shoulder abduction.[46,47] Elbow flexion also relaxes the ulnar collateral ligament, allowing it to bulge laterally and encroaching further into the cubital tunnel.[48] Therefore, decreasing the amount of elbow flexion (ie, 90° instead of 135°) necessary for a specific work-related function, puts less stress on the ulnar nerve. In cubital tunnel syndrome, the ulnar nerve is vulnerable to compression because it penetrates the flexor carpi ulnaris arcade, which is in zone 3 of the medial epicondylar groove. This area is easily compressed by resting the elbows on any firm surface. The extent of ulnar nerve pathology and the precise location of entrapment is readily accomplished via electrodiagnostic testing. Nerve conduction studies in the forearm and across the elbow typically reveal a drop in compound muscle action potential amplitude and/or a decrease in nerve conduction velocity with ulnar nerve stimulation proximal to the site of the lesion.[49] Further localization is accomplished by "inching" the stimulator along the course of the nerve to find the precise segment where the entrapment/compression exists.

Nonsurgical treatment of ulnar nerve pathology at the elbow centers on minimizing the pressure increases around the ulnar nerve with elbow flexion or direct pressure.[50,51] Initially, avoidance of provocative activities and nonsteroidal anti-inflammatory medication can help, although no documented clinical efficacy of nonsteroidals in cubital tunnel syndrome exists.[51] Eisen and Danon[52] followed 30 patients with mild cubital tunnel syndrome both clinically and electrophysiologically for approximately 22 months and found that 90% became asymptomatic. However, they concluded that patients with follow-up electromyography and nerve conduction velocity studies who show an across-elbow conduction velocity of less than 41 m/s and/or motor latency from above the elbow of more than 10.2 ms would probably develop a motor deficit. Ice may be used as a modality, but it is important to keep in mind that the ulnar nerve is subcutaneous and susceptible to cold injury from prolonged ice treatment if not monitored.[53] The application of an anterior splint with the elbow placed between 45° and 70° of flexion and with the wrist supported to relax the flexor carpi ulnaris for several weeks seems to be the best conservative management for cubital tunnel syndrome.[54] No data about the severity of the compression or the length of splint treatment were given, but Dimond and Lister noted an overall improvement rate in 86% of patients followed up for an average of 8.7 months. For patients with mild or intermittent symptoms, Ferlic[55] also favors conservative treatment consisting of patient education about avoiding direct pressure on the nerve and activities involving full elbow flexion or repetitive flexion/extension and a well-padded posterior splint that maintains the elbow in 45° of flexion. Dellon and associates[56] reported on a prospective trial of nonsurgical management of cubital tunnel syndrome in 128 patients followed up at a mean of 58.6 months. For statistical purposes, a successful outcome of the nonsurgical regimen was not having an operation. Of their patients who did not have surgery, 89% had symptoms only, 67% had abnormal sensorimotor thresholds, and 38% had abnormal sensorimotor innervated density. They concluded that a strict nonsurgical regimen be supervised in the initial management of cubital tunnel syndrome.

After any prolonged period of immobilization, inflammatory processes may have subsided but scar tissue formation may have taken place. Joint tissue mobilizations and gentle joint and capsular mobilizations may be necessary to loosen adhesions around the ulnar nerve to allow proper neural function.[14] Icing of the area after soft-tissue mobilizations helps prevent edema and subsequent inflammation about the nerve that can result in scarring. Use of an elbow pad or placing cushions on chair arms may decrease some local direct pressure. Avoidance of recurrent valgus stress and/or elbow flexion by elevating the chair or dropping the desk height theoretically may reduce tension on the nerve. In workers who are attempting to increase their upper body strength and endurance, it is important to emphasize avoiding deep elbow flexion when performing forearm/elbow curls and triceps exercises or bench presses. Similarly, the crank shaft of arm ergometers must be set far enough away from the patient's chest that cycling is performed with moderate elbow flexion on the "pull" stroke and achievement of near full elbow extension during the "push." An easy estimate of good positioning is making sure that the person's elbows never break the plane of the body, ie, they never come back farther than the chest wall/axillary line. Approximately one half of the patients with minimum compression of the ulnar nerve can be expected to recover with this use of elbow pads and icing.[57] Regardless of what conservative treatment is undertaken, recurrence rates of 44% to 75% have been reported in patients with different degrees of severity.[58,59] Avoiding the offending activities and/or ergonomic interventions may decrease recurrence rates.

Basic surgical choices include cubital tunnel release only, anterior transposition of the nerve with fascial sling, medial epicondylectomy, and submuscular transposition.[43] Beyond simple release, all aproaches have in common careful identification of the ulnar nerve proximal to the cubital tunnel, preservation of the medial antebrachial cutaneous nerve branches in the anterior wound, exposure and resection of the medial intermuscular septum, ulnar nerve release through the cubital tunnel, and release of the arch of the flexor carpi ulnaris, allowing mobilization of the nerve.[50]

Summary

Repetitive stress injuries at the elbow are common and cause significant disability in the workplace. Rehabilitation programs for these types of repetitive stress injuries should include acute-phase management of pain and inflammation when present, restoration of proper joint and muscle flexibility and motion, active strengthening programs for weak or imbalanced muscles, using activity-specific types of contractions (eg, eccentric versus concentric), and generalized aerobic conditioning. Ergonomic interventions in the workplace may potentially be beneficial to passively decrease the chronic overload on musculoskeletal structures through proper biomechanical alignment and positioning. Bracing, injections, and surgery are other approaches that may be necessary in the rehabilitation of repetitive stress injuries at the elbow.

References

1. Kibler WB, Chandler TJ, Pace BK: Principles of rehabilitation after chronic tendon injuries. *Clin Sports Med* 1992;11:661–671.
2. Leadbetter WB: Cell-matrix response in tendon injury. *Clin Sports Med* 1992;11: 533–578.
3. Kibler WB, Herring S, Press J: Radiologic imaging in rehabilitation, in Kibler WB, Ilemig S, Press J (eds): *Functional Rehabilitation in Sports Medicine*. Chicago, IL, Aspen Press, in press.
4. Kibler WB: Physiology of exercising muscle, in Reynolds FC (ed): *Instructional Course Lectures 43*. Rosemont, IL, American Academy of Orthopaedic Surgeons, 1994, pp 3–4.
5. Weisner SL: Rehabilitation of elbow injuries in sports. *Phys Med Rehabil Clin North Am* 1994;5:81–113.
6. Boone DC, Azen SP: Normal range of motion of joints in male subjects. *J Bone Joint Surg* 1979;61A:756–759.
7. Elbow joints, in Magee DJ (ed): *Orthopedic Physical Assessment*, ed 2. Philadelphia, PA, WB Saunders, 1992, pp 143–167.
8. Nirschl RP, Morrey BF: Rehabilitation, in Morrey BF (ed): *The Elbow and Its Disorders*, ed 2. Philadelphia, PA, WB Saunders, 1993, pp 173–180.
9. Nirschl RP: Elbow tendinosis/tennis elbow. *Clin Sports Med* 1992;11:851–870.
10. Nirschl RP: Muscle and tendon trauma: Tennis elbow, in Morrey BF (ed): *The Elbow and Its Disorders*, ed 2. Philadelphia, PA, WB Saunders, 1993, pp 537–552.
11. Leach RE, Miller JK: Lateral and medial epicondylitis of the elbow. *Clin Sports Med* 1987;6:259–272.
12. Prentice WE (ed): *Rehabilitation Techniques in Sports Medicine*, ed 2. St. Louis, MO, Mosby Year Book, 1994.
13. Fillion PL: Treatment of lateral epicondylitis. *Am J Occup Ther* 1991;45:340–343.
14. LaFreniere JG: "Tennis elbow:" Reevaluation, treatment, and prevention. *Phys Ther* 1979;59:742–746.
15. Bowling RW, Rockar PA Jr: The elbow complex, in Gould JA III (ed): *Orthopaedic and Sports Physical Therapy*, ed 2. St. Louis, MO, CV Mosby, 1990, pp 463–482.
16. Morrey BF, Regan WD: Tendinopathies about the elbow, in DeLee JC, Drez D Jr (eds): *Orthopaedic Sports Medicine: Principles and Practice*. Philadelphia, PA, WB Saunders, 1994, vol 1, pp 860–881.
17. Muscle injury: Classification and healing, in Reid DC (ed): *Sports Injury Assessment and Rehabilitation*. New York, NY, Churchill Livingstone, 1992, p 85–101.
18. Stratford P, Levy DR, Gauldie S, et al: Extensor carpi radialis tendonitis: A validation of selected outcome measures. *Physiotherapy Canada* 1987;39:250–255.
19. Stratford PW, Levy DR, Gauldie S, et al: The evaluation of phonophoresis and friction massage as treatments for extensor carpi radialis tendinitis: A randomized controlled trial. *Physiotherapy Canada* 1989;41:93–99.
20. Halle JS, Franklin RJ, Karalfa BL: Comparison of four treatment approaches for lateral epicondylitis of the elbow. *J Orthop Sports Phys Ther* 1986;8:62–69.
21. Nirschl RP: Tennis injuries, in Nicholas JA, Hershman EB, Posner MA (eds): *The Upper Extremity in Sports Medicine*. St. Louis, MO, CV Mosby, 1990, pp 827–842.
22. Akeson WH, Amiel D, Woo SL: Immobility effects on synovial joints: The pathomechanics of joint contracture. *Biorheology* 1980;17:95–110.
23. Cyriax JH: The pathology and treatment of tennis elbow. *J Bone Joint Surg* 1936;18:921–940.

24. Kushner S, Reid DC: Manipulation in the treatment of tennis elbow. *J Orthop Sport Phys Ther* 1986;7:264–272.
25. Sobel J, Pettrone F, Nirschl R: Prevention and rehabilitation of racquet sports injuries, in Nicholas JA, Hershman EB, Posner MA (eds): *The Upper Extremity in Sports Medicine*. St. Louis, MO, CV Mosby, 1990, p 843.
26. De Andrade JR, Grant C, Dixon AS: Joint distension and reflex muscle inhibition in the knee. *J Bone Joint Surg* 1965;47A:313–322.
27. Young JL, Press JM: The physiologic basis of sports rehabilitation. *Phys Med Rehabil Clin North Am* 1994;5:9–36.
28. Knapik JJ, Mawdsley RH, Ramos MU: Angular specificity and test mode specificity of isometric and isokinetic strength training. *J Orthop Sports Phys Ther* 1983;5:58–65.
29. Nirschl RP, Sobel J: Conservative treatment of tennis elbow. *Phys Sports Med* 1981;9:43–54.
30. Basmajian JV, De Luca CJ (eds): *Muscles Alive: Their Functions Revealed by Electromyography*, ed 5. Baltimore, MD, Williams & Wilkins, 1985.
31. Stanish WD, Rubinovich RM, Curwin S: Eccentric exercise in chronic tendinitis. *Clin Orthop* 1986;208:65–68.
32. Knott M, Voss DE (eds): *Proprioceptive Neuromuscular Facilitation: Patterns and Techniques*, ed 2. New York, NY, Harper and Row, 1968.
33. Dilorenzo CE, Parkes JC II, Chmelar RD: The importance of shoulder and cervical dysfunction in the etiology and treatment of athletic elbow injuries. *J Orthop Sports Phys Ther* 1990;11:402–409.
34. Press JM, Herring SA, Kibler WB: Rehabilitation of musculoskeletal disorders, in Dillingham T (ed): *Rehabilitation of the Injured Shoulder*. Washington, DC, Borden Institute-United States Army, in press.
35. Wells P: Cervical dysfunction and shoulder problems. *Physiotherapy* 1982;68:66–73.
36. Astrand I, Guharay A, Wahren J: Circulatory responses to arm exercise with different arm positions. *J Appl Physiol* 1968;25:528–532.
37. Burton AK: Grip strength and forearm straps in tennis elbow. *Br J Sports Med* 1985;19:37–38.
38. Groppel JL, Nirschl RP: A mechanical and electromyographical analysis of the effects of various joint counterforce braces on the tennis player. *Am J Sports Med* 1986;14:195–200.
39. Cabrera JM, McCue FC III: Nonosseous athletic injuries of the elbow, forearm, and hand. *Clin Sports Med* 1986;5:681–700.
40. Jobe FW, Nuber G: Throwing injuries of the elbow. *Clin Sports Med* 1986;5:621–636.
41. Leadbetter WB: Corticosteroid injection therapy in sports injuries, in Leadbetter WB, Buckwalter JA, Gordon SL (eds): *Sports-Induced Inflammation: Clinical and Basic Science Concepts*. Park Ridge, IL, American Academy of Orthopaedic Surgeons, 1990, pp 527–545.
42. Calvert PT, Allum RL, Macpherson IS, et al: Simple lateral release in treatment of tennis elbow. *J Roy Soc Med* 1985;78:912–915.
43. Regan WD, Morrey BF: Entrapment neuropathies about the elbow, in DeLee JC, Drez D Jr (eds): *Orthopaedic Sports Medicine: Principles and Practice*. Philadelphia, PA, WB Saunders, 1994, vol 1, pp 844–859.
44. Apfelberg DB, Larson SJ: Dynamic anatomy of the ulnar nerve at the elbow. *Plast Reconstr Surg* 1973;51:79–81.
45. Dangles CJ, Bilos ZJ: Ulnar nerve neuritis in a world champion weightlifter. *Am J Sports Med* 1980;8:443–445.
46. Macnicol MF: Extraneural pressures affecting the ulnar nerve at the elbow. *Hand* 1982;14:5–11.
47. Weinstein SM, Herring SA: Nerve problems and compartment syndromes in the hand, wrist, and forearm. *Clin Sports Med* 1992;11:161–188.
48. Feindel W, Stratford J: The role of the cubital tunnel in tardy ulnar palsy. *Can J Surg* 1958;1:287–300.

49. Kimura J (ed): *Electrodiagnosis in Diseases of Nerve And Muscle: Principles and Practice*, ed 2. Philadelphia, PA, FA Davis, 1989, pp 495–516.
50. Butters KP, Singer KM: Nerve lesions of the arm and elbow, in DeLee JC, Drez D Jr (eds): *Orthopaedic Sports Medicine: Principles and Practice*. Philadelphia, PA, WB Saunders, 1994, vol 1, pp 802–811.
51. Folberg CR, Weiss AP, Akelman E: Cubital tunnel syndrome: Part II. Treatment. *Orthop Rev* 1994;23:233–241.
52. Eisen A, Danon J: The mild cubital tunnel syndrome: Its natural history and indications for surgical intervention. *Neurology* 1974;24:608–613.
53. Glousman RE: Ulnar nerve problems in the athlete's elbow. *Clin Sports Med* 1990;9:365–377.
54. Dimond ML, Lister GD: Abstract: Cubital tunnel syndrome treated by long-arm splintage. *J Hand Surg* 1985;10A:430.
55. Ferlic DC: Clinical assessment and conservative treatment of cubital tunnel syndrome, in Gelberman RH (ed): *Operative Nerve Repair and Reconstruction*. Philadelphia, PA, JB Lippincott, 1991, pp 1055–1061.
56. Dellon AL, Hament W, Gittelshon A: Nonoperative management of cubital tunnel syndrome: An 8-year prospective study. *Neurology* 1993;43:1673–1677.
57. Dellon AL: Review of treatment results for ulnar nerve entrapment at the elbow. *J Hand Surg* 1989;14A:688–700.
58. Wadsworth TG: The external compression syndrome of the ulnar nerve at the cubital tunnel. *Clin Orthop* 1977;124:189–204.
59. Paine KW: Tardy ulnar palsy. *Can J Surg* 1970;13:255–261.

Chapter 34
Overuse Injuries of the Shoulder

Craig L. Levitz, MD
Joseph P. Iannotti, MD, PhD

Labral and Capsular Overuse Injuries

Anatomy and Pathology

The glenoid labrum is a fibrocartilaginous structure that surrounds the glenoid fossa. It deepens the fossa and is the attachment site for the glenohumeral ligaments. DePalma and associates[1] described the labrum as having a glenoid surface that is continuous with the hyaline cartilage of the glenoid cavity and a capsular surface that blends with the capsule. Cooper and associates,[2] in a cadaveric study, recently examined the varied morphology of the glenoid labrum and the patterns of capsular insertion around the rim of the glenoid. The superior and anterosuperior portions of the labrum are loosely attached to the glenoid, and the macroanatomy of this portion of the labrum is likened to the meniscus of the knee. The superior portion of the labrum consistently inserts directly into the biceps tendon, while the inferior portion firmly attaches to the glenoid rim and appears as a fibrous, immobile extension of the articular cartilage. The superior and anterosuperior parts of the labrum have less vascularity than do the posterosuperior and inferior parts, and the vascularity is limited to the periphery of the labrum.

The labrum is firmly attached to the glenoid rim and appears smooth and glistening. With aging or with injury, the gross pathology of the labrum demonstrates a more variable pattern, from being thick and pronounced, to thin and vestigial.[1,3] The relationship of this variation in structure to labral tears and glenohumeral instability is not known.

The glenoid labrum and capsular ligaments play a critical role in preventing excessive translation of the humeral head.[4,5] These tissues stabilize the shoulder, particularly at the extremes of motion. The superior glenohumeral ligament, coracohumeral ligament, and rotator interval capsule serve as the primary restraints to inferior translation of the adducted shoulder. With progressive abduction the middle and inferior glenohumeral ligaments become the main static stabilizers resisting anterior and inferior translation of the humerus.[4]

The labral pathology of overuse injury or aging is characterized by an initial hypertrophy of the labrum.[1] The glenoid ligaments undergo hyperplasia, and the capsule appears to thicken. Along the labral border, the normal smooth surface gives way to tabs, fringes, and villous formation. These changes have been described as paralleling the degree of labral detachment.[1] Repetitive stress of the labral-ligament complex leads to microscopic capsulolabral injury, which with continued use can progress to a glenohumeral ligament tear, or detachment from the labrum. Bigliani and associates[6] have shown that when portions of the inferior glenohumeral ligament are stressed at an average of 5.5

MPa, there is an average strain of 27% at ligament failure. This demonstrates that significant stretching occurs prior to ligament failure. Abrupt failure often occurs at the glenoid insertion, while a steplike pattern is seen with failure in the mid substance of the ligament.[6] Capsular stretching appears to also occur with repetitive overuse, particularly in the competitive overhead-throwing athlete.[7]

Incidence and Epidemiology

The incidence of labral tears has been extensively studied in the throwing athlete. In one series, 100% of throwing athletes who underwent diagnostic arthroscopy for shoulder pain were found to have a labral tear;[8] other studies have yielded similar results.[3] This high incidence of labral tears in the throwing athlete suggests that the pathology may be inevitable with repetitive overload of the shoulder during overhead throwing.

Tears of the glenoid labrum have also been reported in relation to other athletic activities requiring repetitive overhead activity, such as tennis, racquetball, and swimming.[9-12] Sudden avulsion of the labrum can result from a fall on an outstretched arm; in addition, it may be hypothesized that the labrum is susceptible to avulsion secondary to repetitive microtrauma, stretch, or sheer incurred during repetitive use of the shoulder musculature.[3,8,13] Thus, acute labral avulsion might also represent an overuse injury, although one that becomes symptomatic acutely. Further studies are needed to clarify whether repetitive use decreases the load threshold for labral avulsion and whether labral avulsion represents an end-stage overuse injury with an acute presentation.

In contrast to the amount of literature on the throwing athlete, there is a paucity of literature on the incidence of isolated labral tears in industrial workers whose jobs require repetitive overhead motion or shoulder joint loading. Industrial workers may be able to continue working for an extended period of time by altering their biomechanics, whereas in athletes alteration in the biomechanics of the throwing motion is readily apparent. In both groups of patients, continued overuse may lead to instability, impingement, and rotator cuff tears. Early detection of labral tears and prevention of continued overuse could lead to a decreased incidence of more severe overuse injuries.

There is no evidence that extended overhead work causes shoulder joint instability. Work may aggravate existing traumatic instability to the point where a person is no longer able to continue overhead work. It is not known how many patients receive care through workers' compensation for nonwork-related injuries that are aggravated by overhead work or become symptomatic while functioning in the work environment.

Pathophysiology

The capsuloligamentous complex, which includes the glenoid labrum and the glenohumeral ligaments, will respond to overuse with attenuation and elongation. These soft-tissue structures normally provide static stabilization to the shoulder joint. The labrum and capsular ligaments serve to contain the humeral head within the glenoid at the extremes of shoulder rotation. The muscles of the rotator cuff center the humeral head in the glenoid in the midranges of motion and protect the static stabilizers from repetitive stress and physiologic overload. Abnormal translation of the humeral head during shoulder motion can lead to varying degrees of capsular stretch and labral abrasion, depending on the magnitude and duration of force that the static stabilizers need in order to constrain. Excessive laxity of the capsuloligamentous complex can lead to clinical instability.[5,14,15] Initially, attenuation of the static stabilizers leads to mild instability of the shoulder joint and increased demand on the rotator cuff musculature to center the humeral head. This begins as small degrees of sliding but can progress as the rotator cuff muscles fatigue.[16]

When the inferior glenohumeral ligament is stretched or torn and, with repetitive use, there is fatigue and overload of the rotator cuff, the humeral head can translate anteriorly, particularly at the extremes of external rotation and abduction. Rowe[14,15] reported on a group of overhead-throwing athletes with recurrent transient anterior subluxation. Sixty-four percent had a Bankart lesion and 26% had excessive laxity of the capsule (no Bankart lesion). In these patients, secondary impingement of the supraspinatus tendon on the coracoacromial arch can occur, resulting in further pain and weakness of the rotator cuff. Prolonged impingement can lead to inflammatory and degenerative changes in the rotator cuff tendons, which will be described later in this chapter.

The shoulder joint is subjected to a great deal of force during the cocking and acceleration phases of throwing. The humeral head is driven posteriorly during cocking and follow-through and anteriorly during acceleration.[17] The inferior glenohumeral ligament is strained as it tries to stabilize the humeral head during throwing.[5] The muscles of the rotator cuff, particularly the infraspinatus and teres minor, play a critical role in providing anterior glenohumeral stability and reducing the strain on the capsular ligaments during the throwing motion. There is a linear relation between the external rotation of the humerus and the strain of the inferior glenohumeral ligament.[18] Excessive strain can damage the cartilaginous ring of the labrum.[6] Subtle microscopic shearing and degenerative changes can occur within the labrum and capsule that with continued use can develop into labral tears and complete labral detachment from the capsule.[3,8,13] It is unclear whether all labral tears are associated with instability, although there is a wide spectrum of instability symptoms associated with labral pathology.

The superior labral anterior-posterior (SLAP) lesion is a degenerative tear believed to be caused by biceps overload or humeral instability. The anterosuperior labrum is a common location for tears in throwing athletes. There have been few studies examining the effect on the labrum of repetitive throwing or overhead motion. Andrews and associates[3] and Snyder and associates[13] have implicated the tendon of the long head of the biceps as a cause of many of the labral tears seen in overhead-throwing athletes.[3,13] Andrews, Jobe, and Snyder have documented the large forces that the biceps tendon is subjected to during the deceleration phase of throwing, immediately following ball release.[3,8,13,19,20] They hypothesize that repeated eccentric loading of the biceps lifts the labrum off the glenoid, leading to tearing of the glenoid labrum.

Fu and associates[21] demonstrated the role of the long head of the biceps tendon as a restraint to anterior instability. In this study, strain in the inferior glenohumeral ligament did not increase with increasing biceps muscle force and torque, but increased dramatically in the presence of a superior labral tear. These data suggest that the biceps muscle increases the anterior stability of the glenohumeral joint by increasing the shoulder's resistance to torsional stress in the externally rotated, abducted position. Detachment of the superior glenoid labrum decreases the shoulder's resistance to torsion and places a greater demand on the inferior glenohumeral ligament, which can lead to failure and further instability.[6,22]

Relationship of Aging and Repetitive Use

Since DePalma's early work[1] there have been relatively few studies detailing the effects of aging on the capsule and how these effects differ, if at all, from the changes that occur with repetitive use.[1] DePalma observed alterations in the labrum as early as the second decade of life. These changes ranged from minor wrinkling of the labrum and capsular surface to complete detachment of the labrum from the glenoid cavity. These alterations increased with age. Fifty percent of subjects had these changes by the fifth decade of life, and 96% by the eighth decade. DePalma[1] concluded that detachments of the labrum are associated with increasing age. Although it can be said that there are changes of the glenoid and capsular architecture with increasing age, the high incidence of labral and capsular injuries in young athletes whose activity is associated with repetitive use of the shoulder argues against labral and capsular pathology being exclusively a disease of aging. More likely, there is an element of overuse superimposed on the aging process. The contribution of aging and use to labral injury needs to be clarified. Reeves[23] found that the glenohumeral ligaments fail at the glenoid attachments in younger subjects, and in the capsular substance in older subjects, which is the opposite of what is seen in other ligaments, such as the anterior cruciate.[6,23,24] It is also known that collagen composition changes with aging, and the shoulder joint capsule is composed largely of collagen. It would be interesting to compare the collagen in the capsule of a throwing athlete with that of an older industrial worker who performs long hours of overhead work. In summary, understanding of the importance of the labrum in shoulder stabilization has substantially improved over the last two decades with the advent of magnetic resonance imaging (MRI) and arthroscopic surgery. However, the literature relating to overuse injuries of the labrum is dominated by opinions and reviews, without a great deal of hard data. Further studies are needed to define more clearly the etiology of overuse injuries of the labrum and the pathophysiology that transforms a pathologic labral injury into symptomatic instability.

Overuse Syndromes of the Rotator Cuff

Incidence

Rotator cuff tendinopathy (RCT) is a classic example of an overuse injury. Most cases are the result of prolonged or repetitive use of the arms in the overhead position. While a patient with a partial or complete rotator cuff tear may recall a traumatic event at the onset of shoulder pain, the trauma is often not significant enough to result in the tearing of a normal rotator cuff tendon. The trauma often serves to accelerate the disease process or simply results in symptomatic presentation of the ongoing degenerative process that has been initiated by overuse or aging or a combination of the two.

Rotator cuff tears commonly occur in patients older than age 40. Cadaver studies report a varied incidence from 5% to 80%. Partial-thickness tears have a reported incidence of between 15% and 40%, while full-thickness tears are about one third as common. Both types of tears have an increased incidence with increasing age (Figs. 1 and 2).[25-27] Ozaki and associates[28] reported a large increase in the incidence of partial tears beginning at age 60 and of complete tears beginning at age 70. Recently, Sher[29] reported that one third of asymptomatic subjects older than age 60 have a partial or complete rotator cuff tear on MRI. This is the first good noncadaveric study of the true incidence of as-

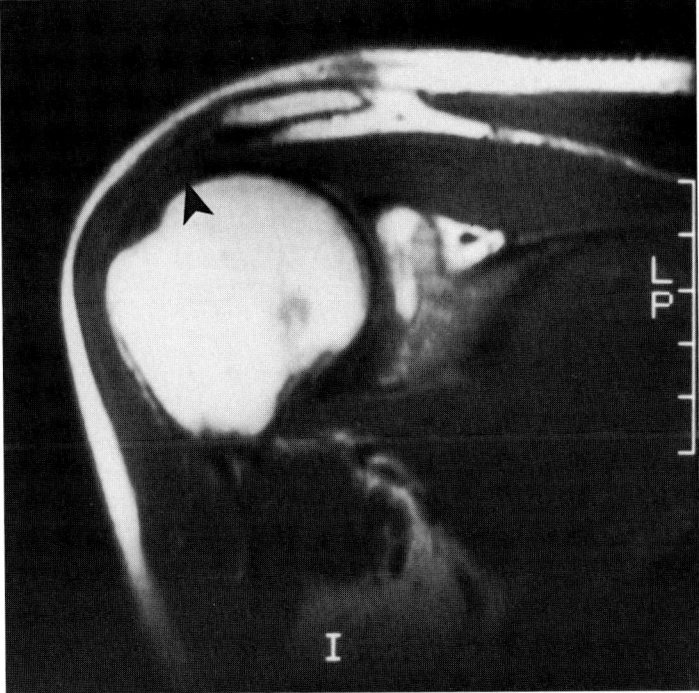

Fig. 1 Magnetic resonance image in axial plane, demonstrating normal anterior capsule and ligament (arrowhead) and posterior labrum and capsule (arrow). This study was performed in a normal 16-year-old male. (Reproduced with permission from Ozaki J, Fujimoto S, Nakagawa Y, et al: Tears of the rotator cuff of the shoulder associated with pathological changes in the acromion: A study on cadavers. *J Bone Joint Surg* 1988;70A:1224–1230.)

ymptomatic rotator cuff tears. The actual incidence is estimated to be somewhat higher secondary to the rigid inclusion criteria.

Pathology

The pathology of rotator cuff tendinitis has been described as a reversible process associated with an inflammatory infiltrate within the subacromial bursa and with increased vascularity and hyperemic changes within the rotator cuff tendons.[30–33] The pathology of rotator cuff tears is variable. The reported findings range from degenerative necrosis and loss of the normal collagen architecture, without a cellular infiltrate or fibroblastic response, to degenerative lesions associated with neovascularization.[30–36] Most partial-thickness cuff tears occur within the substance of the supraspinatus tendon near its insertion site as was classically described by Codman.[33,35] Full-thickness tears may extend to include the infraspinatus, teres minor, and subscapularis and may be associated with subluxation of the biceps tendon from the bicipital groove or a tear of the long head of the biceps tendon. The margins of the tendon in a full-thickness rotator cuff tear may be almost entirely acellular without vascularity, or they can show increased vascularity with a cellular infiltrate. This variety of pathologic processes is thought to result from different pathologic mechanisms.[30–36] It has been hypothesized that the partial cuff tear lesion rep-

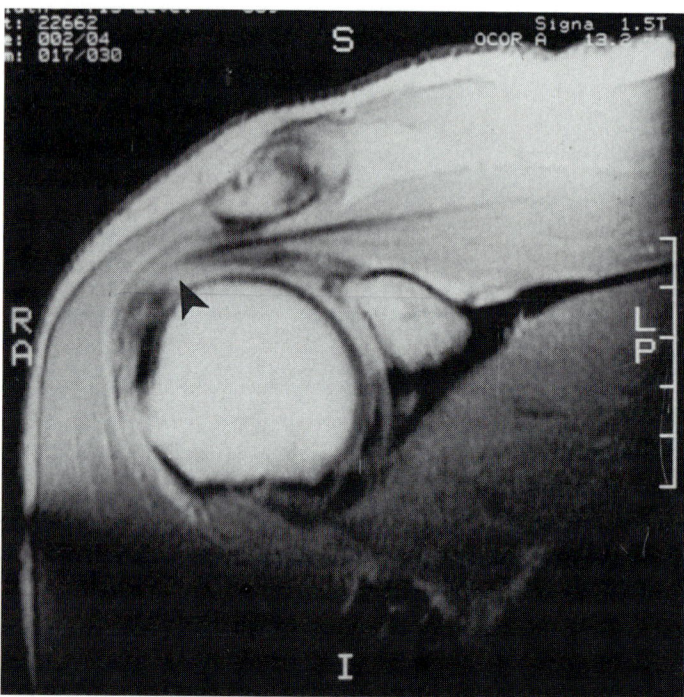

Fig. 2 Magnetic resonance image in axial plane, demonstrating increased signal in anterior labrum (arrowhead) consistent with degeneration. Normal posterior labrum (arrow). This study was performed in an asymptomatic normal 45-year-old athletic male.

resents an early stage of a full-thickness tear, but there has been no documentation to support this claim.[30-36]

There are several theories on rotator cuff pathology and its association with overuse injury. Neer has stated that 95% of rotator cuff tears are associated with impingement.[25-27] Trauma may enlarge the tear, but rarely is it the principal etiologic agent. Rotator cuff disease can result from secondary mechanical impingement as a result of glenohumeral instability from the previously described capsulolabral pathophysiology. Also, primary impingement of the supraspinatus tendon on the coracoacromial arch caused by subacromial outlet narrowing can cause rotator cuff pathology. Chronic abrasions of the rotator cuff from overuse in a patient with primary impingement can result in hypertrophy of the bony and soft tissues of the coracoacromial arch and further narrowing of the subacromial space leading to progressive rotator cuff disease.[21] Neer has classified the changes that occur with rotator cuff impingement into three progressive stages. Stage I is characterized by edema and hemorrhage of the bursae and tendon, stage II by thickening and fibrosis of the bursa and tendons, and stage III by tendon failure and bony changes.[12,26]

Bigliani and associates[37] have correlated developmental and acquired changes in the morphology of the acromion with rotator cuff tears. Patients can be classified as having either a flat, curved, or hooked acromion. There is an established correlation between hooked and curved acromions and rotator cuff tears. This work supports Neer's theory implicating the slope of the acromion in the impingement syndrome. The etiology of this acromial variation is not known, and its relationship to aging and overuse warrants further investigation.

In addition to age-related degeneration and instability, the microvascular pattern of the rotator cuff has been intensely studied. A hypovascular region corresponding to Codman's critical area of the supraspinatus tendon has been described using microinjection techniques in cadavers. Rathbun and Macnab[38] described the influence of arm position on microvascular supply, with a "wringing out" of the vascular supply to the supraspinatus tendon with the arm in the adducted position. Laser Doppler flowmetry has allowed dynamic evaluation of the vascularity of the cuff in living patients with clinical symptoms of rotator cuff tears and impingement syndrome.[39] These data suggest variability in the vascular supply within the tendon substance of a rotator cuff tear or within the rotator cuff tendon in patients with impingement syndrome. Mechanical irritation of the rotator cuff associated with symptomatic supraspinatus outlet impingement may result in hypervascularity of the rotator cuff tendon in the early stages of impingement. This suggests a role for a hyperemic response, as opposed to a hypovascular response, in rotator cuff pathology.

The additive effects of repetitive eccentric muscle contraction on the rotator cuff musculature can lead to tendinitis and rotator cuff tears. The rotator cuff is dependent on the intact static stabilizers and scapular rotators. If these fail, the rotator cuff will be overused to compensate for these abnormalities. When the rotator cuff operates at a biomechanical disadvantage, the sequelae of eccentric overload, repetitive strain, and overuse tendinitis can occur.[21,40,41] Repetitive microtrauma to the supraspinatus tendon is thought to lead to an inflammatory reaction. According to Fu and associates,[21] this consists of transitory vasoconstriction followed by vasodilatation with an influx of acute mediators of inflammation. Continued overuse can lead to chronic inflammation that if unabated can lead to tissue destruction by neutral proteinases. Although this theory may have some merit, there is no data to support it. Further research is necessary to better define the intrinsic tendon changes and rotator cuff deterioration that can occur with overuse injury.

The actual tearing of the rotator cuff is thought to be preceded by a continued cycle of overuse injury without adequate repair, leading to degenerative changes within the cuff that eventually progress to a partial or complete tear. Additional stress can extend or enlarge a preexisting tear, and the onset of pain or weakness may also alert a patient to the presence of a tear. The deep fibers of the cuff near its insertion site on the greater tuberosity is believed to be the most common location of injury.[30-35] These observations support the theory of an inherent vulnerability to failure from overuse at this location.[25]

The throwing athlete frequently presents for evaluation of shoulder pain and dysfunction. The shoulder of the professional baseball pitcher is subject to supranormal demands that can overload the rotator cuff tendon leading to fiber fatigue and breakdown. This has led to the belief that mechanical abrasion is not the only mechanism for complete rotator cuff tears.[41] Hawkins has examined the forces to which the throwing athlete's shoulder is subjected, and he found that these forces can exceed the physiologic limits of the rotator cuff tendon, leading to injury of the tendon. If the rate of injury exceeds the rate of healing, the injury becomes cumulative and progresses to pathology. During throwing, the rotator cuff stabilizes the humeral head in the glenoid fossa and the arm, to protect the static stabilizers. With overuse injury, there is less joint compression, a decreased ability to decelerate the arm in the delayed cocking phase, and eventual anterior excursion of the humerus that can result in instability and secondary impingement.[41,42]

Overuse injuries of the rotator cuff have been reported in many other athletic activities, including cycling, gymnastics, and competitive swimming. Repetitive motion or muscle stress over the horizontal plane is the common denominator.[43,44]

A classic overuse syndrome of the rotator cuff occurs in paraplegic patients. In these patients, the soft-tissue restraints of the shoulder must bear the full body weight. Thirty percent of paraplegics complain of chronic, persistent pain during wheelchair transfers. Most of the pathology involves impingement of the rotator cuff.[45,46] However, these patients exhibit a surprisingly low incidence of degenerative osteoarthritic changes relative to the high incidence of rotator cuff disease. A secondary degenerative arthritis can be seen in paraplegic patients following failure of the soft tissues. The high intra-articular pressure observed in these patients, along with an abnormal distribution of forces across the shoulder joint, appears to lead to soft-tissue injury that results in impingement of the rotator cuff tendons while preserving the bony articulations.[45,46]

Rotator cuff tears in industrial workers are thought to begin as rotator cuff tendinitis. Repetitive overhead work is thought to be the inciting stimulus. Tendinitis that is left untreated leads to degenerative changes in the rotator cuff tendons. This may progress over months to years without producing enough pain to limit activity. Continued neglect progresses to tearing of the cuff. Actual tearing of the tendon is usually associated with a mild traumatic event recalled by the patient. The injury is often attributed to work if the mild trauma occurs at work, though this trauma may have nothing to do with the pathophysiology of the injury.

Rotator Cuff Tears and Aging

The increased incidence of rotator cuff tears with increased age is well known. Almost all the patients in DePalma's and Neer's series were older than age 40, and Neer argues for an atraumatic etiology of rotator cuff tears.[1,25-27] Ozaki and Sher's data show an increased incidence with age as well as a greater incidence of full-thickness tears with increased age.[28,29] Pettersson has characterized some of the degenerative changes that the cuff tendon undergoes with age and makes a case for primary age-related degeneration of the tendon.[47] Examples of a normal rotator cuff MRI from a young person and from an asymptomatic midlife person are shown in Figures 3 and 4. These theories cannot account for the known incidence of rotator cuff tears in young athletes. These injuries occur in relatively young tendons that are subject to excessive overload and overuse that often occurs in association with capsulolabral injury and subtle instabilities. Overuse injury may lead to an acceleration of age-related degeneration of the rotator cuff, or it may cause degeneration of the cuff by an age-independent mechanism. On the other hand, one might hypothesize that rotator cuff disease is a result of the normal aging process and not an actual use-related injury, particularly in the older population. Such a theory would suggest that there may be an infrequent association of work activities with rotator cuff injury. Work may simply be the environment for the mild trauma that draws attention to the age-related degenerative changes. However, this theory would fail to account for the high incidence of rotator cuff disease in young athletes or young workers. We are unaware of any studies that have followed the evolution of asymptomatic changes of the rotator cuff in the work force. In summary, the relationship of overuse injury to known age-related degeneration remains unclear.

Myalgia

Certain shoulder complaints are the result of chronic muscle loading and cannot be classified under any of the aforementioned diagnoses. Trapezius myalgia is the best-described type in the literature. Workers who are required to work with their arms in a constantly elevated position undergo static loading of the shoulder stabilizing muscles and are at risk for fatigue of these muscles and for the aching pain in the belly of the muscle that is characteristic of this disorder. Myalgia is a common cause of long-term sick leave and may have a poor prognosis for return to work.[14,48]

The pathology of myalgia shows inflammation and degeneration of muscle fibers.[14,48] Larson examined a group of patients with localized chronic myalgia severe enough to cause long-term absence from work; this myalgia was the result of static loading of the shoulder during repetitive assembly-line work. The results from open biopsies demonstrated two changes in the interfibrillary network (mitochondria and sarcotubular system) of the trapezius muscle. Type 1 fibers had a moth-eaten appearance and were larger than normal fibers. The moth-eaten appearance is thought to result from sufficient loading to cause an increase in muscle fiber volume. In addition, there was an increase in pathologic ragged red fibers in the area of complaint. This phenomenon is thought to indicate mitochondrial myopathy.[48] A decrease in the energy phosphate content of the muscle fibers has been demonstrated in patients with myalgia and may be a result of depleted energy reserves, hypoxia, and resultant free radical release leading to cellular injury.[49]

Recent work has attempted to determine estimations of muscle load in order to target at-risk occupations. Electromyographic studies have shown lo-

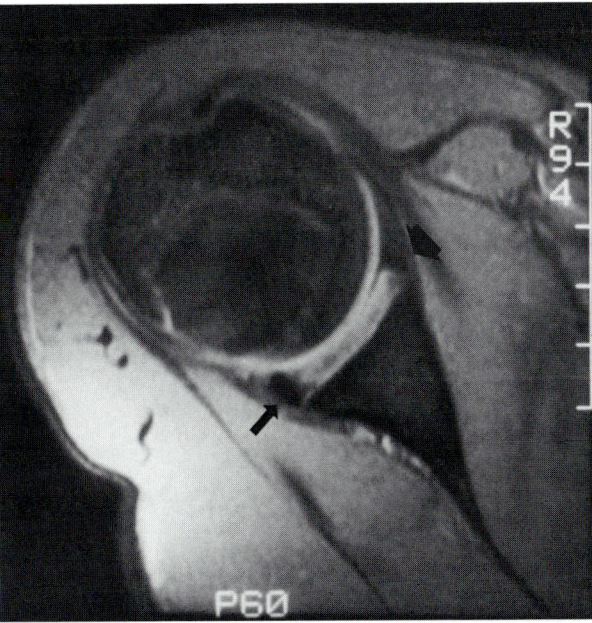

Fig. 3 Magnetic resonance image in 30° coronal oblique plane, demonstrating normal low signal of the supraspinatus tendon (arrowhead). This study was performed in a normal 20-year-old individual.

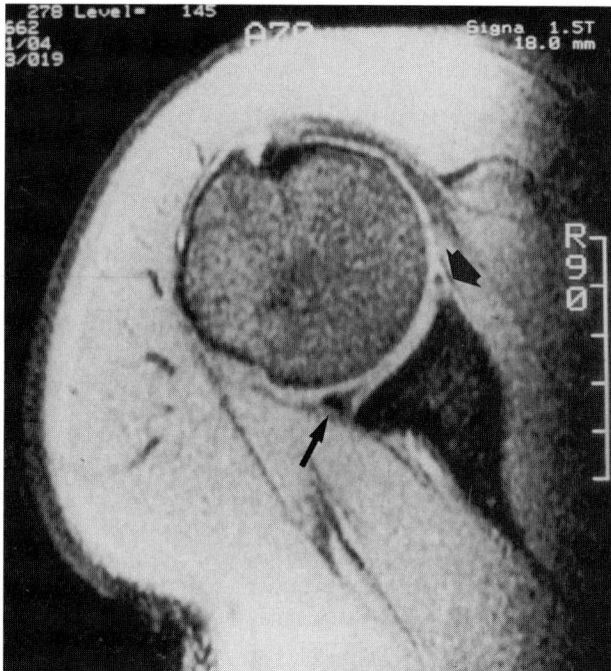

Fig. 4 Magnetic resonance image in 30° coronal oblique plane, demonstrating increased signal intensity of the rotator cuff tendon consistent with asymptomatic degeneration. This study was performed in a normal 45-year-old male athletic.

calized muscle fatigue and high activity in the supraspinatus muscle associated with keeping the arm in an elevated position for a prolonged period. Intramuscular pressure recordings are elevated for the trapezius and deltoid, but not to the level of the supraspinatus and infraspinatus muscles. The work of Jarvholm suggests that prolonged work with the arms elevated will lead to increased intramuscular pressure, which could impede muscle blood flow, resulting in muscle fatigue.[50] Measures to increase local blood flow and to avoid critical amounts of intramuscular pressure warrant further investigation and may aid in the prevention of this syndrome. Enrolling at-risk employees in supervised muscle-strengthening programs may aid in the prevention of this disorder if such programs are initiated prior to the onset of repetitive loading. We are unaware of any controlled studies in which this has been demonstrated to be effective.

A review of the literature did not reveal any studies examining the interrelationship between myalgia and aging.

Degeneration of the Acromioclavicular Joint

Degenerative arthritis of the acromioclavicular joint is a well-recognized entity, but its relationship to overuse and its role in producing shoulder-related disability is unclear. From DePalma's classic work it is known that there is an age-related degenerative change in the acromioclavicular joint beginning in the second decade of life.[51,52] Petersson[52] also observed an age-related narrowing of the acromioclavicular joint space.

The degenerative changes of the acromioclavicular joint are most prominent on the inferior margin of the clavicular side. These changes include marginal bone erosion, which is thought to be secondary to a synovial hyperplasia following entrapment of the synovium with continued use.[53] Petersson followed up his radiologic studies by defining the anatomic basis of the narrowing of the acromioclavicular joint. He described a gradual disintegration of the joint cartilage and disk. The peak incidence of cartilage changes occurs after age 60. The pathologic changes can be correlated with variations in the acromioclavicular fibrocartilaginous disk.[52]

There are two types of disks as described by DePalma[51] and cited by Petersson[52]: the complete disk and the meniscoid disk. Petersson believes that the meniscoid disk is the consequence of regressive changes in a complete disk. He bases this on histologic analysis of meniscoid disks, which consistently revealed signs of degeneration, even in young patients. The joint cartilages were routinely normal in patients with complete disks even if the patients were of advanced age. Petersson concluded from his studies that a gradual deterioration of the acromioclavicular joint is part of the normal aging process and usually not associated with pain or discomfort.

The acromioclavicular disk as described by DePalma and Petersson can be thought of as an anatomic "shock absorber." Others argue that the disk is usually a rather thin structure that provides little protection to the cartilage.[54] It may be reasonable to hypothesize that with overuse this anatomic protection against cartilage wear may undergo an accelerated degeneration.

The most important feature that merits discussion of acromioclavicular joint disease in this chapter is its direct contact with the subacromial bursa and underlying rotator cuff. Degenerative changes of the acromioclavicular joint that appear to be a normal part of the aging process can lead to inflammation and osteophyte formation, which may produce secondary symptoms of subacromial bursitis and rotator cuff tendinitis with consistent use.

In their study of patients with nontraumatic degeneration of the acromioclavicular joint, Worcester and Green[54] found no relation to occupation or heavy labor; however, the patient group was not random.

Posttraumatic osteolysis of the clavicle is known to occur following severe injury. Nontraumatic osteolysis of the distal clavicle associated with overuse is less commonly reported but has been increasingly recognized in the athletic population. Ehricht[55] first reported distal clavicular osteolysis as an overuse injury in an air hammer operator in 1952. Since then, prospective studies have sought to better define the incidence of this overuse syndrome. Twenty-eight percent of elite weightlifters had radiographic evidence of clavicular osteolysis, compared with 0% in a control population in one study.[56] The radiographic findings are similar to those of posttraumatic osteolysis and consist of loss of subchondral bone detail, translucency, and cystic changes in the clavicular bone.[56] Like almost all classic overuse syndromes, symptoms decrease or resolve with cessation of activity. In this case, rest leads to a reparative stage that halts the degeneration of the bone and smoothes the distal clavicle, but degeneration of the clavicle and the associated pain return with resumption of weightlifting. Scavenius described a subset of these patients with the symptoms of nontraumatic distal clavicular osteolysis without radiographic evidence of the syndrome. These patients tended to be younger and had been weight training for fewer years.[56]

In summary, the evidence seems to indicate that acromioclavicular degeneration is a disease of aging. However, once established, repetitive use can lead

Glenohumeral Arthritis

Glenohumeral arthritis does not seem to fit the classic definition of an overuse syndrome. Degenerative changes of the glenohumeral joint most commonly occur following either traumatic injury or alteration in articular mechanics as a result of a pathologic condition.[22] Mow and associates[57] have reported increased joint contact area with overhead elevation of the upper extremity. This suggests that prolonged activity with the arm in the overhead position may lead to accelerated degeneration of the glenohumeral articulation, but there is no hard evidence to support this. The only evidence we were able to find in the literature implicating overuse as the etiology of glenohumeral disease was in the case of a wheelchair-dependent paraplegic patient who developed bilateral osteonecrosis of the humeral heads without any evidence of disease or medical treatment associated with osteonecrosis.[58]

In summary, the literature to date supports the classification of glenohumeral arthritis only as a posttraumatic disease or as the sequela of a pathologic process that alters joint mechanics. Overuse does not seem to affect the glenohumeral bony articulation as long as normal joint mechanics are preserved.

References

1. DePalma AF, Callery G, Bennett GA: Variational anatomy and degenerative lesions of the shoulder joint, in DePalma AF (ed): *Surgery of the Shoulder,* ed 2. Philadelphia, PA, JB Lippincott, 1973, pp 235–271.
2. Cooper DE, Arnoczky SP, O'Brien SJ, et al: Anatomy, histology and vascularity of the glenoid labrum: An anatomical study. *J Bone Joint Surg* 1992;74A:46–52.
3. Andrews JR, Kupferman SP, Dillman CJ: Labral tears in throwing and racquet sports. *Clin Sports Med* 1991;10:901–911.
4. Warner JP, Deng X, Warren RF, et al: Static capsuloligamentous restraints to superior-inferior translation of the glenohumeral joint. *Am J Sports Med* 1992;20:675–685.
5. Turkel SJ, Panio MW, Marshall JL, et al: Stabilizing mechanisms preventing anterior dislocation of the glenohumeral joint. *J Bone Joint Surg* 1981;63A:1208–1217.
6. Bigliani LU, Pollock RG, Soslowsky LJ, et al: Tensile properties of the inferior glenohumeral ligament. *J Orthop Res* 1992;10:187–197.
7. Stenlund B, Goldie I, Hagberg M, et al: Shoulder tendinitis and its relation to heavy manual work and exposure to vibration. *Scand J Work Environ Health* 1993:1:43–49.
8. Andrews JR, Carson WG Jr, McLeod WD: Glenoid labrum tears related to the long head of the biceps. *Am J Sports Med* 1985;13:337–341.
9. Ciullo JV, Stevens GG: The prevention and treatment of injuries to the shoulder in swimming. *Sports Med* 1989;7:182–204.
10. Pink M, Jobe FW, Perry J: Electromyographic analysis of the shoulder during the golf swing. *Am J Sports Med* 1990;18:137–140.
11. Renstrom P: Sports traumatology today. *Ann Chirugiae et Gynaecol* 1991;80:81–93.
12. Collins K, Wagner M, Peterson K, et al: Overuse injuries in triathletes: A study of the 1986 Seafair Triathlon. *Am J Sports Med* 1989;17:675–680.
13. Snyder SJ, Karzel RP, Del Pizzo W, et al: SLAP lesions of the shoulder. *Arthroscopy* 1990;6:274–279.
14. Rowe CR, Zarins B: Recurrent transient subluxation of the shoulder. *J Bone Joint Surg* 1981:63A:863–872.

15. Rowe CR: Recurrent transient anterior subluxation of the shoulder: The "dead arm" syndrome. *Clin Orthop* 1987;223:11–19.
16. Kvitne RS, Jobe FW: The diagnosis and treatment of anterior instability in the throwing athlete. *Clin Orthop* 1993;291:107–123.
17. Howell SM, Galinat BJ, Renzi AJ, et al: Normal and abnormal mechanics of the glenohumeral joint in the horizontal plane. *J Bone Joint Surg* 1988;70A:227–232.
18. Cain PR, Mutschler TA, Fu FH, et al: Anterior stability of the glenohumeral joint: A dynamic model. *Am J Sports Med* 1987;15:144–148.
19. Jobe FW, Moynes DR, Tibone JE, et al: An EMG analysis of the shoulder in pitching: A second report. *Am J Sports Med* 1984;12:218–220.
20. Glousman R, Jobe F, Tibone J, et al: Dynamic electromyographic analysis of the throwing shoulder with glenohumeral instability. *J Bone Joint Surg* 1988;70A: 220–226.
21. Fu FH, Harner CD, Klein AH: Shoulder impingement syndrome: A critical review. *Clin Orthop* 1991;269:162–173.
22. Soslowsky LJ, Flatow EL, Bigliani LU, et al: Quantitation of in situ contact areas at the glenohumeral joint: A biomechanical study. *J Orthop Res* 1992;10:524–534.
23. Reeves B: Experiments on the tensile strength of the anterior capsular structures of the shoulder in man. *J Bone Joint Surg* 1968;50B:858–865.
24. Uhthoff HK, Sarkar K: The effect of aging on the soft tissues of the shoulder, in Matsen FA, Fu FH, Hawkins RJ (eds): *The Shoulder: A Balance of Mobility and Stability*. Rosemont, IL, American Academy of Orthopaedic Surgeons, 1993, pp 269–278.
25. Matsen FA III, Arntz CT: Subacromial impingement, in Rockwood CA, Matsen FA III (ed): *The Shoulder*. Philadelphia, PA, WB Saunders, 1990, p 623–646.
26. Neer CS II: Cuff tears, biceps, lesions and impingement, in Neer CS II (ed): *Shoulder Reconstruction*. Philadelphia, PA, WB Saunders, 1990, pp 73–77.
27. Neer CS II: Impingement lesions. *Clin Orthop* 1983;173:70–77.
28. Ozaki J, Fujimoto S, Nakagawa Y, et al: Tears of the rotator cuff of the shoulder associated with pathological changes in the acromion: A study on cadavers. *J Bone Joint Surg* 1988;70A:1224–1230.
29. Sher J, Uribe JW, Posada A, et al: Abnormal findings on magnetic resonance images of asymptomatic shoulders. *J Bone Joint Surg* 1995;77A:10–15.
30. Uhthoff HK, Sarkar K, Lohr J: Repair in rotator cuff tendons, in Post M, Morrey BF, Hawkins RJ (eds): *Surgery of the Shoulder*. St Louis, MO, Mosby-Year Book, 1990, pp 216–219.
31. Wilson CL, Duff GL: Pathologic study of degeneration and rupture of the supraspinatus tendon. *Arch Surg* 1943;47:121–135.
32. Fukuda H, Hamada K, Yamanaka K: Pathology and pathogenesis of bursal-side rotator cuff tears viewed from en bloc histologic sections. *Clin Orthop* 1990;254:75–80.
33. Codman EA, Akerson IB: The pathology associated with rupture of the supraspinatus tendon. *Ann Surg* 1931;93:354–359.
34. Brewer BJ: Aging of the rotator cuff. *Am J Sports Med* 1979;7:102–110.
35. Codman EA: The pathology of the subacromial bursa and the supraspinatus tendon, in Codman EA (ed): *The Shoulder: Rupture of the Supraspinatus Tendon and Other Lesions in or About the Subacromial Bursa*, supplemental edition. Malabar, FL, RE Kreiger, 1934, pp 65–107.
36. Chansky HA, Iannotti JP: The vascularity of the rotator cuff. *Clin Sports Med* 1991; 10:807–822.
37. Bigliani LU, Ticker JB, Flatow EL, et al: The relationship of acromial architecture to rotator cuff disease. *Clin Sports Med* 1991;10:823–838.
38. Rathbun JB, Macnab I: The microvascular pattern of the rotator cuff. *J Bone Joint Surg* 1970;52B:540–553.
39. Swiontkowski MF, Iannotti JP, Esterhai JL, et al: Abstract: Intraoperative assessment of rotator cuff vascularity using laser Doppler flowmetry. *Orthop Trans* 1989;13:508.

40. Hawkins RJ, Abrams JS: Impingement syndrome in the absence of rotator cuff tear (stages 1 and 2). *Orthop Clin North Am* 1987;18:373–382.
41. Silliman JF, Hawkins RJ: Current concepts and recent advances in the athlete's shoulder. *Clin Sports Med* 1991;10:693–705.
42. Hawkins RJ, Kennedy JC: Impingement syndrome in athletes. *Am J Sports Med* 1980:8:151–158.
43. Jobe FW: Impingement and instability in the athlete, in Rockwood CA Jr, Matsen FA III (eds): *The Shoulder*. Philadelphia, PA, WB Saunders, 1990, pp 963–982.
44. Wadley GH, Albright JP: Women's intercollegiate gymnastics: Injury patterns and "permanent" medical disability. *Am J Sports Med* 1993;21:314–320.
45. Gellman H, Sie I, Waters RL: Late complications of the weight-bearing upper extremity in the paraplegic patient. *Clin Orthop* 1988;233:132–135.
46. Bayley JC, Cochran TP, Sledge CB: The weight-bearing shoulder: The impingement syndrome in paraplegics. *J Bone Joint Surg* 1987;69B:676–678.
47. Pettersson G: Rupture of the tendon aponeurosis of the shoulder joint in anterior inferior dislocation. *Acta Chir Scand* 1942;77(suppl):1–184.
48. Larsson S, Bodegard L, Henriksson KG, et al: Chronic trapezius myalgia: Morphology and blood flow studied in 17 patients. *Acta Orthop Scand* 1990;61:394–398.
49. Mathiassen SE, Winkel J, Sahlin K, et al: Biochemical indicators of hazardous shoulder-neck loads in light industry. *J Occup Med* 1993;35:404–407.
50. Jarvholm U, Palmerud G, Karlsson D, et al: Intramuscular pressure and electromyography in four shoulder muscles. *J Orthop Res* 1991;9:609–619.
51. DePalma AJ: Degenerative changes in the sternoclavicular and acromioclavicular joints in varous decades, in *Surgery of the Shoulder*. Philadelphia, PA, JB Lippincott, 1957, pp 52–108.
52. Petersson CJ: Degeneration of the acromioclavicular joint. *Acta Orthop Scand* 1983;54:434–438.
53. Bullough PG: Pathology and pathogenesis of osteoarthritis, in Matsen FA III, Fu FH, Hawkins RJ (eds): *The Shoulder: A Balance of Mobility and Stability*. Rosemont, IL, American Academy of Orthopaedic Surgeons, 1993, pp 229–237.
54. Worcester JN, Green DP: Osteoarthritis of the acromioclavicular joint. *Clin Orthop* 1968;58:69–73.
55. Ehricht HG: Die ostedys in luteralen llavrulnende nach pressluffs chaden. *Arch Orthop Unfallchir* 1959;50:576–582.
56. Scavenius M, Iversen BF: Nontraumatic clavicular osteolysis in weight lifters. *Am J Sports Med* 1992;20:463–467.
57. Mow VC, Ateshian GA, Spilker AL: Biomechanics of diarthrodial joints: A review of twenty years of progress. *J Biomech Eng* 1993;115:460–467.
58. Barber DB, Gall NG: Osteonecrosis: An overuse injury of the shoulder in paraplegia. Case report. *Paraplegia* 1991;29:423–426.

Chapter 35
Cervicobrachial Disorders

Sidney J. Blair, MD, FACS

This chapter discusses painful disorders of the cervicobrachial region. These disorders are characterized by local pain and discomfort resulting from cumulative trauma in the cervical and shoulder regions. Frequently these disorders are associated with referral patterns to the extremity or to the head region. Signs and symptoms of the various conditions overlap, and ideas about their etiology and treatment are evolving and controversial. This discussion includes the classification, signs, symptoms, physical findings, and treatment of cervicobrachial disorders. Their epidemiology and rehabilitation are discussed in other chapters.

Nerve and Vascular Disorders

Cervical Radiculopathy Secondary to Cervical Spondylosis and Disk Herniation

This is a condition in which the cervical spine tissue progressively degenerates.[1] Degeneration starts in intervertebral disks and subsequently affects the adjacent osseous structures.

The symptoms of cervical spondylosis are insidious and begin gradually. Acute symptoms may occur in patients who previously had asymptomatic cervical spondylosis. Lestini and Wiesel[2] divided the symptoms into five groups: (1) neck pain, (2) headaches, (3) radicular symptoms, (4) spinal cord symptoms, and (5) symptoms of vertebral vascular ischemia. Radicular symptoms and signs will be the focus of this discussion.

Neck pain is usually somewhat mild, occasionally severe, aggravated by activity, worse in the morning, and associated with stiffness with varying degrees of restriction of cervical motion. About 50% of cervical rotation occurs between the atlas and the axis, and is rarely involved in this process.

Radicular symptoms include pain, weakness, and sensory disturbances in the area supplied by the involved nerves. The nerves are compressed by a combination of factors, which include hypertrophic changes and sometimes the extrusion of some intervertebral disk material.

The radicular symptoms are insidious; disability occurs over months or even years. Patients complain of weakness and difficulty with using their hands, as well as dysesthesias and numbness. The signs and symptoms vary and involve sensory changes, motor weakness, and pain. Examinations should include a range of motion of the cervical spine and a replication of pain that is initiated by the patient's active motion. Sensory examination should include light touch, pinprick, or cotton; muscle testing; and testing of deep-tendon reflex changes. Determining precise levels of involvement may be possible using myelography, magnetic resonance imaging (MRI), computed tomography (CT), and electromyography (EMG).

The more common presentations include involvement of the C6 level. Patients complain of pain and numbness in the distribution of the thumb and index finger, with sensory loss in the area. Patients experience weakness of the biceps and wrist extension, and some have reflex loss of the biceps and triceps.

Trauma at the C8 level produces pain and numbness in the distribution of the inner arm, ring finger, and middle finger, with sensory loss in those areas and weakness of the intrinsics. Nonsurgical care includes treatment with a soft collar, mild analgesia, gentle heat, and/or traction for muscle spasm. Surgical management to relieve pressure on the spinal cord and roots can be accomplished by a wide laminectomy or anterior decompression and foraminotomy. Surgical decompression relates to progression of neurologic symptoms.

Thoracic Outlet Syndrome

Neurologic Thoracic Outlet Syndrome The constellation of symptoms characteristic of this syndrome results from the compression of the brachial plexus in the thoracic outlet.[3,4] Thoracic outlet is defined as an area bordered by the first rib, the anterior scalene, and the medial scalene. Narrowing of this outlet can compress the brachial plexus and the brachial artery.

Pain is usually located about the shoulder and the inner aspect of the arm. It is described as burning and is usually worse at night. Paresthesia and numbness are reported in the C8-T1 distribution and can extend along the ulnar border of the forearm and upper arm. Patients complain of fatigue, weakness, and an inability to carry out fine tasks because of a loss of stamina, and there is evidence of wasting of the intrinsic muscles. Physical examination reveals sensory loss in the ulnar distribution of the arm with extension to the forearm and arm. Motor weakness of the intrinsics is detected by active muscle testing.

One of the more reliable tests for diagnosis is a 90° abduction/external rotation of the shoulder. The shoulder should be straight with the elbow, and the elbow flexed to 90°. Many clinicians have abandoned the Adson test. Compression and provocative testing can also be performed.[5] Radiographs, MRI, and CT scans may show a rudimentary cervical rib and an elongated C7 process. Most patients with neurologic thoracic outlet syndrome are treated nonsurgically with exercises, muscle relaxation, and posture reeducation. If there is a rudimentary cervical rib, excision of this process should be performed. At first, rib resection appears to be the procedure of choice for decompression of the thoracic outlet; however, this is a procedure of last resort, and nonsurgical treatment is recommended for the majority of patients.

Arterial Vascular Thoracic Outlet Syndrome (Major) This syndrome is secondary to cervical rib compression, which may be caused by a hypoplastic rib, an elongated C7 transverse process, and an anomalous first thoracic rib. Signs and symptoms include ischemia in the distal extremity and ulceration of the fingers caused by arterial embolization, pain, numbness, cyanosis, major tissue loss, and persistent, unilateral Raynaud's syndrome. Diagnosis is made by palpation for vascular prominence and auscultation for bruits. The pulse should also be checked. Noninvasive vascular examinations should include B mode ultrasound vascular imaging and a Doppler blood flow. Photoplethysmographic tracings should be performed; if these are abnormal, a subclavian arteriogram should be obtained. This disorder is treated by resectioning the abnormal bony structure and repairing the aneurysm with a graft.

Arterial Vascular Thoracic Outlet Syndrome (Minor) This condition is also known as a subcoracoid-pectoralis minor syndrome and has been named the hyperabduction syndrome by Wright.[6] Symptoms and signs include minor elevation of arms associated with obliteration of the pulses, tingling, numbness, and weakness of the arm. The condition is associated with occupations that require arms to be elevated. Treatment stresses the importance of postures that allow arms to be elevated; surgery is indicated only for occupational convenience.

Venous Vascular Thoracic Outlet Syndrome (Effort Thrombosis) This is a nonepisodic condition characterized by spontaneous thrombosis of the subclavian artery and axillary vein. The syndrome is most common in young persons engaged in repetitive vigorous physical activity. Signs and symptoms include arm pain, cyanosis, and swelling. Exercise frequently induces fatigue. The onset of symptoms is sudden, and there is swelling, cyanosis, and dilation of chest and shoulder veins. Thrombosed veins can be seen when palpated. A diagnosis is facilitated with upper extremity phlebography. Treatment includes arm elevation, anticoagulation and thrombolytic therapy, and resection of the first rib.

Double-Crush and Multiple Compression Neuropathy

The double-crush syndrome is characterized by a compression lesion along the course of a single nerve.[7,8] Upton and McComas[9] named the syndrome in 1973 and suggested that proximal compression of a nerve essentially changes its distal portion by lessening its ability to withstand increased distal compression.

Double-Crush Nerve Compression in Thoracic Outlet Syndrome Wood and Biondi[10] studied cases of thoracic outlet syndrome in which the first rib had to be resected. Forty-four percent of the patients had compression of the nerve distally. The most common site of secondary compression was the carpal tunnel.

Cervical Radiculopathy and Carpal Tunnel Syndrome Neck stiffness and radiating arm pain occurs with cervical radiculopathy. In addition, patients experience numbness and tingling in the median nerve distribution as well as thenar atrophy. Fifteen percent of patients with carpal tunnel syndrome complained of pain in the shoulder and neck region.[11] Weakness is another overlapping symptom seen in 20% of carpal tunnel patients.[12] Such patients complain of loss of dexterity and clumsiness. Weakness associated with cervical radiculopathy tends to be related to grasp rather than pinch.

Cervical Radiculopathy and Radial Tunnel Syndrome Osterman[12] conducted a prospective study with refractory lateral epicondolytis and reported that 27% of the patients had electrically proven cervical radiculopathy and 23% had radial tunnel syndrome. Most patients responded to conservative care. Radial tunnel syndrome is defined as a pain syndrome caused by compression of the motor branch of the radial nerve. There is no sensory disturbance, motor loss, or predictable electrophysiologic change.

Muscle Disorders

Tension Neck Syndrome

Tension neck syndrome,[13–15] also called occupational cramp or myalgia, is one of the most common neck and shoulder complaints.[16] This syndrome has a variety of symptoms, such as pain, tenderness and stiffness of muscle, and muscle spasm. Chronic abnormalities of posture is an important etiologic factor. Mannheimer[17] has discussed the major effects of prolonged forward head posture.

Myofascial Pain Syndrome

This is a painful condition in which definite areas generally within muscles or fascia become abnormally active and tend to produce either local or referred pain.[18,19] This condition is characterized by myofascial trigger points, which are defined as hyperexcitable fasciae in the muscles or fascia. The most prominent feature of this syndrome is pain. Patients complain of stiffness (usually in the morning), fatigue, decreased range of motion, and increased sensitivity to cold. In addition, patients sometimes experience depression and disturbed sleep patterns. Soft trigger points have been classified as either active or latent; active trigger points cause referred pain elsewhere in the body. The muscle may demonstrate decreased range of motion and reduced strength. Sometimes there is a referred autonomic phenomenon. A latent trigger point, when present, may show muscular evidence of those changes, but only when there is a local twitch response.

The patient's history reveals an initiating event in the formation of the trigger points, such as an acute strain caused by sudden overloading or an overstretched muscle. It is thought that, once activated, a trigger point can be self-perpetuating. It has been postulated that changes such as muscle tension and vasoconstriction can produce local ischemia or increased vascular permeability, which can cause derangement of the extracellular environment with a resultant increase in sensitivity of the nociceptive elements. The release of mediators such as bradykinin and prostaglandins can cause an increase in sympathetic activity.

After the trigger points have been identified, the patient can be treated by injecting these areas with anesthetic agents. Muscles that contain taut fibers can be recognized as a palpable band that tightens and shortens the muscle. Range of motion and strength decrease. The examiner can elicit a twitch response by rolling his or her fingers over the tight band. A physical therapy program of stretching and strengthening follows treatment of the trigger points.

Multiple Tissue Disorders

Multiple tissue disorders are characterized by involvement of musculoskeletal and neurovascular tissues. Symptoms may be chronic and may be attended by psychologic symptoms.

Refractory Cervicobrachial Pain Syndrome

Cohen and associates[20] in Australia first used the term refractory cervicobrachial pain syndrome to describe the common symptoms of a group of 1,000 patients. The group consisted predominantly of women between 20 and 50 years of age who worked primarily as manual process workers. Their symptoms appeared to develop progressively over periods of time ranging from several months to 5 years. About a quarter of the patients were bilaterally affected. Patients often felt persistent pain locally, which later spread into the neck, pectoral girdle, and arms. Other common symptoms included a deep burning sensation accompanied by hyperpathia, cramping, loss of muscle strength, and vasomotor abnormalities. Examination revealed hypesthesia of the painful limb with allodynia, hyperalgesia of the muscles and joints, sensitivity of the peripheral nerves, abnormal vasomotor and pseudomotor phenomena, and impaired motor function. The patients often showed an antalgic attitude of the affected upper limb with half flexion of the elbow, wrist, and fingers. Commonly, the patients lacked spontaneous movement, had difficulty performing fine movements, and experienced rapid fatigue, spasm, and cramps—all suggesting a dystonic phenomenon.

Dysesthesia was induced by an examination with touch pinprick, two-point discrimination, and vibration intensity. Some of the patients showed clinical signs suggestive of a sympathetic dystrophy and exhibited swelling, unilateral cold, sweating, and blue discoloration.

The results of laboratory investigations were essentially normal. The majority of patients showed changes in anxiety and depression levels that were more marked when painful symptoms had persisted for a long time. Treatment consisted of medication (including analgesics), antidepressant drugs, relaxation, and psychologic programs. In the pathophysiology of this disorder, Cohen and associates[20] hypothesized that there is a central disturbance at nociception induced by a continual afferent barrage from nociceptors in anatomically relevant sites of the neck and upper limb.

Occupational Cervicobrachial Disorders

In 1958, the Japanese first used the term occupational cervicobrachial syndrome.[21,22] In 1972, this syndrome was established by the Japanese Association of Industrial Health as a symptom complex of involuntary pain in the neck and shoulder area. It was found to affect keyboard operators, telephone operators, typists, and others performing repetitive tasks.

This syndrome was subsequently recognized as a new occupational disorder that results from a combination of technological change and increased working speed. Automated activities in the work place relieved physical workloads; the elevated rate of work, however, concentrated the workload in the arm, neck, and shoulder. Mental stress was increased because these monotonous tasks required attention and patience.

The various factors that seemed to cause a problem were (1) a dynamic fraction in repetitive activity; (2) a static fraction; (3) uncomfortable working posture; (4) mental stress from high-speed working; and (5) environmental factors such as noise and low temperature.

In the 1960s when prevalence studies were done, no specific diagnoses were given; more recently, however, diagnoses have been more specific.

Stage I is characterized mainly by subjective symptoms, not necessarily limited to the region of the neck, shoulder, and arm, but without obvious objective findings.

Stage II, in addition to containing the symptoms of stage I, involves muscular induration and/or muscular tenderness in the region of the neck, shoulder, and arm.

Stage III adds some of the following symptoms to those of stage II: (1) increase of the intensity or the extent of muscular induration and/or muscular tenderness; (2) positive neurologic signs; (3) sensory disturbance; (4) decrease of muscle power; (5) percussion pain over the spinal processes; (6) tenderness over the paravertebral region; (7) tenderness along the nerve branch; (8) tremor of the fingers or eyelids; (9) motor disturbance of the neck, shoulder, hand, etc; (10) impairment of peripheral circulatory function; and (11) more severe subjective complaints.

Stage IV adds to the symptoms of stage III a more advanced sensory disturbance. For example, decreased muscle power increases the number of positive neurologic signs. Furthermore, the following specific manifestations may develop subsequent to stage I or II, not necessarily passing through stage III: (1) organic disturbances such as tenosynovitis, tendinitis, or peritendonitis; (2) symptom complex compatible with the cervicobrachial syndrome in orthopaedics; (3) autonomic nervous disturbance (such as Raynaud's phenomenon, blood congestion, equilibrium disturbance, cardia neurosis, etc); and (4) mental symptoms such as emotional instability, difficulty concentrating, sleep disturbance, thinking disturbance, and depression.

Stage V is characterized by worsening of stage IV symptoms so as to obviously disturb not only work but also daily life activities.

The Frozen Shoulder Syndrome and Reflex Sympathetic Dystrophy

Some patients with occupational cervicobrachial disorders present with painful shoulder problems that can be suggestive of frozen shoulder syndrome, adhesive capsulitis, and shoulder-hand syndrome.[5,7,8,12,23,24] Frozen shoulder is a term used to define a clinical syndrome in which the patient has a restricted range of passive and active motion. Patients usually complain of pain that worsens at night and stiffness of the shoulder. A complete physical examination is necessary to rule out other causes of shoulder pain. The sternoclavicular and acromioclavicular joints must be examined. Passive forward elevation and external rotation, active forward elevation, and active internal rotation are measured and muscle strengths should be tested. Radiographs and MRI of the shoulder should be done. Adhesive capsulitis is considered to be a subset of frozen shoulder. There is a contracted, thickened joint capsule that is tightly drawn about the humeral head, with an absence of synovial fluid.

Reflex sympathetic dystrophy, also called shoulder-hand syndrome when limited to the upper extremity,[24] is characterized by diffused swelling, exquisite tenderness, and basal motor changes in the hands and digits of the same extremity as well as the shoulder. Radiographs may reveal a polar osteoporosis of the proximal humeral head. Treatment of the reflex sympathetic dystrophy consists of exercise, pain control, mobilization techniques, and local injections. If these treatments are not successful, mobilization and surgical treatment may be indicated to free up the adhesions.

Pain Dysfunction Syndrome

According to Dobyns,[25] pain dysfunction syndrome "would include all objective and subjective discomfort and all objective and subjective abnormalities of function that afflict the neurovascular and musculoskeletal system." Amadio[26] has discussed the four aspects of pain dysfunction syndrome: local triggers, psychologic factors, systemic factors, and reflex sympathetic dystrophy.

The multiple cervicobrachial disorders show evidence of some autonomic disturbance suggestive of reflex sympathetic dystrophy.[3] Recently, Veldman and associates[27] suggested that the symptoms of reflex sympathetic dystrophy should be considered to be an exaggerated regional inflammatory response rather than a sympathetic disorder.

Neuropeptide studies were conducted on patients at Loyola University Medical Center in Chicago.[16] These patients had symptoms of swelling, stiffness, and pain secondary to cumulative trauma disorders of the upper extremities. Bradykinin and calcitonin gene-related peptide levels were elevated in patients

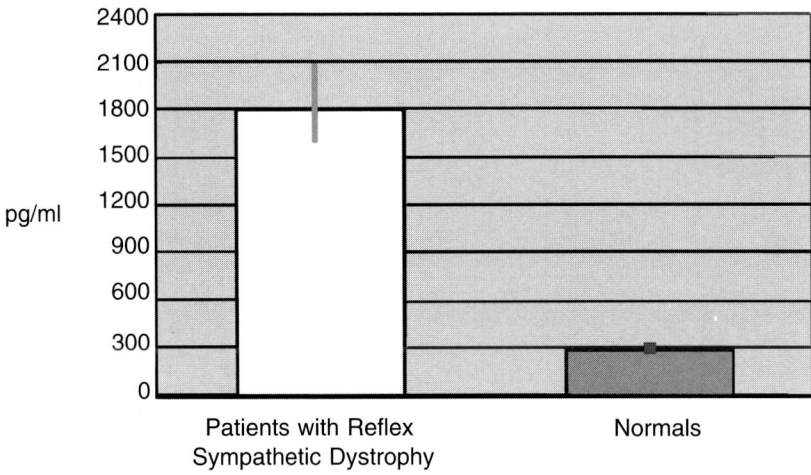

Fig. 1 Bradykinin levels in patients with reflex sympathetic dystrophy.

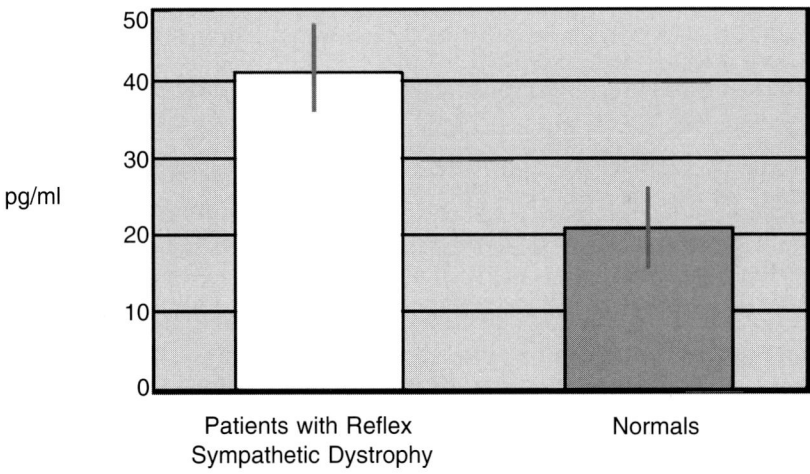

Fig. 2 Calcitonin gene-related peptide in patients with reflex sympathetic dystrophy.

with reflex sympathetic dystrophy, suggesting an inflammatory mechanism to account for the symptoms and signs. Figures 1 and 2 show the levels of bradykinin and calcitonin gene-related peptide in these patients.

Summary

The purpose of this discussion on cervicobrachial disorders was to show various conditions and clinical presentation as well as treatment. As the symptoms increase in severity, patients have multiple tissue involvement and an increase in autonomic symptoms. These signs and symptoms resemble those in patients with reflex sympathetic dystrophy. Neuropeptide studies were performed on a group of patients who complained of chronic pain, swelling, and stiffness of the upper extremities. Bradykinin and calcitonin gene-related peptide were found to be increased in these patients. The significance of these studies is yet to be clarified; however, this type of study might help provide some insight into the pathophysiology of the cumulative trauma disorders.

References

1. Batzdorf V: Spine: Spinal segmental pain and sensory disturbances, in Wiener MA (ed): *Spine and State of the Art Reviews*. Philadelphia, PA, Hanley and Belfus, 1988, pp 565–583.
2. Lestini WF, Wiesel SW: Pathogenesis of cervical spondylosis. *Clin Orthop* 1989;239: 69–93.
3. Sanders RJ: *Thoracic Outlet Syndrome*. Philadelphia, PA, JB Lippincott, 1991.
4. Wilbourn AJ, Porter JM: Thoracic outlet syndromes, in Wiener MA (ed): *Spine and State of the Art Reviews*. Philadelphia, PA, Hanley and Belfus, 1988, pp 597–626.
5. Novak CB, Mackinnon SE, Patterson GA: Evaluation of patients with thoracic outlet syndrome. *J Hand Surg* 1993;18A:292–299.
6. Wright IS: The neurovascular syndrome produced by hyperabduction of the arms. *Am Heart J* 1945;29:1–19.
7. Neviaser TJ: Adhesive capsulitis. *Orthop Clin North Am* 1987;18:439–443.
8. Rizk TE, Pinals RS: Frozen shoulder. *Semin Arthritis Rheum* 1982;11:440–452.
9. Upton A, McComas AS: The double crush nerve entrapment and syndrome. *Lancet* 1973;2:359–362.
10. Wood VE, Biondi J: Double crush nerve compression in thoracic-outlet syndrome. *J Bone Joint Surg* 1990;72A:85–87.
11. Crymble B: Brachial neuralgia and carpal tunnel syndrome. *Br Med J* 1968;3:470–471.
12. Osterman AL: Double crush and multiple compression neuropathy, in Gelberman RH (ed): *Operative Nerve Repair and Reconstruction*. Philadelphia, PA, JB Lippincott, 1991, vol 2, pp 1211–1229.
13. Hagberg M: Shoulder pain-pathogenesis, in Hadler NM (ed): *Clinical Concepts in Regional Musculoskeletal Illness*. Orlando, FL, Grune & Stratton Inc, 1987, pp 191–200.
14. Hagberg M: Neck and shoulder disorders, in Rosenstock L, Cullen M (eds): *Textbook of Clinical Occupational and Environmental Medicine*. Philadelphia, PA, WB Saunders, 1994, pp 356–364.
15. Waris P: Occupational cervico brachial syndrome: A review. *Scand J Work Environ Health* 1979;5(suppl 3):3–14.
16. Kijowski R, Hoppensteadt D, Chinthagada M, et al: Abstract: Studies on the role of neuropeptides in the pathogenesis of cumulative trauma disorders. *FASEB J* 1994; 8A:682.
17. Mannheimer JS: Acute and chronic postural abnormalities as related to craniofacial pain third and upper quarter syndromes. *Dental Clin North Am* 1991;35:185–200.
18. Goldenberg DL: Controversies in fibromyalgia and myofascial pain syndrome, in Arnoff GM (ed): *Evaluation and Treatment of Chronic Pain*, ed 2. Baltimore, MD, Williams & Wilkins, 1992, pp 165–175.
19. Simons DG: Myofascial pain syndromes: Where are we? Where are we going? *Arch Phys Med Rehabil* 1988;69:207–212.
20. Cohen ML, Champion GD, Browne CD: In search of the pathogenesis of refractory cervico-brachial pain syndrome. *Med J Aust* 1992;157:358.
21. Maeda K: Occupational cervicobrachial disorder and its causative factors. *J Human Ergol* 1977;6:193–202.
22. Maeda K, Horiguchi S, Hosokawa M: History of the studies on occupational cervico-brachial disorders in Japan and remaining problems. *J Human Ergol* 1982;11:17–29.

23. Murnaghan JP: Frozen shoulder, in Rockwood CA Jr, Matsen FA III (eds): *The Shoulder*. Philadelphia, PA, WB Saunders, 1990, pp 837–862.
24. Wilson PR: Sympathetically maintained pain: Diagnosis, measurement, and efficacy of treatment, in Stanton-Hicks M (ed): *Pain and the Sympathetic Nervous System*. Boston, MA, Kluwer Academic Publishers, 1990, pp 91–123.
25. Dobyns JH: Pain dysfunction syndrome, in Gelberman RH (ed): *Operative Nerve Repair and Reconstruction*. Philadelphia, PA, JB Lippincott, 1991, vol 2, pp 1489–1495.
26. Amadio PC: Pain dysfunction syndromes. *J Bone Joint Surg* 1988;70A:944–949.
27. Veldman PH, Reynen HM, Arntz IE, et al: Signs and symptoms of reflex sympathetic dystrophy: Prospective study of 829 patients. *Lancet* 1993;342:1012–1016.

Chapter 36

Rehabilitation of the Shoulder After Repetitive Motion Injury

Steven A. Stiens, MD
Barry Goldstein, MD, PhD

Introduction

Musculoskeletal problems are extremely common among both healthy and disabled individuals, accounting for three of the five most common types of ambulatory visits to general practitioners in the United States, according to the National Ambulatory Medical Care Survey of Visits to General and Family Practitioners-1975.[1] Undoubtedly, many complaints related to the musculoskeletal system, such as acute shoulder bursitis, low back pain, ankle sprain, and stiff neck might heal without sequelae. However, many complaints do not resolve, resulting in some level of permanent impairment and disability.

It is more difficult to estimate the incidence of musculoskeletal disability and the expected frequency at which musculoskeletal problems result in permanent impairments and subsequent functional problems. Discriminating early intervention may prevent secondary disability. The challenge for the practitioner is to discern the particular need for rehabilitation and develop a treatment program for each case.

Disability and chronic disease are complex societal issues, and the financial costs related to physical impairments are high for both the individual and society. Unsuccessful prevention and limitations in the rehabilitative process can further compound the problem. In 1986, for example, approximately $140 billion in disability benefits were paid out by business and government in the United States. Claims for workers' compensation alone were $26 billion in 1988 and were expected to climb to $90 billion within 10 years. The Social Security Administration estimated that approximately 12% of the working population had disabilities that significantly limited their ability to work. In real numbers, that is approximately 25 million Americans.[2]

The proportion of disability related to musculoskeletal system injury is great.[3] The National Institute of Occupational Safety and Health has recognized employment related musculoskeletal injuries in their list of the ten leading occupational health problems in the United States.[4] With the rising incidence of upper extremity symptoms, the proportion of shoulder illness is expected to rise as well.

Shoulder injuries, once symptomatic, present challenges that confound the patient, trainer, therapist, physician, and employer. The exact cause is often difficult to identify because of the low sensitivity and specificity of diagnostic tests.[5] Further, many treatment approaches do not fully address the injury's effect on the patient's quality of life. This is particularly true for shoulder overuse and degenerative processes.

In response to the increasing demand for comprehensive rehabilitation services, various treatment techniques, equipment, modalities, and means of delivery have been developed in recent years. However, musculoskeletal complaints remain quite common. Shoulder rehabilitative treatment alone currently contributes to as much as 10% of physiotherapists' case loads in primary care settings.[6]

There are a great variety of interventions to choose from in formulating a rehabilitation program for a given patient's shoulder condition. Detailed treatment plans for use in various shoulder injury patient groups have been promoted.[7–10] The only clear consensus is that prevention should be emphasized and rehabilitation should begin early in the illness process. Rehabilitation in clinical practice is typically eclectic, providing multifaceted, unique treatment plans with multiple modalities that are tailored to an individual patient's needs and goals. These unique solutions to particular patient problems are difficult to generalize. To date, controlled clinical modality-specific studies in relatively homogeneous patient groups are sparse to nonexistent because of the lack of uniform treatment and control groups.[6]

This chapter describes a rehabilitative approach for shoulder overuse injuries. To understand musculoskeletal rehabilitation and apply it to the shoulder, a few general definitions and concepts warrant review.

Rehabilitation Defined

Rehabilitation is an interdisciplinary process (Outline 1) that attempts to "make people able again" by limiting the effects of a shoulder injury on the patient's life activities and self-determination. The objective of the rehabilitative treatment is to eliminate the injury process in the shoulder and minimize shoulder impairment, disability, and handicap (Fig. 1). The injury process directly affects the tissues and, therefore, the physiology of the shoulder thus resulting in dysfunctions at the organ level called impairments. The World Health Organization[11] has defined impairments as any loss or abnormality of psycho-

Outline 1 Interdisciplinary shoulder rehabilitation team

Patient

Family

Physicians

Physical therapist

Occupational therapist

Athletic trainer

Vocational specialist

Employer

Psychologist

Social worker

Recreation therapist

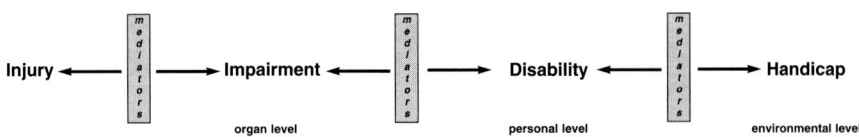

Fig. 1 Relationship of shoulder illness to impairment, disability, and handicap. The interaction of the illness process and the shoulder results in organ-level dysfunctions called impairments. Shoulder impairments interact with all the physical and psychologic characteristics at the personal level to produce task-based dysfunction or disability. Impairments and disabilities interact with the environment to produce handicaps—social or physical environment-related disadvantages resulting from impairments or disabilities that limit an individual's role performance. Mediators are characteristics that allow for compensation to limit the severity of impairments, disabilities, and handicaps.

logic, physiologic, or anatomic structure or function. Because many impairments cannot be fully corrected, personal limitations result due to the person's inability to perform specific tasks. A disability is thus a deficit at the personal level (physical or psychologic characteristics), which prevents the successful completion of a task or activity. A handicap is defined by the interaction between the person (with requisite impairments and disabilities) and the environment. The characteristics of the environment that would contribute to a handicap after a shoulder injury might include height of objects on shelves, weights of items, and attitudes of others regarding the person's disability. All of these factors contribute to the social disadvantage experienced by the person with a shoulder injury that limits full participation in society (Fig. 2).[12] Consequently, for a rehabilitation program to succeed, not only must the site of pathology be treated, but also the subsequent impairments, disabilities, and handicaps. The current approach to rehabilitation of shoulder problems is summarized in Figure 3.

Complex rehabilitation efforts are typically interdisciplinary, involving a variety of professionals who evaluate the patient separately and then share goals as a team. The composition of this team of professionals is defined by the rehabilitation problem and the individual patient's needs. In shoulder rehabilitation, the group (Outline 1) frequently consists of the patient, physical therapist, occupational therapist, athletic trainer, vocational counselor, orthopaedist, physiatrist, family physician, social worker, recreation therapist, and psychologist. This interactive process produces a treatment plan that is negotiated with the patient and leads to the best outcome.[13]

Finally, appreciation of several principles is important to achieve successful rehabilitation. First, the safety and security needs of the individual and family must be addressed immediately. Second, the recognition of economic disincentives is critical in planning resumption of daily activities and work. Third, it is important for the clinician to appreciate that there is no reliably predictable relationship among the variables: illness or injury severity and the degree of impairment, disability or handicap experienced by a particular individual, although in many instances strong associations exist.[14] For example, subacromial bursitis in one person might contribute to greater disability than in another individual because of differences in activity and employment demands. In addition, characteristics of their physical and psychosocial environments may produce varied accommodations. Fourth, disability is mediated within the context of all the functional abilities and personal characteristics of the individual (Fig. 2).[11,12] Fifth, not all shoulder injuries require a formal interdisciplinary

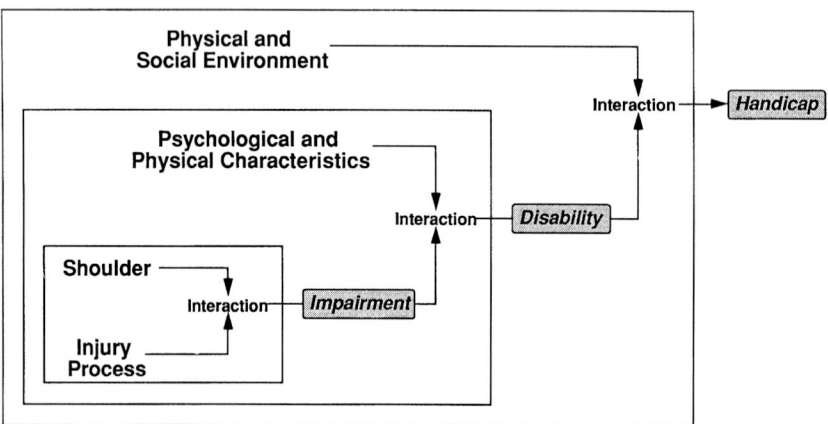

Fig. 2 A shoulder injury's effect on the person. The effects of an injury (impairments) are mediated by the context of the person and the environment. The impairments interacting with the attributes and goals of the whole person define the disability. Impairments and disability interfacing with the environment produce handicap. The rehabilitation process is not linear and involves intervention to minimize the effects of injury in all disablement contexts concurrently. Aspects of intervention can be arbitrarily divided into phases or perspectives of intervention. The phases of emphasis in rehabilitation treatment generally progress from injury resolution (healing) at the tissue level to impairment reduction within organ systems. As improvements are realized, a whole-person emphasis with a task focus emerges.

rehabilitation program; rehabilitation is necessary if significant residual deficits remain after acute treatment. And sixth, successful rehabilitation programs employ positive strategies that involve the patient as an active participant in presenting problems, planning goals, and implementing an independent program.[15]

Rehabilitation Treatment

The beginning of rehabilitative treatment includes functional assessment. The patient's goals for rehabilitation need to be integrated into a plausible plan for improvement. The process of rehabilitation results in changes within many systems: the anatomic site of the injury, associated organ systems, the whole person, the environment, and the community (Fig. 2). Treatment success is finally measured against the original performance and symptomatic tolerance of the activity.

The general steps of the rehabilitation process after shoulder overuse injuries are similarly presented in many studies.[7,10,16] The initial stage of these programs involves pain management because active participation in a rehabilitation program requires a certain degree of comfort. This is followed by therapeutic exercise involving range of motion (ROM) and strengthening programs. Clinical strengthening exercises are subsequently replaced by task-specific training, emphasizing movements that approximate the real task in the vocational or recreational realm. During this process, active patient participa-

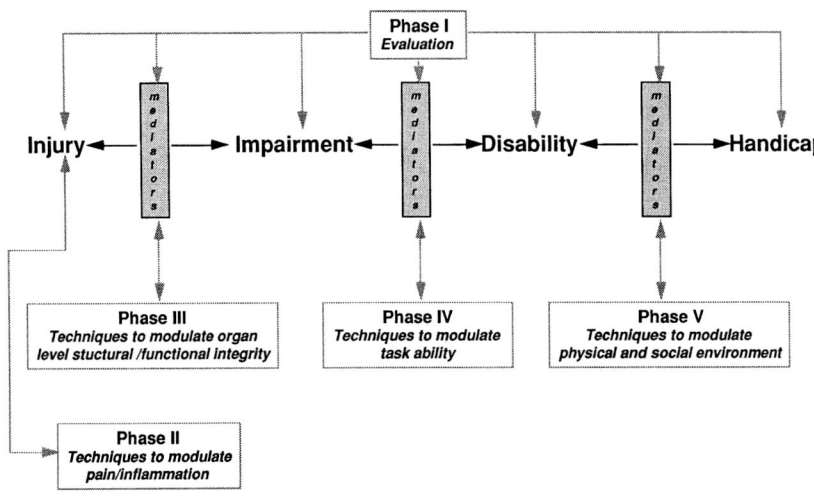

Fig. 3 A model for rehabilitation of the shoulder, representing the relationship between the phases of the shoulder rehabilitation process and shoulder injury, impairment, disability, and handicap. Phase I (Evaluation) begins by emphasizing the assessment and quantification of shoulder injury, functional deficits, task performance and environmental effects. Mediators that allow for adaptive capacity-limiting disablement severity are identified and targeted as foci for therapy. Assessment of task-based activity allows objective assessment of disability as a baseline. The interaction of physical and social environment with the person (including all injuries, impairments, and disabilities) determines handicap. Phase II emphasizes the treatment of the injury itself, limiting tissue damage and reducing pain. Phase III (Therapeutic Exercise) is primarily directed at the organ-based mediators of shoulder impairment, including muscles and ligaments, to reduce impairments such as limited ROM and weakness. Phase IV (skill reacquisition) emphasizes the compensation by the entire person in life or work task activity. Phase V involves environmental enhancement to reduce handicap.

tion and achievement of independence in a home and work program are essential for sustained success.[15] Finally, environmental modifications are employed to minimize extrinsic factors that contribute to shoulder disability.

Phases of the Shoulder Rehabilitation Process

Five phases (Outline 2) can be operationally used to group and order the activities of the shoulder rehabilitation team. These phases overlap chronologically and are emphasized based on the patient's needs as interpreted through ongoing assessment and interdisciplinary interaction. Additionally, because each program is uniquely designed for the patient by the rehabilitation team, not all intervention phases and team members are required by each patient.

Phase I: Evaluation

The evaluation of a shoulder injury begins with a review of the diagnosis (Outline 3). The anatomic locations of the pathology and the contributions to the disease process need to be defined as specifically as possible. The etiology of

Outline 2 The five overlapping phases of shoulder rehabilitation

Phase I	Evaluation
Phase II	Pain and inflammation resolution
Phase III	Therapeutic exercise
Phase IV	Skill reacquisition
Phase V	Environment enhancement

Outline 3 Phase I: Evaluation

History: Intrinsic to extrinsic

Physical examination: Neuromusculoskeletal focus, injury reenactment

Impairment: Strength, ROM, proprioception, instability, reduced smoothness of movement

Disability: Task demonstration, functional assessment

Handicap: Record attitude toward job; workplace environment; video of work activity at the site is helpful

---

the problem is first explored at the mechanistic level to develop an understanding of positions and movements that are contributing to the injury. The patient's perception of the cause of the problem requires careful exploration as well to evaluate his or her concerns and expectations. The circumstances leading to dysfunction should be reviewed in detail, including the acute injury events, training schedule, equipment, and work environment. The physical examination is an aid in developing a differential diagnosis. Provocative activities that evoke symptoms during this examination help to confirm the mechanism of injury.

As a means of sequencing the rehabilitation assessment of the injury process, factors that compound shoulder overuse injury are partitioned into intrinsic and extrinsic contributors to injury (Outline 3).[17,18] Intrinsic factors are located within the body of the patient and are categorized based on the primary site of the pathology (ie, subdeltoid bursitis and acromial spur) and the exacerbating secondary effects of injury (eg, weak shoulder depressors, scapulothoracic adduction contracture, or limitation in lateral thoracic side bending). Although there is controversy as to the mechanisms that mediate overuse injury, the possibility of fatigue of muscular stabilizers of the shoulder needs to be considered as an intrinsic contributor to primary muscle, bone, tendon, and ligament damage from repetitive stresses.[19] Extrinsic factors act on the body from the environment and include the work task itself, tool design, ergonomics, training or work schedules, as well as psychologic stressors.

Sources of pain are identified and categorized by origin: muscle, connective tissue, joint, peripheral nerve or central nervous system. This provides a practical focus for intervention through the use of various modalities in physical therapy.

Frequently, during the examination pain and local tenderness are localized to the neck and shoulder musculature without any evidence of tissue inflammation. Trigger points (hyperirritable spots, frequently in a taut band of muscle, that produce pain in a referral pattern) may be present, most commonly in the trapezius muscles, cervical paraspinals, or shoulder musculature.[20,21] Trigger points can be found in the musculature of patients with the systemic condition fibromyalgia [22] and in patients with localized myofascial pain. Trigger points have been associated with sleep deprivation, fatigue, tendinitis, and decreased spinal fluid serotonin levels. [23]

Shoulder impairments that occur subsequent to injury can compound the overuse injury process. Following an injury, limitations in ROM, strength, kinesthesia,[24] and patterns of dynamic muscle recruitment can affect overall shoulder function.[25] These limitations can be operationally defined through measurement (ie, goniometry and dynamic force assessment) and can be interpreted with respect to their contribution to task performance deficits (disability).

Disability can markedly impact an individual's opportunity to progress along the usual course of personal development, pursue a desired career, and engage in social and community activities. Elements that define a disability are examined within the context of a specific job or task. A clear understanding of the patient's work and daily activity demands is therefore essential.

The causes of handicaps are not always obvious, yet it is extremely important that they be determined so that the focus of intervention is appropriate and effective. By definition, handicaps and their resolution involve environmental factors both physical and interpersonal (eg, ergonomic factors, temporal work demands, relationships to coworkers and to supervisors).

At the completion of evaluation, a baseline is derived through patient history and measurements of impairment, disability, and handicap. This process consideration extends from the history and musculoskeletal examination to functional assessment, which could include isometric dynamometry, dynamic strength testing (Cybex), kinematics, work site assessment, vocational assessment, and estimation of psychologic adjustment.

Gerber[26] has reviewed the currently available clinician-scored systems for functional assessment of the shoulder. It is regrettable that no universal system of functional analysis has been adopted. Some of the available options in ordinal-scored shoulder instruments have included the rating sheet for Bankart repair, the Walch-Duplay rating sheet for anterior instability, the University of California at Los Angeles shoulder rating scale, the American Shoulder and Elbow Surgeons (ASES) shoulder evaluation form, and the Constant Score. The Constant Score includes a subjective (35 points) and an objective (65 points including ROM and strength) assessment and is uniformly applicable across diagnostic categories.[27]

A patient-scored instrument, the "Simple Shoulder Test," was designed as a functionally based outcome assessment tool consisting of 12 questions derived from examination maneuvers, the ASES, and patient complaints as tabulated at the University of Washington.[28,29] The yes/no questions include topics such as pain at rest, ability to carry out functional motions, ability to lift weight in defined movement planes, and the shoulder impairment's effect on full-time work. The instrument is helpful in communicating limitations and achievements of treatment to patients and can be applied across diagnostic groups. For rehabilitative assessment, it lacks discrimination of small functional gains and information on shoulder handicap.

Phase II: Pain and Inflammation Resolution

This phase (Outline 4) can be subdivided into acute and subacute stages. The acute period occurs soon after injury and can last up to 6 weeks if continued active inflammation is present. If there is evidence of acute inflammation, treat-

Outline 4 Phase II: Pain and inflammation resolution

Relative rest, splinting

Analgesics

Topical deep cooling, heat

NSAIDs, steroids

Massage

---

ment involves rest, ice, and nonsteroidal anti-inflammatory drugs (NSAIDs). Immobilization and rest must be used judiciously and only for brief periods to prevent contractures and disuse weakness. The shoulder is particularly susceptible to the development of contractures, muscle strength imbalance, and limited ROM. Subsequently, abnormal movements and forces at the glenohumeral joint are created (obligate translation), resulting in further shoulder pathology. Relative rest is the technique used to reduce the activity to a frequency and intensity that will allow the fastest rate of inflammation resolution and healing while maintaining the maximal overall fitness level possible. A variety of modalities are useful depending on whether the injury and the pain are located in ligament, muscle, nerve, or bone.

During early treatment of a shoulder disorder, a generalized strengthening and aerobic conditioning program should be initiated. General aerobic training is easily maintained with an exercise bicycle or swimming program. Flexibility and strength programs for the unaffected limbs and the distal segments of the affected extremity are essential for maintenance of maximal function. Joints distal to the shoulder and those of other limbs participate in many tasks and can compensate for impairments at the injured shoulder. Isometrics to the distal extremity can retain strength without exacerbation of a proximal injury.

Traumatic injury and subsequent acute inflammation frequently involve the ligaments and the musculotendinous complex. Initial therapy often includes cold application to reduce pain and inflammation. In treating acute bursitis, the use of deep heat is contraindicated because of the risk of exacerbating active swelling.[30] Swelling is limited by direct vasoconstriction and sympathetically mediated reflex vasoconstriction.[31] Cold application has been demonstrated to decrease the swelling of acute trauma in ankle sprains[32] and after total knee arthroplasty.[33] In clinical practice, shoulder injuries respond favorably as well. Destructive enzyme activity of collagenase during the active inflammatory state can be significantly lessened by reducing joint temperatures to between 30°C and 25°C.[34] Furthermore, cold has been demonstrated to decrease pain by reducing muscle spasm[35] and as a segmental counterirritant.[36] Strictly active unresisted ROM is carried out in the acute phase to avoid ligamentous damage and subsequent joint laxity.

Shoulder pain that is referred from the cervical spine because of root compression responds to neck brace immobilization and cervical traction. Inflamed nerve roots entrapped by cervical disks or impinged in the intervertebral foramen can be effectively decompressed on a temporary basis by traction. Although the value of traction remains controversial[37–39] it has been successfully used for centuries in the treatment of cervical disease, low back pain, and peripheral joint problems. Theoretically, traction provides pain relief by passively lengthening intervertebral ligaments and muscles, thereby opening intervertebral foramina and decreasing intradiskal pressure.[39,40] Decompressed nerve roots get improved blood supply for resolution of edema, with resultant improvement in transmission, and axoplasmic flow. Traction can be applied manually or mechanically. To test its value in a given patient, manual traction in the office is advocated. Early trials are gentle and of short duration. If the patient experiences significant relief, a course of home or office mechanical therapy is prescribed. Most protocols recommend that several specific parameters be tailored to the particular patient, depending on the goals of treatment, the underlying pathology, and the patient involved. However, there are no controlled efficacy or clinical studies that compare the various parameters. Parameters include the following: position (body, neck, and joint), angle of traction, weight applied, duration of session, mode of traction (continuous or intermittent), and frequency. Contraindications include hypermobility or ligamentous instability and osteopenia.[41]

The trigger points of myofascial pain respond to a variety of treatments including icing or vapocoolant spray, stretch, acupressure, lidocaine injection, and dry needling (sterile needle insertion into the taut muscle band). Low-level laser therapy has not been demonstrated to be of any benefit.[42] Patients with myofascial pain require special attention to sleep quality and regular aerobic exercise. Sleep quality can be enhanced with tricyclic dosing at bedtime: amitriptyline 25 to 50 mg, with an increase of 25 mg per week to a maximum dose of 150 mg.

In the subacute stage, deep heat applied with ultrasound successfully increases blood flow to the tissues and increases distensibility with stretch for maintenance of range. Ultrasound is inaudible acoustic mechanical vibrations of high frequency. Therapeutic frequencies range from 0.8 to 1 MHz.[30] As the waves hit tissue interfaces, there is resultant interference and heat production for tissue absorption. This modality has become the standard form of deep heat utilized in physiotherapy. Uncontrolled past studies reported successful results in the treatment of chronic bursitis with ultrasound.[43,44] However, the effect of ultrasound on supraspinatus tendinitis, subacromial bursitis and adhesive capsulitis in 20 patients was evaluated in a double-blind randomized study.[45] No significant reduction in pain nor increased ROM could be demonstrated. The specific indications for the modality are as yet undefined but repeated use for periods longer than a few weeks in patients with fixed contracture or chronic bursitis has not been substantiated. Although use of ultrasound to reduce spasm, increase circulation, and increase tissue distensibility as an adjunctive part of a comprehensive shoulder rehabilitative program has been quite successful in clinical practice.

Inflammation can also be treated pharmacologically with local or systemic therapy. Aspirin and the other NSAIDs are often considered the first line of treatment of inflammatory problems (eg, bursitis, tendinitis, and arthritis). The NSAIDs inhibit the cyclo-oxygenase enzyme and exert their primary effects by inhibiting prostaglandin and thromboxane synthesis. Although NSAIDs are not as powerful as corticosteroids in reducing inflammation, they are associated with less serious side effects and offer the added advantage of analgesia. Newer NSAIDs (eg, diflunisal, etodolac, and nabumetone) have doses of once or twice per day.

Steroid injection into a joint or bursa or over a synovial sheath offers several advantages over oral anti-inflammatory medications. First, removal of excess fluid may provide an immediate decrease in symptoms. Second, there is a limitation of the systemic side effects of steroids and analgesics. And third, aspiration of fluid allows bursa decompression and diagnostic tests to be performed. Indications for shoulder arthrocentesis include treatment of osteoarthritis and rheumatoid arthritis of the glenohumeral, acromioclavicular, and sternoclavicular joints, subacromial bursitis, and supraspinatus tendinitis. In an investigation of corticosteroid injections for shoulder bursitis and adhesive capsulitis, intrabursal and intra-articular injections of methylprednisolone produced a reduction in pain but had no effect on the course of shoulder motion recovery.[46] Selective focal application of steroid injection can contribute significantly if applied in the context of a comprehensive shoulder rehabilitation program.

Phonophoresis, first described by Fellinger and Schmid,[47] is the attempt to propel substances across membranes using the ultrasound beam and the mechanical massage of the applicator at the skin surface. The technique is most often used to deliver cortisone in an ointment medium that also acts as a coupling medium for the ultrasound. The depth of penetration of the steroid medication with phonophoresis was explored by Davick and associates[48] in dogs. There was no evidence that the cortisol went any deeper than the epidermis. The combination of 10% cortisol and ultrasound produced a greater depth of penetration than surface cortisol application alone but the difference was clinically insignificant because delivery did not cross the dermis with either technique. The problems of steroid molecule size and lipid solubility in tissues over joints limit the success with clinically significant drug delivery using physical and electric modalities.

Phase III: Therapeutic Exercise

This phase involves the following three basic components: ROM exercises, strengthening, and kinesthetic awareness training (Outline 5). The effective use of therapeutic exercise in the treatment of overuse shoulder injuries depends on a clear understanding of four factors: (1) an accurate diagnosis; (2) functional limitations; (3) treatment potential of the involved tissues; and (4) the relationship between the underlying pathology, impairment, and resulting disability.

Adaptation Range of motion and strengthening may play important roles in the treatment of overuse injuries by stimulating adaptive changes at the tissue level. Many overuse injuries result in dense connective tissue injuries (labrum, capsule, tendons, and ligaments). There is a growing body of literature that supports adaptation and strengthening of collagenous tissues as a result of ten-

Outline 5 Phase III: Therapeutic exercise*

Range of motion recovery

Strength increase

  Resistance to motion
  Type of contraction (isometric, isotonic, eccentric)
  Specific muscle groups
  Open versus closed kinetic chain

Proprioceptive training

Aerobics

---

*Modulate with mode, intensity, frequency, and duration

sile forces. The release of distractive forces from the Achilles tendon supports the adaptation hypothesis. After sectioning of the Achilles tendon, collagen was found to disaggregate, only to reform after tendon repair. Proteoglycans also changed, from sulfated to nonsulfated types after the release of distractive forces, and back to sulfated molecules after repair.[49] Other investigations have demonstrated similar changes in connective tissue structure to meet new functional demands. In exercised versus nonexercised animals, mean collagen diameter, fibril number, and fibril cross-linking were all found to increase in tendons and ligaments from exercised animals.[50,51] Thus, increases in anatomic and mechanical properties have been demonstrated in connective tissues in response to increased tensile forces.

The ability of muscle to adapt has also been demonstrated and appears to be somewhat specific. High resistance increases strength; resistance that allows repeated repetition improves endurance.[52] Therefore, the best exercise for the task approximates the task itself. However, recent research suggests that whereas specificity is important, exercise types may not be as mutually exclusive in achieving specific results as was once believed.[53–56] An exercise program should be designed with specific tissue and functional goals in mind. Therefore, to increase strength, low-repetition, high-resistance exercises are prescribed. To increase endurance, high-repetition, low-resistance exercises are best. Recently, some interchangeability between these regimens has been demonstrated.

Range of Motion All soft and osseous tissues surrounding a joint demonstrate viscoelastic properties. By definition, these properties are time dependent and show sensitivity to rate of loading and deformation. A viscoelastic material deforms with time even when it is subjected to a constant applied load. Eventually, the change in deformation will stop and a steady state will be reached. The longer a load is applied, the greater the deformation until that steady state is achieved. The rate of deformation also depends on the magnitude of the applied load. Finally, the time-dependent properties of a material depend on physical properties (such as temperature). These properties are important to consider when attempting to increase range of joint motion with prolonged stretch.

A certain degree of flexibility is essential to allow for the greatest efficiency of the musculoskeletal system. This is particularly true of the shoulder joint. Many of the stabilizing mechanisms of the shoulder (eg, glenohumeral concavity compression and glenohumeral balance) depend on a full range of shoulder motion.

To increase flexibility, connective tissues must be lengthened. Indeed, in the shoulder with restricted ROM it is the periarticular connective tissues and collagenous tissues within and around muscles that are usually shortened (rather than the contractile elements of muscles). These connective tissues are composed fundamentally of collagen and proteoglycans. Stretching of collagenous tissues requires a linear deformation (elongation) of the collagen fibers. There are two types of elongation: elastic and plastic. Elastic elongation occurs when the elongation produced by loading is followed by a recovery to resting length when the load is removed. No permanent lengthening or increase in range of motion will result from this type of stretching. Plastic elongation is achieved when the elongation is maintained after removal of the load.

Plastic elongation is the mechanism necessary to increase ROM. It is maximized by applying a prolonged stretch with the tissues warmed to between 42°C and 45°C. Superficial heat will not sufficiently warm the periarticular connective tissues. Bouncing stretch, heat without stretch, and short duration stretching are also ineffective in increasing flexibility at the shoulder, often leading to microscopic tears.

Establishment of a normal ROM at the shoulder requires normal flexibility at the four joints of the shoulder. Most ROM exercises are directed at the glenohumeral joint, whereas other joints of the pectoral girdle are often neglected. It is essential that normal flexibility of all joints (including the scapulothoracic articulation) is achieved.

Range of motion exercises are prescribed to either maintain normal range or regain lost flexibility (Outline 6). Because of the propensity of the shoulder joint to undergo contracture, early and aggressive management is undertaken to maintain normal motion. Pain, muscle spasm, guarding, altered biomechanics, weakness, and muscle imbalance all might result in progressive loss of ROM.

Many types of ROM exercises are available. First, passive ROM exercises involve no active muscle contraction. Passive "ranging" by a therapist, gravity, the patient, or continuous passive motion (CPM)[57] are all examples of this type of exercise. Codman[58] first advocated the use of a gravity-eliminated position in which pendular, circumferential movements of the upper extremity are performed. Others have modified Codman's idea to minimize muscular activation and optimize painless, passive ROM activities. Passive ROM exercises are particularly effective early in a rehabilitation program and when there is significant joint pain. Demonstration by a therapist is necessary to avoid the application of excessive force and resultant joint laxity from overstretching. Planes of motion must be carefully defined and mechanisms for prolonged patient maintenance of stretch devised. Second, active-assisted ROM exercises are used as the patient progresses in the rehabilitation program. These exercises involve some active contraction of the shoulder muscles. Facilitation by active muscle contraction is probably important if the tightness is related to muscles (as opposed to capsular or ligamentous contractures).[59] Finally, many types of equipment can be used in ROM exercise programs. Weights and pulleys, for example, are frequently prescribed, particularly if there is significant contracture. The risk in using equipment is that patients will often overstretch parts of the shoulder joint that are already flexible, resulting in joint laxity, while the tight areas become even tighter.

If full ROM cannot be achieved by the above methods, manipulation techniques can be useful. Mobilization techniques of the shoulder for treatment of adhesive capsulitis vary considerably, from the use of constant tension following heating of the periarticular structures to arthrographic capsular disten-

Outline 6 Principles of maintaining or increasing flexibility

Prolonged stretch

Static stretch

Several short stretching sessions per day

Warming of the tissues to be stretched (deep heating)

Cooling down in the stretched position

Avoidance of bouncing

Avoidance of overstretching and laxity

sion,[60] to violent manipulation of the shoulder during general anesthesia. There is little research comparing the efficacy and outcome after restoring shoulder motion with the different types of mobilization protocols. Overvigorous mobilization can produce adverse effects, particularly ligamentous and bony injury with resultant hypermobility.

Strengthening Techniques for building muscle strength are important in the management of instability and weakness. There are several types of strengthening exercises and programs. Unfortunately, there is little research comparing one approach with another in shoulder rehabilitation.

In general, strengthening programs employ high-resistance loads against which a muscle must work. Strength gains from exercise stem from two components: a learning effect and muscle hypertrophy. Learning to more efficiently recruit motor units accounts for much of the increase in force capability during the early stages of an exercise program and involves increased synchrony of motor unit recruitment.[56] As repetitive overloads continue, muscle cells hypertrophy. As muscle fibers increase in size and contractile mass, each cell is able to generate more tension as compared to the preexercised state.

There are many factors to be considered in designing a strengthening program. The resistance to motion can be of different types (eg, isometric, isotonic, or isokinetic), each offering certain advantages and disadvantages. There are also different types of contractions that can be employed. Shortening (concentric) contractions develop the lowest muscle tension, lengthening (eccentric) contractions develop the highest tension, and isometric contractions produce intermediate levels of tension. Different muscle groups can be targeted for strengthening with an anatomic focus (anterior versus posterior muscles) or a functional focus (shoulder stabilizers, positioners, depressors). Strengthening can be performed by varying the degrees of freedom of a limb (eg, open versus closed kinematic chains). Finally, resistance to motion can be applied manually by a therapist or trainer, by using weights, or through the use of various types of equipment.

Resistance to motion The resistance to motion can be of three types: isometric, isotonic, and isokinetic. Isometric contractions result in no external movement or change in the joint angle. These exercises are started early in the rehabilitation program targeting glenohumeral stabilizers, scapular elevators, and scapular stabilizers. Isometrics offer several advantages: they are easy to perform and require no equipment; injury secondary to these exercises is rare; and they require no joint motion (this is particularly important in an immobilized limb or when joint motion is painful). One particular contraindication is the rise in blood pressure during isometric exercises.

Isotonic exercises involve moving a constant load through a full ROM. The velocity of movement can vary. Low-resistance, high-repetition exercises are started early in a rehabilitation program, initially using below-shoulder-level exercises. Gradually, resistance is increased. DeLorme and Watkins[61] developed the hypothesis that resistive exercises can be used to increase strength in rehabilitative programs. There have been many studies and modifications of strengthening regimens since DeLorme's original work. It is now generally believed that strength can be improved by many types of protocols and exercises, as long as they are carried out to the point of muscle fatigue. Isotonic exercises that involve eccentric contractions are added late in the rehabilitation program because the highest tension and force develop with eccentric contractions.[62] The advantages of isotonic exercises include low cost, effectiveness, and availability. Exercises can be performed with free weights, pulleys, or against resistance from surgical tubing. As heavier weights and eccentric exercises are prescribed, caution must be used to avoid repeated shoulder injury.

Isokinetic exercises are exercises with constant angular velocity as the muscle shortens or lengthens. The load and force are variable. An advantage of this type of exercise is that the person can generate maximal force at all angles of joint range. Strength gains are related to the maximal torque[54,63] generated during training. Training at slow velocities generates the greatest torque. A disadvantage of isokinetic exercise is the reliance on special expensive equipment.

Types of contraction Strengthening exercises can be performed using one of three types of contraction: concentric, isometric, and eccentric. Concentric contractions are shortening contractions (eg, biceps contraction while lifting a barbell against gravity in a "curl") and develop the lowest muscle tensions. Therefore, concentric contractions are used in the early stages of a rehabilitation program. As mentioned previously, isometric contractions result in no external movement (eg, serratus anterior contraction when trying to push a fixed object). The force developed is intermediate between concentric and eccentric contractions yet isometric exercises are the least effective method of building strength. The advantages of this type of exercise include no joint movement (an advantage with degenerative or inflammatory conditions) and the strengthening of short stabilizers of the shoulder. Finally, eccentric contractions develop the highest muscle tensions. Strengthening with eccentric contractions can be very effective with proper dosing.[64] This mode of strengthening has particular relevance to shoulder problems because static shoulder stabilizers frequently fail during eccentric activities.[65]

Strengthening of specific muscle groups Strengthening of specific muscle groups reportedly improves dynamic stability in shoulders with weakness and/or instability. Matsen and associates,[28] for example, emphasize strengthening of muscle groups that elevate the shoulder in compensation for rotator cuff tears. Jobe and Pink[8] emphasize treatment of four functional groups of muscles: glenohumeral protectors, scapulohumeral pivoters, humeral positioners, and propeller muscles. For instability, Burkhead and Rockwood[66] prescribed a specific set of progressive resistance exercises designed to strengthen the deltoid and rotator cuff muscles. The relative efficacy of these different types of strengthening programs for shoulder overuse injuries is unknown.

The specific exercises to use in shoulder strengthening have been evaluated with electromyography to document the fullest recruitment. Townsend and associates[67] evaluated the glenohumeral stabilization musculature (rotator cuff muscles, pectoralis major, latissimus dorsi, and deltoid) with fine wire electrodes and found four exercises that were the most challenging (ie, generated more than 50% of the maximum voluntary contraction). These included (1) elevation in the scapular plane with thumbs down, (2) shoulder flexion, (3) horizontal abduction with arms externally rotated, and (4) the seated press-up. (Scapulothoracic depression lifting the trunk off the chair with a handgrip on the seat and elbows extended). These exercises are recommended as a succinct glenohumeral stabilizer strengthening protocol. A similar study evaluated the scapular stabilizers (upper, middle, and lower trapezius, levator scapula, rhomboids, pectoralis minor, and middle to lower serratus anterior), and recommended the following four exercises as part of a core scapular muscle strengthening program: (1) scaption (scapular plane elevation); (2) rowing; (3) push-up with a plus (full push-up with elbow extension followed by scapulothoracic depression to raise the body further off the floor); and (4) press-up.[68]

Kinematic chain The upper limb can be used in an open or closed chain. The chain consisting of the joints and linking segments can be described as open when the hand is moving freely in space with or without holding an object. Swimming and the use of free weights are examples of open kinematic chain exercises. Open chain exercises allow for position and inertial feedback as objects are moved through space. A closed kinetic chain occurs when the hand has contact with an immovable object and upper extremity movement produces movement of the body (ie, push-up). The use of the open kinematic chain is advocated to strengthen proximal, scapular muscles, whereas the closed chain is thought to strengthen glenohumeral muscles more effectively.[8,69] A balance of open- and closed-chain exercises should be included in each patient's program to address impairments and functional goals.

Phase IV: Skill Reacquisition

This phase involves the reacquisition of skills required for routine activities of daily living and identification of specialized activities desired by the individual for employment or unique avocational pursuits (Outline 7). Following a review of physical capacity, current skill level, learning ability, and psychologic functioning, implementation of task-focused activity can begin. This phase considers shoulder range, strength, and kinesthesia and applies them together to task-based activities. A combination of independent exercise prescription and on-site treatment extends the performance to the work/avocational environment with the help of therapists (physical, occupational, and recreational), athletic trainers, and counselors (vocational and psychologic).

Neuromuscular Control Training Proprioception or kinesthesia can be described as the ability to accurately perceive the relative position and mass of body parts. Dynamic proprioception extends awareness to velocity, direction, and momentum. These techniques bring the patient a step closer to putting pain-free range and strength to functional use, and they provide the perceptual foundation for dynamic neuromuscular control techniques. Kinesthetic deficits in injured shoulders have been demonstrated as compared to contralateral controls and normal shoulders.[24] Specific training with an awareness of this deficit successfully reduces the recurrence of first-time shoulder dislocation.[70]

Motor control requires involuntary associated movements, organized subcortically, that contribute to a well-learned skill.[71] There is clear evidence that the patterns of shoulder muscle use vary with training.[72] Although certain

Outline 7 Phase IV: Skill reacquisition

Proprioceptive neuromuscular facilitation

Plyometrics

Successive approximation

Task modification

Endurance training

movements that make up different tasks may be the same, patterns of muscle recruitment differ. This is true for different sports and is demonstrated in dynamic electromyographic recordings with certain activities.[73]

Rehabilitative approaches to the refinement of neuromuscular control build on dynamic kinesthesia adding active movement with successive approximation of the activity goal. The variety of these techniques is wide and expanding. One frequently used technique is proprioceptive neuromuscular facilitation (PNF), which builds on the observations of Sherrington and Kabat[74] that sensory feedback regarding position and reflex stimulation by the therapist during patterned movement can refine the sequence of motor unit recruitment, improving movement quality.[74] The effectiveness of PNF techniques for improving dynamic muscle contraction, such as stretching before movement, has been substantiated.[75] Specific indications for PNF shoulder rehabilitation are yet to be defined but would likely include static and dynamic kinesthetic deficits or reduced fluency of dynamic movement.

Occasionally, sports or job-related tasks require explosive-reactive movement. Another technique to refine dynamic proprioception is plyometrics "jump training," which has its roots in eastern Europe. Plyometrics can be simply defined as quick, powerful movements preceded by a prestretching (eccentric contraction) of the muscles to activate the stretch-shortening cycle. Plyometric exercises are designed to increase power by linking sheer strength with speed of movement. Spindle afferents are stimulated, increasing extrafusal fiber contraction in response to the stretch. The technique attempts to increase the excitability of the receptors in the motor pathways to the muscle, thereby enhancing voluntary contraction force.[75] There is also a significant component of stored elastic energy that contributes to the concentric contraction.[75] These exercises train the neuromuscular system to react quickly and forcefully during stretch-shortening actions. The exercises should try to duplicate any rapid movement with an intensity that is equal to or greater than normal. These rapid and forceful exercises require great flexibility and agility. Complete healing, normal ROM, great strength, and coordination are prerequisites for plyometric exercises. The risk of injury is high with these activities. These techniques therefore require close supervision by a therapist to develop proper technique and prevent reinjury.

Activity-Specific Training Although general coordination and strengthening exercises offer a great base on which to build, they cannot surpass activity-specific training to develop proper technique and eliminate poor technique in the prevention of future injuries. In sports or work, the final coordination exercises need to resemble the ultimate goal activity. If the activity is complex, it can be broken down and practiced in component parts that are easier to master. The goal activity can be successively approximated by adding the components. Through repetition, accuracy and endurance are achieved.

Phase V: Environmental Enhancement

Studies of the physical demands of various occupations have confirmed a positive association between workload exposure and musculoskeletal disorders requiring disability pensions.[2] It is also clear that workers in certain occupations, such as directory assistance operators in the telecommunications industry, are particularly susceptible to upper extremity pain in the workplace. However, there are no ergonomic descriptors that can fully account for the endemic involvement of operators as compared with workers in other occupations.[76]

Other factors in addition to the mechanics of the job demand consideration. A broad database is therefore required to fully assess the relationship between the individual and the occupation. The interdisciplinary conference of the rehabilitation team can combine important perceptions of the patient's effectiveness with life goals in the family, at work, and in the community. This synthesis is particularly effective in defining areas for intervention and treatment. Human factors analysis is effective in the identification of disparities between demands generated by the design of the environment and occupational tasks, and the capacity of the worker to meet the job demands.[77–79] Visits to the work site by occupational therapists and the other rehabilitation team members allow for an ergonomic assessment of the tools, immediate work space, and tasks of the occupation. The overall sequence and scheduling of tasks and operations can be examined. Modifications (Outline 8) can be suggested to change the work position, reduce overhead work, or reapportion activities to be balanced between the right and left limbs. Ergonomic deficiencies often are attributable to one of three general causes: machines and tools, handling of materials, and the movement subcomponents that make up the work tasks.[80] General approaches include the elimination of demand for extreme reach,[81] static posture, excessive force, faulty man-machine interaction, stress concentration, one-task jobs, and temperature extremes.[80] Modification of the environment is not universally successful in solving the problem of upper extremity pain but the greatest success occurs with careful attention to the specific characteristics of the environment that exacerbate symptoms.[76]

In addition, psychosocial and physical aspects of the work environment determine the opportunity that the person has to produce quality work. Rehabilitation psychology can be helpful to patients who need to explore the effect of their work environment on their resting muscle tension. Specific strategies for intervention that allow a person to effectively resolve conflicts and negotiate responsibilities with supervisors enhance relationships. The eventual goal is maximal patient understanding and control over the modifiable aspects of the home, work, and avocational environment.

Acknowledgments

The consultation and perspective that Jessie Peters, PhD, MD,[12] provided regarding the structure of the relationship between impairments, disabilities, and handicaps as illustrated in the figures is greatly appreciated. His synthesis of disablement terminology within the focus of our rehabilitation phases, as depicted in the figures, brings theory to practice!

Outline 8 Phase V: Environmental enhancement

Tool fit and use
Task frequency, order, variety
Workstation design: Posture and position variety
Psychosocial work environment
Home
Community

The work of Debra Roberts, unit assistant, in obtaining references and clerical refinement of the manuscript should also be recognized. Her assistance with our access to the literature allows us a perspective that constantly improves the quality of care.

References

1. Barker L, Burton J, Zieve P: *Principles of Ambulatory Medicine.* Baltimore, MD, Williams & Wilkins, 1982, pp 1–15.
2. Harris LA: *The ICO Survey of Disabled Americans.* New York, NY, ICO, 1986.
3. National Institute for Occupation Safety and Health: *Proposed National Strategy For The Prevention Of Musculoskeletal Injuries.* DHHS (NIOSH) Publication No 89–129. Washington, DC, 1986.
4. Eva V, Lars A, Evy F, et al: Disability pensions due to musculo-skeletal disorders among men in heavy occupations: A case-control study. *Scand J Soc Med* 1992;20:31–36.
5. Lehto TU, Helenius HY, Alaranta HT: Musculoskeletal symptoms of dentists assessed by a multidisciplinary approach. *Commun Dent Oral Epidemiol* 1991;19:38–44.
6. Beckerman H, Bouter LM, van der Heijden GJ, et al: Efficacy of physiotherapy for musculoskeletal disorders: What can we learn from research? *Br J Gen Pract* 1993;43:73–77.
7. Ellenbecker TS, Derscheid GL: Rehabilitation of overuse injuries of the shoulder. *Clin Sports Med* 1989;8:583–604.
8. Jobe FW, Pink M: Classification and treatment of shoulder dysfunction in the overhead athlete. *J Orthop Sports Phys Ther* 1993;18:427–432.
9. McLaughlin TM: Strength/power training for baseball pitchers, in Zarins B, Andrews JR, Carson WG Jr (eds): *Injuries to the Throwing Arm.* Philadelphia, PA, WB Saunders, 1985, pp 293–304.
10. Scheib JS: Diagnosis and rehabilitation of the shoulder impingement syndrome in the overhand and throwing athlete. *Rheum Dis Clin North Am* 1990;16:971–988.
11. World Health Organization: *The International Classification of Impairments, Disabilities and Handicaps: A Manual Relating to the Consequences of Disease.* Geneva, World Health Organization, 1980.
12. Peters J: Human experience in disablement: The imperative of ICIDH (International Classification of Impairment Disability and Handicap). *Disabil Rehabil*, in press.
13. Dean BZ, Geiringer SR: Physiatric therapeutics: 6. The rehabilitation team/behavioral management. *Arch Phys Med Rehabil* 1990;71:S275–S277.
14. Badley E, Lee J, Wood P: Patterns of disability related to joint involvement in rheumatoid arthritis. *Rheumatol Rehabil* 1979;18:105–109.
15. Levoska S, Keinanen-Kiukaanniemi S: Active or passive physiotherapy for occupational cervicobrachial disorders? A comparison of two treatment methods with a 1-year follow-up. *Arch Phys Med Rehabil* 1993;74:425–430.
16. Pink M, Jobe FW: Shoulder injuries in athletes. *Clin Management* 1991;11:39–47.
17. Renstrom P, Johnson RJ: Overuse injuries in sports: A review. *Sports Med* 1985;2:316–333.
18. Herring SA, Nilson KL: Introduction to overuse injuries. *Clin Sports Med* 1987;6:225–239.
19. Frankel VH, Nordin M (eds): *Basic Biomechanics of the Skeletal System.* Philadelphia, PA, Lea & Febiger, 1980.
20. Travel J, Rinzler S: The myofacial genesis of pain. *Postgrad Med* 1952;11:425–434.
21. Travel J, Simons D: *Myofascial Pain and Dysfunction: The Trigger Point Manual.* Baltimore, MD, Williams & Wilkins, 1983.

22. Wolfe F, Smythe HA, Yunus MB, et al: The American College of Rheumatology 1990 criteria for the classification of fibromyalgia: Report of the Multicenter Criteria Committee. *Arthritis Rheum* 1990;33:160–172.
23. Waylonis G, Ronan P, Gordon C: A profile of fibromyalgia in occupational environments. *Am J Phys Med Rehabil* 1994;73:112–115.
24. Blasier RB, Carpenter JE, Huston LJ: Shoulder proprioception: Effect of joint laxity, joint position, and direction of motion. *Orthop Rev* 1994;23:45–50.
25. Kronberg M, Brostrom LA, Nemeth G: Differences in shoulder muscle activity between patients with generalized joint laxity and normal controls. *Clin Orthop* 1991;269:181–192.
26. Gerber C: Integrated scoring systems for the functional assessment of the shoulder, in Matsen FA, Fu FH, Hawkins RJ (eds): *The Shoulder: A Balance of Mobility and Stability*. Rosemont, IL, American Academy of Orthopaedic Surgeons, 1994, pp 531–550.
27. Constant CR, Murley AH: A clinical method of functional assessment of the shoulder. *Clin Orthop* 1987;214:160–164.
28. Matsen FA III, Lippitt SB, Sidles JA, et al (eds): *Practical Evaluation and Management of the Shoulder*. Philadelphia, PA, WB Saunders, 1994.
29. Lippit SB, Harryman DT, Matsen FA: A practical tool for evaluating function: The simple shoulder test, in Matsen FA, Fu FH, Hawkins RJ (eds): *The Shoulder: A Balance of Mobility and Stability*. Rosemont, IL, American Academy of Orthopaedic Surgeons, 1994, pp 501–518.
30. Lehmann JF, de Lateur BJ: Diathermy and superficial heat, laser, and cold therapy, in Kottke FJ, Lehmann JF (eds): *Krusen's Handbook of Physical Medicine and Rehabilitation*, ed 4. Philadelphia, PA, WB Saunders, 1990, pp 283–367.
31. Perkins J, Li M, Hoffman F: Sudden vasoconstriction in denervated or sympathectomised paws exposed to cold. *Am J Physiol* 1948;155:165–178.
32. Basur RL, Shephard E, Mouzas GL: A cooling method in the treatment of ankle sprains. *Practitioner* 1976;216:708–711.
33. Hecht PJ, Bachmann S, Booth RE Jr, et al: Effects of thermal therapy on rehabilitation after total knee arthroplasty: A prospective randomized study. *Clin Orthop* 1983;178:198–201.
34. Harris ED Jr, McCroskery PA: The influence of temperature and fibril stability on degradation of cartilage collagen by rheumatoid synovial collagenase. *N Engl J Med* 1974;290:1–6.
35. Ottoson D: The effects of temperature on the isolated muscle spindle. *J Physiol* 1965;180:636–648.
36. Bini G, Cruccu G, Hagbarth KE, et al: Analgesic effect of vibration and cooling on pain induced by intraneural electrical stimulation. *Pain* 1984;18:239–248.
37. Cyriax J: Treatment by manipulation, massage, and injection, in *Textbook of Orthopaedic Medicine*. London, UK, Balliere Tindall, 1982, pp 164–171.
38. Colachis S, Strohm B: A study of traction forces and angle of pull on vertebral interspaces. *Am J Phys Med Rehabil* 1965;46:820–830.
39. Calliet R: *Neck and Arm Pain*, ed 3. Philadelphia, PA, FA Davis Co, 1991.
40. Swezey RL: The modern thrust of manipulation and traction therapy. *Semin Arthritis Rheum* 1983;12:322–331.
41. Geiringer S, Kincaid C, Rechtien J: Traction, manipulation, and massage, in DeLisa J (ed): *Rehabilitation Medicine: Principles and Practice*. Philadelphia, PA, JB Lippincott, 1988, pp 276–295.
42. Thorsen H, Gam AN, Svensson BH, et al: Low level laser therapy for myofascial pain in the neck and shoulder girdle: A double-blind cross-over study. *Scand J Rheumatol* 1992;21:139–141.
43. Bearzy HJ: Clinical applications of ultrasonic energy in treatment of acute and chronic subacromial bursitis. *Arch Phys Med Rehabil* 1953;34:228–231.
44. Lehmann JF, Erickson DJ, Martin GM, et al: Comparison of ultrasonic and microwave diathermy in the physical treatment of periarthritis of the shoulder. *Arch Phys Med Rehabil* 1954;35:627–634.

45. Downing DS, Weinstein A: Ultrasound therapy of subacromial bursitis: A double blind trial. *Phys Ther* 1986;66:194–199.
46. Rizk TE, Pinals RS, Talaiver AS: Corticosteroid injections in adhesive capsulitis: Investigation of their value and site. *Arch Phys Med Rehabil* 1991;72:20–23.
47. Fellinger K, Schmid J: *Klink und Therapie des Chronischen Gelenkrheumatismus.* Vienna, 1954.
48. Davick JP, Martin RK, Albright JP: Distribution and deposition of tritiated cortisol using phonophoresis. *Phys Ther* 1988;68:1672–1675.
49. Flint M: Interrelationships of mucopolysaccharide and collagen in connective tissue remodelling. *J Embryol Exp Morph* 1972;27:481–495.
50. Vilarta R, Vidal BC: Anisotropic and biomechanical properties of tendons modified by exercise and denervation: Aggregation and macromolecular order in collagen bundles. *Matrix* 1989;9:55–61.
51. Woo S, Ritter MA, Amiel O, et al: The biomechanical and biochemical properties of swine tendons: Long term effects of exercise on the digital extensors. *Connect Tissue Res* 1980;7:177–183.
52. Hunter-Griffin LY (ed): *Athletic Training and Sports Medicine*, ed 2. Park Ridge, IL, American Academy of Orthopaedic Surgeons, 1991, pp 775–789.
53. Robinson M, Braverman S: Exercise: Principles, methods, and prescription, in Buschbacher R (ed): *Musculoskeletal Disorders: A Practical Guide for Diagnosis and Rehabilitation.* Boston, MA, Andover Medical Publishers, 1994, pp 52–61.
54. Esselman PC, de Lateur BJ, Aquist AD, et al: Torque development inisokinetic training. *Arch Phys Med Rehabil* 1991;72:723–728.
55. de Lateur B, Lehmann J, Fordyce W: A test of the DeLorme axiom. *Arch Phys Med Rehabil* 1968;49:245–248.
56. de Lateur B, Lehmann J: Therapeutic exercise to develop strength and endurance, in Kottke F, Stillwell G, Lehmann J (eds): *Krusen's Handbook of Physical Medicine and Rehabilitation.* Philadelphia, PA, WB Saunders, 1990, pp 480–519.
57. Gebhard JS, Kabo JM, Meals RA: Passive motion: The dose effects on joint stiffness, muscle mass, bone density, and regional swelling: A study in an experimental model following intra-articular injury. *J Bone Joint Surg* 1993;75A:1636–1647.
58. Codman EA (ed): *The Shoulder: Rupture of the Supraspinatus Tendon and Other Lesions in or About the Subacromial Bursa.* Boston, MA, Thomas Todd, 1934.
59. Moore MA, Hutton RS: Electromyographic investigation of muscle stretching techniques. *Med Sci Sports Exerc* 1980;12:322–329.
60. Rizk TE, Gavant ML, Pinals RS: Treatment of adhesive capsulitis (frozen shoulder) with arthrographic capsular distension and rupture. *Arch Phys Med Rehabil* 1994;75:803–807.
61. DeLorme TL, Watkins AL: Techniques of progressive resistance exercise. *Arch Phys Med Rehabil* 1948;29:263–273.
62. Stanish WD, Rubinovich RM, Curwin S: Eccentric exercise in chronic tendinitis. *Clin Orthop* 1986;208:65–68.
63. Moffroid MT, Whipple RH: Specificity of speed of exercise. *Phys Ther* 1970;50: 1692–1700.
64. Komi PV, Rusko H: Quantitative evaluation of mechanical and electrical changes during fatigue loading of eccentric and concentric work. *Scand J Rehabil Med* 1974;3(suppl):121.
65. Litchfield R, Hawkins R, Dillman CJ, et al: Rehabilitation for the overhead athlete. *JOSPT* 1993;189:433–441.
66. Burkhead WZ, Rockwood CA Jr: Treatment of instability of the shoulder with an exercise program. *J Bone Joint Surg* 1992;74A:890–896.
67. Townsend H, Jobe FW, Pink M, et al: Electromyographic analysis of the glenohumeral muscles during a baseball rehabilitation program. *Am J Sports Med* 1991;19:264–272.
68. Moseley JB Jr, Jobe FW, Pink M, et al: EMG analysis of the scapular muscles during a shoulder rehabilitation program. *Am J Sports Med* 1992;20:128–134.
69. Davies GJ, Dickoff-Hoffman S: Neuromuscular testing and rehabilitation of the shoulder complex. *JOSPT* 1993;18:449–458.

70. Aronen JG, Regan K: Decreasing the incidence of recurrence of first time anterior shoulder dislocations with rehabilitation. *Am J Sports Med* 1984;12:283–291.
71. Payton OD, Hirt S, Newton RA (eds): *Scientific Basis For Neurophysiologic Approaches to Therapeutic Exercise: An Anthology*. Philadelphia, PA, FA Davis, 1977.
72. Shadmehr R, Mussa-Ivaldi FA: Adaptive representation of dynamics during learning of a motor task. *J Neurosci* 1994;14:3208–3224.
73. Glousman R: Electromyographic analysis and its role in the athletic shoulder. *Clin Orthop* 1992;288:27–34.
74. Engle R: Proprioceptive neuromuscular facilitation for the shoulder, in Andrews J, Wilk K (eds): *The Athletic Shoulder*. New York, NY, Churchill Livingstone, 1994, pp 451–467.
75. Bosco C, Komi PV: Potentiation of the mechanical behavior of the human skeletal muscle through pre-stretching. *Acta Physiol Scand* 1979;106:467.
76. Hadler NM: Arm pain in the workplace: A small area analysis. *J Occup Med* 1992;34:113–119.
77. Czaja SJ, Weber RA, Nair SN: A human factors analysis of ADL activities: A capability-demand approach. *J Gerontol* 1993;48:44–48.
78. Falkenburg SA, Schultz DJ: Ergonomics for the upper extremity. *Hand Clin* 1993;9:263–271.
79. Stock S: Workplace ergonomic factors and the development of musculoskeletal disorders of the neck and upper limbs: A meta-analysis. *Am J Ind Med* 1991;19:87–107.
80. Ayoub M: Ergonomic deficiencies: III. Root causes and their correction. *J Occup Med* 1990;32:455–460.
81. Yasukouchi A, Arai K: Effects of the direction and distance of horizontal arm movements on local muscular strain: A fundamental study on the teller workplace in a bank. *Ann Physiol Anthropol* 1993;12:341–350.

Chapter 37

Overview of Complete Patient Management in Upper Extremity Repetitive Motion Disorders

Glenn Pransky, MD, MOccH
Jay Himmelstein, MD, MPH

Introduction

Occupational upper extremity disorders are the fastest-growing cause of work-related injuries[1] and may soon surpass low back disorders as the most frequent category of problems leading to work disability in U.S. manufacturing plants.[2] Treatment, rehabilitation, and indemnity costs have increased dramatically over the past 10 years. For example, indemnity and medical costs per case of work-related upper extremity disorder in New York state more than doubled from 1986 to 1992.[3] This dramatic increase has prompted responses by insurers, employers, equipment manufacturers, regulators, and (to a lesser extent) the medical community.

Interventions have included changes in tools and organization of work and institution of worker selection, exercise and fitness programs, intensive case management, splints and vitamins, medical management protocols, regulations, and standards. The principles of successful patient management strategies for occupational upper extremity disorders (especially those caused by repetitive motion) will be examined, based on experiences drawn from a variety of related disorders, and other conditions affecting work capacity.

Sources of Information Relevant to Upper Extremity Disorder Management Programs

Various sources of information (Outline 1) are helpful in developing a successful approach to patients with upper extremity disorders. Although the scientific literature on comprehensive approaches to occupational upper extremity disorders is sparse, the current lay and business literature is replete with successful approaches to rehabilitation and prevention of these problems.[3] These reports are usually descriptions of successful interventions at a single plant.[4] There has been little scientific evaluation to determine effectiveness in returning patients to work or in preventing disability; however, the consistency of positive findings across sites with multifactorial interventions is important, and has influenced proposed Occupational Safety and Health Administration (OSHA) regulations.[5]

Two investigations published in the medical literature followed patients with disabling, chronic upper extremity disorders through comprehensive, multidis-

Outline 1 Sources of information on comprehensive upper extremity disorders programs

---

Upper extremity studies
 Comprehensive program outcome studies
 Comprehensive program reports (medical and lay literature)
 Condition-specific studies (prospective, controlled; cross-sectional)
 Treatment-specific studies (ultrasound, injection, and so on)

Occupation-specific studies
 Athletes
 Musicians

Low back pain studies
 Comprehensive program outcome studies
 Diagnosis and workplace-specific investigations

Cardiac treatment outcome studies

Disability outcome studies

Regulations (OSHA Meatpacking) and standards (ANSIZ365 Committee)

---

ciplinary treatment programs, focusing on return to work as a primary outcome.[6,7] Only one included a matched control group. Many studies followed patients with specific upper extremity diagnoses; more than 60 addressed the carpal tunnel syndrome, and a dozen each focused on treatments for lateral epicondylitis, ulnar neuritis, and cervical syndromes. Several included placebo controls or randomization to alternative treatments, but few studies evaluated return to work as an outcome—most merely inquired about patient satisfaction, symptoms, and limited objective clinical measures, with only a few months of follow-up.

Upper extremity work in industry can be intensive and physically exhausting, requiring significant job-specific skills, strength, and dexterity. Many workers have been appropriately described as industrial athletes. The literature on sports injuries[8] and performance-related upper extremity disorders in musicians offers valuable suggestions for management of occupational upper extremity problems. Although published studies are uncontrolled, investigator experience and length of follow-up are considerable, and the outcomes of primary interest (successful return to athletic competition or musical performance) are analogous to successful return to work.

Regardless of cause, work disability is multifactorial in origin, representing a summation of physiologic, attitudinal, social, motivational, legal, employer-specific, and cultural influences.[9] This complexity is similar to that for low back pain, in which a multifaceted, multidisciplinary program is necessary for successful return to work for patients with chronic, disabling problems.[10] In fact, this program was patterned after a successful intervention targeted to low back pain. Controlled studies in this area are few in number,[11,12] but descriptions of successful programs illustrate those elements that their directors believe are most important in achieving a high level of success.[13]

Investigations of outcome after cardiac bypass surgery and myocardial infarction have a strong tradition of examining return to work as a major outcome. These studies have the advantages of large and diverse patient populations and reasonably long follow-up.[14] Diagnosis-independent studies of work-related disability are also relevant.[15]

Clarifying the Goals and Outcomes of Treatment and Rehabilitation

Before a discussion of what constitutes a successful comprehensive program can begin, the goals and outcomes of importance must be clarified, recognizing that each participant in the process may have different expectations and desires. There are five major types of outcome addressed in management of repetitive motion occupational upper extremity disorders: symptoms, function, work ability and status, cost, and prevention of reinjury.

Symptoms

Symptoms are the primary reason patients seek treatment, and the focus is often on the degree of relief from pain and other symptoms as the most important outcome. Unreasonable expectations of complete absence of pain have resulted in prolonged low back disability.[16] Similar problems have been encountered in an investigation of 120 individuals referred for chronic work-related upper extremity disorders. Usually, absence of pain is less important to employers or insurers, who are more concerned with function, work status, and cost.

Function

In many hand-intensive occupations, the presumption may be valid that returning to usual hand-intensive activities at work implies near-normal function and a reasonable level of pain relief or control. However, workers may desire the ability to perform tasks at home that may be far more demanding than those performed at work. Preliminary results from our prospective study of more than 200 carpal tunnel surgery patients, evaluated for more than a year after initial evaluation, has shown that although the majority were able to return to work, many had persistent, significant limitations in ability to perform activities about the house or were forced to discontinue hobbies.

Return to Work

The literature on treatment of occupational conditions has focused on work resumption or retention as the outcome of greatest importance. Certainly, this result is a primary concern for employers and insurers, and it is usually desired by physicians and other health care providers. It is consistent with traditional views of a normal societal role. The cardiac rehabilitation literature suggests that in older workers who perceive limited employment options in their future regardless of disability, the condition may create a welcome opportunity to obtain an early disability retirement.[17] Although cardiac bypass surgery provides a physiologic correction of the disabling condition, it is associated with a net loss of employment, most often in those with lower incomes, lower socioeconomic status, and a belief that work was a major contributing factor to their illness.[18] Workers with upper extremity disorders may also have significant concerns about reinjury, and an important (although not always explicit) outcome for them may include sufficient workplace changes to prevent reinjury.[19] The family may also want the patient to stay away from a job that they perceive as dangerous, or they may become used to having the disabled worker available for child care.[20]

Cost

Employers and insurers more often address cost as a central focus for evaluating alternative strategies for occupational upper extremity disorder management. However, workers are relatively unconcerned about costs (compared to the employer and insurer), and are more interested in optimal treatment and pursuit of diagnostic tests. Workers' compensation insurers seek to return an employee to work as soon as possible, with the least expensive but most rapidly effective treatment. In contrast, private health insurance seeks to avoid any expenses associated with work-related conditions. The resulting conflicts may create difficulties for a worker in obtaining necessary treatment for conditions that are aggravated but not caused by work, as well as interesting variations in approved treatment between insurers. For example, a workers' compensation insurer may favor endoscopic carpal tunnel surgery (faster return to work), whereas private health insurance may choose to reimburse only for an open procedure if it is less expensive. Cost considerations will be seen in a completely different light by a patient's lawyer, who may advise staying out of work until the case is settled in order to maximize the settlement. Federal programs, in the interests of controlling costs and providing health care for all, may seek to limit the extent of services for some, or may not incorporate workers' compensation, creating further impetus for providers to label conditions as occupational.

Prevention of Reinjury and Disability

The most effective occupational injury management programs link early recognition of work-related conditions to ergonomic changes in the workplace, in order to prevent development of similar disorders. The ergonomic job modifications needed to permit a worker with an occupational upper extremity disorder to return to work safely will usually decrease risk of injury for asymptomatic individuals performing the same job. Therefore, a measure of program success should include level of employee feedback on suggested changes, number of changes implemented, trend in numbers of new injuries over time, and rates of reinjury.

These considerations may be new to those who have recently started treating occupational upper extremity disorders. Their importance has been recognized for decades by those involved in chronic low back pain and cardiac rehabilitation research, who strongly suggest that the goals and expectations of treatment must be openly addressed by the medical provider early on in the treatment process. A truly comprehensive program will help patients, employers, and insurers define reasonable expectations, including minimizing (but not necessarily eliminating) symptoms, maximizing function, preventing unnecessary disability, controlling costs, and preventing reinjury.

A Complete Upper Extremity Disorder Patient Management Program

Successful upper extremity disorder programs described in the literature have a number of common features, similar to interventions for low back pain, upper extremity disorders in musicians and athletes, and cardiac disability. They are based on a model of occupational upper extremity disorders, that links the progression of illness through increasing severity and symptoms and decreasing function, eventually resulting in work disability (Fig. 1). The characteristics and intensity of intervention parallel the severity and extent of impact of the disorder. The following three types of intervention may not always be distinct; they are described separately to clearly illustrate program elements. A complete upper extremity disorder management program would include the resources to provide each type of intervention.

Primary Intervention

Much of the lay literature on workplace-based programs targeting occupational upper extremity disorders has focused on primary intervention—that is, those activities that occur at a plant once a worker develops symptoms. Successful programs encourage early symptom reporting by employees, presence of on-site personnel trained in initial evaluation and treatment, recognition and correction of causative ergonomic factors, and appropriate medical referral, if needed.[6,21] One approach has become codified in the OSHA Ergonomics Program Management Guidelines for Meatpacking Plants (OSHA 3123), and it may receive support for broader implementation through the proposed OSHA industry-wide Ergonomic Standard and the American National Standards Institute (ANSI) Ergonomics Standard. The meatpacking guideline requires follow-up to determine whether treatment was effective, referral of an individual with positive symptoms or findings on physical examination to a physician, and an adequate trial of conservative therapy before surgery.

Successful programs include a consistent management response that acknowledges a worker's concerns and that emphasizes prevention, remediation, and accommodation rather than discriminating between work-related and non-occupational conditions.[22] There is considerable controversy regarding the proportion of occupational upper extremity disorder cases that are actually caused by work; some argue that the numbers are low,[23] while others argue that the majority of cases would not have been present without the repetitive, forceful, and awkward activities in the workplace.[24,25] The low back pain literature sug-

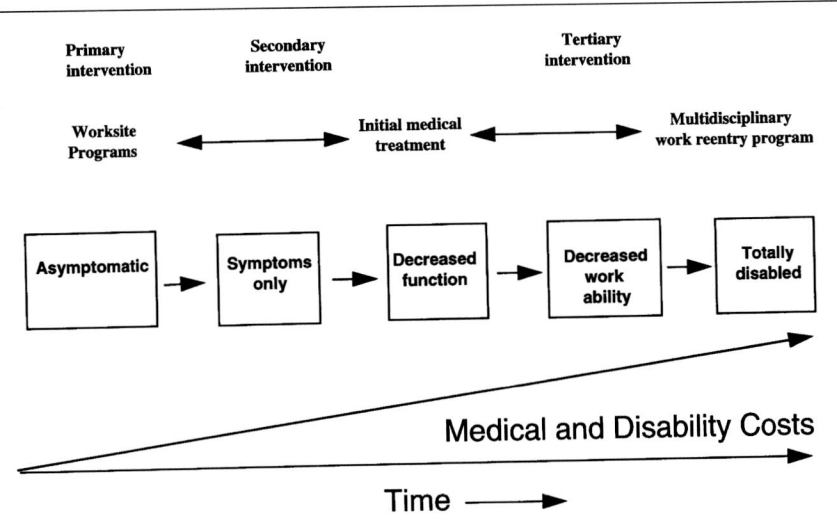

Fig. 1 Evolution and management of upper extremity disorders.

gests that both viewpoints may be partially correct. Because low back disability[26] or carpal tunnel syndrome[27] will affect 3% to 10% of the population during a lifetime, and the incidence is much higher for nondisabling upper extremity pain,[28] both of these disorders will always be encountered in working populations. Certain jobs, such as meatpacking, have occupational upper extremity disorder injury rates that approach 40% per year, with clear linkage between diagnoses and job activities. In contrast, the prevalence of upper extremity complaints in other employment may be similar to that in the general population, with social factors and medical overtreatment contributing to elevated job-specific disability rates.[29,30] In either case, an affected employee may suffer prolonged work absence, with associated expenses for treatment and wage replacement and employer costs for lost skills and replacement workers. These expenses may be similar in both the workers' compensation and the private insurance systems. A proactive approach with early accommodation, specific ergonomic modifications, appropriate treatment, and periodic reevaluation may result in considerable overall savings, certainly more than can be gained by focusing on separating work-related from nonoccupational disorders.

Secondary Intervention: Integrated Medical Treatment

Patients with occupational upper extremity disorders who have persistent symptoms and loss of function should be referred to a physician, ideally one familiar with the ergonomic, psychosocial, and demographic characteristics of the workplace. A few hours spent touring a facility provides the treating physician with a much clearer picture of job activities and greatly increases credibility with employers, insurers, and patients. Ideally, this should occur early so that the physician can see the patient perform tasks associated with symptoms. Slow-speed videotape analysis[31] and ergonomic checklists[32] can be used to efficiently collect data needed to detect significant ergonomic problems. Though some basic ergonomic training may be necessary for a physician to accurately interpret this data, several texts[33] and videotapes[34] are helpful.

This information must be combined with a thorough evaluation of the patient, including a detailed history of the problem. Although upper extremity disorders caused by work, athletics, or musical performance can result from the cumulative effect of years of ergonomically stressful activities, an acute precipitant has usually increased symptoms and brings the patient to the office.[35] Because the sensitivity and specificity of most physical examination maneuvers is limited, the importance of positive findings should not be overrated. Often, the degree of positivity (time to positive Phalen's test, degree of grip strength difference between hands, amount of elbow flexion required to elicit finger tingling, and so on) may be more important than discriminating between presence or absence of a finding.

Diagnostic testing by physicians has been extensively studied in low back pain, where the majority of tests are not helpful, but are ordered in response to patient demands for a specific diagnosis.[36] Similar considerations apply to hand radiographs in simple nontraumatic conditions, nerve conduction studies without clear-cut physical findings of nerve entrapment, and shoulder films in myofascial syndromes, where the likelihood of false-positive tests may be high.[37] Preventive patient education may be helpful here.

A plethora of therapeutic options is available for occupational upper extremity disorders, with surprisingly little scientific basis for choice of regimen.[38] Wide variations in surgery rates for similar populations in different regions suggests that overutilization of treatment, without scientifically based selection, is common.[29,39] The sports medicine literature suggests that a short period of anti-inflammatory measures and rest is often beneficial. Ultrasound may have advantages over placebo treatment, but it is often difficult to separate treatment effect from the natural history. Modality treatment is followed by gradual, supervised activity resumption.[40] Physical therapy for athletes begins with flexion, supported by modalities, and progresses to isometric and then active strength training. Splinting is occasionally useful, as long as the job does not require forceful exertions against the movement limitation imposed by the device.

Frequent contact with the employer assures both the physician and the patient that alternative duty assignments are appropriate, informs the employer that the patient's condition is legitimate, and reinforces reasonable expectations from treatment. Although comprehensive, highly integrated treatment programs may be required for more severe cases (to be discussed later), the informed physician, working closely with a physical or occupational therapist familiar with ergonomics and the workplace, can effectively manage the majority of these early-stage, nondisabled patients. Early discussion of the patient's expectations with respect to symptoms, function (on and off the job), and work has been essential in directing therapeutic planning in low back pain,[41] and is equally important in upper extremity disorders. Preventive interventions should be considered throughout the evaluation and treatment process, to decrease the likelihood of recurrence or similar injuries to coworkers;[42] the ergonomic changes necessary for accommodation and avoidance of reinjury will usually prevent future injuries in coworkers.

Tertiary Intervention: Multidisciplinary Programs for Disabled Workers

Work absence in occupational upper extremity disorders may result from more severe conditions, worker concerns, lack of alternative work or accommodations at the workplace, and other factors.[43] Low back disability research suggests that work absence is usually independent of severity of physical findings and diagnosis, and often depends on psychosocial factors.[44] The disability research literature suggests that better results in long-term work outcome occur if work disability is minimized at the outset. In patients with cardiac disease or low back pain, musicians, and athletes, longer time away from work activities is correlated with a lower likelihood of eventual return to employment or performance. This does not mean that complete rest is always contraindicated; frequently, there must be relative rest of the affected area for a period of time. Again, alternative job activities and accommodations in the workplace can often obviate the need for prolonged work absence while resting the injured area.

A subset of these patients require surgical or other therapeutic interventions, such as injections or carpal tunnel release. The medical literature has few controlled studies to guide treatment selection, postsurgical rehabilitation program, or projections of expected work capacity at medical end-result. Reports from centers for treatment of musicians or athletes suggest that surgery should be reserved for specific, confirmed diagnoses; many of these patients will get better and return to former activities. Nonspecific problems, including regional pain syndromes, dystonia, and myofascial syndromes, usually become worse after surgery; thus, patient selection is critical.[45] The long-term advantages of physical therapy over rest are still unknown, and it is not known how to determine when, and in what jobs, a patient can safely return to modified or full duty after surgery (such as carpal tunnel surgery).

Most of these patients will not benefit from a purely medical approach, and are more appropriate candidates for an integrated, multidisciplinary intervention. Intensive low back pain programs often accept patients after 3 months of work absence, but find that efforts to return patients after 2 years out of work are unsuccessful. The program team may include physicians, psychologists, occupational and physical therapists, ergonomists, and vocational rehabilitation experts.[13] Each case is coordinated by a case manager. Only one program for chronic occupational upper extremity disorder patients has been evaluated in comparison with a control population, as described by Feuerstein and associates in 1993. This program achieved a 58% return-to-work rate in comparison with a control group, who had a 40% return-to-work rate. Similar programs for musicians begin with rest to control inflammation and symptoms, followed by intensive rehabilitation that includes strengthening as well as ergonomics (posture, technique), counseling, and development of a conditioning and flexibility program, with more than 80% success in return to performance.[45]

Physical conditioning programs for these patients may be more successful if based upon actual work activities, thereby providing an opportunity to reestablish skills required to do the job. This requires knowledge of the workplace, the actual job that the patient will resume, and ability to effectively simulate the required tasks. Although less quantitative, the validity and predictive ability of work simulation to measure actual work capacity is usually much better than standardized testing measures.[46] In the cardiac setting, work simulation provides essential positive reinforcement to the patient that it is safe to return to work.[47] Therapists must clearly understand the etiology of the condition and its relation to work activities, and they should be willing to provide adequate and timely feedback to employers, insurers, and physicians.[48]

Retraining has been most effective in preventing reinjury in sign-language interpreters[49] and musicians,[45] in whom technique variations account for substantial injuries. Activity-specific conditioning, stretching, and training are important in maintaining recovery. Several investigators suggest that this approach might be fruitful with occupational upper extremity disorders,[50] although these programs have had less dramatic success with low back pain.[51]

Interface Between Rehabilitation Programs and the Workplace

Traditional medical models for chronic occupational upper extremity disorders and low back pain have been sequential. Here the patient first receives diagnosis-specific treatment, primarily directed toward symptom relief, and often without much consideration of work activities. Once a medical end-result is reached, rehabilitation (often directed by a nurse employed by the workers' compensation carrier) begins, and this may be the first time that the patient's concerns about work ability, reinjury, and function are addressed. Finally, if work-specific physical retraining cannot restore function to the level needed to return to the former job, vocational rehabilitation experts perform a skills inventory and job search. The sequential approach leads to excessive delays in resolution and increased expense, especially in those patients who have multiple reasons (physical, vocational, psychosocial) for not returning to work.[52]

Because patients with occupational upper extremity disorders from repetitive trauma may be even less likely to be able to return to their jobs, the sequential approach may be even less appropriate for them than it is for patients with low back pain. Cardiac rehabilitation programs have recently begun to integrate work-related rehabilitation, interface with the workplace, and even vocational evaluation as early as 3 days after an infarct has occurred. This concurrent approach is much more successful in addressing a broad range of patient, family, and employer concerns. In occupational upper extremity disorders, employers often question the likelihood of return to a former job, the types of ergonomic changes required to accommodate, and the chances of re-injury. Although a lack of scientific data precludes definitive answers in most cases,[53] clarifying these issues early and including the patient in the discussion will often improve the ultimate chances for safe return to work.[54]

Summary

Comprehensive approaches to upper extremity disorders are appearing in industry, outpatient clinic, and intensive treatment settings. Although many appear to be successful, controlled studies are rarely conducted, because programs are constantly evolving to meet the changing needs of industry, insurance providers, and workers. In contrast to low back pain, the value of many treatments of upper extremity disorders has not been compared with that of placebos, and much less is known about methods for determining when work can be safely resumed. Studies of these aspects are critical to developing the most effective approach for these disorders.

References

1. Bureau of Labor Statistics: *Occupational Injuries and Illnesses*. Washington, DC, United States Department of Labor, 1993.
2. Roughton J: Cumulative trauma disorders: The newest business liability. *Professional Safety* 1993;38:29–35.
3. Kohn JP, Friend MA: Quality and ergonomics: The team approach to the occupational people factor. *Professional Safety* 1993;38:39–42.
4. Pipinich RE: Ergonomics: A high priority at Lockheed Fort Worth facility. *Industrial Engineering* 1993;25:20–22.
5. Hales TR, Bertsche PK: Management of upper extremity cumulative trauma disorders. *AAOHN J* 1992;40:118–128.
6. Feuerstein M, Callan-Harris S, Hickey P, et al: Multidisciplinary rehabilitation of chronic work-related upper extremity disorders: Long-term effects. *J Occup Med* 1993;35:396–403.
7. Flinn-Wagner S, Maldonicky A, Goodman G: Characteristics of workers with upper extremity injuries who make a successful transition to work. *J Hand Therapy* 1990;3:51–55.
8. Herring SA, Nilson KL: Introduction to overuse injuries. *Clin Sports Med* 1987;6:225–239.
9. Gay DA, Wong DW: Predicting rehabilitation outcomes from clinical and statistical data: A probability model. *Int J Rehabil Res* 1988;11:11–19.
10. Feuerstein M: A multidisciplinary approach to the prevention, evaluation, and management of work disability. *J Occup Rehabil* 1991;1:5–12.
11. Mayer TG, Gatchel RJ, Mayer H, et al: A prospective two-year study of functional restoration in industrial low back injury: An objective assessment procedure. *JAMA* 1987;258:1763–1767.
12. Hazard RG, Fenwick JW, Kalisch SM, et al: Functional restoration with behavioral support: A one-year prospective study of patients with chronic low-back pain. *Spine* 1989;14:157–161.
13. Rosomoff HL, Rosomoff RS: Comprehensive multidisciplinary pain center approach to the treatment of low back pain. *Neurosurg Clin N Am* 1991;2:877–890.

14. Russell RO Jr, Abi-Mansour P, Wenger NK: Return to work after coronary bypass surgery and percutaneous transluminal angioplasty: Issues and potential solutions. *Cardiology* 1986;73:306–322.
15. Tate DG: Workers' disability and return to work. *Am J Phys Med Rehabil* 1992; 71:92–96.
16. Waddell G: A new clinical model for the treatment of low-back pain. *Spine* 1987; 12:632–644.
17. Fitzgerald TE, Tennen H, Affleck G, et al: The relative importance of dispositional optimism and control appraisals in quality of life after coronary artery bypass surgery. *J Behav Med* 1993;16:25–43.
18. Maeland JG, Havik OE: Psychological predictors for return to work after myocardial infarction. *J Psychosom Res* 1987;31:471–481.
19. McFarlane AC: The longitudinal course of posttraumatic morbidity: The range of outcomes and their predictors. *J Nerv Ment Dis* 1988;176:30–39.
20. Fordyce WE: Behavioral factors in pain. *Neurosurg Clin N Am* 1991;2:749–759.
21. Millar JD: Valuing, empowering employees vital to quality health & safety management. *Occup Health Saf* 1993;62:100–101.
22. Pransky GS, Snyder TB, Himmelstein JS: Organizational factors and cumulative trauma disorders, in Sauter SL, Moon S (eds): *Psychosocial Aspects of Office-Related Cumulative Trauma Disorders*, in press.
23. Nathan PA, Keniston RC: Carpal tunnel syndrome and its relation to general physical condition. *Hand Clin* 1993;9:253–261.
24. Armstrong TJ, Buckle P, Fine LJ, et al: A conceptual model for work-related neck and upper-limb musculoskeletal disorders. *Scand J Work Env Health* 1993;19:73–84.
25. Luopajarvi T, Kuorinka I, Virolainen M, et al: Prevalence of tenosynovitis and other injuries of the upper extremities in repetitive work. *Scand J of Work Env Health* 1979;5(suppl 3):48–55.
26. Biering-Sorensen F: A prospective study of low back pain in a general population: I. Occurrence, recurrence and aetiology. *Scand J Rehabil Med* 1983;15:71–79.
27. Stevens JC, Sun S, Beard CM, et al: Carpal tunnel syndrome in Rochester, Minnesota, 1961–1980. *Neurology* 1988;38:134–138.
28. Kelsey JL (ed): *Epidemiology of Musculoskeletal Disorders*. New York, NY, Oxford University Press, 1982.
29. Hadler NM: Arm pain in the workplace: A small area analysis. *J Occup Med* 1992;34:113–119.
30. Hocking B: Letter: "Repetition strain injury" in Telecom Australia. *Med J Aust* 1989;150:724.
31. Feuerstein M, Hickey PF: Ergonomic approaches in the clinical assessment of occupational musculoskeletal disorders, in Turk DC, Melzack R (eds): *Handbook of Pain Assessment*. New York, NY, Guilford Press, 1992, pp 71–99.
32. Keyserling WM, Armstrong TJ, Punnett L: Ergonomic job analysis: A structured approach for identifying risk factors associated with over-exertion injuries and disorders. *Appl Occ Env Hyg* 1991;6:353–363.
33. Putz-Anderson V (ed): *Cumulative Trauma Disorders: A Manual for Musculoskeletal Diseases of the Upper Limbs*. London, UK, Taylor and Francis, 1988.
34. National Institute of Occupational Safety and Health: Videotape: *The Finest Tools*. Cincinnati, OH, National Institute of Occupational Safety and Health, 1988.
35. Fry HJ: The treatment of overuse injury syndrome. *Md Med J* 1993;42:277–282.
36. Volinn E, Turczyn KM, Loeser JD: Theories of back pain and health care utilization. *Neurosurg Clin N Am* 1991;2:739–748.
37. Redmond MD, Rivner MH: False positive electrodiagnostic tests in carpal tunnel syndrome. *Muscle Nerve* 1988;11:511–518.
38. Spitzer WO, Leblanc FE, Dupuis M, et al: Scientific approach to the assessment and management of activity-related spinal disorders: A monograph for clinicians. Report of the Quebec Task Force on Spinal Disorders. *Spine* 1987;12 (suppl 2):S1–S59.

39. Wennberg JE, Freeman JL, Culp WJ: Are hospital services rationed in New Haven or over-utilized in Boston? *Lancet* 1987;1:1185–1189.
40. Kiefhaber TR, Stern PJ: Upper extremity tendinitis and overuse syndromes in the athlete. *Clin Sports Med* 1992;11:39–55.
41. Bigos SJ, Battie MC: Acute care to prevent back disability: Ten years of progress. *Clin Orthop* 1987;221:121–130.
42. Kilbom A: Intervention programs for work-related neck and upper limb disorders: Strategies and evaluation. *Ergonomics* 1988;31:735–747.
43. Novek J, Yassi A, Spiegel J: Mechanization, the labor process, and injury risks in the Canadian meat packing industry. *Int J Health Serv* 1990;20:281–296.
44. Bigos SJ, Battie MC, Spengler DM, et al: A prospective study of work perceptions and psychosocial factors affecting the report of back injury. *Spine* 1991;16:1–6.
45. Amadio PC, Russotti GM: Evaluation and treatment of hand and wrist disorders in musicians. *Hand Clin* 1990;6:405–416.
46. Bear-Lehman J, Abreu BC: Evaluating the hand: Issues in reliability and validity. *Phys Ther* 1989;69:1025–1033.
47. Ewartk CK, Taylor CB, Reese LB, et al: Effects of early postmyocardial infarction exercise testing on self-perception and subsequent physical activity. *Am J Cardiol* 1983;51:1076–1080.
48. King J: An integration of medicine in industry. *J Hand Ther* 1990;3:45–50.
49. Feuerstein M, Fitzgerald TE: Biomechanical factors affecting upper extremity disorders cumulative trauma in sign language interpreters. *J Occ Med* 1992;34:257–264.
50. Kilbom A, Persson J: Work technique and its consequences for musculoskeletal disorders. *Ergonomics* 1987;30:273–279.
51. Deyo RA, Cherkin D, Conrad D, et al: Cost, controversy, crisis: Low back pain and the health of the public. *Ann Rev Pub Health* 1991;12:141–156.
52. Curtis NM: Managed care and workers' compensation. *Hand Clin* 1993;9:373–377.
53. Christiansen C: Continuing challenges of functional assessment in rehabilitation: Recommended changes. *Am J Occup Ther* 1993;47:258–259.
54. Sandstrom J, Esbjornsson E: Return to work after rehabilitation: The significance of the patient's own prediction. *Scand J Rehab Med* 1986;18:29–33.

Directions for Future Research

For the clinical and epidemiologic literature to be more consistent and meaningful, there must be agreement on the definitions and diagnoses of repetitive motion disorders. Definitions for repetitive motion disorders that identify the tissues which are injured and the nature of the injuries and case definitions for clinical and epidemiologic studies should be standardized.

Short, practical testing methods can be applied to large numbers of workers in order to identify those with early stage disorders who would benefit from early intervention. Such test methods would be valuable in tracking the effectiveness of preventive or therapeutic efforts. These simple tests should correlate with the early signs and symptoms of repetitive motion disorders and with more-detailed clinical examinations using explicit diagnostic criteria. If a small constellation of signs and symptoms are found to be predictive of a more-complete clinical examination, this short battery of tests would be very useful in surveillance and control efforts. If correlated with long-term outcomes, such tests could be applied to large groups of workers in order to direct and evaluate both medical management and ergonomic interventions.

Depending on the purpose of the research investigation, three levels of diagnostic accuracy may be appropriate. Level 1 concerns general surveillance (easily obtained, low cost, moderate specificity and high sensitivity, and probable diagnosis). Level 2 concerns nonsurgical therapy (unable to work and greater specificity than above). Level 3 concerns presurgical diagnosis (most costly, highest specificity, and extensive testing, including possible workplace simulation). These definition should be more fully defined and endorsed by appropriate professional organizations.

In all clinical studies there is a need for improved and standardized outcome measures for repetitive motion disorders. One important current concept in outcome assessment is the appropriate use of patient expectation and patient perspectives in addition to physical and laboratory examinations. Clinical studies must be anatomic site and disorder specific (eg, the clinical findings on treatment of carpal tunnel syndrome may not necessarily be transferred to other upper extremity conditions).

Most aspects of clinical diagnosis, treatment, and rehabilitation for repetitive motion disorders require extensive additional evaluation to establish optimal approaches. The following future research topics are broad representations of some areas that could be studied.

Conduct studies on the diagnosis of repetitive motion disorders.

There is currently a broad range of physical tests and diagnostic evaluations (such as sensibility testing, nerve conduction, and imaging studies) that can be performed on patients presenting with signs and/or symptoms of repetitive motion disorders. Functional capacity testing is described more specifically in the next future research topic. Because of the large number of cases that can be successfully evaluated and treated with minimal testing, it would be important for cost containment purposes to define more clearly which tests should be performed and at what stage of disease progression. The simplified tests proposed above may also be part of such a clinical evaluation. Clinical studies could be conducted in a large health maintenance organization (HMO) setting with direct referral from an industrial or work setting having a high incidence of repetitive motion disorders. Outcome measures must include patient and work status in both the short- and long-term stages following initial patient identification.

Establish improved measures of functional capacity.

Functional capacity evaluation is often used to measure progress in treating patients with repetitive motion disorders. Three of the methods are (1) force/strength testing by computerized devices, (2) performance of standardized tasks, and (3) observation during simulated work activities. The last method, while less quantitative, may be a more accurate predictor of ability to return to work. The flaw of this method may be that it is only applied over a short period of time and not an 8-hour real work setting.

A prospective study should be performed to compare the value of these functional assessments to predict successful return to work with reduced reinjury over a long-term follow-up. Special effort could be made to avoid referral and selection bias as well as confounding clinical, provider, insurance, and workplace factors. A large study of this type may be expensive to conduct.

Conduct studies on therapeutic and rehabilitative interventions.

There is a great need for further clinical studies to define optimal therapy and rehabilitation in each of the repetitive motion disorders of the upper extremity. Even basic issues, such as exercise and conditioning versus rest and immobilization, have not been studied rigorously to determine the proper balance between these approaches. There is very little information regarding the training of the health care provider (eg, occupational nurse, family practitioner, general orthopaedist, or hand surgeon) and the impact of the health care setting (eg, HMO or private practice) on the treatment and outcomes for these patients. In a similar manner, many states have developed algorithms to be followed in work compensation cases. These protocols have not been tested for clinical efficacy or cost effectiveness.

Both intrinsic and extrinsic risk factors must be controlled to avoid biasing the outcomes. Intrinsic risk factors include psychosocial factors, body mass index, age, cultural background, anatomic abnormalities, physical condition, avocations, metabolic conditions, smoking, and substance abuse. Extrinsic factors in the workplace and home activity include level of force, posture, repetition, and cumulative exposure. All of these factors must be incorporated in the context of a well-designed investigation that utilizes all of the features expected in epidemiologic and clinical studies. Outcome variables must be carefully selected to assess short- and long-term measures of patient health and work status. Clearly, a multidisciplinary team must be gathered to undertake such a complex task. These clinical studies will be expensive and require substantial federal commitment to support these endeavors. Therefore, investigators should identify interventions that are likely to have a large public health impact.

Determine which work and recreational activities are safe following therapy.

Following appropriate therapy and rehabilitation, many patients expect to be able to return to their previous work or recreational activities. There is little in the way of scientific evidence to guide ergonomic changes or activity limitations for specific repetitive motion conditions; for example, it is not clear when patients can return to repetitive gripping jobs after surgery for carpal tunnel syndrome, and the maximum amount and frequency of gripping that is compatible with long-term safe job retention are not known. Clinical studies of the medical and work/sport interface could be conducted using the sound scientific principles described above.

Clinical Questions

On June 20-22, 1994, a workshop was held on the topic of Repetitive Motion Disorders of the Upper Extremity. This workshop was sponsored by the National Institute of Arthritis and Musculoskeletal and Skin Diseases, the National Institute for Occupational Safety and Health, the National Center for Medical Rehabilitation Research, National Institute of Child Health and Human Development, the Orthopaedic Research and Education Foundation, the Center for VDT and Health Research, and the Public Health Services Advisory Committee on Employment of Persons With Disabilities. A group of leading basic and clinical scientists gathered to discuss the state of knowledge and directions for future research in this field. These internationally recognized experts were asked to address six practical clinical questions that a layperson might ask a physician regarding these conditions.

The answers are summarized below. A few common concepts are contained in many of the answers. Although this may be somewhat repetitious, each answer can be understood independently without extensive reference to other answers.

Question #1: Doctor, what are the early symptoms of these conditions?

It is normal to have a small amount of occasional pain or discomfort in the upper extremity. As people get older, it is more common to experience periodic pain or discomfort. When episodes are separated by a month or more, do not last for more than a few days, and are not caused by a specific activity, these mild pains should not be a cause for concern.

Symptoms of a repetitive motion disorder may include pain, aching, stiffness, fatigue, weakness, and numbing and/or tingling. In many conditions, nighttime pain occurs as the disorder progresses; in other cases, the symptoms may start with nighttime pain. Frequent recurrence of the symptoms, especially after performing specific work or recreational activities, is a possible indication of the early stages of a repetitive motion disorder. Another important sign may be a decrease in functional ability to perform tasks in the workplace or during leisure. It is very likely that any early symptoms will significantly improve with proper rest, activity modification, and therapy.

Question #2: Doctor, I have some mild occasional pain. Can I prevent this from becoming permanent?

If you can describe your upper extremity pain as being very mild and occurring only occasionally, it may be normal and probably would require no specific action on your part. If the symptoms appear to be progressive, that is, the pain worsens and occurs more frequently following certain work or home activities, then it is time to take some action. It is advisable at this point to seek medical assessment and specific recommendations for your symptoms. Early intervention is an important key to successfully preventing further progress toward a permanent condition. Your physician will help to distinguish between activity-related fatigue and/or mild irritation of musculoskeletal tissues as compared to repetitive motion disorders that have become chronic.

You should try to identify the specific work, sports, or home activities that seem to precede the pain or other symptoms. If you can identify a probable cause, you should attempt to reduce the frequency, duration, or manner in which the activity is performed. Reduce your pain-inducing activities as much as you can. Do not immobilize or splint a painful area without the specific recommendation of a physician. You may be able to reduce the finger or hand force required by using assistive devices or by changing the relative position of your hands or arms to be less stressful. You should take short but frequent breaks. If possible, switch between different tasks to avoid repeating the same loading pattern continuously. Try to develop and maintain a high level of general fitness and health.

By acting early, in conjunction with your physician's advice, it is very likely that your condition will not become permanent.

Question #3: Doctor, what are the medical tests to evaluate my condition?

Your physician will obtain a complete medical history of your current and past symptoms and any other factors that may be related to your problem. It is important to distinguish between symptoms caused by a single injury and those resulting from a repetitive motion disorder. You will receive a thorough neurologic and musculoskeletal physical examination. Your doctor will try to isolate the location of any painful tissues in your neck or upper extremity. In some cases, the painful site may be removed from the source of the problem. For example, pain in the elbow region may be caused by, or reproduced by, motions and forces applied to the fingers and wrist. This direct evaluation by a well-qualified physician may be all the testing required to make an initial diagnosis of the problem and prescribe proper treatment.

In some cases, your physician may initially or subsequently recommend that additional testing be performed. Potential medical tests include radiography, magnetic resonance imaging (MRI), electromyography (EMG), nerve conduction velocity (NCV), computed tomography (CT), bone scan, psychophysical testing, and laboratory testing. It is not likely that all of these diagnostic procedures will be recommended. Your doctor will indicate what tests are needed to more accurately assess and treat your particular condition.

Question #4: Doctor, what is the correct treatment for my condition and will I need surgery?

Your doctor will thoroughly evaluate the nature of your symptoms and the possible role of work or recreational activities in causing the problem. The required treatment will be specific for your situation. You may be treated by several medical and rehabilitation specialists to enhance your recovery.

Some of the common elements for treatment of repetitive motion disorders of the upper extremity include reduced activity, activity modification, part-time use of splints, heat and/or cold, pain relievers, anti-inflammatory medication, and cortisone injections. Physical or occupational therapy may be recommended to increase the flexibility and strength of the upper extremity. It is important to realize that you are an active contributor to the recovery process. You should carefully follow the specific treatment advice provided.

For most individuals, the treatments outlined above will relieve the symptoms and allow a return to full or nearly full activity. In some cases, temporary or permanent modification of work or recreational activities is required to relieve the pain and keep it from recurring. Surgery is indicated only if nonsurgical treatments fail to relieve symptoms and if a specific anatomic problem is the cause. Surgery may permit improvement, but the injured tissues will not be fully normal and special care should be taken to avoid future reinjury.

Question #5: Doctor, can I continue at my work or recreational activity?

The level of injury will determine the initial ability to return to work or recreational activity. If the injury is minor, the symptoms minimal, and there is no anatomic loss of tissue integrity, you may be able to continue to perform your work tasks or sport with small modification of activity level and a simple treatment program.

If the symptoms are more severe, the intensity and duration of the activity must be greatly reduced and a more thorough treatment initiated. Accommodation at the work site with consultation between you, your physician, and your employer will allow an early return to the job with gradual return to normal activities as your symptoms improve and function returns. For recreational activities you may need to seek professional coaching to reduce the mechanical overloads caused by improper form. Your diligence in following the treatment and rehabilitation program is key to assuring the earliest possible return to normal activities. The specific strategy for each medical condition and each work or recreational activity is different. In most cases, you will probably be able to continue your previous activities. In a small number of cases, it may not be possible to return to your work or recreational activity.

In all cases, establishing and/or maintaining a healthy lifestyle is very important for your well-being and for your recovery. If your upper extremity symptoms do not permit continuing your favorite exercise, substitute another form of conditioning until the disorder improves.

Question #6: Doctor, will I recover completely and how long will it take?

You are likely to recover completely in about 4 to 6 weeks from the symptoms related to repetitive upper extremity usage. Early diagnosis and treatment help assure this positive outcome. In many cases, some temporary reduction or alteration in your work or recreational activities may be required.

If the extent of the injury is severe or if it is left untreated for a long time, the outcome may be less successful. Some patients have substantial improvement, but are not fully functional at the same level of performance as before the repetitive motion injury. In these cases, a permanent change in activities may be required. In a few cases, the work or recreational activities cannot be modified and these activities must be totally avoided. If work environment modifications or alternative employment are required, they can be established best with the full cooperation of the patient, the doctor, and the employer.

In the full range of clinical outcomes, from minimal to severe residual deficit in function or other symptoms, your compliance with the treatment and rehabilitation program is crucial for achieving the best possible results.

Index

Page numbers in italics refer to figures or figure legends.

A

Abductor pollicis longus 436–*440*
Achilles tendinitis 251–252
    epidemiology 217
Acromioclavicular joint, degeneration of 502–504
Adenosine triphosphate (ATP) 287–289, 295
    in muscle protein turnover 332–333
Age
    and carpal tunnel syndrome 425–426, 431
    and cervical spine degeneration 36
    and connective tissue 166
    and neck disorders 31
    and rotator cuff tears 500
    and the shoulder 496
    and skeletal muscle regeneration 319–320
    and trigger finger 439
Aggrecan 206–208
Allen's test 22
American National Standards Institute (ANSI) Ergonomics Standard 540, 543
Anatomy
    abductor pollicis longus 436–*438*
    abnormalities and carpal tunnel syndrome 425
    axon 381, 383–385
    cubital tunnel *456–457*
    and de Quervain's disease 436–*438*
    elbow 134–135
    extensor carpi ulnaris *443–444*
    extensor pollicis brevis 436–437
    ligament 185–198, 218–219
    nerve 359–376, 381–387
    shoulder 145–149, 493–494
    tendon and ligament 185–198, 218–219
    wrist 138–139, 427 (*see also* Wrist)
Animal models
    of gene regulation in dorsal root ganglion 399–405
    and muscle pain 407, 409
    on muscle protein turnover 326
    and tendon loading 208–210
Arcade of Fröhse 372–*373*
Arcade of Struthers 370
Arthritis, glenohumeral 38–39, 154–156, 504
Axillary nerve anatomy 364–365
Axonotmesis, definition 374, 388
Axons 359–362
    anatomy and function 381, 383–385

B

Biochemisty, tendon and ligament 219–221
Biomechanics (*see also* Physical stressors)
    in computer keyboard operation 103–104, 107–108
    elbow 133–142
    finger model 100–101
    hand and wrist models 111–120
    of muscle injury 339–347
    in piano playing 100–107
    shear forces and nerve compression 388
    shoulder 145–157
    of soft tissue 161–171
    of tendon 166–168, 208–210, 231–242
Blood supply
    and compression 388–389
    of nerves 385–386
    of tendons and ligaments 192–193, 211–213
    tendon 219
Borg
    CR-10 scale 52–53, 56–57
    RPE scale 51–53, 55
Brachial plexus
    anatomic mousetraps 366–368
    anatomy 361–363
Bursae 197, 269

C

Calcium
 activated proteases 317, 332
 ions 232–235, 238–239, 331–332
 overload 344–347
Capitate *114*, 427
Capsaicin 399–404, 408, 411–412
Carpal tunnel syndrome 7–13, 99–100
 and carpal tunnel pressure 123–131
 in computer users 107–108
 definition 123, 421
 diagnosis 421–424
 and Linburg syndrome *442*
 as a model for nerve compression 391–393
 risk factors 112–*113*, 424–429
 in women 376
 workers' compensation for 421
 as a work-related disorder 421–431
Cervical disk herniations 32–33
Cervicobrachial disorders 507–514
 muscle 509–510
 nerve and vascular 507–509
 occupational (OCD) 37–38, 511–512
 thoracic outlet syndrome 32, 35, 367, 508–509
Classification
 of nerve injury 373–374, 387–388
 Sunderland 373–374, 387–388
Collagen, ligament 219–220
Compartment syndrome 21
Computer keyboard operation 3–4, 43–47
 and fingertip force 103–104, 107–108
 and psychosocial factors 65–74
Constant Score shoulder evaluation form 523
Contact stress 89, 92–93, *113*–114
Corticosteroids 486, 525–526
Crimp, definition 218
Cubital tunnel syndrome 455–463
 anatomy 456–457
 diagnosis 457–458
 grading 459
 rehabilitation of 487–488
 treatment 458–461
Cytokines
 in ligament and tendon healing 248, 255
 interleukin-1 (IL-1) 324, 326–330
 and muscle protein turnover 326–327, 334

D

De Quervain's disease 435–439, 445, 450
 and retaining ligaments 195
Desmin *303, 305*–307

 and contraction-induced muscle injury 345
 and Z-band connections 306
Diabetes
 and compressive neuropathies 376, 381
 and Dupuytren's contracture 23
 risk factor for carpal tunnel syndrome 425
Diagnosis
 of carpal tunnel syndrome 421–424
 of cubital tunnel syndrome 457–458
 of de Quervain's disease 435–437
 of Linburg syndrome 441–442
Dorsal root ganglion, gene regulation in 399–405
Double crush syndromes 389–390, 509
Dupuytren's contracture 23

E

Eccentric
 contractions 301–308, 340–347, 530
 exercise 323–*325*, 330
Elbow
 anatomy 134–135
 biomechanics 133–142
 pain 23–26
 tendinosis 253
 tennis 138–139, 372, 467–478
Electromyography 87, 89
 for carpal tunnel syndrome 424
 and measuring force 90–91
 for muscle disorders 115
 for the shoulder 149
Entheses 187–*191*, 198
Epicondylitis 15, 18–20
 lateral 138–139, 479–486 (see also Tennis elbow)
 medial 487
Epidemiology
 carpal tunnel syndrome 3
 epicondylitis 18–19
 labral tears 494
 neck disorders 31–36, 39–40
 shoulder disorders 36–40
 tendon and ligament overuse injuries 217–218
 tennis elbow 469
 tenosynovitis 16–17
Epineurium 381–382, *384*–385
Epitenon, definition 187, 236
 tendon cells 231–242
Evans splint *441*
Exercise
 effect on synovial membrane 265–267
 effect on tendons and ligaments 223–224

and muscle injury 323–334
and protein metabolism 324–326
therapeutic shoulder 526–531
types of 529, 530
Extensor carpi ulnaris 443–444
Extensor digitorum 443
Extensor pollicis longus 443

F
Fascicles
definition 187, 197, 360, 362, 384–385
factor in nerve compression 381–382
and endoneurial fluid pressure 386
patellar tendon 219
Fatigue, muscle 294–299
Fatty acid oxidation 289
Finger
model 100–101
postures 102, 105–108
Finkelstein test 436–437
Flexor carpi radialis 442–443
Flexor carpi ulnaris 443, 456

G
Ganglion 22
dorsal root 399–405
Gender differences 273 (see also Men; Women)
Gene regulation in DRG neurons 399–405
Glenohumeral
anatomy, articular 145–146
arthritis 38–39, 154–156, 504
instability 151–154
Glucose metabolism 287–289
Goniometry 87, 89, 95
Growth factors
in Achilles tendon 252
and inflammation 248, 250, 255
for tendons 234–236, 239–242
Guyon's canal 13
ganglion in 22
and ulnar artery thrombosis 22
and ulnar nerve entrapment 371

H
Hamate 114, 427
Hand
models 111–120
position 426–427
tendons 253
History of medicine 4
carpal tunnel pressure, measuring 123
cubital tunnel syndrome 455
de Quervain's disease 436
epidemiologic studies 7
tennis elbow 467, 472–473

tenosynovitis 13
Human studies
on eccentric exercise 324–326
on motor unit recruitment 292–294
on pain 407, 409–412
on tendon fibrocartilage 211–213
Hyperalgesia 407–408
Hypothenar hammer syndrome 22

I
Industries requiring repetitive motion 3, 10, 18, 24 (see also Occupations)
automobile manufacturing 3, 438–439
engineering 18
forestry 24
garment 10, 24
hospital 24
meat-packing plants 3, 18
newspaper 24
Inflammatory processes 247–258
in exercise-induced muscle injury 323–334
Intersection syndrome 438–440
Intraneural microstimulation (INS) 409–412

J
Job
content, varying 59
rotation 118–119

K
Kienböck's disease 20
Kiloh Nevin syndrome 369

L
Ligament
anatomy 185–198, 218–219
development 193–194
glenohumeral 146–149
healing 168–171, 224–226, 247–249
and inflammation 247–251, 253–258
overuse injuries 217–218, 253–254
retaining 195–197
tensile properties of 161–166
Linburg syndrome 441–442

M
Maximum voluntary contraction (MVC) 49
in a cold environment 15
and muscle fatigue 295–297
in video display terminal users 70
Median nerve
anatomic mousetraps 368–370
anatomy 363–364
compression 9

Median nerve (*continued*)
  mechanical stress to 114–115
Men
  cervical herniated disks in 32
  intersection syndrome in 439
Mesenchymal syndrome 248, 468
Metabolism
  skeletal muscle 287–289
  tendon and ligament 221–224
  whole body protein 324–326
Microneurography 409–412
Motor units 289–295
Muscle (*see also* Skeletal muscle)
  and anterior interosseous syndrome 370
  biceps brachii *368*
  disorders 115–116, 509–510
  elbow joint 134–138
  fatigue 50, 294–299
  flexor carpi ulnaris *371*
  hand 138–139
  injury, contraction-induced 339–347
  pain, studies of 407–412
  and posterior syndrome 373
  pronator teres *135*, 368–369
  protein turnover 326–334
  strengthening shoulder 530–531
  supinator 373
  wrist 138–139
Muscle fatigue 50, 294–299
  and injury 298–299
Muscle injury
  contraction-induced 339–347
  mechanics of 301–302
  wrist extensor 308–309
Myalgia 501–502
Myofascial pain syndrome 510

N
Nerve injury
  and anatomic mousetraps 366–373
  and compression, pathophysiology of 381–393
  in the hand and wrist 114–115
  peripheral 373–376
Nerves
  axillary *362*, 364–365
  brachial plexus 361–363, 366–367
  median 114–115, 362–364, 368–369
  microvascular system in 385–386
  peripheral 359–376
  posterior interosseous 373–374
  radial *362*, 365, 372–373
  synovium 267
  ulnar *362*, 364, 370–371
Neurapraxia, definition 374, 387
Neurons 359–360
  dorsal root ganglion 399–405

Neutrophils and muscle protein turnover 327–328
Neurotmesis 388
Nociceptors 408–412
  characterization of 416
  definition 409
Node of Ranvier 360, *384*
Nonsteroidal anti-inflammatory drugs
  in rehabilitation 451
  for shoulder pain 523–525
  for tendon entrapment syndromes 436
Nordic Questionnaire 4

O
Occupational Safety and Health Administration (OSHA) 539
  Ergonomics Program Guidelines for Meatpacking Plants 540, 543
Occupations
  carpenters 99
  cash register operators 35, 37–38
  chain saw operators 429
  and cross-sectional studies of carpal tunnel syndrome 10–12
  dancers 217, 366
  data entry 34–35, 39 (*see also* Video display unit operators)
  dentists 33–34, 36, 39
  forestry workers 24, 36, 428
  frozen food workers 10, 429
  garment workers 10, 24, 38, 99, 429
  with high-speed repetitive tasks 359, 369–370
  housework 436
  meatcutters/carriers/packers 13, 16–19, 22–25, 33–36, 39, 99, 429
  miners 33–34, 36
  newspaper employees 22, 24, 66
  pianists 100–107
  pizza cutters 371
  poultry processors 429
  scissor makers 16, 34–35, 39
  sign language interpreters 26, 217
  ski-manufacturer workers 10, 429
  supermarket checkers 26, 38, 99
  urologists 35
  welders 38–39
Olecranon bursitis 22
Osteoarthritis, glenohumeral 38–39, 154–156, 504

P
Pain
  cervicobrachial 510–511
  dysfunction syndrome 512
  muscle 407–412
  myofascial 510

neck 32–36
receptors 408–412, 416
shoulder 523–526
tendon 444
upper extremity 23–26
Paratenon, definition 187
Patient education 481
Perceived exertion 49–62
acceptability scaling 53–54
and job content, varying 59
rating scales 51–53
Peritendinitis 13–16
Phalen's test 22, 423
in carpal tunnel syndrome 10, 12
Phonophoresis 526
Physical stressors 87–95
contact stress 89, 92–93, *113*–114
duration 89, 92–94, *113*
force 89–92, *113*
measurement of 87–93, 95
posture 58–59, 89, 92, 94–95 (*see also* Posture)
repetition 87–90, *113*
temperature 89, 93
vibration 89, 93 (*see also* Vibration)
and work requirements 93–95
Piano playing 100, *102*–*103*
biomechanical forces in the fingers during 104–108
Posterior interosseous nerve *373*–*374*
syndrome 13
Posture
finger 102, 105–108
in video display operators 116–118
working 58–59, 92, 94–95
wrist 112–*113*, 125–127, *129*
Pronator syndrome 368–369
Proprioceptive neuromuscular facilitation 532
Proteoglycan
ligament 220
tendon 205–213
Psychosocial factors
in VDU operators 65–74
work organization 66–70, 79

R
Racquetball 3
Radial nerve *362*
anatomic mousetrap 372–373
anatomy 365
entrapments 13
groove *134*
neurapraxia 470
Radial tunnel syndrome 13
Raynaud's phenomenon 428, 512
Reflex sympathetic dystrophy 512–*513*
Rehabilitation

defined 518–520
of muscular overuse syndrome 452
of nerve entrapment at the wrist 451–452
phases of 449
of repetitive trauma at the elbow 479–489
shoulder 517–533
of tendinitis at the wrist 450–451
and the workplace 546–547
Retinacular
reconstruction 438–*439*
retaining ligaments 195–196
Risk factors (*see also* Physical stressors)
biomechanical 112–*113*, 119
for carpal tunnel syndrome 112–*113*, 424–429
for cervical herniated disks 32–33
computer keyboard operation 43–47
posture, working 58–59, 89, 92, 94–95 (*see also* Posture)
psychosocial 65–74
smoking 32–33
vibration 20 (*see also* Vibration)
Rotator cuff
disease 149–151
tendinitis 38–39, 496–500
Running
downhill *325*, 329–330
marathon 343

S
Satellite cell 313–320
Schwann cells 359–362
and acute compression injury 375–376
anatomy *383*–*384*
Seddon's classification 373–374
Semmes-Weinstein monofilament test 424
Shoulder
anatomy 145–149
assessment systems 523
biomechanics 145–157
evaluation forms 523
frozen 512
overuse injuries of 493–504
rehabilitation 517–533
Sign language interpreters 217
Skeletal muscle 287–299 (*see also* Muscle)
fatigue 40, 294–299
fiber types 285, 289
injury, contraction-induced 285, 339–347
metabolism 287–289
motor units 289–294
regeneration 313, 316–320
Z-bands 302, 306–308, 324–*325*, 327, 332–333

Smoking, cigarette
    and carpal tunnel syndrome 425
    and cervical disk herniations 32–33
Stressors, physical 88, 89
    contact stress 89, 92–93, 113
    force 90–92
    posture 58–59, 92, 94–95 (see also Posture)
    repetition 87–90
    temperature 93
    vibration 26, 93 (see also Vibration)
    work duration 92–93
Sunderland's classification 373–374
Synovial sheaths 197
Synovium
    exercise and 265–267
    lining cells 268–269
    medications and 272–273
    nerves 267–268
    normal 263–273

T
Tendon
    anatomy 185–198, 218–219
    biomechanical loads 140–142, 208–210, 231–242
    biomechanics of injury 166–168
    development 193–194
    fibrocartilage in 205–213
    growth factors 234–236, 239–242
    healing 168–171, 224, 241–242, 247–249
    hypovascularity 211–213
    and inflammation 247–258
    overuse syndromes 249–253
    pain without entrapment 444
    patellar 252–253
    predicting disorders in 113–116
    proteoglycan 205–213
    syndromes 13–15, 435–445
    tensile properties of 161–166
Tennis elbow 372, 467–478
    and enthesopathy 189
    etiology 285, 467–470
    postsurgical protocol 475–477
    and racket size 138–139, 141
    surgery for 471–477
Tenosynovitis 435, 444–445 (see also Tendon, syndromes)
    and physical stressors 13–17
Tension neck syndrome 32–35, 509–510
Thoracic outlet syndrome 32, 35
    arterial vascular 508–509
    neurologic 367, 508
    venous vascular 509
Thumb, trigger 439–441
Tinel's sign 22, 423
    and carpal tunnel syndrome 10

Trapezium 114
Trapezoid 114
Trigger finger 439–441

U
Ubiquitin 332–333
Ulnar artery 427
    thrombosis 22
Ulnar nerve
    anatomic mousetraps 370–371
    anatomy 364, 427, 456
    in situ release of 460

V
Vascularity
    and low pressure compression 388–389
    of the nerve trunk 385–386
    in synovium 263–265
    of tendons and ligaments 192–193, 198, 211–213
Vibration 93
    and bone and joint pathology 20
    and carpal tunnel syndrome 8–9, 12, 428–429
    and cervical herniated disks 32–33
    and muscle injury 309–311
Vibrometry 423
Video display unit (VDU) operators 4, 43–47
    biomechanical loads in 116–118
    and psychosocial factors 65–74
von Willebrand factor 266–267

W
Wallerian degeneration 374–375
Waris classification 32–33
WATTSMART motion measurement system 101, 107
Women
    and de Quervain's disease 435–436
    and tendon pain 444
    and tension neck syndrome 33
    and trigger finger 439
Workers' compensation
    for carpal tunnel syndrome 421, 428–431
    claims, cost of 517
    and an employee's return to work 542
    occupational injuries versus occupational diseases 3
    for sprains and strains 83
Wrist
    models 111–120
    muscle disorders in 115–116
    nerve disorders in 114–115 (see also Carpal tunnel syndrome; Median nerve)

pain 23–26
posture 112–*113*, 116–118, 125–127, *129*
tendons 113–116, 253

Wrist extensor
muscle injury 308–309
passive stretching of 482

Z

Z-band damage
and calcium-activated neutral proteases 317, 332
and eccentric exercise 302, 306–308, 324–*325*, 333
and neutrophils 327